CRITICAL CONCEPT
MASTERY SERIES
Chest Imaging Cases

CRITICAL CONCEPT MASTERY SERIES
Chest Imaging Cases

Zachary Healy, MD, PhD
Assistant Professor
Division of Pulmonary and Critical Care Medicine
Department of Medicine
Duke University Hospital
Durham, North Carolina

New York   Chicago   San Francisco   Athens   London   Madrid   Mexico City
Milan   New Delhi   Singapore   Sydney   Toronto

1 2 3 4 5 6 7 8 9   LCR   26 25 24 23 22 21

ISBN 978-1-260-45789-6
MHID 1-260-45789-3

The editors were Amanda Fielding, Julie Grishaw, and Christina M. Thomas.
The production supervisor was Richard Ruzycka.
Project management was provided by Tasneem Kauser, KnowledgeWorks Global Ltd.
The cover designer was W2 Design.

Library of Congress Cataloging-in-Publication Data

Names: Healy, Zachary, author.
Title: Chest imaging cases / Zachary Healy.
Other titles: Critical concept mastery series.
Description: New York : McGraw Hill, [2022] | Series: Critical concept mastery series | Includes bibliographical references and index. | Summary: "The Critical Concept Mastery Series is meant to help advanced students and residents master concepts that are frequently seen but difficult to conquer using a case-based approach. This case series on thoracic diseases was developed to provide a framework for the evaluation of patient's presenting with clinical syndromes and associated abnormalities on chest imaging"—Provided by publisher.
Identifiers: LCCN 2021019660 | ISBN 9781260457896 (trade paperback) | ISBN 9781260457902 (ebook)
Subjects: MESH: Thoracic Diseases—diagnostic imaging | Radiography, Thoracic | Diagnosis, Differential | Examination Questions | Atlas | Case Reports
Classification: LCC RD536 | NLM WF 18.2 | DDC 617.540754—dc23
LC record available at https://lccn.loc.gov/2021019660

CONTENTS

Contributor .... *vii*

Preface.. *ix*

Introduction 1

Case 1.. 21

Case 2.. 33

Case 3.. 43

Case 4.. 55

Case 5.. 65

Case 6.. 79

Case 7.. 89

Case 8.. 101

Case 9.. 111

Case 10.. 123

Case 11.. 133

Case 12.. 151

Case 13.. 161

Case 14.. 171

Case 15.. 181

Case 16.. 191

Case 17.. 207

Case 18.. 221

Case 19.. 229

Case 20.. 237

Case 21.. 251

Case 22.. 261

Case 23.. 275

Case 24.. 285

Case 25.. 295

Case 26.. 307

Case 27.. 319

Case 28.. 333

Case 29.. 351

Case 30.. 359

Case 31.. 369

Case 32.. 383

Case 33.. 395

Case 34.. 409

Case 35.. 421

Case 36.. 433

Case 37.. 445

Case 38.. 459

Case 39.. 473

Case 40.. 487

Case 41.. 503

Case 42.. 527

Case 43.. 547

Case 44.. 565

Case 45.. 573

Case 46.. 585

Case 47.. 599

Case 48.. 611

Case 49.. 617

Case 50.. 631

Case 51.. 647

Index.. *675*

CONTRIBUTOR

Caitlin Welch, MD
Attending Physician
Pulmonary and Critical Care
Mid Coast Hospital
Brunswick, Maine

PREFACE

This case series on thoracic diseases was developed to provide a framework for evaluating patients presenting with clinical syndromes and associated abnormalities on chest imaging. Such evaluation requires careful integration of the patient's clinical presentation (ie, symptoms, physical examination findings), pertinent radiographic findings, laboratory values, medical history, environmental and occupational history, medication exposure, and histopathologic findings to identify the underlying etiology. Rarely is a diagnosis established based on imaging findings in the absence of these clinical aspects.

Although each case will include interpretation of thoracic ("chest") radiographic images, this text is not intended to provide a comprehensive introduction to chest radiography. There are numerous such textbooks available, such as *Basic Radiology*, 2nd edition, by authors Michael Y.M. Chen, Thomas L. Pope, and David J. Ott. This case series assumes some basic knowledge of chest imaging. The introduction and the first case will, however, provide some background on chest imaging, a framework for classifying abnormalities, and a review of basic anatomy and terminology that will be used in the cases to follow.

A few recommendations:

- When encountering a patient with abnormalities on chest imaging, clinicians often overlook a crucial step in evaluation: comparing current imaging with prior imaging. Although obtaining copies of studies from other facilities or providers may be tedious or time consuming, it is a vitally important step to identify acute and chronic issues and prevent unnecessary diagnostic and invasive procedures.

- When ordering a radiology study, clinicians should provide the radiologist with the necessary information to ensure the appropriate protocol is applied (this is particularly true for computed tomography studies). There are generally two sections on current electronic medical record systems that must be completed to request a study. First, there is usually a diagnostic indication associated with an ICD-10 code that is primarily used for billing purposes, for example, "acute hypoxemic respiratory failure." The second section is usually a free-form textbox that allows the ordering clinician to communicate pertinent medical history to the radiologist. When completed appropriately, this section allows the radiologist to ensure that the appropriate study has been selected and that the study is protocoled appropriately. It also has other benefits: (1) it helps ensure that the radiologist will address specific clinical questions in the interpretation, (2) it provides the necessary background to determine the appropriate differential diagnoses, and (3) it may help guide further recommendations from the radiologist on further imaging or diagnostic studies.

- It is encouraged to not only read the interpretation or summary section on radiology reports but also to read and review the findings section carefully. This section will often direct the ordering clinician to specific images within specific studies that reveal various abnormalities. There also may be additional information in the findings section that should be addressed outside of the immediate context of the patient's presenting clinical syndrome.
- If the case is complicated, or if one is not sure of the appropriate study to order for a specific question, a discussion with the radiologist before ordering the study is also helpful.
- It is highly encouraged to discuss the results of studies with the interpreting radiologist, particularly if there is a thoracic imaging specialist available. Often, there are nuances or findings that may be described in the interpretation or findings that may be of interest.
- It is also encouraged to discuss the pathology results with the pathologist because this can greatly aid in one's understanding of disease pathogenesis as well as the imaging abnormalities seen.
- Another great learning opportunity is participation in multidisciplinary committees (MDCs) or multidisciplinary teams (MDTs). These committees typically consist of physicians and staff members from various divisions or departments who meet regularly to discuss the evaluation and treatment of patients who will require care from these various providers. Many academic centers have such committees for the management of organ-specific malignancy, and this has been shown to improve patient outcomes. This is especially true in lung cancer, where thoracic oncology MDCs—typically consisting of a thoracic surgeon, a medical oncologist, a radiation oncologist, a pathologist, a radiologist, and a pulmonologist—have been associated with an up to 10% increase in 5-year survival in retrospective studies. There may also be MDCs for other nononcologic diseases, such as interstitial lung disease, pulmonary hypertension, and lung transplantation, among others, for which additional education is possible.

Zach Healy

INTRODUCTION

BACKGROUND ON (PLAIN) CHEST RADIOGRAPHY

Luckily, the plain chest radiograph ("x-ray") is relatively straight-forward. The most common study is posteroanterior (PA) and lateral chest films, which provide two views of the thoracic cavity. The first is the PA film, with the source at the patient's back and the detector on the patient's anterior chest. The lateral film is typically taken with the source on the patient's right side and the detector on the patient's left side and requires the patient to stand. It is the standard and preferred method of chest radiography. However, many patients in the hospital are unable to undergo a PA and lateral study and will have an anteroposterior (AP) study instead. AP units are portable, so patients do not have to travel for the study, and the unit comes to the patient. The source is aimed at the anterior chest, and the detector is placed on the patient's posterior chest (back). Patients may also have decubitus films performed to examine for the presence of free-flowing pleural effusions.

APPROACH TO CHEST RADIOGRAPHY

There are different systematic approaches to viewing and interpreting chest radiographs. Although most are quite similar, the underlying principle is to use a consistent approach to interpretation to prevent missing key findings. Below is a general approach to the interpretation of chest radiographs (**STUDY** your **ABC**s so you don't get an **F**):

STUDY

- Is this a PA and lateral, AP, or lateral decubitus film?
  - Recall that on AP films, the heart and mediastinal borders will appear larger than on PA films.
  - AP films are often plagued by poor inspiratory effort or low lung volumes, which can give the false appearance of increased opacities.
- What was the indication for the study?
- Is the patient information correct?
- Is the date of the study correct?
- Are there prior images for comparison?
  - This can be situation-dependent.
    - If something acute has occurred, you may want to compare the image with the most recent chest radiograph before the acute event.
    - If you are monitoring for improvement or a more subacute worsening, you may want to compare the image with an image obtained several days ago because there may be incremental changes and much about the trajectory can be gained from comparison with these films.
    - If you are looking at a nodule or mass, you may want to review a chest radiograph from several months or even years ago to look for changes.

- Is there any digital enhancement of the film?
  - Many of the chest images acquired today are digital and may undergo algorithm-based enhancements, depending on the indication. This is typically indicated somewhere on the chest radiograph, and you may see some of these throughout the cases presented here. Some examples are discussed below.
    - Bone suppression – This removes the ribs and clavicles from the image and can improve the detection of soft tissue and parenchymal abnormalities.
    - Confirm/enhanced – This enhances artificial lines or other medical devices.
    - Compare – This is a mode that highlights areas of the lung parenchyma that have an increased or decreased density between studies.
- Exposure/penetration
  - Are the intervertebral discs of the thoracic spine visible?
- Inspiratory effort (**VERY IMPORTANT**)
  - Ideally, the top of the diaphragm should be located between the posterior eighth and tenth ribs on the left. There may be a one-half rib-space elevation of the right hemidiaphragm because of the liver.
  - Visualization of less than seven posterior ribs is concerning for either poor inspiratory effort or restriction.
- Rotation (particularly important on AP films)
  - When the patient is perpendicular to the source, the clavicular heads should be equidistant from the spinous processes.

AIRWAY (CENTRAL)

- Is the trachea midline down to the level of the carina, or is there deviation present?
- Is there narrowing of the trachea at any point?
- Are the carina and the left and right mainstem bronchi visible? The right mainstem is generally more visible than the left.
- Are the mainstem bronchi narrowed or occluded, or is a foreign body present?

AIRWAY (DISTAL)

- Symmetry and attenuation (*dark – air, white – x-ray–absorbing material*)
  - Both bilaterally and unilaterally (ie, within a lung, between the upper and lower regions of the lung parenchyma). DON'T FORGET the apices above the clavicles, which are often overlooked.
    - Is there a noticeable loss of volume?
    - Are the hilar structures symmetric and clearly visible, or are they enlarged or hazy?
    - Are there differences in the appearance of bronchovascular bundles as you move proximal to distal?
      - Is there peribronchial "cuffing"?
        - This generally indicates bronchial wall thickening due to increased interstitial fluid and or local atelectasis.
      - Is there "cephalization" of the upper lobes?
        - Typically, the bronchovascular bundles are not clearly visible in the upper lobes due to reduced overall blood flow to zone I of the lung, whereas they are more visible in the lower lungs where there is increased blood flow.

Cephalization is a term stolen from evolutionary biology and here refers to increased visualization of the vascular bundle in the upper lobes (cephalad).

- Are there lung markings visible throughout and extending to the pleura?
  - If not, is this due to increased air or fluid present between the parietal and visceral pleura?
- Are there any areas of increased or decreased density/attenuation? (Some examples that will be covered in these cases are shown in **Images I-1** and **I-2**.)
  - If the answer is yes to any of the following questions, how are they distributed?
    - Focal, multifocal, or diffuse?
    - Perihilar/central, peripheral, or diffuse?
    - Diffuse or upper- or lower-lobe predominant?
  - Are the opacities interstitial in appearance? (linear, reticular, nodular)
  - Are there focal nodules or masses? (cavitary, air-fluid levels, compression of other structures)
  - Are there alveolar opacities?
  - Are there cystic lesions?
  - Are there areas of consolidation?
  - Are the fissures visible? (abnormal)
  - Are there air bronchograms?
  - Is there evidence of bronchiectasis or bronchial wall thickening?

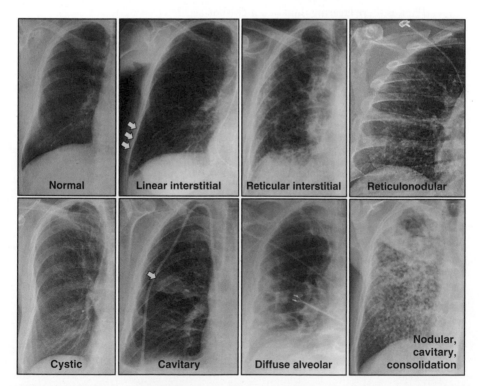

Image I-1 • Examples of different abnormalities associated with increased or decreased attenuation on chest radiographs.

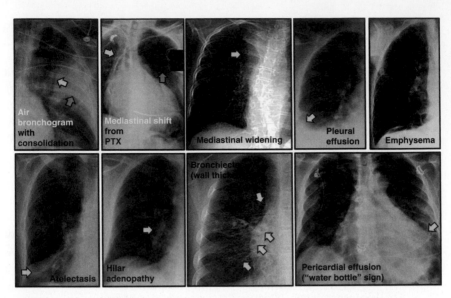

Image I-2 • Additional examples of abnormalities seen on chest radiography.

- Trace the borders of the lungs all the way around.
  - Are the costophrenic angles visible and sharp?
    - If not, is there layering fluid or a meniscus sign?
    - Are the sulci symmetric, or is there a deep sulcus sign?
  - Are the diaphragms clearly visible and crisp?
    - Is there free air under the diaphragm (not the gastric bubble)?
  - Do the diaphragms have the appropriate appearance?
    - Is the right hemidiaphragm slightly more elevated than the left (½ rib space approximately)?
  - Are the heart borders clearly visible?
    - On the lateral film, does the spine become clearer as you move caudally, or is there a "spine" sign indicating a retrocardiac opacity?

BONY STRUCTURES (AND SOFT TISSUE)

- Check for obvious asymmetry, lucency, or discontinuity in the ribs (posterior and anterior), the clavicles, and the vertebral bodies.
- Are there any obvious abnormalities in the soft tissues?
  - Subcutaneous emphysema?
  - Masses?
  - Lines, drains, or tubes?

CARDIAC

- Trace the borders of the mediastinum.
  - Is the border widened? If so, can you determine if it is anterior, middle, or posterior?
  - Is the mediastinum shifted? If so, is there a lesion or other pathology pushing the mediastinum or volume loss pulling the mediastinum?

- Trace the heart borders.
  - Is the shape of the heart normal?
    - If not, which portion of the heart is abnormal?
  - Are the dimensions of the heart normal?
    - PA – The cardiac silhouette should occupy no more than 50% of the thoracic width.
    - AP – The more proximal location of the heart to the beam path causes projection of the heart, and the heart will appear enlarged compared with PA film.
  - Is the position of the heart normal?
    - Two-thirds of the heart is visible left of the left border of the spine, and one-third is visible right of the left border.
      - Is there evidence of right ventricle (RV) enlargement?
      - Is there evidence of left ventricle (LV) enlargement?
- Trace the heart borders.
  - Is there a change in density along the heart borders?
    - This may suggest infiltrate is present.
  - Is there a "waterbag" or "water bottle" sign? This is the appearance of the heart as an old-fashioned red rubber water bag one might see used as an ice pack in old cartoons. Alternatively, it could be described as the appearance of a balloon being filled with water.
    - This may represent a pericardial effusion.
- Are the aortic arch and pulmonary trunk visible?
  - Are either enlarged or displaced?

FOREIGN OBJECTS

- Observe and note the presence of foreign objects
  - Are there foreign objects present in soft tissue?
  - Are there implantable medical devices, including pacemakers or implantable cardioverter-defibrillators?
  - Are there other medical devices? Consider the following possibilities:
    - Nasogastric or orogastric tubes
    - Oxygen or ventilator circuit tubes
    - Suction devices (including subglottic suction ports)
    - Electrocardiogram (ECG) leads, stickers, or telemetry devices
    - Endotracheal or tracheostomy tubes
    - Central venous or pulmonary artery catheters
    - Sternal wires
    - Artificial valve rings
    - Endobronchial valves or coils
    - Chest or thoracostomy tubes
    - Mediastinal drains
    - Pericardial catheters or drains
    - Other surgical drains

One of the more important concepts to understand is to avoid overreading chest radiographs. Outside of some obvious cases, such as pneumothorax, mucous plugging, or massive pulmonary effusion, most diagnoses are not going to be obtained by interpreting a chest radiograph alone. Often, additional imaging studies (echocardiogram, point-of-care ultrasound, chest computed tomography [CT]) are required to either confirm or further characterize the abnormalities seen on plain chest radiography. Rather, look for some basic patterns on the chest radiograph that can help narrow a differential diagnosis. These abnormalities can be further classified by their number, size, distribution, location, and margins.

These basic patterns include the following, and some examples are shown in **Images I-1** and **I-2**.

- "Airspace" or "alveolar" opacities: These are confluent areas of hazy or ill-defined opacities in which the air of the alveoli and terminal bronchioles is replaced by other radiodense material, such as fluid, blood, inflammatory cells, or debris.
- Interstitial opacities: These may be more linear (Kerley A, B, and C lines), reticular or net-like in appearance, reticulonodular (net-like with small nodules present along the lines), nodular, or miliary (diffuse nodular opacities).
- Nodules, masses, and consolidation: These refer to opacities that completely obscure the underlying lung tissue. There may be air bronchograms present. The difference between a nodule and mass is the size. Nodules are less than 3 cm in the greatest dimension, while masses are 3 cm or larger in the greatest dimension. Both nodules and masses are examples of consolidation, though in some cases, the term *consolidation* is used rather than *nodule* or *mass*, particularly when the lesion is poorly defined. These lesions are further characterized by the number, location, size, margins, and composition (eg, calcifications, cavitation, presence of fat).
- Lesions associated with decreased attenuation: Decreased lung markings may indicate emphysematous changes, the presence of blebs (collection or air between the lung and visceral pleura), or bullae (coalescence of blebs into a larger cystic or cavitary lesion). A cyst is a thin-walled lesion in the lung parenchyma. Cysts are thin-walled lesions, while cavities are thick-walled lesions.
- Airway abnormalities: These include shifting or obstruction or opacification of the airways as well as bronchiectasis or bronchial wall thickening.
- Pleural and diaphragmatic abnormalities: These include diaphragmatic flattening, hemidiaphragm elevation, pneumothoraces, pleural effusions, pleural thickening, and pleural calcifications.
- Mediastinal abnormalities: These include widening and the presence of masses as well as a shift of the mediastinal compartment. The latter may help differentiate between volume loss and volume-occupying processes.
- Lymphadenopathy: This includes hilar and mediastinal adenopathy.

Background on CT of the chest. First, reacquaint yourself with the image reconstruction planes in CT. Images are acquired in the axial plane (horizontal or transverse; images are shown from caudal to cranial) and may be reconstructed in sagittal (longitudinal; images shown from the right to the left side of the body) and coronal (frontal plane; images shown from anterior to posterior).

CT of the chest is a bit more complex than plain chest radiography. Without going into too much detail, CT scans are predominantly performed in either sequential or volumetric modes. Previously, CT scans were performed in sequential mode (often termed "conventional") with a linear beam ("fan" beam) of electrons and a linear series of detectors. This produced images of a certain thickness (ie, slice thickness, which is the thickness of the linear arrangement of detectors). The slice thickness is the axial "resolution" of a scan. After a discrete set of images was taken at one axial location, the patient was moved a specified distance, and another series of images was taken. The distance the patient was moved was called the *slice increment*. So, if the slice is 2 mm thick and the patient was moved 4 mm between images, there would be approximately 2 mm of space on each side of the slice that is not imaged. This 2-mm area that was not imaged was termed the *gap*. Sequential CT scans were performed in contiguous mode (the slice is the same thickness as the increment, leaving no gap), in overlap mode (where the slice thickness is larger than the increment), or with a gap, as described previously. If a gap was present, this indicated areas that were not imaged, and if coronal or sagittal reconstructions were recreated, these gap areas would need to be artificially reconstructed using an algorithm, so this was not typically done. Spiral CT is as described: the patient was continuously moved through the scanner as images were continuously collected, creating a spiral or helical series of images. High-resolution CT was CT performed with high resolution (1-mm slice thickness) with minimal or no gap present.

The vast majority of modern CT scanners use volumetric imaging, with a cone beam of electrons and square-shaped detectors (often termed *multidetector CT* [MDCT]). This creates a two-dimensional image rather than the one-dimensional image of conventional CT. Volumetric CT images provide more detail with more overlap and less overall radiation exposure. This significantly increases the sensitivity for lung nodule detection and allows for the generation of axial, coronal, and sagittal reconstructions. Coronal and sagittal reconstructions are useful for differentiating upper- and lower-lobe predominant disease processes as well as central versus peripheral lesions. Similar to plain chest radiography, CT scans of the chest can be digitally processed and enhanced. Some examples include vessel suppression (suppresses the appearance of blood vessels, particularly helpful to identify lung nodules), compare (optimizes comparisons between current and prior CT images for comparison of nodules or masses), maximal intensity projection (MIP; again useful for nodule detection), minimal intensity projection (MinIP; useful for airway abnormalities), and virtual bronchoscopy (creates a three-dimensional map of the airways for navigational bronchoscopy or surgical planning). Sequential CT scanning is performed in rare cases, typically where specific areas of interest are being investigated, as it can reduce radiation exposure in these circumstances.

Additionally, there are different protocols that may be used during CT. Noncontrasted CT of the chest is the workhorse for the evaluation of interstitial lung disease (ILD), while contrasted CT scans of the chest are useful in the evaluation of vascular abnormalities (ie, pulmonary embolism [PE]), nodule/mass evaluation (including lesion enhancement and lymph node abnormalities), and in bleeding or trauma. CT scans are traditionally performed with the patient in the supine position with the arms above the head (if possible) and in full inspiration with a breath hold.

Here are just some of the more common protocols for non- and contrast-enhanced CT scans:

- **Noncontrasted CT scans**
  - Standard protocol
  - ILD-protocol. This is used in patients with suspected ILD and includes the following noncontrasted studies:

- Standard volumetric CT performed in the supine position during inspiration with a breath hold and high-resolution (1- to 1.25-mm slice thickness) axial, sagittal, and coronal reconstructions.
- Expiratory scan performed supine during a breath hold after full expiration. The posterior border of the trachea should be bowed. This is used to investigate air trapping (ie, hypersensitivity pneumonitis [HP]), small airways disease, and tracheobronchomalacia.
- Prone inspiratory scan performed in a prone position at full inspiration with a breath hold. This is used to differentiate between gravity-dependent changes in lung density and those due to early ILD (eg, subpleural reticulations, early honeycomb changes).
- Low-dose CT (LDCT). This is the method used most often for patients with expected repeated CT exposure, utilizing one-tenth to one-fifth the total radiation dose of a standard CT scan. This is most commonly used in lung cancer screening.
- Ultra-low-dose CT (ULDCT). This is a new method that may be useful for lung nodule follow-up as well.
- Cine CT. This is a protocol that is particularly useful for the evaluation of dynamic airway collapse (tracheobronchomalacia).
- **Contrasted CT scans**
  - Routine contrasted CT studies are used for the evaluation of soft tissue, including nodules, masses, and lymph nodes. This typically requires a delay of 50 to 70 seconds after contrast injection for optimal enhancement.
  - CT angiography: This includes protocols for CT of the pulmonary artery (CTPA), CT of the aorta and its branches (CTA), split-bolus scan (examining pulmonary arteries and systemic arteries [specific bronchial arteries]) in patients with hemoptysis, and the triple rule-out (PE, aortic aneurysm, and coronary artery dissection/disease).
  - Functional CT: This is a dynamic multiphase study that looks for temporal changes in contrast enhancement during the study.

Positron-emission tomography (PET) is another form of imaging used extensively in the evaluation of thoracic malignancy. It is most commonly performed in tandem with CT and is termed *PET-CT*. The PET portion of the study requires intravenous injection of a radioactive carbohydrate, fluorodeoxyglucose (^{18}FDG). When ^{8}FDG is metabolized, the radioactive component (^{18}F) is trapped inside the cell. Cells with high metabolic activity (ie, malignant cells) take up more ^{18}FDG and appear "hot" on imaging. This will be covered in the cases to follow. PET-CT requires the patient to fast before the study, and the intravenous injection is performed about 3 hours before image acquisition.

Approach to CT of the chest findings. A complete review of CT abnormalities is well beyond the scope of this text. However, here is a basic review of some of the terminology and a basic system of interpretation, similar to that provided previously for chest radiography.

First, it is important to discuss the secondary pulmonary lobule (shown in **Image I-3**). The second pulmonary lobule is the smallest functional unit of the lung, and it provides a good basis for the interpretation of abnormalities seen on CT imaging of

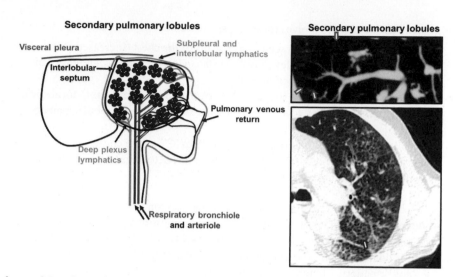

Image I-3 • Secondary pulmonary lobule. This is the smallest functional unit of the lung, and it is the basis for interpretation of CT of the chest.

the chest. The secondary pulmonary lobule consists of a pulmonary arteriole, venule, and respiratory "preterminal" bronchiole (and associated lymphatics) as well as all the acini that are serviced by this bronchovascular bundle (typically 20–30 acini with about 2000 alveoli per acini). The secondary pulmonary lobule is bound by an inter-lobular septum, and the shape of the unit on axial imaging is typically that of a poly-hedron or hexagon. This is most classically broken down into three separate segments.

- **The centrilobular structure** (the structures are in the center of the lobule) includes the bronchovascular bundle (pulmonary arteriole, preterminal bronchiole, and lymphatics) and the peribronchovascular interstitium (ie, the soft tissue immedi-ately surrounding the bronchovascular bundle).
- **The lobular parenchyma** includes the alveoli and the alveolar septum and the surrounding interstitium (containing the pulmonary capillaries). This is where gas exchange occurs.
- **The interlobular septum** contains the subpleural and interlobular septa, lymphat-ics, and pulmonary veins.

This will be discussed throughout the text to connect imaging and histopathologic changes with disease pathogenesis.

The classification of abnormalities on CT of the chest and how these changes relate to potential underlying ILD or other disease pathogenesis has been extensively discussed in the literature. Any of the review articles listed in the references section of this introduction provide practical approaches on how to use abnormal findings seen on CT of the chest to narrow the differential diagnosis. Two good examples are the papers by Pipavath and Godwin (2004) and the more recent publication by Gruden et al. (2020). Such approaches will also be addressed in each case. However, please remember that despite many of these disease processes having "classic" or "typical" findings on chest imaging, many may pres-ent with various abnormalities on CT of the chest.

In general, the approach involves these steps:

1. Determine the abnormalities seen on CT scans of the chest (increased attenuation, decreased attenuation, nodules/masses, cysts/cavitary lesions, adenopathy, airway abnormalities, vascular abnormalities).
2. Determine the distribution (upper lobe, lower-lobe predominant, focal/diffuse, central/peripheral, relative to secondary lobular structure [centrilobular/panlobular/paraseptal/subpleural]).
3. Determine the chronicity of the abnormalities on CT of the chest.
4. Integrating clinical and laboratory characteristics, determine if these characteristics fit a specific pattern consistent with ILD.

Here is a basic structure to describe abnormalities seen on CT of the chest:
- **Abnormalities associated with increased attenuation**. Primarily ground-glass opacities (GGOs) and consolidation (see **Image I-4** for some basic examples)
  - GGOs do not obscure the underlying lung architecture.
    - Mosaic pattern – heterogenous attenuation of lung parenchyma
      - Mosaic attenuation may be due to heterogeneous areas of GGO or air trapping
        - This can be differentiated using expiratory imaging (identified air trapping) and the presence or absence of airway abnormalities (bronchial wall thickening).
        - Air trapping can be seen in hypersensitivity pneumonitis (HP), respiratory bronchiolitis–associated ILD (RB-ILD), desquamative interstitial pneumonia (DIP), bronchiolitis obliterans, respiratory bronchiolitis, and chronic obstructive pulmonary disease (COPD).
        - Mosaic attenuation due to GGO can be seen in many conditions, including atypical or viral pneumonia, *Pneumocystis jirovecii* pneumonia (PJP), organizing pneumonia (OP; including drug toxicity), radiation pneumonitis, eosinophilic pneumonia (EP), acute respiratory distress syndrome (ARDS), and early in acute interstitial pneumonia (AIP).

Increased interlobular thickening (reticulation)

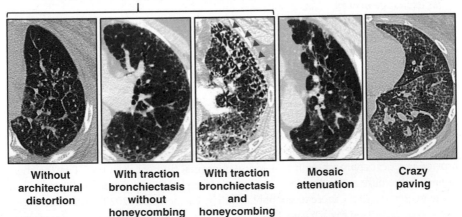

| Without architectural distortion | With traction bronchiectasis without honeycombing | With traction bronchiectasis and honeycombing | Mosaic attenuation | Crazy paving |

Image I-4 • Examples of abnormalities associated with increased attenuation seen on CT of the chest.

- Mosaic perfusion is the enlargement of pulmonary arterioles, typically in the case of pulmonary hypertension (HTN), particularly in chronic thromboembolic pulmonary HTN (CTEPH).
- "Crazy paving," the presence of interlobular septal thickening with GGO, may be seen in a number of conditions as well, including pulmonary alveolar proteinosis (PAP), ARDS, cellular form of nonspecific interstitial pneumonia (NSIP), viral infection, PJP, drug-induced pneumonitis, pulmonary edema, invasive mucinous adenocarcinoma, alveolar sarcoidosis, pulmonary veno-occlusive disorder (PVOD), lipoid pneumonia, atypical infection, pulmonary hemorrhage (including diffuse alveolar hemorrhage [DAD]), and chronic eosinophilic pneumonia (CEP; particularly early in the disease process).
- Consolidation obscures the underlying lung architecture.
  - Air-bronchograms may be present.
    - Focal/multifocal: May be due to infection, primary lung cancer, atelectasis, or ARDS.
      - Be sure to understand the difference between multifocal and diffuse.
    - Diffuse: May be due to sarcoidosis, AIP, or ARDS.
- **Abnormalities associated with decreased attenuation**. This primarily includes emphysematous changes, blebs, bullae, cysts, and cavitary lesions (see **Image I-5**).
  - Decreased attenuation may be due to centrilobular and paraseptal emphysema (typically seen in COPD), alpha-1-antitrypsin deficiency, bronchiolitis obliterans (BO), or respiratory bronchiolitis (RB).
  - No visible wall with associated abnormalities in the airways (bronchial wall thickening) is more likely BO, RB, or emphysema. This may also be seen in pulmonary Langerhans cell histiocytosis (PLCH).
  - Cysts are thin-walled structures with decreased central attenuation. These may be seen in lymphangioleiomyomatosis (LAM), lymphocytic interstitial pneumonia (LIP), PLCH, pulmonary amyloidosis, and cystic fibrosis (CF).

Centrilobar and paraseptal emphysema   **Panlobular emphysema**

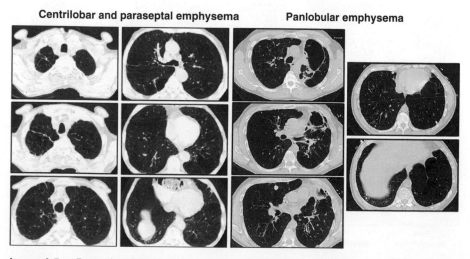

Image I-5 • Examples abnormalities associated with decreased attenuation seen on CT of the chest.

- Cavitary lesions are thick-walled structures with decreased central attenuation. These may be seen in fungal infections, mycobacterial infections, nocardiosis, PLCH, pulmonary abscesses, allergic bronchopulmonary aspergillosis (ABPA), coal workers' pneumonoconiosis (in association with nodules, sarcoidosis, collagen-vascular disease (notably, granulomatosis with polyangiitis and rheumatoid arthritis), and cystic fibrosis (CF).
- **Interstitial or "reticular" abnormalities**. These terms are often used interchangeably. These changes can be seen in many conditions, including any of those associated with chronic fibrosis (idiopathic pulmonary fibrosis [IPF], asbestosis, CWP, CF, poorly controlled PAP, fibrotic complications from ARDS, radiation fibrosis, drug toxicity, HP, NSIP, CVD-associated pulmonary fibrosis) (see **Image I-4**).
  - Peribronchovascular thickening may be seen in cardiogenic pulmonary edema, sarcoidosis, and lymphangitic carcinomatosis.
  - Interlobular septal thickening is the same as peribronchovascular thickening and represents the first stages of fibrosis.
  - Traction bronchiectasis (represents architectural distortion) represents the progression of fibrosis.
  - Honeycomb changes represent end-stage fibrosis.
- **Presences of nodules or masses**. These are further described by the size, number, distribution, composition, density, and margins of the lesion (see **Image I-6**).
  - "Tree-in-bud" nodules are representative of infection (classically seen in *Mycobacterium avium* complex, or MAC) and aspiration.
  - Nodules along the lymphatics (both peribronchovascular and interlobular) may be consistent with sarcoidosis, silicosis, CWP, and lymphangitic carcinomatosis.

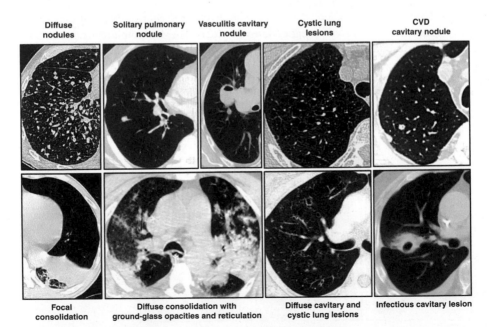

| Diffuse nodules | Solitary pulmonary nodule | Vasculitis cavitary nodule | Cystic lung lesions | CVD cavitary nodule |

| Focal consolidation | Diffuse consolidation with ground-glass opacities and reticulation | Diffuse cavitary and cystic lung lesions | Infectious cavitary lesion |

Image I-6 • Examples of abnormalities associated with nodules, masses, consolidation, cysts, and cavitary lesions seen on CT of the chest.

- Nodules predominantly along the bronchovascular tree may be associated with hemorrhage, vasculitis (classically GPA), rheumatoid arthritis (RA), respiratory bronchiolitis (RB), and lymphoma, especially lymphomatoid granulomatosis (LyG).
- Randomly distributed nodules may be seen in miliary tuberculosis, disseminated fungal infections, PLCH, primary neoplasms (particularly invasive mucinous adenocarcinoma), metastatic disease, lymphoma, sarcoidosis, and septic emboli.
- **Presence of airway abnormalities**. Some abnormalities may include:
  - Bronchial wall thickening
  - Bronchiectasis
    - This may be cylindrical, varicose, or cystic in appearance. It may be seen in diffuse panbronchiolitis, CF, non-CF bronchiectasis, or chronic infections. Traction bronchiectasis may be seen in any condition with architectural distortion.
  - Airway malacia
  - Airway obstruction or compression due to a mass
  - Airway nodularity
    - This may be seen in amyloidosis, sarcoidosis, tracheobronchopathia osteochondroplastica (TPO), GPA, *Mycobacterium* tuberculosis (MTB), papillomatosis, and primary malignancy.
  - Stenosis or strictures
  - Discontinuity
  - Tracheoesophageal fistulas
  - Bronchopleural fistulas
- **Pericardial or pleural abnormalities**. Note that conditions that affect the lung may also affect the pericardium, such as SLE, RA, sarcoidosis, and malignancy.
  - Pleural effusions
    - These may be seen in many conditions and will be discussed at length. They may be simple or complicated (contain loculations).
  - Hemothorax
  - Empyema
  - Pneumothoraces
  - Pericardial effusions
  - Pleural thickening
- **Lymphadenopathy**. This may be reactive (infection, inflammatory conditions, edema) or result from malignancy.
  - Hilar and mediastinal adenopathy
- **Vascular abnormalities**. If possible, characterize:
  - Pulmonary emboli
  - Tumor emboli
  - Pulmonary artery enlargement
  - RV-to-LV ratio
  - Central venous access placement

A QUICK WORD ON BRONCHOSCOPY

The capabilities of bronchoscopy, both diagnostic and therapeutic, continue to evolve. A number of different diagnostic procedures, aside from simple visual inspection ("airway examination"), may be performed using bronchoscopy, including bronchoalveolar lavage (BAL), endobronchial brushing, endobronchial biopsies, transbronchial biopsies (guided by either fluoroscopy, radial endobronchial ultrasound [R-EBUS], or CT-assisted virtual bronchoscopy images), transbronchial needle aspiration (either anatomy-guided or linear endobronchial ultrasound [L-EBUS]), and cryobiopsy. A standard bronchoscopy (18F) has a distal tip diameter of 5.9 mm and a working channel of 2.8 mm (ie, port through which tools may be advanced). The bronchoscopy may be advanced either via the nasopharyngeal or oropharyngeal passages (or via tracheostomy or laryngectomy site) through the vocal cords and into the trachea. An airway examination is then performed by visually inspecting the trachea, carina, and mainstem and lobar bronchi as well as the segmental and subsegmental bronchi bilaterally. This is generally as far as the bronchoscope can advance for visualization (to the fourth generation of approximately 15-18 leading to the terminal bronchi and alveoli). BAL is performed by "wedging" the bronchoscopy into one of these bronchi, injecting sterile water or saline through the working channel (usually 30-60 mL at a time) and suctioning the solution back through the working channel into a sputum trap. This may be sent for cytology, microbiology, and cell count studies, in addition to other molecular studies that are under research investigation. Importantly, note the difference between cytology (which looks for atypical cells typically in solution) and histopathology (which looks at intact tissue specimens).

The term *endobronchial* means that the procedure is done under direct visualization within the airway. An endobronchial biopsy is performed using forceps on tissue under direct visualization and sent for histopathology, and endobronchial brushing is performed by advancing a small brush with a protective sheath out of the working port on the bronchoscope into an airway of interest, advancing the brush from the protective sheath, literally brushing the airway, and then retracting the brush into the protective sheath. This is typically sent for cytology studies, though it could be sent for microbiology studies as well. If desired, endobronchial needle aspiration could also be performed by sticking a small-bore needle (usually 20 gauge or less) into a lesion and aspirating material to send for cytology studies.

The term *transbronchial* indicates that a procedure is performed through the bronchial wall. The most common procedures are transbronchial biopsy using forceps and transbronchial needle aspiration (TBNA). Transbronchial biopsy is performed by passing forceps through the working channel into the lung and taking small biopsy specimens (approximately 2.5 mm^2). These are very small pieces that, in the best case, contain alveoli, interstitium, terminal bronchioles, and small vascular structures. These are sent for histopathology and, if the sample is appropriate, can undergo immunohistochemistry (IHC), staining for infectious organisms, or molecular testing. Transbronchial needle aspiration is performed by passing a needle through a bronchial wall into a structure of interest, aspirating material from the structure, and is sent for cytology. These procedures may be done under direct visualization (TBNA of a lymph node) using anatomic markings, using fluoroscopy, using virtual bronchoscopy or navigational bronchoscopy, or using endobronchial ultrasound equipment (EBUS). Virtual bronchoscopy was briefly discussed previously and uses a CT scan, specialized software, and often specialized equipment to provide a three-dimensional map of the airways to allow for biopsy of peripheral lesions. These images are often adjusted for respiratory variation as well.

Endobronchial ultrasound may be performed in one of two ways: linear or radial. These terms refer to how the ultrasound beam is oriented. In linear ultrasound, a specialized bronchoscope (usually larger, about 7 mm in distal diameter) is passed into the trachea with an ultrasound probe at the distal end of the scope. It is primarily used to identify vascular and lymphatic structures under the bronchial wall and allow for transbronchial needle aspiration under ultrasound visualization. Radial EBUS is a different procedure that is performed using a standard bronchoscope. A small radial EBUS probe is passed through the working channel into the airway of interest. The radial EBUS probe rotates at a very high speed, producing a two-dimensional view of the tissue surrounding the airway wall. This is primarily used for localizing a peripheral lesion to a specific airway. The airway or target can then be marked visually or on fluoroscopy, or alternatively, a special sheath can be passed into the airway through which smaller pair of forceps may be advanced to biopsy the lesion. This allows for transbronchial biopsy to be performed and sent for histopathology as well molecular, IHC, or infectious studies if necessary.

These are the more common diagnostic methods in bronchoscopy to date. One of the more common misconceptions is the utility of bronchoscopy for the diagnosis of ILD. Transbronchial biopsy produces small fragments of tissue that often lack all the architectural information necessary to make a diagnosis of ILD. There are exceptions, however, that vary by disease process. In some cases, the combined information from BAL, transbronchial biopsy, the clinical presentation, laboratory studies, and imaging findings may be sufficient to decide on a formal diagnosis. In other cases, a surgical lung biopsy may be necessary. The utility of these various procedures to aid in or definitively diagnose thoracic disease will be covered throughout these cases.

Cryobiopsy is a relatively new method of transbronchial lung biopsy that utilizes cryogenic forceps to essentially snap-freeze tissue during a biopsy, preventing some of the architectural ("crush") distortion that can occur with standard transbronchial biopsy techniques. Cryobiopsy remains controversial. Although it offers the potential for greater diagnostic yield (up to 85% compared with likely 20% with standard techniques) in ILD owing to the preservation of tissue architecture and large biopsy specimen size (15-25 mm^2), it is associated with the increased risk of pneumothorax (5%) and bleeding (5%-20%), depending on the indication. As with all of the aforementioned techniques, the yield of cryobiopsy likely varies not only according to indication but also to operator expertise.

Some common indications for bronchoscopy include but are not limited to:
- Persistent atelectasis (to examine for evidence of an obstructing lesion in the airway); nonresolving parenchymal abnormalities (eg, nonresolving consolidation thought to be pneumonia); evaluation for infection or abnormal lesions in immunocompromised hosts; lung transplant surveillance; evaluation of centrally located nodules or masses; evaluation of thoracic adenopathy, hemoptysis, stridor, or central airway wheezing; tracheobronchomalacia; airway nodularity; concern for tracheoesophageal fistula (TEF); central airway stenosis or discontinuity (eg, anastomoses in lung transplant); foreign bodies; burn injury; chest trauma; mucous plugging; and airway clearance for patients unable to do so on their own.

Most of the newer technology developed over the last 10 years has focused on improving diagnostics in the evaluation of lung cancer, enabling biopsy of more peripheral lesions. In terms of ILD, the use of bronchoscopy for diagnosis has been limited to those conditions with centrilobular disease involvement, including sarcoidosis, GPA, HP, lymphangitic carcinomatosis, eosinophilic pneumonia, PLCH, and, occasionally, organizing pneumonia (eg, drug toxicity). BAL can be diagnostic in malignancy and may aid in the diagnosis of PAP, DAH (serial BAL), berylliosis, asbestosis, silicosis, CWP, and lipoid pneumonia, among others. Bronchoscopy can also be used to rule out certain conditions (particularly infection), which may help to narrow a differential diagnosis. Again, in each case in this text, the utility of bronchoscopy will be addressed.

The decision to proceed with biopsy requires carefully weighing the risk of the procedure with the potential diagnostic or therapeutic benefit. Aside from the bronchoscopy-related complications (infection, bleeding, pneumothorax), careful consideration must be put toward patient-related risk factors, including the patient's level of hypoxemia and potential respiratory reserve, the presence of central airway stenosis or narrowing, the patient's American Society of Anesthesiologists (ASA) class, the risk factors for conscious sedation or general anesthesia, and bleeding issues (eg, thrombocytopenia, recent use of antiplatelet or anticoagulation agents, uremia). Consider the type of sedation and the length of the procedure. Finally, also consider the risk to the staff performing the procedure because bronchoscopy produces aerosols. All these factors must be balanced against the potential yield of the procedure, not only to confirm a diagnosis but also to rule out other causes. Please keep this in mind during the evaluation of these cases as well as in clinical practice.

Similar to the aforementioned risk-benefit discussion, keep these issues in mind when considering referring a patient for a surgical lung biopsy. Although a lung biopsy may be the only way to establish a truly definitive diagnosis in some cases, it must be weighed against not only the procedural risk but also the risk for an acute exacerbation or "flare-up" of existing ILD. This was recently reviewed by Raj et al. (2017) in the journal *Chest*. Although a formal discussion of surgical lung biopsy is outside the scope of this text, the decision to send a patient for a surgical lung biopsy often comes down to the question of "Will this change the patient's management?"

Note: Although not specifically covered in this case series, bronchoscopy can be used in a therapeutic manner in a number of ways. This includes foreign body removal, whole lung lavage in PAP, repositioning of an endotracheal tube or placement of a double-lumen endotracheal tube, percutaneous tracheostomy guidance, awake fiberoptic intubation, laser resection, argon plasma coagulation, cryoablation, bronchial thermoplasty, endobronchial valve or coil placement, airway balloon dilation or stent deployment, endobronchial blockade in the event of bleeding, photodynamic therapy, brachytherapy (ie, placement of radioactive seeds), and airway clearance.

References

Bango-Álvarez A, Ariza-Prota M, Torres-Rivas H, et al. Transbronchial cryobiopsy in interstitial lung disease: experience in 106 cases - how to do it. ERJ Open Res. 2017;3.

Barbas CS, Capelozzi VL, Hoelz C, et al. Impact of open lung biopsy on refractory acute respiratory failure. J Bras Pneumol. 2006;32:418.

Bilfinger TV, Albano D, Perwaiz M, et al. Survival outcomes among lung cancer patients treated using a multidisciplinary team approach. Clin Lung Cancer. 2018;19:346.

Bradley B, Branley HM, Egan JJ, et al. Interstitial lung disease guideline: the British Thoracic Society in collaboration with the Thoracic Society of Australia and New Zealand and the Irish Thoracic Society. Thorax. 2008;63:v1.

Chen AC, Feller-Kopman D. Cryobiopsy: a work in progress. Ann Am Thorac Soc. 2017;14:827.

Churg A, Wright JL, Tazelaar HD. Acute exacerbations of fibrotic interstitial lung disease. Histopathology. 2011;58:525.

Costabel U, Uzaslan E, Guzman J. Bronchoalveolar lavage in drug-induced lung disease. Clin Chest Med. 2004;25:25.

Dickoff C, Dahele M. The multidisciplinary lung cancer team meeting: increasing evidence that it should be considered a medical intervention in its own right. J Thorac Dis. 2019;11:S311.

Ensminger SA, Prakash UB. Is bronchoscopic lung biopsy helpful in the management of patients with diffuse lung disease? Eur Respir J. 2006;28:1081.

Ernst A, Feller-Kopman D, Becker HD, Mehta AC. Central airway obstruction. Am J Respir Crit Care Med. 2004;169:1278.

Ernst A, Silvestri GA, Johnstone D, American College of Chest Physicians. Interventional pulmonary procedures: guidelines from the American College of Chest Physicians. Chest. 2003;123:1693.

Flaherty KR, King TE Jr, Raghu G, et al. Idiopathic interstitial pneumonia: what is the effect of a multidisciplinary approach to diagnosis? Am J Respir Crit Care Med. 2004;170:904.

Fruchter O, Fridel L, El Raouf BA, et al. Histological diagnosis of interstitial lung diseases by cryo-transbronchial biopsy. Respirology. 2014;19:683.

Gershman E, Fruchter O, Benjamin F, et al. Safety of cryo-transbronchial biopsy in diffuse lung diseases: analysis of three hundred cases. Respiration. 2015;90:40.

Gotway MB, Reddy GP, Webb WR, Elicker BM, Leung JW. High-resolution CT of the lung: patterns of disease and differential diagnoses. Radiol Clin North Am. 2005;43:513.

Griffin CB, Primack SL. High-resolution CT: normal anatomy, techniques, and pitfalls. Radiol Clin North Am. 2001;39:1073.

Gruden JF, Naidich DP, Machnicki SC, Cohen SL, Girvin F, Raoof S. An algorithmic approach to the interpretation of diffuse lung disease on chest CT imaging: a theory of almost everything. Chest. 2020;157:612.

Hetzel J, Eberhardt R, Herth FJ, et al. Cryobiopsy increases the diagnostic yield of endobronchial biopsy: a multicentre trial. Eur Respir J. 2012;39:685.

Hetzel J, Maldonado F, Ravaglia C, et al. Transbronchial cryobiopsies for the diagnosis of diffuse parenchymal lung diseases: expert statement from the Cryobiopsy Working Group on Safety and Utility and a call for standardization of the procedure. Respiration. 2018;95:188.

Iftikhar IH, Alghothani L, Sardi A, et al. Transbronchial lung cryobiopsy and video-assisted thoracoscopic lung biopsy in the diagnosis of diffuse parenchymal lung disease. A meta-analysis of diagnostic test accuracy. Ann Am Thorac Soc. 2017;14:1197.

Johannson KA, Marcoux VS, Ronksley PE, Ryerson CJ. Diagnostic yield and complications of transbronchial lung cryobiopsy for interstitial lung disease. A systematic review and metaanalysis. Ann Am Thorac Soc. 2016;13:1828.

Ketai L, Washington L. Radiology of acute diffuse lung disease in the immunocompetent host. Semin Roentgenol. 2002;37:25.

Kilinç G, Kolsuk EA. The role of bronchoalveolar lavage in diffuse parenchymal lung diseases. Curr Opin Pulm Med. 2005;11:417.

Lee YC, Wu CT, Hsu HH, et al. Surgical lung biopsy for diffuse pulmonary disease: experience of 196 patients. J Thorac Cardiovasc Surg. 2005;129:984.

Leslie KO, Gruden JF, Parish JM, Scholand MB. Transbronchial biopsy interpretation in the patient with diffuse parenchymal lung disease. Arch Pathol Lab Med. 2007;131:407.

Lettieri CJ, Veerappan GR, Helman DL, et al. Outcomes and safety of surgical lung biopsy for interstitial lung disease. Chest. 2005;127:1600.

Maldonado F, Danoff SK, Wells AU, et al. Transbronchial cryobiopsy for the diagnosis of interstitial lung diseases: CHEST guideline and expert panel report. Chest. 2020;157:1030.

Meyer KC, Raghu G, Baughman RP, et al. An official American Thoracic Society clinical practice guideline: the clinical utility of bronchoalveolar lavage cellular analysis in interstitial lung disease. Am J Respir Crit Care Med. 2012;185:1004.

Meyer KC. The role of bronchoalveolar lavage in interstitial lung disease. Clin Chest Med. 2004;25:637.

Nishino M, Itoh H, Hatabu H. A practical approach to high-resolution CT of diffuse lung disease. Eur J Radiol. 2014;83:6.

Nishino M, Washko GR, Hatabu H. Volumetric expiratory HRCT of the lung: clinical applications. Radiol Clin North Am. 2010;48:177.

Pannu J, Roller LJ, Maldonado F, et al. Transbronchial cryobiopsy for diffuse parenchymal lung disease: 30- and 90-day mortality. Eur Respir J. 2019;54.

Papazian L, Doddoli C, Chetaille B, et al. A contributive result of open-lung biopsy improves survival in acute respiratory distress syndrome patients. Crit Care Med. 2007;35:755.

Pipavath S, Godwin JD. Imaging of interstitial lung disease. Clin Chest Med. 2004;25:455.

Poletti V, Hetzel J. Transbronchial cryobiopsy in diffuse parenchymal lung disease: need for procedural standardization. Respiration. 2015;90:275.

Poletti V, Ravaglia C, Gurioli C, et al. Invasive diagnostic techniques in idiopathic interstitial pneumonias. Respirology. 2016;21:44.

Qureshi RA, Ahmed TA, Grayson AD, et al. Does lung biopsy help patients with interstitial lung disease? Eur J Cardiothorac Surg. 2002;21:621.

Raj R, Raparia K, Lynch DA, Brown KK. Surgical lung biopsy for interstitial lung diseases. Chest. 2017;151:1131.

Raju S, Ghosh S, Mehta AC. Chest CT signs in pulmonary disease: a pictorial review. Chest. 2017;151:1356.

Ravaglia C, Bonifazi M, Wells AU, et al. Safety and diagnostic yield of transbronchial lung cryobiopsy in diffuse parenchymal lung diseases: a comparative study versus video-assisted thoracoscopic lung biopsy and a systematic review of the literature. Respiration. 2016;91:215.

Ravaglia C, Wells AU, Tomassetti S, et al. Transbronchial lung cryobiopsy in diffuse parenchymal lung disease: comparison between biopsy from 1 segment and biopsy from 2 segments - diagnostic yield and complications. Respiration. 2017;93:285.

Romagnoli M, Colby TV, Berthet JP, et al. Poor concordance between sequential transbronchial lung cryobiopsy and surgical lung biopsy in the diagnosis of diffuse interstitial lung diseases. Am J Respir Crit Care Med. 2019;199:1249.

Seaman DM, Meyer CA, Gilman MD, McCormack FX. Diffuse cystic lung disease at high-resolution CT. AJR Am J Roentgenol. 2011;196:1305.

Seaman DM, Meyer CA, Kanne JP. Occupational and environmental lung disease. Clin Chest Med. 2015;36:249.

Sharp C, McCabe M, Adamali H, Medford AR. Use of transbronchial cryobiopsy in the diagnosis of interstitial lung disease-a systematic review and cost analysis. QJM. 2017;110:207.

Sheth JS, Belperio JA, Fishbein MC, et al. Utility of transbronchial vs surgical lung biopsy in the diagnosis of suspected fibrotic interstitial lung disease. Chest. 2017;151:389.

Stone E, Rankin N, Kerr S, et al. Does presentation at multidisciplinary team meetings improve lung cancer survival? Findings form a consecutive cohort study. Lung Cancer. 2018;124:199.

Troy LK, Grainge C, Corte TJ, et al. Diagnostic accuracy of transbronchial lung cryobiopsy for interstitial lung disease diagnosis (COLDICE): a prospective, comparative study. Lancet Respir Med. 2020;8:171.

Ussavarungsi K, Kern RM, Roden AC, et al. Transbronchial cryobiopsy in diffuse parenchymal lung disease: retrospective analysis of 74 cases. Chest. 2017;151:400.

Webb WR. Thin-section CT of the secondary pulmonary lobule: anatomy and the image—the 2004 Fleischner lecture. Radiology. 2006;239:322.

Welker L, Jörres RA, Costabel U, Magnussen H. Predictive value of BAL cell differentials in the diagnosis of interstitial lung diseases. Eur Respir J. 2004;24:1000.

CASE 1: BASIC ANATOMY

We will begin with a brief review of the anatomy on chest radiographs and CT scans. This is not intended to replace basic anatomy education or radiology training but to provide a brief review before delving into chest cases.

Identify the following structures on a normal chest radiograph shown in Image 1-1.

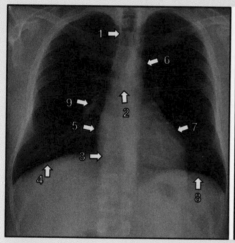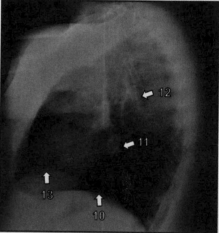

Image 1-1 • Normal chest radiograph.

A. Carina
B. Spine
C. Right atrium and right heart border
D. Lower pulmonary vascular bundle
E. Left ventricle and left heart border
F. Right hemidiaphragm
G. Left hemidiaphragm
H. Right hilum
I. Trachea
J. Aortic knob
K. Upper pulmonary vascular bundle and left mainstem bronchi

QUESTIONS

Q1-1: Structure 1?

Q1-2: Structure 2?

Q1-3: Structure 3?

Q1-4: Structure 4?

Q1-5: Structure 5?

Q1-6: Structure 6?

Q1-7: Structure 7?

Q1-8: Structure 8?

Q1-9: Structure 9?

Q1-10: Structure 10?

Q1-11: Structure 11?

Q1-12: Structure 12?

Q1-13: Structure 13?

Next, identify the following anatomic structures on mediastinal windows of the CT scan in Image 1-2.

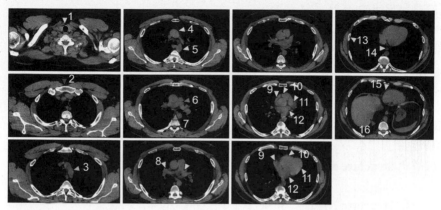

Image 1-2 • Normal chest CT scan, mediastinal window (without contrast).

A. Thoracic duct
B. Superior vena cava (SVC)
C. Ascending aorta
D. Descending aorta
E. Aortic arch
F. Trachea
G. Carina
H. Right mainstem
I. Left mainstem
J. Main pulmonary artery
K. Right and left main pulmonary arteries
L. Pericardium
M. Right atrium
N. Left atrium
O. Right ventricle
P. Left ventricle
Q. Thymus
R. Thyroid gland
S. Esophagus
T. Rib
U. Liver
V. Spleen
W. Sternum

Q1-14: Structure 1?

Q1-15: Structure 2?

Q1-16: Structure 3?

Q1-17: Structure 4?

Q1-18: Structure 5?

Q1-19: Structure 6?

Q1-20: Structure 7?

Q1-21: Structure 8?

Q1-22: Structure 9?

Q1-23: Structure 10?

Q1-24: Structure 11?

Q1-25: Structure 12?

Q1-26: Structure 13?

Q1-27: Structure 14?

Q1-28: Structure 15?

Q1-29: Structure 16?

Q1-30: What is the smallest functional unit of the lung termed?
A. Lobule
B. Secondary lobule
C. Tertiary lobule
D. Lobe
E. Segment
F. Subsegment

Q1-31: How many lobes and segments are there in the right lung?

A. 2 lobes, 8 segments
B. 3 lobes, 8 segments
C. 2 lobes, 10 segments
D. 3 lobes, 10 segments
E. 3 lobes, 9 segments

Q1-32: How many lobes and segments are there in the left lung?

A. 2 lobes, 8 segments
B. 3 lobes, 8 segments
C. 2 lobes, 10 segments
D. 3 lobes, 10 segments
E. 2 lobes, 9 segments

Q1-33: Into how many compartments is the mediastinum traditionally divided?

A. Two
B. Three
C. Five
D. Six
E. One

Q1-34: Which statement is false regarding AP chest radiographs?

A. They are commonly used in the intensive care unit (ICU).
B. Supplementary views are not often performed.
C. They are adequate to determine the positioning of central venous catheters and endotracheal tubes.
D. Compared with PA films, they better magnify mediastinal structures such as the heart.
E. Compared with PA films, they are more sensitive for the detection of small pneumothoraces and pleural effusions.

ANSWERS

Q1-1: I
Trachea

Rationale: It is always important to examine the trachea, both in terms of diameter and path. A trachea that is deviated may indicate an external mass, whereas a trachea that is narrowed may represent an internal mass, stricture, or other pathology (eg, foreign body).

Q1-2: A
Carina

Rationale: The carina represents the point at which the trachea divides into the right and left main stem bronchi. The right mainstem bronchi quickly divide into the right upper lobe bronchus and the bronchus intermedius, which serves the right middle and right lower lobes.

Q1-3: B
Spine

Rationale: It is always important to identify the bony structures of the thorax, including the clavicles, ribs, and spine. The clavicles can significantly aid in determining if a patient is rotated. The ribs provide anatomic landmarks. The spine images may demonstrate scoliosis or kyphosis, both of which can contribute to restrictive lung disease.

Q1-4: F
Right hemidiaphragm

Q1-5: C
Right atrium and right heart border

Rationale: This is particularly important when looking for adequate placement of a central venous catheter or peripherally inserted central catheter (PICC) line. Also, when the right heart border becomes hazy, this may represent pathology in the right middle lobe, which sits anterior to the right heart border.

Q1-6: J
Aortic knob

Q1-7: E
Left ventricle and left heart border

Rationale: Measurement of the left heart border on posteroanterior (PA) films can provide information regarding cardiomegaly.

Q1-8: G
Left hemidiaphragm

Rationale: Examination of the hemidiaphragm and the costophrenic angle (ie, where the pleural and diaphragm meet) can provide important information regarding hyperinflation, hemidiaphragmatic paralysis, pleural effusions, and subtle pneumothoraces (ie, deep sulcus signs).

Q1-9: H
Right hilum

Rationale: The right and left hilum are important areas to identify the presence of hilar adenopathy. Additionally, patients with pulmonary hypertension (HTN) or pulmonary edema may have enlargement/engorgement of the vasculature and lymphatics in this region.

Q1-10: G
Left hemidiaphragm

Rationale: Note the left hemidiaphragm is more caudal to the right hemidiaphragm because of the presence of the liver. Additionally, note that the space immediately caudal to the left hemidiaphragm demonstrates a clear view of the spine. A left lower lobe infiltrate will often present with a positive "spine sign," reducing the clarity with which one would see the spine on a lateral film.

Q1-11: D
Lower pulmonary vascular bundle

Q1-12: K
Upper pulmonary vascular bundle and left mainstem bronchi

Q1-13: F
Right hemidiaphragm

Rationale: Note the right hemidiaphragm is elevated anteriorly because of the liver.

Q1-14: F
Trachea

Q1-15: W
Sternum

Q1-16: E
Aortic arch

Q1-17: C
Ascending aorta

Q1-18: D
Descending aorta

Q1-19: J
Main pulmonary artery

Q1-20: S
Esophagus

Q1-21: K
Right and left main pulmonary artery

Q1-22: M
Right atrium

Q1-23: O
Right ventricle

Q1-24: P
Left ventricle

Q1-25: N
Left atrium

Q1-26: T
Rib

Q1-27: S
Esophagus

Q1-28: L
Pericardium

Q1-29: U
Liver

Q1-30: B
Secondary lobule

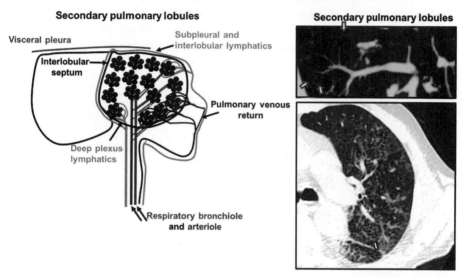

Image 1-3 • Secondary pulmonary lobule. The secondary pulmonary nodule is considered the smallest individual working unit of the lung, serviced by one common pulmonary arteriole and bronchiole and consisting of 20 to 40 alveoli. The structure is surrounded by interlobular septa, which hold the structure together and are a key component when examining radiographic abnormalities. These are the smallest structures visible on chest CT, typically around 0.5 to 1 cm. The centrilobular structures are the airways, lymphatics, and vasculature leading to the center of the lobule, while the interlobular structures consist of veins and lymphatics. The lung "parenchyma" is contained within the interlobular septa and around the centrilobular structures. This terminology aids greatly in defining the various pathologic conditions that can affect the lung.

Q1-31: D
3 lobes, 10 segments

Rationale: The right lung consists of the right upper lobe (RUL) (anterior, apical, posterior segments), the right middle lobe (RML) (medial, lateral segments), and the right lower lobe (RLL) (superior, anterobasal, lateral basal, posterior basal, medial basal). Note the location of the major and minor fissures. On the right, the major fissure separates the RUL and the RMLs from the RLL, while the minor fissure separates the RUL and the RMLs.

Q1-32: E
2 lobes, 9 segments

Rationale: The left lung consists of 2 lobes, the left upper and the left lower lobes as shown in **Image 1-4**. The left upper lobe (LUL) consists of 2 segments, an apicoposterior segment and an anterior segment. The left lower lobe (LLL), like the right lower lobe, has 5 segments (superior, anterior basal, medial basal, lateral basal, and posterior basal). Although the anterior and medial basal segments of the lower lobe (and the lateral and basal segments) may have a common segmental bronchus in some patients, they are separate segments. The left lung also contains the lingua, which is not considered a lobe, but it does have 2 segments (inferior and superior).

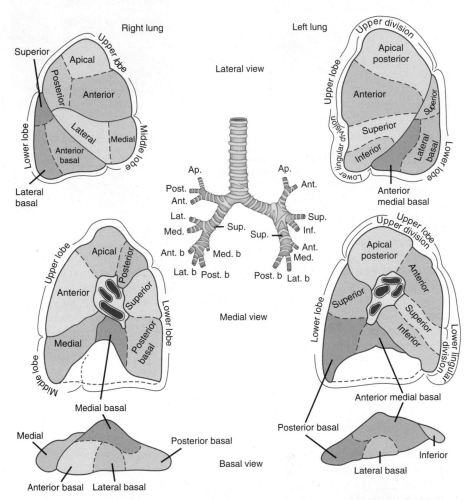

Image 1-4 • Lobes, segments, and subsegments of the human lung. (*Reproduced with permission from Doherty GM. Current Diagnosis & Treatment: Surgery, 13th ed. New York, NY: McGraw Hill; 2010.*)

The lobes of the lung are divided by the major and minor fissures (**Images 1-5 and 1-6**).

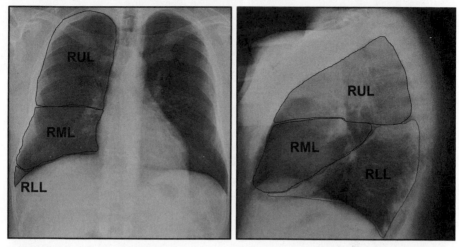

Image 1-5 • The RUL and RML are separated by the minor fissure, while the RUL and RLL are divided by the major fissure.

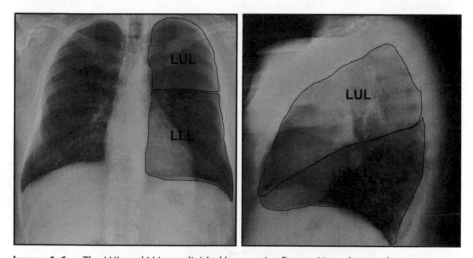

Image 1-6 • The LUL and LLL are divided by a major fissure. Note that on the postero-anterior (PA) films above there is considerable overlap between the segments that is not possible to display here. This is why the lateral films are particularly important to identify anatomic locations for lesions.

Q1-33: B
Three

Rationale: The mediastinum is classically divided into three compartments as shown in **Image 1-7** (anterior, middle, and posterior); however, some texts divide the anterior mediastinum into two segments (superior, containing the thyroid, and anterior). There are several cases that relate to the mediastinal compartments.

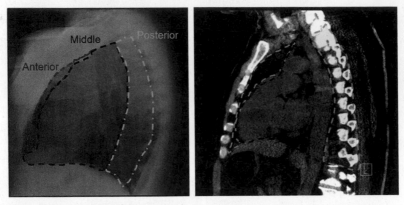

Image 1-7 • Mediastinal compartments. Again, note that the mediastinal compartment, like the lobes of the lung, is best examined on lateral or coronal images as opposed to PA or anteroposterior (AP) films.

> ## Q1-34: E
> **Compared with PA films, they are more sensitive for the detection of small pneumothoraces and pleural effusions**

Rationale: Compared with PA films, AP films offer less sensitivity for pneumothoraces (see "**Image 1-8** deep sulcus sign") and pleural effusions. They also provide less resolution overall, and the mediastinal structures (notably the heart) are enlarged. Supplementary views are not often performed, though lateral decubitus and lordotic films can be attempted. It is commonly used in the ICU and the emergency department (ED) when patients cannot travel or stand for imaging. It is adequate for views of common ICU apparatuses such as central venous catheters, endotracheal tubes, and nasogastric tubes.

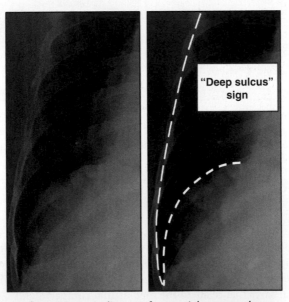

Image 1-8 • Deep sulcus sign, an indicator of potential pneumothorax.

CASE 2

An 18-year-old male college soccer player who is otherwise healthy is referred to your office by his primary care physician because of "an abnormal chest x-ray." The patient initially developed a dry cough approximately 6 months ago, which was thought to be due to exercise-induced asthma. The cough did not improve with an albuterol inhaler or inhaled corticosteroid, and the patient has now developed some dyspnea with exertion and a productive cough. The patient underwent further testing, which included a chest radiograph. His vital signs are T 37.2°C, HR 52, BP 123/76, RR 13, saturating 97% on room air. His electrocardiogram (ECG) shows only sinus bradycardia. He denies any fevers, chills, sweats, hemoptysis, weight loss or weight gain, vision issues, lightheadedness, or dizziness. His pulmonary examination demonstrates bronchial breath sounds on the right and some dullness. He has a wet-sounding cough that is partially cleared with a deep cough. He has no family history of rheumatologic disease or malignancy. He did have childhood asthma, but this resolved spontaneously when he was approximately 12 years old. He takes only ibuprofen or acetaminophen on an as-needed pro re nata (PRN) basis. He has no reported allergies. Over the last week, he has developed low-grade fevers and night sweats.

His chest x-ray (CXR) is shown in Image 2-1:

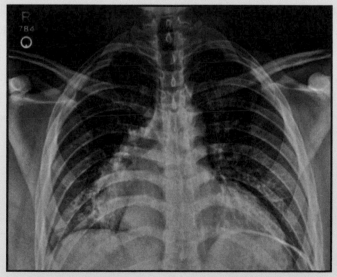

Image 2-1 • Enhanced chest radiograph for the patient in **Case 2** (AP film).

QUESTIONS

Q2-1: How would you describe the abnormalities on the chest radiograph in Image 2-1?

A. Diffuse cystic and nodule opacities
B. Mass or consolidation in the right lower lobe or mediastinum
C. Pneumomediastinum
D. Right-sided hydropneumothorax
E. Diaphragmatic flattening and loss of lung markings in the upper lobes bilaterally

Q2-2: The patient undergoes a CT scan of the chest as well as positron emission tomography (PET)-CT. These images are shown in Image 2-2.

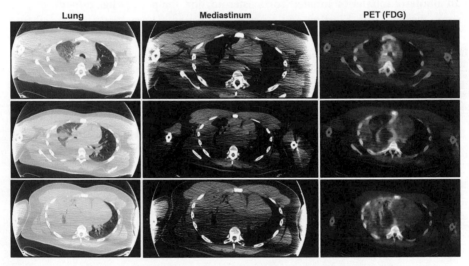

Image 2-2 • CT (lung and mediastinal windows) and associated PET-CT images. FDG, fluorodeoxyglucose.

How would you describe the abnormalities present on the CT and PET-CT scans shown in Image 2-2?

A. Right anterior mediastinal mass with associated atelectasis and pleural effusion
B. Right middle mediastinal mass with associated atelectasis and pleural effusion
C. Right posterior mediastinal mass with associated atelectasis and pleural effusion
D. Pneumothorax
E. Pericardial effusion

Q2-3: What are the cranial and caudal anatomic boundaries of the mediastinum?

A. Cranial – Thyroid gland; Caudal – Diaphragm
B. Cranial – Thoracic inlet; Caudal – Peritoneum
C. Cranial – Larynx; Caudal – Peritoneum
D. Cranial – Thoracic inlet; Caudal – Diaphragm
E. Cranial – Larynx; Caudal – Diaphragm

Q2-4: What are the anterior and posterior anatomic boundaries of the middle mediastinal compartment?

A. Anterior – Sternum; Posterior – 1 cm posterior to the anterior surface of the vertebral bodies

B. Anterior – Anterior surface of the pericardium; Posterior – Anterior surface of the descending thoracic aorta

C. Anterior – Anterior surface of the pericardium; Posterior – 1 cm posterior to the anterior surface of the vertebral bodies

D. Anterior – Sternum; Posterior – Posterior surface of the pericardium

E. Anterior – Anterior surface of the pericardium; Posterior – Posterior surface of the pericardium

Q2-5: Which structure is not present in the middle mediastinum?

A. Pericardium
B. Esophagus
C. Thymus
D. Trachea
E. Ascending aorta
F. Aortic arch
G. Descending aorta
H. Vagus nerve
I. Paratracheal and mediastinal lymph nodes
J. Azygous vein
K. Thoracic duct
L. Superior vena cava (SVC)

Q2-6: Which structures are included in the differential diagnoses for middle mediastinal masses? Select all that apply.

A. Thymoma
B. Teratoma
C. Hiatal hernia
D. Diaphragmatic hernia
E. Descending aortic aneurysm
F. Germ cell tumor
G. Meningocele
H. Bronchogenic cyst
I. Enteric cyst
J. Pericardial cyst
K. Lymphoma
L. Epidural abscess

Q2-7: Because the PET-CT scan demonstrated hypermetabolic uptake in the middle mediastinal mass, the patient undergoes video-assisted thoracoscopic surgery. The pleural fluid studies are consistent with an empyema, frozen sections performed in the operative suite demonstrate no evidence of malignancy, and the mass is not consistent with lymphoid tissue. What is the most likely diagnosis?

A. Infected bronchogenic cyst
B. Infected enteric cyst
C. Infected pericardial cyst
D. Infectious aortitis
E. Thoracic duct obstruction

ANSWERS

Q2-1: B
Mass or consolidation in the right lower lobe or mediastinum

Rationale: Unfortunately, this patient did not have a PA and lateral film. On this more limited AP film, one can see a mass or consolidation projecting over the posterior right lower lobe with widening of the mediastinum (**Image 2-3**). The consolidation appears posterior to the heart and pericardium in this view, though a lateral film would have been particularly helpful to localize the lesion. The borders of the mass appear somewhat jagged in this image as well. There may be some atelectasis in the right middle lobe. There is perhaps some overall volume loss. There are no pneumothoraces or hydropneumothoraces present. Pneumomediastinum would appear translucent rather than as an opaque consolidation. There are no cystic lesions, and there is no diaphragmatic flattening or other changes consistent with emphysema.

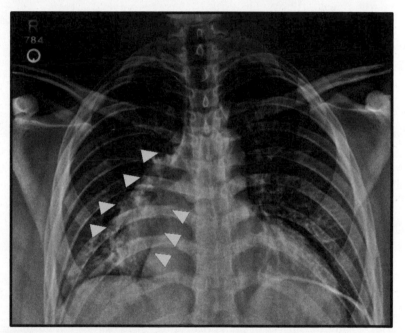

Image 2-3 • Consolidation/mass posterior to the pericardium/heart.

Q2-2: B
Right middle mediastinal mass with associated atelectasis and pleural effusion

Rationale: As this is a noncontrasted CT of the chest, the margins of the mass are difficult to delineate without the added benefit of the PET-CT scan. One can see that there is a heterogeneous fluid collection in the right pleural space as well as some associated atelectasis in the right middle lobe particularly (**Image 2-4**). The PET-CT demonstrates a middle mediastinal mass, with a hypermetabolic wall and a non-FDG avid center, indicating that there is some central necrosis present that has yet to cavitate. There are also possibly some hypermetabolic lymph nodes present, but they are difficult to make out on the PET-CT. There is some increased uptake in the vertebral bodies as well, though there are no obvious lytic lesions on CT. There is no apparent pneumothorax or pericardial fluid. This question focuses primarily on identifying the boundaries of the mediastinal compartments because this significantly aids in determining the most likely diagnosis.

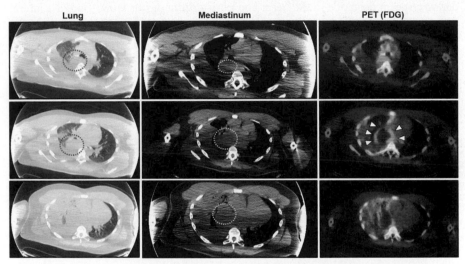

Image 2-4 • Note the hypermetabolic wall of the mass and the hypometabolic (black) center of the lesion (illuminated by white arrows). The white circles identify the mass on CT, which is difficult to discern from the complex fluid collection/pleural effusion.

Q2-3: D
Cranial – Thoracic inlet; Caudal – Diaphragm

Rationale: This will be further discussed in **Question Q2-4.**

Q2-4: C
Anterior – Anterior surface of the pericardium; Posterior – 1 cm posterior to the anterior surface of the vertebral bodies

Rationale: The mediastinum is the space contained within the following anatomic structures: cranially, thoracic inlet; caudally, diaphragm; left, left pleural cavity; right, right pleural cavity; anteriorly, sternum; posteriorly, vertebral bodies (inclusive of vertebral bodies and associated structures). The mediastinum may be further subdivided into three or four categories: anterior, middle, and posterior (**Image 2-5**), with superior being used in some classification systems. In 2017, the International Thymic Malignancy Interest Group (ITMWG) proposed a revised, three-compartment classification for mediastinal masses that is based on natural anatomic boundaries and is overall better suited to classification via cross-sectional imaging. We will use this classification system for the cases in this text. One primary difference between this current classification system and some prior systems is the border between the middle and posterior mediastinum. Some prior classification systems have used the posterior border of the pericardium or anterior border of the descending thoracic aorta; this often meant that benign cystic structures (eg, bronchogenic cysts) could be classified as either middle or posterior, despite arising from the same anatomic structures. The current system obviates these issues by using the vertebral bodies as the border between the middle and posterior compartments.

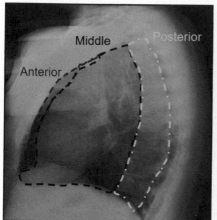 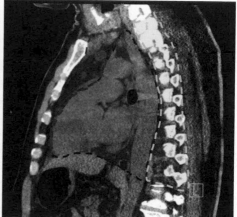

Image 2-5 • Mediastinal compartments.

TABLE 2-1 • Mediastinal Compartments Definitions			
	Cranial/Caudal	Left/Right	Anterior/Posterior
Mediastinum	Cranial – thoracic inlet Caudal – diaphragm	Left and right pleural cavities	Anterior: Sternum Posterior: Transverse processes
Compartment			
Anterior *(prevascular)*	Cranial – thoracic inlet Caudal – diaphragm	Left and right pleural cavities	Anterior: Sternum Posterior: Anterior aspect of the pericardium as it wraps around the heart, not a linear plane
Middle *(visceral)*	Cranial – thoracic inlet Caudal – diaphragm	Left and right pleural cavities	Anterior: Anterior mediastinum as defined above. Posterior: Mark a point 1 cm posterior to the anterior margin of each vertebral body, and draw a line connecting the dots
Posterior *(paravertebral)*	Cranial – thoracic inlet Caudal – diaphragm	Left and right pleural cavities	Anterior: Middle mediastinum as defined above Posterior: Line drawn down the posterior aspect of the transverse processes of the spine

Texts that use the superior mediastinum often define it by the following borders: left and right pleural spaces, thoracic inlet to the level of an imaginary plane drawn from the sternal angle to approximately the upper portion of the T4 vertebral body. The superior mediastinum contains the thymus/thymic remnants, possibly portions of the thyroid if substernal, the superior vena cava, the brachiocephalic veins, the aortic arch (and associated branches), the thoracic duct, the anterior portion of the esophagus, and the trachea. It contains paratracheal and mediastinal lymph nodes as well. It also contains the vagus, phrenic, left recurrent pharyngeal, and autonomic nerves. These structures are split among the various compartments in a three-compartment model.

Q2-5: C
Thymus

Rationale: The structures of the middle mediastinum include the pericardium, heart, aorta, trachea, mainstem bronchi, the pulmonary trunk (trunk of the pulmonary arteries and veins), esophagus, phrenic and vagus nerves, left recurrent laryngeal nerve, the SVC, the azygos vein, the thoracic duct, and numerous hilar and mediastinal lymph nodes. The thymus, thyroid (if substernal component), brachiocephalic vessels, fat, and lymph nodes make up the anterior compartment, while the vertebral bodies, paravertebral soft tissue, spinal ganglia, sympathetic chain, and portions of the spinal arteries make up the posterior mediastinum.

Structures Contained in the Mediastinal Compartments		
Anterior	Middle	Posterior
• Thymus • Brachiocephalic vein • Lymph nodes • Fat	• Pericardium • Heart • Aorta (ascending, arch, descending) • SVC • Thoracic duct • Azygous vein • Pulmonary vascular trunk • Lymph nodes • Esophagus • Trachea and mainstem bronchi	• Spinal ganglia • Sympathetic chain • Proximal intercostal arteries/nerves • Spinal cord • Paravertebral soft tissue • Lymph nodes • Portions of spinal arteries

Q2-6: C; D; E; H; I; J; K
Hiatal hernia; Diaphragmatic hernia; Descending aortic aneurysm; Bronchogenic cyst; Enteric cyst; Pericardial cyst; Lymphoma

Rationale: Thymomas, teratomas, and germ cell tumors are more common in the anterior mediastinum; meningocele and epidural abscesses are in the posterior mediastinum. The remaining pathologic processes should be included in the differential diagnoses of a middle mediastinal mass.

The new classification system for the mediastinal compartments provides the following differential diagnoses:

Differential Diagnosis for Mediastinal Masses		
Anterior	Middle	Posterior
Thymoma (approximately 50%)	Lymphoma	Neurogenic tumor (eg, neurofi-
Teratoma	Bronchial cyst	broma, neural sheath tumors)
Germ cell tumor (seminoma,	Pericardial cyst	Meningocele
non-seminoma)	Enteric cyst	Paravertebral abscess
Lymphoma	Granulomatous disease	Extramedullary hematopoiesis
Carcinoma (thyroid)	(eg, sarcoidosis)	Discitis/osteomyelitis
Substernal goiter	Aortic pathology	
Lipoma	Diaphragmatic hernia	

Q2-7: A
Infected bronchogenic cyst

Rationale: The most common cause of middle mediastinal masses is lymphadenopathy. This may be due to granulomatous disease, reactive in response to infection/inflammation/volume overload, or related to malignancy (lymphoma, metastatic lung cancer, small cell lung cancer). Because lymphadenopathy and malignancy have been eliminated, the next most likely diagnosis would be a bronchogenic cyst. Bronchogenic cysts arise as duplication cysts during initial lung budding during the first trimester. The location of the lesion here is classic for bronchogenic cysts in the right subcarinal region. Patients may be asymptomatic, with the lesion having been discovered incidentally, or patients may present with symptoms of dyspnea, cough, chest pain, and recurrent infection. In this case, the patient's bronchogenic cysts became infected, leading to the development of empyema. Although a simple cyst can often be monitored via imaging without the need for resection, patients with more complex cyst characteristics, evidence of infection, or cysts that are causing significant symptoms will require resection.

The clinical presentation of patients with mediastinal masses varies significantly and is dependent on several factors, including whether the mass is benign or malignant (and if malignant, from which tissue it originates), the size of the mass, and the anatomic location of the mass. Patients with larger masses may experience symptoms simply from the mass/volume effect of the lesions, which can lead to potentially life-threatening complications through constriction or obstruction of the airways/bronchi, blood vessels, heart, and nerves. Patients with malignant lesions may experience constitutional symptoms commonly associated with malignancy or paraneoplastic symptoms (eg, thymoma-associated myasthenia gravis). Patients with small, benign masses may be entirely asymptomatic, and the mass is discovered incidentally.

Similarly, the imaging of mediastinal masses varies widely depending on the pathology. In terms of the diagnostic workup, a thorough history and physical examination are followed by appropriate imaging studies. CT is often the first imaging modality chosen, given its availability. Contrasted CT is often helpful because it will differentiate vascular structures from lymph nodes and more clearly define anatomic structures. It may also aid in identifying which vascular structures are supplying a particular mass or lesion. Often, magnetic resonance imaging (MRI) is required. MRI is more effective at characterizing the composition of tissue structures (cystic versus solid versus fat), and can better delineate if a mass is compressing or invading other structures, which may be necessary to determine the most appropriate treatment. MRI is particularly useful in the posterior mediastinum, where the spine and nervous system are involved. PET-CT is of somewhat limited utility in the mediastinum, due in part to a higher propensity for false-positive results. However, PET-CT is often performed because it can identify distant sites of disease that may be more amenable to biopsy and that may provide more staging information. For patients with suspected thyroid cancer or substernal goiter, a technetium uptake scan may also be helpful.

Some lesions that can be identified with imaging alone include:

- Cystic lesions – well-circumscribed, homogeneous, fluid-attenuated lesions – Duplication cysts (bronchogenic, enteric, pericardial)
- Enhancing masses on CT – paragangliomas, pheochromocytomas (extra-adrenal), Castleman disease (nonclonal lymphoid hyperplasia), metastatic carcinomas (renal, thyroid, melanoma, choriocarcinoma, sarcoma)
- Esophageal lesions – cancer, polyp, lipoma
- Cardiac masses (angiosarcomas)

References

Carter BW, Benveniste MF, Madan R, et al. ITMIG classification of mediastinal compartments and multidisciplinary approach to mediastinal masses. Radiographics 2017;37:413.

Carter BW, Betancourt SL, Benveniste MF. MR imaging of mediastinal masses. Top Magn Reson Imaging. 2017;26:153.

Chira RI, Chira A, Mircea PA, Valean S. Mediastinal masses-transthoracic ultrasonography aspects. Medicine (Baltimore). 2017;96:e9082.

Duwe BV, Sterman DH, Musani AI. Tumors of the mediastinum. Chest. 2005;128:2893.

Juanpere S, Cañete N, Ortuño P, et al. A diagnostic approach to the mediastinal masses. Insights Imaging. 2013;4:29.

Laurent F, Latrabe V, Lecesne R, Zennaro H, Airaud JY, Rauturier JF, Drouillard J. Mediastinal masses: diagnostic approach. Eur Radiol. 1998;8:1148.

Nakazono T, Yamaguchi K, Egashira R, Mizuguchi M, Irie H. Anterior mediastinal lesions: CT and MRI features and differential diagnosis. Jpn J Radiol. 2021;39:101.

Prosch H, Röhrich S, Tekin ZN, Ebner L. The role of radiological imaging for masses in the prevascular mediastinum in clinical practice. J Thorac Dis. 2020;12:7591.

Su S, Colson YL. Overview of benign and malignant mediastinal diseases. In: Adult Chest Surgery, 2nd ed, Sugarbaker DJ, Bueno R, Colson YL, et al (Eds), McGraw-Hill Education, New York 2015. p. 1234.

Thacker PG, Mahani MG, Heider A, Lee EY. Imaging Evaluation of Mediastinal Masses in Children and Adults: Practical Diagnostic Approach Based on A New Classification System. J Thorac Imaging. 2015;30:247.

Whitten CR, Khan S, Munneke GJ, Grubnic S. A diagnostic approach to mediastinal abnormalities. Radiographics. 2007 May;27:657.

CASE 3

A 55-year-old White man with a history of primary HTN and hyperlipidemia, currently taking lisinopril and simvastatin, presents to the office as a referral from his primary care physician for a "mass" on a chest radiogram. The patient has no other medical history and no family history of malignancy, lung disease, or rheumatologic disease. He notes that he has been more fatigued recently, particularly at the end of the day, and this is associated with some blurry vision. He attributes this to working longer hours and not getting restful sleep. He also has not been to the optometrist in several years and suspects he may simply need new glasses. The chest radiograph was performed as part of an executive health evaluation because of insurance requirements for his investment business. It is the first chest radiograph he has had performed in approximately 25 years when he was involved in a skiing accident. His laboratory values are all within normal range. His physical examination is entirely unremarkable. His vital signs are all within normal limits. He is saturating 100% O_2 on room air, with no tachypnea, no cyanosis, and no clubbing.

The patient provides a CD with the following images:

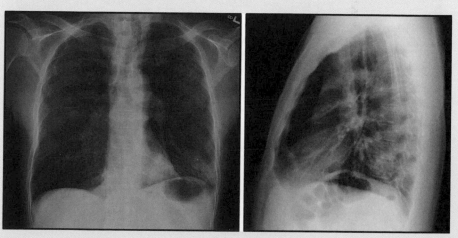

Image 3-1 • Chest radiograph of the patient in **Case 3**.

QUESTIONS

Q3-1: What is the primary abnormality present in the chest radiograph in Image 3-1?

A. Hyperinflation with diaphragmatic flattening
B. Tram-track bronchial wall-thickening concerning for bronchiectasis
C. Bilateral hilar adenopathy
D. Cardiomegaly
E. Tracheal deviation

Q3-2: The patient is in Case 3 undergoes a CT scan of the neck and chest because of the abnormalities identified.

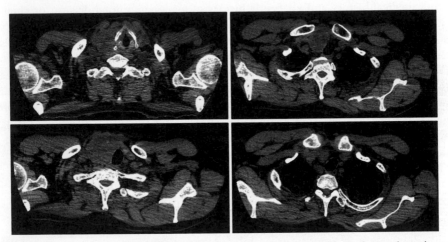

Image 3-2 • CT scan of the neck and chest for the patient in **Case 3**. Mediastinal windows only are shown. The esophagus can just be made out posterior to the trachea in the most inferior image of the CT scan (bottom right).

What is the primary abnormality on the CT scan shown in Image 3-2?

A. Heterogenous mass in the right anterior mediastinum
B. Heterogenous mass in the right middle mediastinum
C. Heterogenous mass in the right posterior mediastinum
D. Right lung mass causing mediastinal shift to the left
E. Sternal osteomyelitis

Q3-3: What are the borders of the thoracic inlet?

A. The plane formed by the sternal notch, the second ribs bilaterally, and the T2 vertebral body.
B. The plane formed by the sternum, the fourth ribs bilaterally, and the T4 vertebral body.
C. The plane formed by the manubrium, the first ribs bilaterally, and the T1 vertebral body.
D. The plane between the scalene muscles, the clavicle, and the first rib.

Q3-4: What are the anatomic structures of the anterior mediastinum?

A. Vascular structures, lymph nodes, pericardium, esophagus, trachea
B. Lymph nodes, brachiocephalic veins, fat, thymus
C. Spinal ganglia, paravertebral soft tissue, proximal intercostal arteries
D. Thymus, Heart, Esophagus, Pulmonary vascular trunk

Q3-5: What is the likely diagnosis?

A. Teratoma
B. Thyroid carcinoma
C. Lymphoma
D. Thymoma
E. Thymic cyst

Q3-6: Which laboratory testing would be most helpful to confirm the diagnosis of a thymoma?

A. Cancer antigen 19-9 (CA 19-9)
B. Thyroid-stimulating hormone
C. Serum calcium, ionized calcium, and parathyroid hormone
D. Serum alpha-fetoprotein (AFP) and beta-human chorionic gonadotropin (bHCG)
E. Anti-acetylcholinesterase receptor antibodies

Q3-7: From which embryonic structure does the thymus develop?

A. Pharyngeal arch 3
B. Pharyngeal arch 4
C. Pharyngeal pouch 2
D. Pharyngeal pouch 3

Q3-8: Aside from myasthenia gravis, what other complications are often associated with thymomas?

A. Thrombocytosis
B. Hypergammaglobulinemia
C. Lymphopenia
D. Pure red cell aplasia
E. Aplastic anemia
F. Paroxysmal nocturnal hemoglobinuria

Q3-9: Which imaging modality is most sensitive to determine if a thymoma has invaded local tissue structures?

A. Contrasted CT scan
B. MRI
C. Technetium-99 uptake scan
D. Ultrasonography
E. Arteriogram

Q3-10: What is the diagnostic yield of ultrasound-guided core percutaneous core needle biopsy for the diagnosis of thymoma?

A. 25%
B. 35%
C. 50%
D. 65%
E. 95%

ANSWERS

Q3-1: E
Tracheal deviation

Rationale: Although there does seem to be some possible flattening of the diaphragm, there is an appropriate number of rib spaces present, and there is no evidence of hyperlucency in the upper lobes. There is no evidence of tram-track bronchiectasis or hilar adenopathy, and the heart is entirely normal. There is a significant deviation of the trachea to the left just above the sternoclavicular joint, between the first and second ribs (**Image 3-3**). This is the most significant abnormality present in **Image 3-1**.

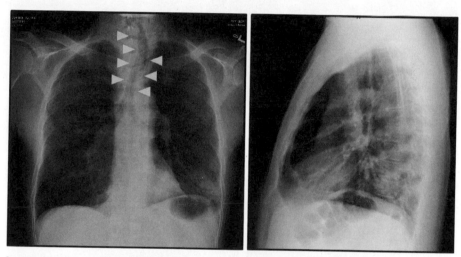

Image 3-3 • Note the tracheal deviation on the left. This is concerning for a possible mass.

Q3-2: A
Heterogenous mass in the right anterior mediastinum

Rationale: Here, we can see a well-circumscribed mass in the anterior mediastinal compartment abutting the trachea and causing tracheal deviation without significant external compression (**Image 3-4**). The mediastinal compartments are demonstrated in **Image 3-5** as well. The anterior mediastinum is bordered posteriorly (and posteroinferiorly) by the anterior pericardium; this is not a linear plane but rather is contoured by the shape of the pericardium, so anything anterior and above the pericardium is contained in the anterior mediastinum. There is no evidence of a lung mass in this image, nor is there evidence of sternal osteomyelitis (stranding or enhancement in sternum). The anterior mediastinum contains a small portion of the upper trachea.

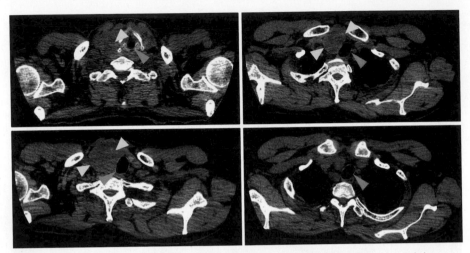

Image 3-4 • Note the mass present in the paratracheal space (*white arrows*) and the deviation of the trachea as a result of the mass effect (*gray arrows*).

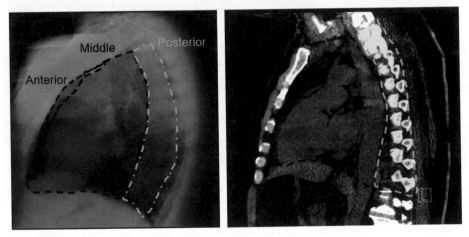

Image 3-5 • Mediastinal compartments.

The mediastinum is the space contained within the following anatomic structures: cranially, thoracic inlet; caudally, diaphragm; left, left pleural cavity; right, right pleural cavity; anteriorly, sternum; posteriorly, vertebral bodies (inclusive of vertebral bodies and associated structures). The mediastinum may be further subdivided into three or four categories: anterior, middle, and posterior, with superior being used in some classification systems. In 2017, the International Thymic Malignancy Interest Group (ITMWG) proposed a revised, three-compartment classification for mediastinal masses that is based on natural anatomic boundaries and is overall better suited to classification via cross-sectional imaging. We will use this classification system for the cases in this text. One primary difference between this current classification system and some prior systems is the border between the middle and posterior mediastinum. Some classification systems have used the posterior border of the pericardium or the anterior border of the descending thoracic aorta; this often meant that benign cystic structures (eg, bronchogenic cysts) could be classified as either middle or posterior, despite arising from the same anatomic structures. The current system obviates these issues by using the vertebral bodies as the border between the middle and posterior compartments.

TABLE 3-1 • Mediastinal Compartments Definitions			
	Cranial/Caudal	Left/Right	Anterior/Posterior
Mediastinum	Cranial – thoracic inlet Caudal – diaphragm	Left and right pleural cavities	Anterior: Sternum Posterior: Transverse processes
Compartment			
Anterior *(prevascular)*	Cranial – thoracic inlet Caudal – diaphragm	Left and right pleural cavities	Anterior: Sternum Posterior: Anterior aspect of the pericardium as it wraps around the heart, not a linear plane
Middle *(visceral)*	Cranial – thoracic inlet Caudal – diaphragm	Left and right pleural cavities	Anterior: Anterior mediastinum as defined above Posterior: Mark a point 1 cm posterior to the anterior margin of each vertebral body, and draw a line connecting the dots
Posterior *(paravertebral)*	Cranial – thoracic inlet Caudal – diaphragm	Left and right pleural cavities	Anterior: Middle mediastinum as defined above Posterior: Line drawn down the posterior aspect of the transverse processes of the spine

Texts that use the superior mediastinum often define it by the following borders: left and right pleural spaces and the thoracic inlet to the level of an imaginary plane drawn from the sternal angle to approximately the upper portion of the T4 vertebral body. The superior mediastinum contains the thymus/thymic remnants, possibly portions of the thyroid if substernal, the superior vena cava, the brachiocephalic veins, the aortic arch (and associated branches), the thoracic duct, the anterior portion of the esophagus, and the trachea. It contains paratracheal and mediastinal lymph nodes as well. It also contains the vagus, phrenic, left recurrent pharyngeal, and autonomic nerves. These structures are split among the various compartments in a three-compartment model.

Q3-3: C
The plane formed by the manubrium, the first ribs bilaterally, and the T1 vertebral body

Rationale: The thoracic inlet is the cranial or superior border of the mediastinum. It is an imaginary plane drawn between the superior border of the manubrium and the superior portion of the T1 vertebral body, and it is bordered laterally on both the right and left by the first ribs. The thoracic outlet is described in answer D. A vast number of structures travel through the thoracic inlet, including the trachea, esophagus, thoracic duct, sympathetic trunk, and multiple arterial, venous, and nerve structures.

Q3-4: B
Lymph nodes, brachiocephalic veins, fat, thymus

Structures Contained in the Mediastinal Compartments		
Anterior	Middle	Posterior
• Thymus • Brachiocephalic vein • Lymph nodes • Fat	• Pericardium • Heart • Aorta (ascending, arch, descending) • SVC • Thoracic duct • Azygous vein • Pulmonary vascular trunk • Lymph nodes • Esophagus • Trachea and mainstem bronchi	• Spinal ganglia • Sympathetic chain • Proximal intercostal arteries/nerves • Thoracic spinal cord • Paravertebral soft tissue • Lymph nodes • Portions of spinal arteries

Q3-5: D
Thymoma

Rationale: The CT scan shows a well-circumscribed mass with a likely fat component. Thymomas are the most common pathology causing anterior mediastinal masses. The patient's symptoms of fatigue and blurry vision (likely double vision) at the end of the day would be concerning for myasthenia gravis, which complicates approximately 30% of thymomas. Although this patient's CT scan shows no calcifications, thymomas often contain punctate calcifications. A teratoma is a tumor with a heterogeneous composition and may contain fat, bone, hair, muscle, and teeth. Goiters and thyroid carcinomas are typically lobulated in nature, while lymphomas are typically more abnormal in shape. A thymic cyst would not produce symptoms of myasthenia gravis.

Q3-6: E
Anti-acetylcholinesterase receptor antibodies

Rationale: Laboratory studies may be supportive but are rarely diagnostic in the evaluation of mediastinal masses. If a substernal thyroid goiter is suspected, thyroid function testing would be useful. For patients with a suspected thymoma, the presence of anti-acetylcholinesterase receptor antibodies should be obtained. For patients with a suspected germ cell tumor, AFP and bHCG are typically sent; these studies can help to differentiate seminomas from nonseminomas (approximately 50% to 70% positive for elevated levels of both AFP and bHCG). Hypercalcemia may indicate a parathyroid adenoma, granulomatous disease, or a lymphoma. Elevated lactate dehydrogenase (LDH) and uric acid levels may indicate a lymphoma, while hypoglycemia may indicate a sarcoma or teratoma. Elevated cortisol levels may indicate a carcinoid tumor.

Q3-7: D
Pharyngeal pouch 3

Rationale: Arch 3 produces the internal carotid artery and cranial nerve (CN) IX, while arch 4 leads to the development of the right subclavian artery, the vagus nerve, and the pharyngeal and laryngeal musculature. Pouch 2 leads to the supratonsillar fossa; pouch 3 (and 4) leads to the thymus and parathyroid gland.

Q3-8: D
Red cell aplasia

Rationale: Red cell aplasia is most often seen a paraneoplastic syndrome associated with thymoma and is effectively cured with thymectomy. Thymomas are associated with a wide range of autoimmune complications including Lambert-Eaton syndrome, Morvan syndrome, systemic lupus erythematosus (SLE), bullous pemphigoid, mysositis, encephalitis, paraneoplastic cerebellar degeneration, and stiff person syndrome, among others.

Q3-9: B
MRI

Rationale: CT is often the first imaging modality chosen during the evaluation of a mediastinal mass because of its availability. A contrasted CT scan is often helpful because it will differentiate vascular structures from lymph nodes and more clearly define anatomic structures. It may also aid in identifying which vascular structures are supplying a particular mass or lesion. Often, MRI is required. MRI is more effective at characterizing the composition tissue structures (cystic vs solid vs fat) and can better delineate if a mass is compressing or invading other structures, which may be necessary in determine the most appropriate treatment. This is particularly important for staging thymomas, and it is also particularly useful in the posterior mediastinum, where the spine and nervous system are involved. Positron Emission Tomography-Computed Tomography (PET-CT) is of somewhat limited utility in the mediastinum, due in part to a higher propensity for false-positive results. However, PET-CT is often performed because it can identify distant sites of disease that may be more amenable to biopsy and it may provide more staging information. For patients with suspected thyroid cancer or substernal goiter, a technetium uptake scan may also be helpful.

For thymomas, staging is the most important determinant of survival. This is accomplished using the Masaoka staging system: (I) intact thymic capsule; (II) capsular invasion into the mediastinal fat or pleura; (III) macroscopic invasion into adjacent organs or vessels; and (IV) dissemination into the thoracic cavity (IVa) or distant disease (IVb).

Q3-10: E
95%

Rationale: For anterior and posterior masses, ultrasound or CT-guided percutaneous biopsy offers a high diagnostic yield (70%), with nearly a 100% yield in thymomas.

However, as is typical with lymphomas (particular in the anterior mediastinum, where fibrosis or sclerosis may be present in the nodes of Hodgkin lymphoma), the yield is less than 20%. When this biopsy is attempted, a clinician should always use a core needle rather than a fine-needle for aspiration, as this increases the diagnostic yield from 60% to between 80% and 90%. For middle mediastinal masses, or some anterior masses, ultrasound-guided biopsy via the esophagus (EUS) or bronchial tree (EBUS) may be viable options if a mass or lymph node rests in close proximity to these structures. If not, mediastinoscopy or video-assisted thoracoscopic surgery (VATS) is often required.

Most mediastinal masses will require tissue sampling to obtain a definitive diagnosis. This may be done at the time of resection if necessary, or a preresection biopsy may be necessary in cases of malignancy. If the structures are purely cystic on imaging, the masses likely do not require biopsy because they are very likely to be benign and the decision on resection will depend on the clinical symptoms induced by the mass. Some other lesions that may be identifiable at imaging include thyroid goiter and pure lipomas. A combination of CT and PET can often identify germ cell neoplasms and lymphomas. A combination of laboratory findings and imaging can often identify a parathyroid adenoma. However, if there is soft tissue characteristics present (other than those homogenous cases described above) or any doubt regarding the diagnosis, the mass will likely require a biopsy.

Some lesions that can be identified with imaging and other noninvasive studies alone include:

- Cystic lesions – well-circumscribed, homogeneous, fluid-attenuated lesions – Duplication cysts (bronchogenic, enteric, pericardial)
- Enhancing masses on CT – paragangliomas, pheochromocytomas (extra-adrenal), Castleman disease (nonclonal lymphoid hyperplasia), metastatic carcinomas (renal, thyroid, melanoma, choriocarcinoma, sarcoma)
- Esophageal lesions – cancer, polyp, lipoma
- Cardiac masses (angiosarcomas)

References

Carter BW, Benveniste MF, Madan R, et al. ITMIG classification of mediastinal compartments and multidisciplinary approach to mediastinal masses. Radiographics. 2017;37:413.

Carter BW, Betancourt SL, Benveniste MF. MR imaging of mediastinal masses. Top Magn Reson Imaging. 2017;26:153.

Chira RI, Chira A, Mircea PA, Valean S. Mediastinal masses-transthoracic ultrasonography aspects. Medicine (Baltimore). 2017;96:e9082.

Duwe BV, Sterman DH, Musani AI. Tumors of the mediastinum. Chest. 2005;28:2893.

Juanpere S, Cañete N, Ortuño P, et al. A diagnostic approach to the mediastinal masses. Insights Imaging. 2013;4:29.

Laurent F, Latrabe V, Lecesne R, Zennaro H, Airaud JY, Rauturier JF, Drouillard J. Mediastinal masses: diagnostic approach. Eur Radiol. 1998;8:1148.

Nakazono T, Yamaguchi K, Egashira R, Mizuguchi M, Irie H. Anterior mediastinal lesions: CT and MRI features and differential diagnosis. Jpn J Radiol. 2021;39:101.

Prosch H, Röhrich S, Tekin ZN, Ebner L. The role of radiological imaging for masses in the prevascular mediastinum in clinical practice. J Thorac Dis. 2020;12:7591.

Su S, Colson YL. Overview of benign and malignant mediastinal diseases. In: Adult Chest Surgery, 2nd ed, Sugarbaker DJ, Bueno R, Colson YL, et al. (Eds), McGraw-Hill Education, New York 2015. p. 1234.

Thacker PG, Mahani MG, Heider A, Lee EY. Imaging evaluation of mediastinal masses in children and adults: Practical diagnostic approach based on a new classification system. J Thorac Imaging. 2015;30:247.

Whitten CR, Khan S, Munneke GJ, Grubnic S. A diagnostic approach to mediastinal abnormalities. Radiographics. 2007;27:657.

CASE 4

A 44-year-old man with refractory HTN is admitted to the hospital for medical management. He has been experiencing anxiety, palpitations, and episodes of diaphoresis intermittently for the last 2 to 3 months. He was seen by his primary care provider, and his thyroid-stimulating hormone (TSH) was within normal limits. The remainder of his laboratory studies were also normal. He was started on amlodipine for his elevated BP and was sent for some basic studies. His vital signs are reported as T 99.0°F, BP 197/111, HR 99, RR 12, and O₂ saturation 99% on room air. The patient states that he is unsure of any significant family history because he was adopted as a baby. He works for a security company but works behind a desk monitoring security camera feeds and has no exposures. He also takes medication for gastroesophageal reflux disease (GERD). He has no allergies and no other occupational or environmental exposures. He has no other apparent medical history.

The ED physician reports that the patient's CXR was abnormal and needs follow-up.

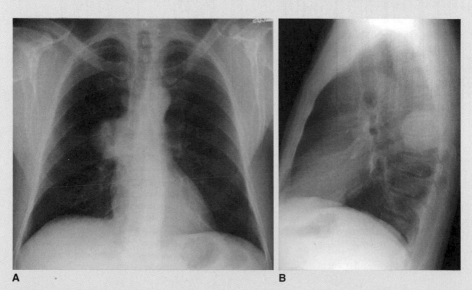

A   B

Image 4-1 • Chest radiograph for the patient in **Case 4**. (*Reproduced with permission from Chen MYM, Pope TL, Ott DJ: Basic Radiology, 2nd ed. New York, NY: McGraw Hill; 2011.*)

QUESTIONS

Q4-1: What is the primary abnormality identified in the chest radiograph Image 4-1?

A. A poorly circumscribed mass in the anterior mediastinum
B. A well-circumscribed mass in the right lung
C. A well-circumscribed mass in the middle mediastinum
D. A well-circumscribed mass in the posterior mediastinum
E. A poorly circumscribed mass in the posterior mediastinum
F. A well-circumscribed mass in the anterior mediastinum

Q4-2: What is the best imaging modality to further evaluate the mass in question?

A. Noncontrasted CT scan
B. Contrasted CT scan
C. MRI
D. PET-CT
E. Technetium-99 scan
F. Gallium bone scan
G. Ultrasonography

Q4-3: Which structures are not contained in the posterior mediastinum? Select all that apply.

A. Thoracic spine
B. Spinal ganglia
C. Proximal intercostal arteries
D. Distal intercostal arteries
E. Descending thoracic aorta
F. Superior vena cava
G. Thoracic duct
H. Azygous vein
 I. Sympathetic chain

Q4-4: What are differential diagnoses for posterior mediastinal masses?

A. Teratoma, goiter, lymphoma
B. Schwannoma, meningocele, neuroblastoma
C. Pericardial cyst, atrial myxoma

Q4-5: On examination, you notice the following dermatologic findings (Image 4-2).

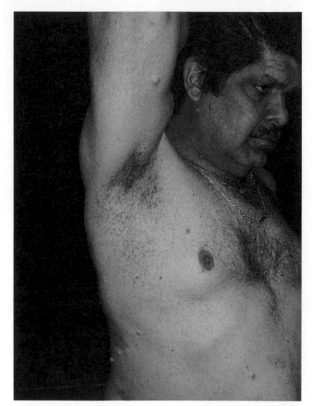

Image 4-2 • Findings on dermatologic examination of the patient in **Case 4**. (*Reproduced with permission from Usatine RP, Smith MA, Mayeaux EJ, et al: The Color Atlas and Synopsis of Family Medicine, 3rd ed. New York, NY: McGraw Hill; 2019. Photo contributor: Richard P. Usatine, MD.*)

What is the most likely diagnosis for the patient's mediastinal mass?

A. Schwannoma
B. Lymphoma
C. Duplication cyst
D. Neurofibroma
E. Bronchogenic cyst
F. Diaphragmatic hernia

Q4-6: What laboratory test should be ordered next to determine the etiology of the patient's presenting symptoms?

A. Free T4 and T3
B. Parathyroid hormone (PTH) and ionized calcium
C. Serum metanephrines and 5-HIAA
D. Serum aldosterone and cortisol
E. Procalcitonin

Q4-7: Mutations of the neurofibromin gene causing NF1 are associated with increased activity of which tumor gene?

A. BRCA
B. Bcr-Abl
C. p53
D. Retinoblastoma
E. Ras
F. Bcl2

ANSWERS

Q4-1: D
A well-circumscribed mass in the posterior mediastinum

Rationale: Here we have a standard PA and lateral image (**Image 4-3**). There is a mass present along the right heart border. It is well circumscribed. The right heart border remains visible, indicating that the mass lies posterior to the right atrium and the great vessels. On the lateral view, the mass is obscuring the vertebral column, indicating that it likely originates from the posterior mediastinum.

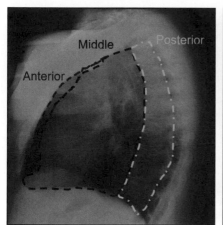 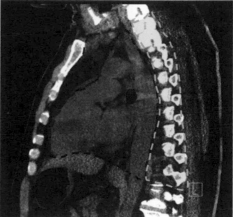

Image 4-3 • Mediastinal compartments.

Mediastinal masses may be benign or malignant, with the likelihood of malignancy depending on age, mass location, and presence or absence of symptoms. Mediastinal masses may arise from mediastinal structures (either those present at birth or resulting from abnormalities during development) or from metastatic disease from malignancies arising elsewhere.

The mediastinum is the space contained within the following anatomic structures: cranially, thoracic inlet; caudally, diaphragm; left, left pleural cavity; right, right pleural cavity; anteriorly, sternum; posteriorly, vertebral bodies (inclusive of vertebral bodies and associated structures). The mediastinum may be further subdivided into three or four categories: anterior, middle, and posterior, with superior being used in some classification systems. In 2017, the International Thymic Malignancy Interest Group (ITMWG) proposed a revised, three-compartment classification for mediastinal masses that is based on natural anatomic boundaries and is overall better suited to classification via cross-sectional imaging. We will use this classification system for the cases in this text. One primary difference between this current classification system and some prior systems is the border between the middle and posterior mediastinum. Some prior classification systems have used the posterior border of the pericardium or anterior border of the descending thoracic aorta; this often meant that benign cystic structures (eg, bronchogenic cysts) could be classified as either middle or posterior, despite arising from the same anatomic structures. The current system obviates these issues by using the vertebral bodies as the border between the middle and posterior compartments.

Mediastinal Compartments Definitions			
	Cranial/Caudal	Left/Right	Anterior/Posterior
Mediastinum	Cranial – thoracic inlet Caudal - diaphragm	Left and right pleural cavities	Anterior: Sternum Posterior: Transverse processes
Compartment			
Anterior (*prevascular)*	Cranial – thoracic inlet Caudal – diaphragm	Left and right pleural cavities	Anterior: Sternum Posterior: Anterior aspect of the pericardium as it wraps around the heart, not a linear plane
Middle (*visceral)*	Cranial – thoracic inlet Caudal – diaphragm	Left and right pleural cavities	Anterior: anterior mediastinum as defined above Posterior: Mark a point 1 cm posterior to the anterior margin of each vertebral body, and draw a line connecting the dots
Posterior (*paravertebral)*	Cranial – thoracic inlet Caudal – diaphragm	Left and right pleural cavities	Anterior: Middle mediastinum as defined above Posterior: Line drawn down the posterior aspect of the transverse processes of the spine

Q4-2: C
MRI

Rationale: MRI is the preferred imaging technique for masses in the posterior mediastinum. This will be discussed further in this case. Here, the patient underwent an MRI scan demonstrating a well-circumscribed paraspinal tumor associated with the neural foramen (**Image 4-4**).

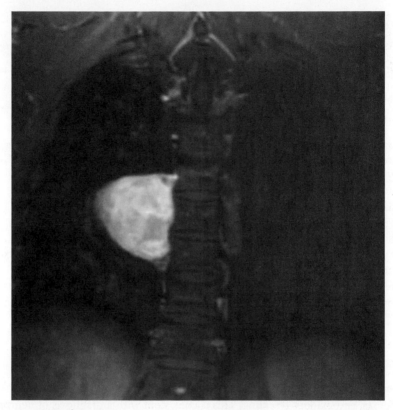

Image 4-4 • MRI of paraspinal mass in **Case 4**. (*Reproduced with permission from Chen MYM, Pope TL, Ott DJ: Basic Radiology, 2nd ed. New York, NY: McGraw Hill; 2011.*)

Q4-3: D; E; F; G; H
Distal intercostal arteries; Descending thoracic aorta; Superior vena cava; Thoracic duct; Azygous vein

Rationale: Although a small portion of the azygous vein is contained in the posterior mediastinum, the majority of the vessel is contained in the middle mediastinum. These structures are all contained in the middle mediastinum.

Structures Contained in the Mediastinal Compartments		
Anterior	Middle	Posterior
• Thymus • Brachiocephalic vein • Lymph nodes • Fat	• Pericardium • Heart • Aorta (ascending, arch, descending) • SVC • Thoracic duct • Azygous vein • Pulmonary vascular trunk • Lymph nodes • Esophagus • Trachea and mainstem bronchi	• Spinal ganglia • Sympathetic chain • Proximal intercostal arteries/nerves • Spinal cord • Paravertebral soft tissue • Lymph nodes • Portions of spinal arteries

Q4-4: B
Schwannoma, meningocele, neuroblastoma

Rationale: The posterior mediastinum consists of the thoracic spine, the associated spinal ganglia and the sympathetic chain, servicing arteries and veins, associated lymph nodes, and paraspinal soft tissue. The differential diagnoses for posterior mediastinal masses include the following:

Differential Diagnosis for Mediastinal Masses		
Anterior	Middle	Posterior
Thymoma (approximately 50%)	Lymphoma	Neurogenic tumor (eg, neurofibromatosis)
Teratoma	Bronchial cyst	Meningocele
Germ cell tumor (seminoma, nonseminoma)	Pericardial cyst	Paravertebral abscess
	Enteric cyst	Extramedullary hematopoiesis
Lymphoma	Granulomatous disease (eg, sarcoidosis)	Discitis/osteomyelitis
Carcinoma (thyroid)	Aortic pathology	
Substernal goiter	Diaphragmatic hernia	
Lipoma		

Q4-5: D
Neurofibroma

Rationale: The patient has classic dermatologic findings of café-au-lait spots, neurofibromas, and axillary freckling. This is consistent with a diagnosis of neurofibromatosis (NF) type 1. Patients with NF type 1 develop tumors during adolescence or adulthood. These patients may also have HTN, short stature, macrocephaly, scoliosis, and learning disorders (attention deficit hyperactivity disorder). Some patients may have involvement of the optic nerve leading to vision issues. Patients also have an increased risk of developing other forms of malignancy, including leukemia.

Neurogenic tumors are the most common cause of posterior mediastinal masses under the new classification system, accounting for approximately 60% to 70% of masses. Schwannomas and neurofibromas both arise from the intercostal nerve sheath. These two etiologies account for the vast majority of neurogenic tumors in the posterior mediastinum, while ganglioneuromas (arising from the sympathetic thoracic spinal ganglia) are the most common lesion in young adults. Other causes of posterior mediastinal masses include paravertebral abscesses and meningoceles.

Q4-6: C
Serum metanephrines and 5-HIAA

Rationale: The patient's presenting symptoms of anxiety, diaphoresis, HTN, and palpitations could be consistent with a number of disorders, including hyperthyroidism, pheochromocytoma, alcohol withdrawal, insulinoma, and intestinal carcinoid tumor, among others. Given the patient's history of NF1, common complications include pheochromocytoma, hyperparathyroidism, and carcinoid tumors of the intestine. Of these, the patient's symptoms are most consistent with either a pheochromocytoma or a carcinoid tumor (though the patient lacks GI symptoms). Given the patient's normal TSH, hyperthyroidism is unlikely (A). He does not have symptoms classic of hyperparathyroidism (B). There is no evidence of infection (E).

Q4-7: E
Ras

Rationale: NF1 is a negative regulator of the Ras oncogene. Patients with NF1 have a defective NF1 protein, leading to excessive Ras activity and unregulated cell division.

References

Carter BW, Benveniste MF, Madan R, et al. ITMIG classification of mediastinal compartments and multidisciplinary approach to mediastinal masses. Radiographics. 2017;37:413.

Carter BW, Betancourt SL, Benveniste MF. MR imaging of mediastinal masses. Top Magn Reson Imaging. 2017;26:153.

Chira RI, Chira A, Mircea PA, Valean S. Mediastinal masses-transthoracic ultrasonography aspects. Medicine (Baltimore). 2017;96:e9082.

Duwe BV, Sterman DH, Musani AI. Tumors of the mediastinum. Chest. 2005;128:2893.

Juanpere S, Cañete N, Ortuño P, et al. A diagnostic approach to the mediastinal masses. Insights Imaging. 2013;4:29.

Laurent F, Latrabe V, Lecesne R, Zennaro H, Airaud JY, Rauturier JF, Drouillard J. Mediastinal masses: diagnostic approach. Eur Radiol. 1998;8:1148.

Nakazono T, Yamaguchi K, Egashira R, Mizuguchi M, Irie H. Anterior mediastinal lesions: CT and MRI features and differential diagnosis. Jpn J Radiol. 2021;39:101.

Prosch H, Röhrich S, Tekin ZN, Ebner L. The role of radiological imaging for masses in the prevascular mediastinum in clinical practice. J Thorac Dis. 2020;12:7591.

Su S, Colson YL. Overview of benign and malignant mediastinal diseases. In: Adult Chest Surgery, 2nd ed, Sugarbaker DJ, Bueno R, Colson YL, et al. (Eds), McGraw-Hill Education, New York 2015:1234.

Thacker PG, Mahani MG, Heider A, Lee EY. Imaging evaluation of mediastinal masses in children and adults: Practical diagnostic approach based on a new classification system. J Thorac Imaging. 2015;30:247.

Whitten CR, Khan S, Munneke GJ, Grubnic S. A diagnostic approach to mediastinal abnormalities. Radiographics. 2007;27:657.

CASE 5

A 77-year-old man with Parkinson disease and presumed chronic recurrent aspiration presents with hypoxia and a persistent cough. His caregiver is present and provides the history. He has had frequent and recurrent cases of pneumonia over the past 2 years that have been ascribed to aspiration. He has an 80–pack-year smoking history. He has no known family history of malignancy, rheumatologic disease, or pulmonary disease. He has been taking increasing doses of anticholinergics to help with oral secretions. He is admitted to the hospital with suspected aspiration pneumonia and started on antibiotics. His initial chest radiograph demonstrates consolidation in the right lower lobe but good aeration of the right upper lobe. This morning, the patient's oxygenation worsened, and the patient became more tachypneic. His white blood cell (WBC) count is 5.5 ×10^9, and the remainder of his laboratory studies are normal. His vital signs are T 36.5°C, BP 110/60, RR 22, and O$_2$ saturation 87% on room air, 93% on 4 L NC. His repeat chest radiograph is shown in Image 5-1.

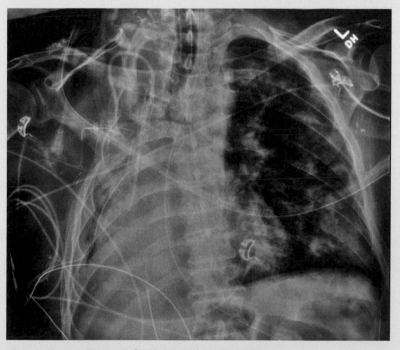

Image 5-1 • Chest radiograph for the patient in Question 5-1.

QUESTIONS

Q5-1: What is the likely diagnosis?

A. Aspiration pneumonia
B. Pleural effusion
C. Pneumothorax
D. Atelectasis
E. Pulmonary embolism

Q5-2: What is the likely cause of the patient's atelectasis?

A. External compression of the airway due to enlarging lymph nodes
B. Mucous plug in the right mainstem bronchus
C. Mucous plug in the bronchus intermedius
D. Mucous plug in the trachea
E. Mass in the right mainstem bronchus

Q5-3: What is the subtype of atelectasis in this patient?

A. Obstructive atelectasis
B. Adhesive atelectasis
C. Passive atelectasis
D. Cicatrization atelectasis

Q5-4: Which patient would be expected to have the most developed airway collaterals?

A. An infant
B. An 8-year-old child
C. A 45-year-old man with no medical problems
D. A 65-year-old man with no medical problems
E. A 65-year-old man with Global Initiative for Chronic Obstructive Lung Disease (GOLD) class C chronic obstructive pulmonary disease (COPD)

Q5-5: What is the best treatment approach for the patient?

A. Antibiotics to cover community-acquired organisms
B. Antibiotics to cover hospital-acquired organisms
C. Antibiotics to cover multidrug-resistant organisms
D. Systemic glucocorticoids
E. Bronchoscopy
F. Chest physiotherapy and airway clearance
G. Bronchial stent placement

Q5-6: A 66-year-old woman presents with new-onset dyspnea. She had a normal chest radiograph 3 months ago. Over the last 2 to 3 weeks, she has noticed worsening dyspnea on exertion after experiencing a fall at home. She takes warfarin for atrial fibrillation and aspirin for nonobstructive coronary artery disease. Which subtype of atelectasis is present in the following radiograph?

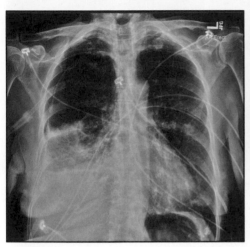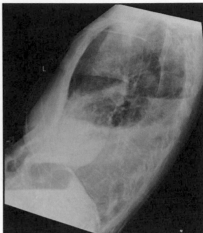

Image 5-2 • Chest radiograph for the patient in **Question 5-6**.

A. Right-sided relaxation (passive) atelectasis
B. Right-sided obstructive atelectasis
C. Right-sided subsegmental atelectasis
D. Left-sided cicatrization atelectasis
E. Left-sided adhesive atelectasis
F. Left-sided compressive atelectasis

Q5-7: Which segment of the lung is atelectatic in the following films?

Q5-7-1: Image 5-3?

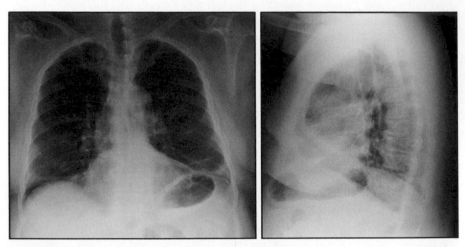

Image 5-3 • Chest radiograph for the patient in **Question 5-7-1.**

A. Right upper lobe
B. Right middle lobe
C. Right lower lobe
D. Left upper lobe
E. Left lower lobe or lingula

Q5-7-2: Image 5-4?

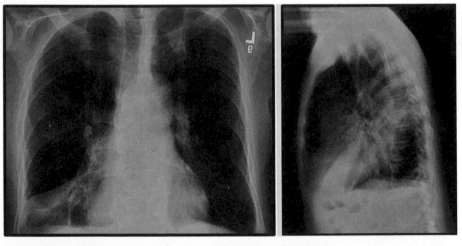

Image 5-4 • Chest radiograph for the patient in **Question 5-7-2.**

A. Right upper lobe
B. Right middle lobe
C. Right lower lobe
D. Left upper lobe
E. Left lower lobe

Q5-7-3: Image 5-5?

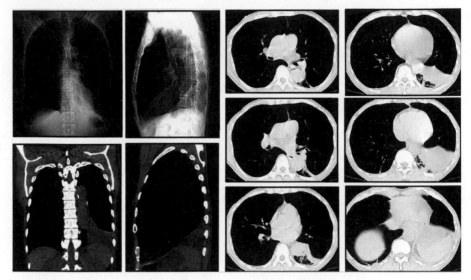

Image 5-5 • Chest imaging for **Question 5-7-3**.

A. Right upper lobe
B. Right middle lobe
C. Right lower lobe
D. Left upper lobe
E. Left lower lobe

Q5-7-4: Image 5-6?

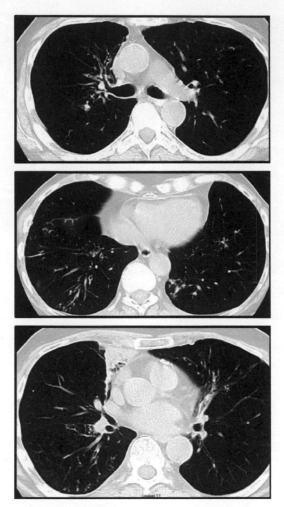

Image 5-6 • Chest CT for the patient in **Question 5-7-4**.

A. Right upper lobe, apical subsegment
B. Right middle lobe, medial subsegment
C. Right middle lobe, lateral subsegment
D. Right lower lobe, posterior subsegment
E. Left upper lobe
F. Left lower lobe, medial subsegment

Q5-7-5: Image 5-7?

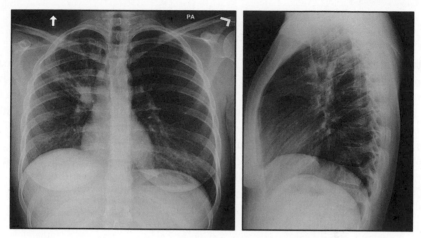

Image 5-7 • Chest radiograph for the patient in **Question 5-7-5**.

A. Right upper lobe
B. Right middle lobe
C. Right lower lobe
D. Left upper lobe
E. Left lower lobe

Q5-8: Which subtype of atelectasis is displayed in Image 5-8?

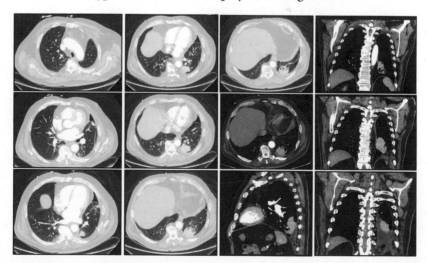

Image 5-8 • Chest CT imaging for **Question 5-8**.

A. Compressive/passive atelectasis
B. Obstructive atelectasis
C. Rounded atelectasis
D. Cicatrization atelectasis

ANSWERS

Q5-1: D
Atelectasis

Rationale: Atelectasis is the loss of lung volume due to collapse. There is a near-complete loss of aeration in the right lung, with volume loss in the left chest as evidenced by the shift of the trachea to the right. The combination of volume loss on the right and a near white-out of the lung suggests that the cause of the abnormalities seen is atelectasis. Pneumothorax and pleural effusion are space-occupying lesions that would be associated with a mediastinal shift to the left rather than the right. Aspiration pneumonia does not typically result in complete loss of lung aeration in all three lobes of the right lung, and when it does, it is usually not associated with any mediastinal shift unless there is associated atelectasis. A pulmonary embolism typically does not present with significant changes on plain chest radiographs, though it may be associated with pleural effusion or wedge-shaped infarcts.

Q5-2: B
Mucous plug in the right mainstem bronchus

Rationale: The patient has a history of frontotemporal dementia and has demonstrated an inability to clear his airway appropriately as he has experienced multiple episodes of pneumonia. Given that the patient's initial chest radiograph on admission demonstrated some aeration in the right lung, the change seen here is rather acute and unlikely due to either a mass in the right mainstem bronchi or progressive external compression of the right mainstem bronchus. The pattern of abnormalities suggests likely compression of the right mainstem bronchi because there is essentially no aeration of the right lung; if the plug occurred more distally in the bronchus intermedius, the RUL should still be aerated. A mucous plug in the trachea would be associated with bilateral findings (and likely would be terminal if not cleared rapidly).

Q5-3: A
Obstructive atelectasis

Rationale: Obstructive atelectasis is due to blockage of the airway, in this instance by a mucous plug. The development of atelectasis in obstructive atelectasis depends on the degree of collateralization. The more proximal the occlusion, the more likely one is to see obstructive (resorptive) atelectasis because collateralization occurs more frequently between alveoli within adjacent subsegments than those in adjacent segments or lobes (interlobar fissures are often incomplete and may therefore contain some collaterals).

Q5-4: E
A 65-year-old man with GOLD class C COPD

Rationale: Collateral airflow between alveoli occurs via three pathways: the pores of Kohn (small communications between adjacent pulmonary alveoli), the canals of Lambert (accessory connections between terminal bronchioles and alveoli), and the fenestrae of Boren (essentially holes through alveolar walls). The pores of Kohn and canals of Lambert are present at birth in a small number and develop with age; therefore, infants and children have poor collateralization. Of the adults, COPD is associated with the development of fenestrae of Boren, which are not present in non-diseased alveoli. This additional conduit for collateral airflow means that patients with COPD tend to have more significant collateral airflow potential.

Q5-5: F
Chest physiotherapy and airway clearance

Rationale: As the patient is not in extremis, the best treatment for the patient's obstructive atelectasis would be chest physiotherapy and airway clearance. Bronchoscopy is generally reserved for patients in whom the aforementioned is ineffective or for patients in extremis. Unfortunately, bronchoscopy does not solve the underlying problem that led to the patient developing atelectasis (poor airway clearance) and only treats the immediate problem and is therefore generally only temporizing. Bronchoscopy is indicated if there is concern for an endobronchial mass causing an obstruction. Bronchial stent placement is certainly not indicated for a patient without an obstructive mass or stenosis, and it is associated with reduced airway clearance and increased risk of mucous plugging. Patients with stents require aggressive pulmonary airway clearance regimens ("pulmonary toilet"), including albuterol and hypertonic saline nebulizers two to three times daily, the use of acapella valves or flutter valves, and regular exercise (or chest physiotherapy). Although antibiotics may be indicated, the specific antibiotics should be dictated by the patient's risk factors, severity of illness, prior culture data, and local susceptibilities. Antibiotics also will not immediately solve the acute issue of atelectasis (though with time, they may reduce airway secretions). Systemic steroids may be useful for severe community-acquired pneumonia, but that is not the primary issue in this case.

Q5-6: A
Right-sided relaxation (passive) atelectasis

Rationale: This is an example for passive atelectasis, which is atelectasis resulting from a space-occupying process in the pleural space. In this film, there is a moderate right-sided pleural effusion and associated volume loss on the right. Note that many texts will combine compressive and passive atelectasis into one category. Passive (relaxation) atelectasis occurs when the contact between the visceral and parietal pleura is disrupted and the lung is not exposed to the traditional negative intrathoracic pressure (ie, free-flowing pleural effusion, pneumothorax, hemothorax; see **Image 5-9** for an example), whereas compressive atelectasis occurs when an intrathoracic lesion directly compresses the lung (ie, loculated pleural effusion, pleural or intraparenchymal tumor, elevated hemidiaphragm), resulting in a reduced forced vital capacity (FVC).

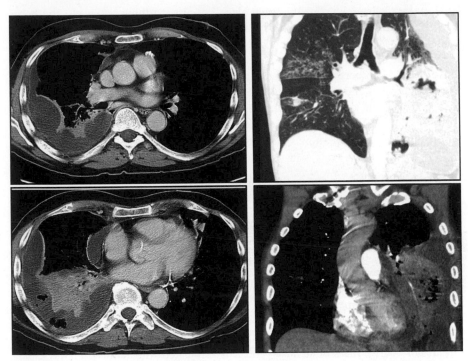

Image 5-9 • A patient with an empyema leading to loss of contact between the visceral and parietal pleural and resultant passive atelectasis of the neighboring lung.

It is often difficult to separate the two processes, and they may often present together and exist on a spectrum. For instance, a massive pleural effusion resulting from a lung malignancy may initially give rise to passive atelectasis, while the tumor itself causes compressive atelectasis. Some texts may refer to compressive atelectasis as arising only from processes occurring in the lung (ie, lung mass or cavity lesion), separating passive and compressive atelectasis more fully. Obstructive atelectasis is due to airway obstruction (either by mucus, foreign objects, or a mass/lesion). Cicatrization is atelectasis due to lung scarring, such as may be seen in radiation fibrosis or sarcoidosis. Adhesive atelectasis is atelectasis resulting from a lack or dysfunction of pulmonary surfactant, such as may be seen in acute respiratory distress syndrome (ARDS) or radiation pneumonitis. Replacement atelectasis is due to physical replacement of the alveolar space with tumor. Plate-like atelectasis is seen commonly in patients in the hospital and is due to poor ventilation, commonly from a lack of physical activity. This is in large part why incentive spirometry is used. Plate-like atelectasis may be described as discoid, segmental, or linear.

Q5-7-1: E
Lingula

Rationale: See **Image 5-10**. This may be left lower lobe or lingular collapse, depending on individual anatomy, but it is more likely lingular atelectasis. This is consistent with plate-like atelectasis.

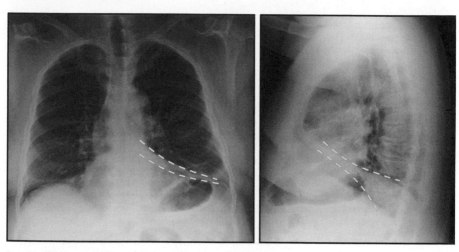

Image 5-10 • Left lower lobe or lingular collapse.

Q5-7-2: B
Right middle lobe

Rationale: See **Image 5-11**.

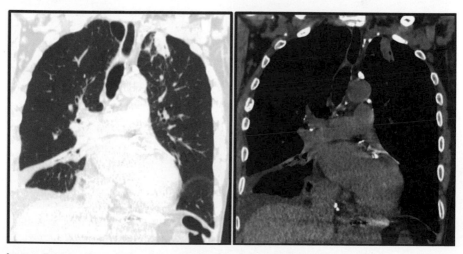

Image 5-11 • Chest CT for the patient in **Question 5-7-2**.

Q5-7-3: E
Left lower lobe

Rationale: Note the elevation of the left hemidiaphragm in response to the volume loss.

Q5-7-4: B
Right middle lobe, medial subsegment

Rationale: This is an example of atelectasis in the right middle lobe, medial subsegment. Note the location directly adjacent to the mediastinum.

Q5-7-5: A
Right upper lobe

Rationale: See **Images 5-12** and **5-13**. Note that the patient has an apparent mass in the right upper lobe perihilar region with distal atelectasis. This is a classic case of obstructive atelectasis. Features of right upper lobe collapse may include an increased density along the medial aspect of the right mediastinum/spine, elevation of the minor fissure (horizontal fissure), and deviation of the upper trachea to the right. Left upper lobe atelectasis is more difficult to identify on plain films because it tends to form a thin sheet along the left hilar border (see **Image 5-14**). This is usually identified on lateral films, where there is increased haziness of density along the retrosternal space (between the sternum and cardiac borders in the upper lateral lung space).

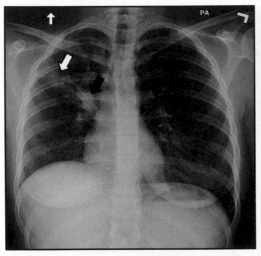 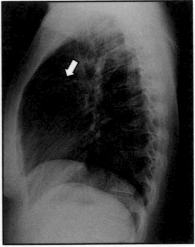

Image 5-12 • Annotated chest radiograph for **Question 5-7-5**, demonstrating a perihilar mass (black arrow) with distal collapse of the lung (obstructive atelectasis, *white arrow*).

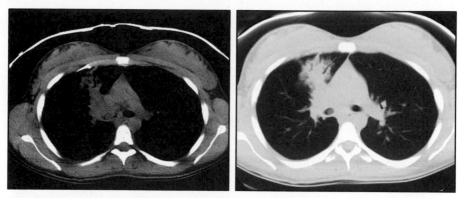

Image 5-13 • Chest CT scan for **Question 5-7-5**, demonstrating an endobronchial mass (mediastinal window, left) and resultant volume loss with air bronchograms in the right upper lobe.

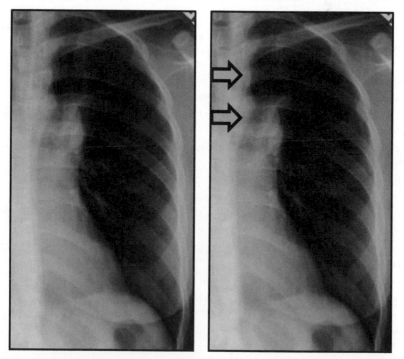

Image 5-14 • A patient with left upper lobe atelectasis. Note the very slight opacity along the left hilum as well as the sight shift of the mediastinum to the left, indicating volume loss. Additionally, there is likely a mass in the left hilum.

Q5-8: C
Rounded atelectasis

Rationale: This is an example of rounded atelectasis, a finding that is commonly associated with asbestos exposure. Note there is the presence of an associated pleural effusion here as well, which is also a potential complication of asbestos exposure (benign asbestos-related pleural effusions [BAPE]). However, rounded atelectasis may also develop in patients with histoplasmosis, sarcoidosis, chronic congestive heart failure, pulmonary infarction, or prior empyema/parapneumonic effusions. On CT, the atelectasis appears rounded rather than plate-like or discoid and abuts the pleura. There is usually pleural thickening or an effusion (or both). Air bronchograms may be present. This most commonly involves the lower lobes, specifically the posterior subsegments. This is thought to arise from local pleuritis or inflammatory pleural effusions, causing the pleura to thicken. The lung is compressed and appears to curl in a concentric fashion. This can lead to a "comet tail" or "crow's feet" appearance of the bronchovascular bundle serving the atelectatic lung (see bottom left image in **Image 5-8**).

References

Ashizawa K, Hayashi K, Aso N, Minami K. Lobar atelectasis: diagnostic pitfalls on chest radiography. Br J Radiol. 2001;74:89.

Gurney JW. Atypical manifestations of pulmonary atelectasis. J Thorac Imaging. 1996;11:165.

Kattan KR, Wlot JF. Cardiac rotation in left lower lobe collapse. "The flat waist sign". Radiology. 1976;118:275.

Kottler NE, Stark P, Levin DL. The challenge of combined lobar atelectasis. Contemp Diagnostic Radiol. 2004;27:1.

Partap VA. The comet tail sign. Radiology. 1999;213:553.

Proto AV. Lobar collapse: basic concepts. Eur J Radiol 1996;23:9.

Stark P, Leung A. Effects of lobar atelectasis on the distribution of pleural effusion and pneumothorax. J Thorac Imaging. 1996;11:145.

Stathopoulos GT, Karamessini MT, Sotiriadi AE, Pastromas VG. Rounded atelectasis of the lung. Respir Med. 2005;99:615.

Webber M, Davies P. The Luftsichel: an old sign in upper lobe collapse. Clin Radiol. 1981;32:271.

Westcott JL, Cole S. Plate atelectasis. Radiology. 1985;155:1.

Woodring JH, Reed JC. Types and mechanisms of pulmonary atelectasis. J Thorac Imaging. 1996;11:92.

CASE 6

A 66-year-old man presents to your clinic for worsening dyspnea on exertion over the past several years. The patient first noted some mild dyspnea on exertion approximately 3 years ago but believed this was due to some weight gain and inactivity. However, over the next 24 months, despite attempts to exercise more frequently, he feels as though his exercise tolerance has only continued to decrease. Over the last few months, he has begun to feel short of breath with some of his normal daily activities, including walking from the car to the front door. He presented to an urgent care facility a few days ago and had a chest radiograph that was described as abnormal. A referral was made for an outpatient pulmonary visit. The patient was noted to be saturating 92% O_2 on room air at rest and desaturated to 86% with activity and was thus prescribed 2 L/min supplemental O_2 with activity. The patient was also sent for a noncontrasted CT scan before his appointment in your clinic. The patient has a history of diabetes mellitus (DM) type 2, gastroesophageal reflux disease (GERD), and hypertension. He smokes two to four cigarettes a day and has a 45–pack-year smoking history. He drinks one to two alcoholic beverages a day but has no history of alcohol dependence or withdrawal. He served in the Navy from 1959 to 1963 in a shipyard. After retiring from the Navy, he worked as an automotive mechanic for 10 years before opening his own auto repair shop, at which time he transitioned to working in an office. He has no known environmental exposure.

The patient's vital signs are T 97.7°F, HR 99, BP 102/56, RR 21, O2 saturation 93% on room air at rest, 87% on room air with activity, and 94% with 2 L/min supplemental O2 with activity. His chest radiograph and chest CT scan are shown in Images 6-1, 6-2, and 6-3.

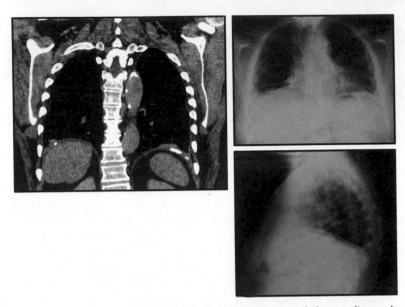

Image 6-1 • Noncontrasted CT scan (mediastinal window) and chest radiographs (PA and lateral views) for the patient in **Question 6-1**.

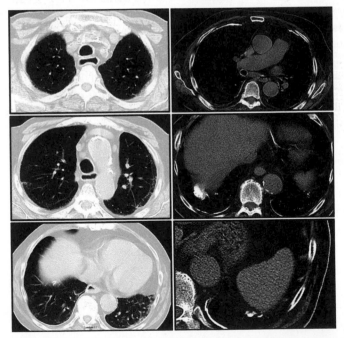

Image 6-2 • CT scan (left, lung window; right, mediastinal window) for the patient in **Question 6-1**.

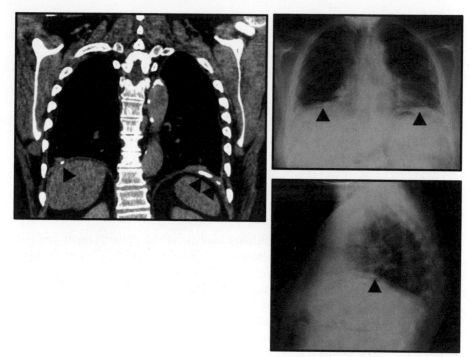

Image 6-3 • Annotated images displayed in **Image 6-1**, with the black arrows identifying calcified pleural plaques for the patient in **Case 6**.

QUESTIONS

Q6-1: Which abnormalities are in the patient's chest imaging shown in Images 6-1 and 6-2? Select all that apply.

A. Pneumothorax
B. Pneumomediastinum
C. Pleural plaques (calcifications)
D. Calcified lymph nodes
E. Aortic calcifications
F. Subpleural interlobular and intralobular septal thickening
G. Cavitary lung lesions
H. Honeycomb changes

Q6-2: You order a number of additional studies for the patient, including pulmonary function testing, a 6-minute walk distance (6MWD), a home O_2 titration study, and a number of laboratory studies. Unfortunately, after the initial visit, the patient did not schedule these additional tests and is lost to follow-up. He returns to the clinic approximately 24 months later when his symptoms have worsened. He has continued to smoke in the interval. He presented to an outside hospital with worsening hypoxemia a few weeks ago, and a pulmonary consultant ordered a CT scan, which is shown in Image 6-4.

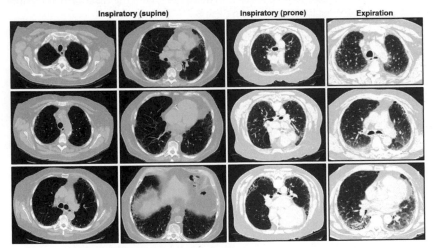

Image 6-4 • Chest CT obtained from the outside hospital facility for the patient in **Case 6**.

Which abnormalities are in the chest CT shown in Image 6-4?

A. Air trapping in a mosaic pattern
B. Lower-lobe predominant interlobular and intralobular septal thickening
C. Honeycombing
D. Parenchymal bands
E. Cystic lung lesions
F. Upper-lobe predominant interlobular and intralobular septal thickening
G. Rounded atelectasis

Q6-3: The patient undergoes a bronchoscopy with bronchoalveolar lavage (BAL) at an outside hospital, and the following specimen is obtained on cytology (Image 6-5). Additionally, the patient's laboratory studies include a negative evaluation for rheumatologic conditions, a negative HIV antibody study, normal immunoglobulin levels, and an appropriate response to the pneumonia vaccination the patient received the year prior. What is the most likely diagnosis?

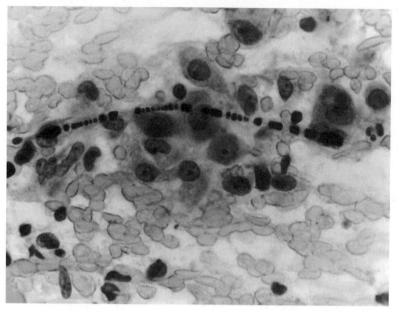

Image 6-5 • Cytology sample obtained from BAL performed for the patient in **Case 6**. *(Reproduced with permission from Reisner H. Pathology: A Modern Case Study, 2nd ed. New York, NY: McGraw Hill; 2020.)*

A. Pulmonary histoplasmosis
B. Pulmonary blastomycosis
C. Asbestosis
D. Non-small cell lung cancer
E. Pulmonary nocardiosis
F. Coal-worker pneumonoconiosis

Q6-4: What is the typical latency period between asbestos exposure and the development of asbestosis?

A. Days to weeks
B. Weeks to months
C. 3 to 5 years
D. 10 years
E. 20 to 30 years

Q6-5: Which factor increases the risk of developing asbestosis in a patient with prior asbestos exposure?

A. Vitamin C supplementation
B. Smoking tobacco use
C. Alcohol use
D. Supplemental O_2 use
E. Diabetes mellitus

Q6-6: What is the most common pulmonary function testing (PFT) abnormality in patients with asbestosis?

A. Increased residual volume (RV)/total lung capacity (TLC) ratio (hyperinflation)
B. Expiratory airflow obstruction (decreased forced expiratory volume [FEV1]/forced vital capacity [FVC] ratio)
C. Reduced diffusing capacity of carbon monoxide (DLCO)
D. Isolated reduced expiratory reserve volume (ERV)
E. Isolated reduced vital capacity (VC)

Q6-7: Which is NOT a primary component of the treatment plan for asbestosis?

A. Smoking cessation
B. Early detection and avoidance of further exposure
C. Supplemental O_2 therapy as needed for resting or exercise-induced hypoxemia
D. Systemic glucocorticoids
E. Pulmonary rehabilitation
F. Age- and condition-appropriate vaccinations
G. Lung transplantation
H. Whole lung lavage (WLL)

ANSWERS

Q6-1: C; E; F

Pleural plaques (calcifications); Aortic calcifications; Subpleural interlobular and intralobular septal thickening

Rationale: The chest films and the mediastinal window images of the chest CT scan reveal calcified lesions on the parietal pleura abutting the diaphragm (**Image 6-6**). These abnormalities are referred to as *pleural plaques*. Additionally, one can see that there are concentric calcifications around the aortic arch, which is a common finding as patients get older. Most importantly, there are lower-lobe predominant, subpleural (ie, immediately adjacent to the visceral pleura) abnormalities, with linear densities parallel to the pleura and interlobular and intralobular septal thickening. This almost has the appearance of a "crazy paving" pattern; however, there is a paucity of ground glass. Additionally, there is central sparing, as these lesions are predominantly along the subpleural regions (periphery) of the lung. There is no evidence of honeycomb changes or cavitary lung lesions at this stage.

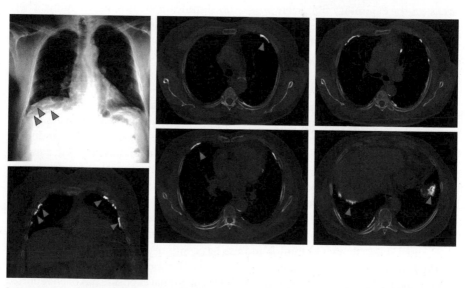

Image 6-6 • Additional examples of pleural plaques. These linear or nodular opacities occur in the parietal pleura. Pleural plaques are often found bilaterally in the parietal pleura, adjacent to the ribs or on the diaphragm. The costophrenic angles are usually spared. Plaques may also form on any parietal mesothelial surface. The visceral pleura is not involved.

Q6-2: B; C; D

Lower-lobe predominant interlobular and intralobular septal thickening; Honeycombing; Parenchymal bands

Rationale: The CT scan is referred to as an *interstitial lung disease (ILD)-protocol CT scan*, which includes three separate patient positions, and all images are non-contrasted. The patient has a standard inspiratory-supine study (left two columns), followed by an expiratory-supine study (far right) and an inspiratory-prone study (third column from left). Each of these studies has a particular point of interest. The inspiratory-supine study is the standard CT position. Here we can see a lower-lobe predominant process. In the upper lobes, there are subtle subpleural reticulations (intralobular and interlobular septal thickening), which become more prominent in the lower lobes. Additionally, there are more dense bands in the parenchyma that appear to stretch to the pleura, termed *parenchymal bands* (most notably in the most caudal image). However, note that honeycomb changes are difficult to evaluate here, though there is a hint of this at the right lung base. The inspiratory-prone film is used to better evaluate the dependent portions of the lung, where volume loss during supine positioning can hide such changes. Here, on the inspiratory-prone image, there are distinct honeycomb changes on the right. The expiratory-supine study, when compared with the inspiratory-supine study, is used to determine if air trapping is present. On expiration, the lung volume decreases, and the radio-dense structures of the lung are in closer approximation. This has the effect of making the lung appear more radiopaque. When there is air trapping, the air is trapped in specific areas of the lung during expiration, and these areas will continue to appear as radiotranslucent areas on the expiratory film. Here we see no significant areas of air trapping. There are no cystic lung lesions, and there is no evidence of atelectasis.

Q6-3: C
Asbestosis

Rationale: The cytology specimen demonstrates a classic asbestos body. The asbestos fibers are transparent on light microscopy but are coated by iron particles, which appear yellowish-brown on light microscopy. Asbestos bodies are a classic finding in patients with asbestos-related lung disease. The presence of asbestos bodies in a patient with a history of likely or confirmed exposure (eg, naval shipyards) and a slowly progressive interstitial pneumonia/fibrosis points to a diagnosis of asbestosis. Asbestos is composed of fibers of hydrate magnesium silicates, which in individual fiber form are highly respirable and can deposit in small airways and the alveoli. Asbestos is primarily used as a fire retardant in insulation. The use of asbestos has decreased dramatically in the United States, though its mining and use has continued in much of the developing world. Patients are most commonly exposed to asbestos fibers as a consequence of occupation, though second-hand exposure or nonoccupational exposure has been reported to cause disease. Industries where asbestos is still regularly used include textiles (particularly the manufacturing of fire-retardant materials such as fireman jackets), cement manufacturing, astronautical engineering, pipe-welding and insulation, shipbuilding, and the manufacture of brake pads. Patients may also be exposed during the process of mining and milling the fibers for use in the aforementioned industries. Asbestos fibers may either be straight (amphibole) or serpentine (eg, chrysotile), with the former believed to the primary toxic form. Currently, more than 90% of applications requiring asbestos use serpentine fibers. In this image, one can see an amphibole fiber.

The pathology does not demonstrate any fungal elements, nor is there evidence of non-small cell lung cancer (note the uniform nuclei). Coal-worker pneumoconiosis is marked by the presence of carbon-laden macrophages.

Importantly, asbestos is associated with a number of potential pleural and parenchymal abnormalities.

Asbestosis is a slowly progressive, lower-lobe predominant fibrotic lung disease that preferentially affects the periphery of the lung (subpleural) with central sparing. This topic will be further explored in the following section.

Q6-4: E
20 to 30 years

Rationale: The latency period for the development of asbestosis from the initial exposure is typically 20 to 30 years, though the latency period is inversely proportional to the cumulative dose exposure (time-dose product).

Q6-5: B
Smoking tobacco use

Rationale: Smoking tobacco use increases not only the risk of developing asbestosis but also increases the rate of progression of the disease. Asbestos fibers are removed from the lung by mucociliary clearance, which is hampered by smoking tobacco use. Smoking cessation is an important intervention for patients at risk for asbestosis. It has been hypothesized that vitamin C may counteract the effects of asbestos-related inflammation via the reduction of reactive O_2 species. There have been no studies relating alcohol use or diabetes mellitus to asbestosis. Supplemental O_2 therapy may be used in patients with resting or exercise hypoxemia.

Q6-6: C
Reduced diffusing capacity of carbon monoxide (DLCO)

Rationale: A reduced DLCO is the most common abnormality seen in patients with asbestosis. Patients often also demonstrated evidence of restrictive lung disease, with a reduced TLC, VC, and RV. Often, a reduction in VC may precede the reduction in TLC or RV. An increased RV/TLC and expiratory airflow obstruction are commonly seen in patients with COPD. An isolated reduced ERV is often seen in patients with obesity because of reduced chest wall compliance.

Q6-7: D
Systemic glucocorticoids

Rationale: There is no evidence supporting the use of systemic glucocorticoids or other immunosuppressive medications in the treatment of asbestosis. It is possible that future studies may point to the use of antifibrotic agents in patients with asbestosis, though data are currently lacking. Unlike idiopathic pulmonary fibrosis, there is generally a lack of large fibroblast foci, which suggests that such therapy may not be as effective in asbestosis. All of the other answers are viable treatment options for patients with asbestosis. A lung transplant is an option for patients who develop end-stage lung disease as a result of asbestosis. Smoking cessation, early detection of disease, and avoidance of further exposure are likely the most important aspects of treatment. There is no evidence for whole lung lavage in the treatment of asbestosis.

References

A physician's guide to asbestos-related diseases. Council on Scientific Affairs. JAMA. 1984;252:2593.

Aberle DR, Balmes JR. Computed tomography of asbestos-related pulmonary parenchymal and pleural diseases. Clin Chest Med. 1991;12:115.

Aberle DR, Gamsu G, Ray CS, Feuerstein IM. Asbestos-related pleural and parenchymal fibrosis: detection with high-resolution CT. Radiology. 1988;166:729.

Baur X, Woitowitz HJ, Budnik LT, et al. Asbestos, asbestosis, and cancer: The Helsinki criteria for diagnosis and attribution. Critical need for revision of the 2014 update. Am J Ind Med. 2017;60:411.

Centers for Disease Control and Prevention (CDC). Asbestosis-related years of potential life lost before age 65 years – United States, 1968-2005. MMWR Morb Mortal Wkly Rep. 2008;57:1321.

Fujimoto N, Gemba K, Aoe K, et al. Clinical Investigation of Benign Asbestos Pleural Effusion. Pulm Med. 2015;2015:416179.

Hillerdal G. Rounded atelectasis. Clinical experience with 74 patients. Chest. 1989;95:836.

Hourihane DO, McCaughey WT. Pathological aspects of asbestosis. Postgrad Med J. 1966;42:613.

Kato K, Gemba K, Fujimoto N, et al. Pleural irregularities and mediastinal pleural involvement in early stages of malignant pleural mesothelioma and benign asbestos pleural effusion. Eur J Radiol. 2016;85:1594.

Kilburn KH, Warshaw RH. Airways obstruction from asbestos exposure. Effects of asbestosis and smoking. Chest. 1994;106:1061.

Markowitz SB, Levin SM, Miller A, Morabia A. Asbestos, asbestosis, smoking, and lung cancer. New findings from the North American insulator cohort. Am J Respir Crit Care Med. 2013;188:90.

Mossman BT, Gee JB. Asbestos-related diseases. N Engl J Med. 1989;320:1721.

O'Reilly KM, Mclaughlin AM, Beckett WS, Sime PJ. Asbestos-related lung disease. Am Fam Physician. 2007;75:683.

Roggli VL, Gibbs AR, Attanoos R, et al. Pathology of asbestosis – An update of the diagnostic criteria: Report of the asbestosis committee of the college of american pathologists and pulmonary pathology society. Arch Pathol Lab Med. 2010;134:462.

Schwartz DA, Fuortes LJ, Galvin JR, et al. Asbestos-induced pleural fibrosis and impaired lung function. Am Rev Respir Dis. 1990;141:321.

Sebastien P, Armstrong B, Monchaux G, Bignon J. Asbestos bodies in bronchoalveolar lavage fluid and in lung parenchyma. Am Rev Respir Dis. 1988;137:75.

Sette A, Neder JA, Nery LE, et al. Thin-section CT abnormalities and pulmonary gas exchange impairment in workers exposed to asbestos. Radiology. 2004;232:66.

Wagner GR. Asbestosis and silicosis. Lancet. 1997;349:1311.

CASE 7

You are called to see a 33-year-old woman on the hematologic malignancy service. She was diagnosed with Hodgkin lymphoma approximately 9 months ago and completed her chemotherapy approximately 5 months ago. Her regimen included doxorubicin, bleomycin, vinblastine, and dacarbazine. She had a complete remission. However, on her routine follow-up imaging, she was noted to have some abnormalities. Additionally, she developed a dry cough and some mild dyspnea a few weeks ago. She was admitted to the hospital for evaluation of these abnormalities.

The chest imaging is shown below (Image 7-1), in which (A) is a pretreatment CXR and (B) is the CXR on admission:

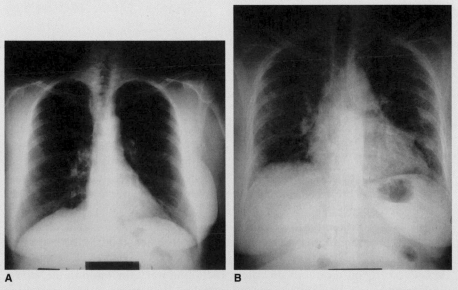

A   B

Image 7-1 • Chest radiographs for the patient in Question 7-1. (*Reproduced with permission from Grippi MA, Elias JA, Fishman JA, et al: Fishman's Pulmonary Diseases and Disorders, 5th ed. New York, NY: McGraw Hill; 2015.*)

QUESTIONS

Q7-1: How would you describe the abnormalities on the CXR?

A. Consolidative opacities

B. Pneumothorax

C. Linear opacities

D. Pleural effusions

E. Cavitary lesions

Q7-2: The patient has a viral panel sent on admission that is negative. She subsequently undergoes a bronchoscopy with bronchoalveolar lavage (BAL). The BAL has a negative viral panel and negative sputum culture, there are no fungi on a potassium hydroxide (KOH) stain, and the silver stain is negative. There is slight eosinophilia on the BAL. Which is the most likely diagnosis for this patient?

A. Invasive aspergillus

B. Cytomegalovirus (CMV) pneumonitis

C. Bleomycin-induced lung injury

D. Doxorubicin-induced lung injury

E. Pneumocystis pneumonia

F. Dacarbazine-induced lung injury

G. Vinblastine-induced lung injury

Q7-3: Which of the following is NOT a risk factor for bleomycin-induced lung injury/toxicity?

A. High concentrations of supplemental O_2

B. Concomitant radiation therapy to the chest

C. Renal dysfunction/failure

D. Use of bronchodilators

Q7-4: A 66-year-old man presents to the clinic for evaluation of abnormalities on his CXR. He has a history of HTN, chronic obstructive pulmonary disease (COPD), and pancreatitis. Approximately 3 years ago, he was hospitalized in the ICU for necrotizing pancreatitis, during which time he developed a number of complications, including ARDS, kidney failure, atrial fibrillation, and ventilator-associated pneumonia. He recovered after a 2-month hospital stay. He has otherwise been well since then and has regularly met with his primary care physician. He is currently on several medications, including warfarin, amlodipine, carvedilol, amiodarone, spironolactone, and ursodiol. He has noted some worsening dyspnea over the last few months, as well as a dry cough. His CXR prior to the hospitalization 3 years ago was largely unremarkable except for some borderline cardiomegaly. Upon presentation, his CXR and CT scan of the chest are as shown in Images 7-2 and 7-3:

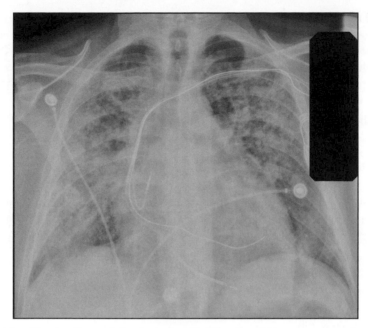

Image 7-2 • Chest radiograph for the patient in **Question 7-4**.

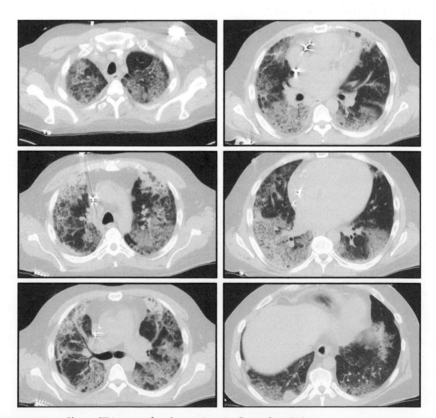

Image 7-3 • Chest CT images for the patient in **Question 7-4**.

The patient is admitted to the hospital for hypoxemia (82% on room air), and he undergoes an extensive evaluation. A bronchoscopy reveals no infectious cause for the abnormalities, with notes of abundant CD8+ T cells and occasional "foamy" macrophages present on BAL. A right heart catheterization is performed, which reveals pulmonary capillary wedge pressure (PCWP) of 8 mm Hg. What is the most likely explanation for the patient's CT scan abnormalities?

A. Cardiogenic pulmonary edema
B. Lymphangitic spread of pancreatic adenocarcinoma
C. Amiodarone toxicity
D. Adenovirus infection

Q7-5: What is the first abnormality identifiable on pulmonary function testing (PFT) in amiodarone toxicity?

A. Reduced forced vital capacity (FVC)
B. Reduced diffusing capacity of carbon monoxide (DLCO)
C. Reduced total lung capacity (TLC)
D. Increased forced expiratory volume (FEV1)/FVC ratio
E. Increased vital capacity (VC)

Q7-6: Which factor is NOT associated with an increased risk of pulmonary toxicity from amiodarone use?

A. Older age
B. Higher daily dosage
C. Preexisting thyroid disease
D. Preexisting pulmonary disease
E. Renal disease
F. Male sex assigned at birth
G. High levels of supplemental O_2

Q7-7: An 80-year-old woman is referred for evaluation of dyspnea and an abnormal chest radiograph. She has a history of COPD, ischemic cardiomyopathy, and dementia. She does not smoke. She was started on prophylactic oral antibiotics about 1 year ago for recurrent urinary tract infections. She has been reporting some joint pain and a rash. Her blood work shows a normal WBC count with slight peripheral eosinophilia.

Her chest imaging is as follows:

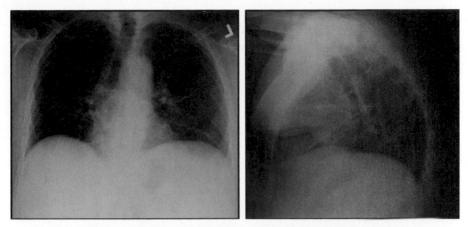

Image 7-4 • Chest radiographs (PA and lateral) for the patient in **Question 7-7**.

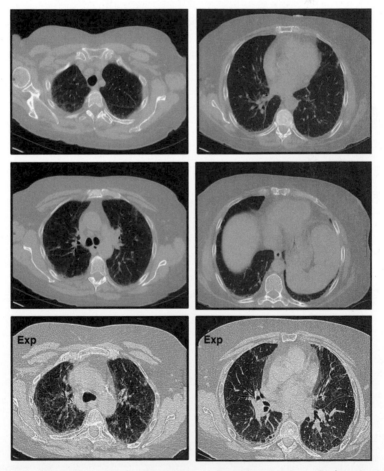

Image 7-5 • Chest CT images for the patient in **Question 7-7**. Exp – End-expiration CT images.

She undergoes a bronchoscopy, which was negative for any infectious cause. Your colleague reviews the chart and makes a diagnosis of drug-induced lung injury. Which aspect of her history pointed the colleague in that direction?

A. COPD
B. Ischemic cardiomyopathy
C. Frontotemporal dementia
D. Chronic urinary tract infections

ANSWERS

Q7-1: C
Linear opacities

Rationale: There are increased linear interstitial opacities in the bilateral lower lobes, more prominently along the periphery. Also note the reduced lung volumes bilaterally. Note that the high-resolution chest CT image (**Image 7-6**) from the same patient, taken at the same time, demonstrates a mix of ground-glass opacities, as well as nodular and linear interstitial opacities. The involvement is much larger than would be anticipated by the plain film alone.

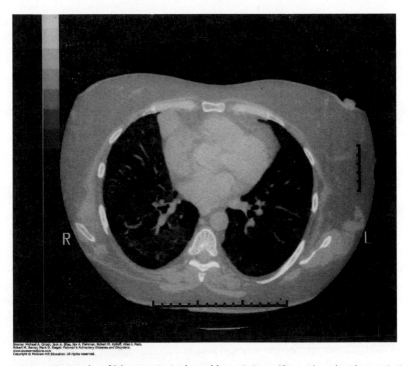

Image 7-6 • Example of bleomycin-induced lung injury. (*Reproduced with permission from Grippi MA, Elias JA, Fishman JA, et al: Fishman's Pulmonary Diseases and Disorders, 5th ed. New York, NY: McGraw Hill; 2015.*)

Q7-2: C
Bleomycin-induced lung injury

Rationale: Bleomycin commonly causes lung injury in a dose-dependent manner, developing in a subacute fashion weeks to 6 months following exposure. It can progress to acute respiratory distress syndrome (ARDS) and lung fibrosis in up to 10% of patients with acute toxicity.

Bleomycin-induced lung injury presents with a dry cough and dyspnea. On occasion, patients may also report low-grade fevers. Bleomycin has been associated with organizing pneumonia, eosinophilic pneumonia, and interstitial pneumonitis, which is most common and most severe.

Chest radiographs generally reveal bibasilar infiltrates, though the pattern on imaging is highly variable. CT is a more sensitive means of detecting abnormalities associated with toxicity.

Bleomycin-induced lung injury is often a diagnosis of exclusion. Bronchoscopy is used to evaluate for infection.

Treatment of bleomycin-induced lung injury includes withholding further treatment with bleomycin, and in the case of severe pneumonitis, administration of corticosteroids is recommended.

Q7-3: D
Use of bronchodilators

Rationale: Risk factors for pneumonitis include higher cumulative doses, supplemental O_2 use, prior radiation therapy to the chest, renal dysfunction, advanced age, and tobacco use.

Q7-4: C
Amiodarone toxicity

Rationale: This patient has a history of atrial fibrillation that started 3 years ago and was likely initiated on amiodarone. There is no evidence of decompensated congestive heart failure on the catheterization with a normal PCWP, and his BAL is negative for an infectious cause (adenovirus). There is currently no indication that the patient has pancreatic cancer based on the vignette (no weight loss, fevers, abdominal pain, jaundice). The BAL findings of a CD8+ lymphocytic process are consistent with alveolitis; however, the presence of foamy macrophages is seen in most patients on amiodarone without lung toxicity, so this is not specific for lung toxicity. A true diagnosis would require a lung biopsy with demonstration of interstitial lymphocytes infiltrates, fibrosis, and alveolar distortion on a background of macrophages with lamellar bodies.

Although amiodarone pulmonary toxicity can occur at any time during treatment, it most commonly occurs in a subacute manner between 6 and 24 months of therapy. Patients usually present with a nonproductive cough and progressive dyspnea. Constitutional symptoms like weight loss, fevers, and fatigue may accompany the pulmonary symptoms. Imaging may show patchy or diffuse pulmonary infiltrates. Infiltrates are generally bilateral. There may also be ground-glass opacities. There are no specific laboratory data to help diagnose amiodarone pulmonary toxicity. Amiodarone pulmonary toxicity is a diagnosis of exclusion. Amiodarone should be discontinued in the setting of pulmonary toxicity. As with other drug-induced pulmonary toxicities, the mainstay of therapy is systemic corticosteroids. Corticosteroids are often required for months because of the long half-life of amiodarone. At the start of amiodarone therapy, patients should have a chest radiograph and pulmonary function testing done to establish a baseline.

Q7-5: B
Reduced DLCO

Rationale: An impairment in the diffusion capacity is the first abnormality seen on PFT. Over time, patients may also develop restrictive physiology.

Q7-6: C
Preexisting thyroid disease

Rationale: Preexisting thyroid disease is not a known risk factor for the development of pulmonary toxicity from amiodarone, though amiodarone is associated with thyroid, liver, and lung toxicity. All the other risk factors listed predispose patients on amiodarone to pulmonary toxicity.

Q7-7: D
chronic urinary tract infections

Rationale: The patient's history is most consistent with nitrofurantoin-induced lung injury. Risk factors predisposing to the development of lung injury from nitrofurantoin include age and the presence of comorbid cardiopulmonary disease.

Nitrofurantoin-induced lung injury may present in an acute, subacute, or chronic fashion. The diagnosis may be made weeks to years after starting on the medication. The presentation of this toxicity is highly variable.

A Quick Note on Drug-induced lung toxicity.

As the number of approved pharmacologic and biologic drugs increase over time, the number of drugs associated with the development of lung disease continued to increase. While some of the more common causes were discussed above – chemotherapeutic agents, amiodarone, and nitrofurantoin – the list of drugs that have been associated with pulmonary complications or adverse events is considerable. This includes, but is certainly not limited to, anti-neoplastic agents, small molecule inhibitors, biologic agents such as monoclonal antibodies, antibiotics, cardiovascular drugs, non-steroidal anti-inflammatory drugs (NSAIDs), anticoagulants, anti-platelet agents, anti-hypertensives, and anti-viral medications. Additionally, the spectrum of disease that may be caused by different drugs is also extensive, ranging from the more typical pneumonitis discussed above to fibrosis, obliterative bronchiolitis, non-cardiogenic pulmonary edema, alveolar hemorrhage, and organizing pneumonia. A number of references have been provided below that can provided additional information should one desire. Pneumotox.com is a particularly useful website – which is also available as a app for smart-phones and computers – that was developed in 1997 to provide a free, evidence-based database of drug-induced lung disease publications or reports. This database may be organized by either the drug name or the pattern of lung disease encountered. This is an excellent resource for clinicians who suspect a potential drug-related adverse event.

References

Akoun GM, Cadranel JL, Blanchette G, et al. Bronchoalveolar lavage cell data in amiodarone-associated pneumonitis. Evaluation in 22 patients. Chest. 1991;99:1177.

Camus P, Dijon F. Pneumotox.com. The drug-induced respiratory disease website. Accessed on April 12th, 2021.

Camus P, Fanton A, Bonniaud P, et al. Interstitial lung disease induced by drugs and radiation. Respiration. 2004;71:301.

Dhokarh R, Li G, Schmickl CN, et al. Drug-associated acute lung injury: a population-based cohort study. Chest. 2012;142:845.

Kabbara WK, Kordahi MC. Nitrofurantoin-induced pulmonary toxicity: A case report and review of the literature. J Infect Public Health. 2015;8:309.

Leger P, Limper AH, Maldonado F. Pulmonary toxicities from conventional chemotherapy. Clin Chest Med. 2017;38:209.

Livanios K, Karampi ES, Sotiriou A, et al. Nitrofurantoin-induced acute pulmonary toxicity. Respirol Case Rep. 2016;4:25.

Martin WJ 2nd, Rosenow EC 3rd. Amiodarone pulmonary toxicity. Recognition and pathogenesis (Part I). Chest. 1988;93:1067.

Martin WJ 2nd, Rosenow EC 3rd. Amiodarone pulmonary toxicity. Recognition and pathogenesis (Part 2). Chest. 1988;93:1242.

Mendez JL, Nadrous HF, Hartman TE, Ryu JH. Chronic nitrofurantoin-induced lung disease. Mayo Clin Proc. 2005;80:1298.

Nacca N, Bhamidipati CM, Yuhico LS, Pinnamaneni S, Szombathy T. Severe amiodarone induced pulmonary toxicity. J Thorac Dis. 2012;4:667.

Nebeker JR, Barach P, Samore MH. Clarifying adverse drug events: a clinician's guide to terminology, documentation, and reporting. Ann Intern Med. 2004;140:795.

Okayasu K, Takeda Y, Kojima J, et al. Amiodarone pulmonary toxicity: a patient with three recurrences of pulmonary toxicity and consideration of the probable risk for relapse. Intern Med. 2006;45:1303.

Ott MC, Khoor A, Leventhal JP, et al. Pulmonary toxicity in patients receiving low-dose amiodarone. Chest. 2003;123:646.

Ozkan M, Dweik RA, Ahmad M. Drug-induced lung disease. Cleve Clin J Med 2001;68:782.

Poletti V, Poletti G, Murer B, et al. Bronchoalveolar lavage in malignancy. Semin Respir Crit Care Med. 2007;28:534.

Possick JD. Pulmonary toxicities from checkpoint immunotherapy for malignancy. Clin Chest Med. 2017;38:223.

Sleijfer S. Bleomycin-induced pneumonitis. Chest. 2001;120:617.

Snyder LS, Hertz MI. Cytotoxic drug-induced lung injury. Semin Respir Infect. 1988;3:217.

Standertskjöld-Nordenstam CG, Wandtke JC, Hood WB Jr, et al. Amiodarone pulmonary toxicity. Chest radiography and CT in asymptomatic patients. Chest. 1985;88:143.

Tanoue LT, McArdle J, Possick J. Pulmonary toxicity related to chemotherapeutic agents. In: Grippi MA, Elias JA, Fishman JA, et al., eds. *Fishman's Pulmonary Diseases and Disorders.* 5th ed. McGraw-Hill; 2015. https://accessmedicine.mhmedical.com/content.aspx?bookid=1344&sectionid=81191694

Wolkove N, Baltzan M. Review: amiodarone pulmonary toxicity. Can Respir J. 2009;16:43.

Zitnik, RJ. Drug-induced lung disease: antiarrhythmic agents. J Respir Dis. 1996;17:254.

CASE 8

A 55-year-old man presents to the office reporting progressive dyspnea. He has a history of HTN and gout. He notes that the onset of symptoms was perhaps 2 years ago, but it was rather insidious, so he cannot be sure. At first, he noticed only dyspnea with heavy exertion, which he attributed to his age, but over the past year, this has progressed to include dyspnea with mild activity such as walking to his car on level ground. He is a never-smoker. He has no family history of pulmonary disease, rheumatologist disease, or malignancy. He denies any lower extremity edema, chest pain, or diaphoresis. He has noticed a mild nonproductive cough.

On examination, his body mass index (BMI) is 27 kg/m^2. His vitals are HR 95, BP 110/80, RR 12, O$_2$ saturation 94% on room air. His ambulatory O$_2$ saturation is 92% after 1000 feet, with an HR of 133.

QUESTIONS

Q8-1: His PFTs are as follows:

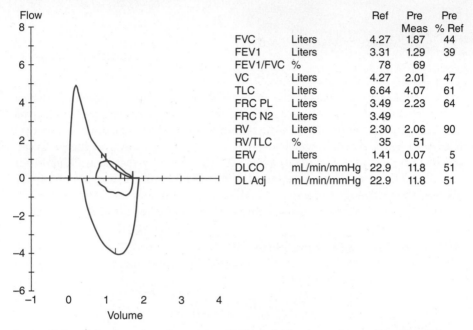

		Ref	Pre Meas	Pre % Ref
FVC	Liters	4.27	1.87	44
FEV1	Liters	3.31	1.29	39
FEV1/FVC	%	78	69	
VC	Liters	4.27	2.01	47
TLC	Liters	6.64	4.07	61
FRC PL	Liters	3.49	2.23	64
FRC N2	Liters	3.49		
RV	Liters	2.30	2.06	90
RV/TLC	%	35	51	
ERV	Liters	1.41	0.07	5
DLCO	mL/min/mmHg	22.9	11.8	51
DL Adj	mL/min/mmHg	22.9	11.8	51

Image 8-1 • Pulmonary function testing (PFT) results for the patient in **Question 8-1**.

Which abnormalities are present in this patient?

A. Expiratory airflow obstruction
B. Restrictive lung physiology
C. Reduced O_2 diffusion
D. Extrathoracic airway obstruction
E. A and B
F. B and C
G. A, B, and C
H. A and D
I. A and C
J. A, C, and D
K. A, B, and D

Q8-2: The patient has a CXR and CT scan from his primary care physician, and the images are shown in Image 8-2.

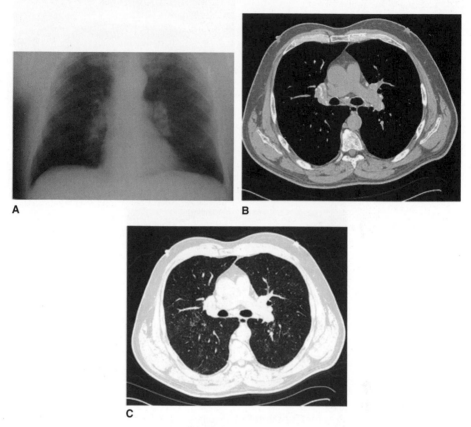

A   B

C

Image 8-2 • Chest images for **Question 8-2**. (*Reproduced with permission from Grippi MA, Elias JA, Fishman JA, et al: Fishman's Pulmonary Diseases and Disorders, 5th ed. New York, NY: McGraw Hill; 2015.*)

On the chest film, what is the correct order of lung zone involvement, from most severe to least severe?

A. Lower lung fields > mid-lung fields > upper lung fields
B. Upper lung fields > lower lung fields > mid-lung fields
C. Upper lung fields > mid-lung fields > lower lung fields

Q8-3: Which disease process is NOT commonly associated with involvement of the upper lung fields early in the disease, compared with the lower lung fields?

A. Sarcoidosis
B. Hypersensitivity pneumonitis (HP)
C. Idiopathic pulmonary fibrosis (IPF)
D. Emphysema

Q8-4: Which abnormalities are present on the CT images shown in Image 8-3?

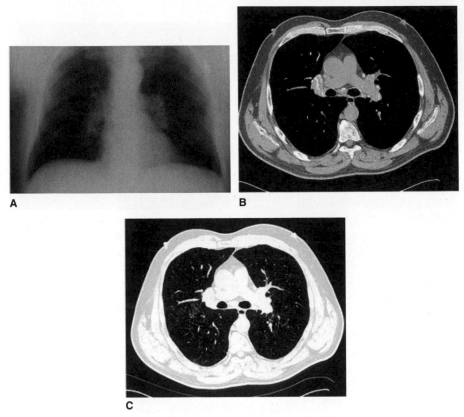

Image 8-3 • Chest images for **Question 8-4**. (*Reproduced with permission from Grippi MA, Elias JA, Fishman JA, et al: Fishman's Pulmonary Diseases and Disorders, 5th ed. New York, NY: McGraw Hill; 2015.*)

A. Reticular interstitial opacities with honeycombing
B. Cavitary lung lesions with air-fluid levels
C. Cystic lung lesions
D. Nodular interstitial opacities with hilar adenopathy

Q8-5: The patient's occupational history shows that he worked as a machinist for a company that has been manufacturing fluorescent light bulbs for the last 30 years. What is the most likely diagnosis?

A. Sarcoidosis
B. Silicosis
C. Byssinosis
D. Berylliosis
E. Asbestosis

Q8-6: Which procedure is necessary to make a diagnosis of berylliosis? Choose one procedure.

A. Open lung biopsy
B. Bronchoscopy with bronchoalveolar lavage fluid sent for silver staining
C. Bronchoscopy with transbronchial biopsy with neutron activation analysis on tissue specimen
D. Bronchoscopy with transbronchial biopsy and bronchoalveolar lavage fluid for CD4/CD8 T-cell ratio
E. Bronchoscopy with transbronchial biopsy and bronchoalveolar lavage fluid for CD4+ Lymphocyte proliferation test
F. Serum precipitins

Q8-7: Match the following symptoms to the beryllium-induced disorder:

A. Erythematous skin papule with vesiculations
B. Cough, chest pain, dyspnea, burning eyes, sore throat, hemoptysis
C. Exertional dyspnea, clubbing, chest pain, weight loss, hepatosplenomegaly, adenopathy
D. Diaphoresis, HTN, flushing, fever, diarrhea, confusion

Disorders:

Q8-7-1: ____ **CBD**

Q8-7-2: ____ **Acute berylliosis**

Q8-7-3: ____ **Beryllium dermatitis**

ANSWERS

Q8-1: G
(A) Expiratory air flow obstruction, (B) Restrictive lung physiology, and (C) Reduced O$_2$ diffusion

Rationale: The patient clearly has restrictive physiology, with reductions in the TLC, VC, and FVC. There is also clearly a reduction in the DLCO, which is a measure of the ability of O$_2$ to diffuse across the epithelial–endothelial barrier between the alveoli and the pulmonary capillary bed. And although the patient's FEV1/FVC is borderline for significant airflow obstruction according to some guidelines (FEV1/FVC less than 70% or less than lower limit of normal for age-appropriate control), it is always important to look at the expiratory flow loop (particularly in patients with restrictive lung disease). This patient's PFTs show reduced flow at lower lung volumes (ie, convex or "scooped" shape to the curve), as opposed to a straight line from the end of inspiration to the end of expiration. Despite the FEV1/FVC ratio being close to 70% predicted, the loop is suggestive of significant expiratory flow obstruction. This pattern is occasionally referred to as "pseudonormalization." Therefore, this patient also has some expiratory airflow obstruction. There is no abnormality on the inspiratory flow loop to suggest an extrathoracic airway obstruction.

Q8-2: B
Upper lung fields > Lower lung fields > Mid-lung fields

Rationale: The upper lung fields appear predominantly involved, followed by the mid-lung fields, and then the lower lung fields.

Q8-3: C
Idiopathic pulmonary fibrosis (IPF)

Rationale: IPF is more commonly associated with involvement of the lung bases early in the disease process. Alternatively, more airway-centric disease processes (sarcoidosis, HP) typically show involvement of the upper lobes early in the disease process. However, though unusual, IPF can have atypical presentations with diffuse involvement early in the disease process as well.

Q8-4: D
Nodular interstitial opacities with hilar adenopathy

Rationale: In **Image 8-3B** (chest/mediastinal window), one can see calcifications of the hilar (station 7) and mediastinal (stations 10-12) lymph nodes, which are enlarged. On the lung window in **Image 8-3C**, one can see small nodules along the septal lines, almost with the appearance of ground glass in areas where the nodules are finer, and linear interstitial opacities as well. This is a nodular interstitial pattern commonly seen in granulomatous lung diseases such as sarcoidosis. This pattern can be seen in a number of interstitial lung diseases as well as some types of infectious or inflammatory diseases.

Q8-5: D
Berylliosis

Rationale: Although all the answer options listed can have a similar radiographic appearance and clinical presentation, the patient's occupational history points toward chronic berylliosis or chronic beryllium disease (CBD). The etiology of sarcoidosis remains unclear (some point toward possible chronic infection), but some occupations, such as deck grinders working on military aircraft carriers, have a significantly increased risk of sarcoidosis, suggesting a possible occupational etiology. Byssinosis is associated with cotton exposure, asbestosis with asbestos exposure, and silicosis with exposure to silicon dust.

Q8-6: E
Bronchoscopy with transbronchial biopsy and bronchoalveolar lavage fluid for CD4+ Lymphocyte proliferation test

Rationale: There are two requirements for a diagnosis of berylliosis: tissue evidence of granulomatous lung disease and evidence of beryllium hypersensitivity. Bronchoscopy with transbronchial biopsy would be sufficient to obtain tissue to diagnose granulomatous lung disease. Demonstration of beryllium hypersensitivity is best performed in BAL fluid, though it can also be performed using blood samples if necessary. The BAL cell count would show a significant proportion of CD4+ lymphocytes, which would proliferate in response to beryllium exposure (CD4+ lymphocyte proliferation test). In terms of testing, an open lung biopsy would be overly aggressive at this point, given the potential morbidity. A bronchoscopy without biopsy or a blood test alone, while able to demonstrate beryllium hypersensitivity, would not confirm the diagnosis of granulomatous lung disease, leaving other possible causes (such as infection) in the differential diagnosis. A serum precipitins test is used in the diagnosis of hypersensitivity pneumonitis (antibody test), representing a different form of hypersensitivity reaction. A CD4/CD8 T-cell ratio has been proposed to aid in the diagnosis of sarcoidosis, though it lacks the necessary sensitivity and specificity. Inductively coupled plasma (ICP) and electrothermal atomic absorption spectroscopy (ETASS) or neutron activation analysis (NAA) can be employed to look for evidence of beryllium in lung tissue (and help differentiate what metal or elemental exposures a patient has experienced), but it does not confirm hypersensitivity per se. For example, a patient with granulomatous disease and prior beryllium exposure but **without** beryllium hypersensitivity would carry a diagnosis of sarcoidosis rather than berylliosis. Berylliosis is a granulomatous disorder caused by exposure to beryllium metal aerosols. Up to 10% to 15% of workers exposed to beryllium metals or salts may develop a hypersensitivity to beryllium. Exposure to beryllium dust or aerosol is most common in the following areas of manufacturing: ceramics, fluorescent light bulbs, nuclear and aerospace engineering, dental alloys, and electronics.

Q8-7-1: C

Q8-7-2: B

Q8-7-3: A

Rationale: Answer D contains symptoms associated with serotonin syndrome. Chronic berylliosis is a more indolent disorder characterized by hepatosplenomegaly as well as the classic symptoms seen in idiopathic interstitial pneumonia (exertional dyspnea, clubbing, pulmonary cachexia). The CD4+ hypersensitivity leads to involvement of the reticuloendothelial system (RES) involving the liver, spleen, and lymph nodes. Initially, chest imaging will typically show bilateral, upper-lobe predominant micronodular opacities along the bronchovascular bundles, consistent with an airway-centric disease process. Patients may also have hilar adenopathy and mild interlobular septal thickening. Ground-glass opacities may also be present. The micronodules may also coalesce and appear to form larger nodules, such as those seen in silicosis. As the disease progresses, patients may develop more severe interstitial fibrosis (interlobular and interlobar septal thickening), honeycombing, and associated traction bronchiectasis. These latter changes may be diffuse or lower-lung predominant. Mediastinal and hilar adenopathy are often seen at this later stage of disease.

Acute berylliosis is associated more commonly with symptoms of influenza (fever, cough, chest pain, sore throat) but may also be associated with hemoptysis, which is usually nonmassive. Beryllium dermatitis is a skin-limited disease associated with erythematous skin papules with vesiculations. Note that CBD can result from acute berylliosis. The abnormalities on chest imaging in acute berylliosis are generally milder, with hilar adenopathy and a nodular interstitial pattern. Patients with hemoptysis may develop more of an alveolar pattern on chest imaging.

The primary treatment in all forms of beryllium-related disease is removing the patient from further exposure. In patients with more significant disease, oral corticosteroids, appropriate vaccination, smoking cessation, and O_2 therapy may be initiated. Steroids are typically started at 0.5 to 1 mg prednisone equivalent per day and tapered slowly over the ensuing 3 to 6 months. In patients unable to discontinue steroids, methotrexate has been used as a steroid-sparing agent.

References

Balmes JR, Abraham JL, Dweik RA, et al. ATS Ad Hoc Committee on Beryllium Sensitivity and Chronic Beryllium Disease. An official American Thoracic Society statement: diagnosis and management of beryllium sensitivity and chronic beryllium disease. Am J Respir Crit Care Med. 2014;190:e34.

Boffetta P, Fordyce TA, Mandel JS. A mortality study of beryllium workers. Cancer Med. 2016;5:3596.

Cummings KJ, Deubner DC, Day GA, et al. Enhanced preventive programme at a beryllium oxide ceramics facility reduces beryllium sensitisation among new workers. Occup Environ Med. 2007;64:134.

Cummings KJ, Stefaniak AB, Virji MA, Kreiss K. A reconsideration of acute Beryllium disease. Environ Health Perspect. 2009;117:1250.

Fireman E, Haimsky E, Noiderfer M, Priel I, Lerman Y. Misdiagnosis of sarcoidosis in patients with chronic beryllium disease. Sarcoidosis Vasc Diffuse Lung Dis. 2003;20:144.

Fontenot AP, Amicosante M. Metal-induced diffuse lung disease. Semin Respir Crit Care Med. 2008;29:662.

Harber P, Su J, Alongi G. Beryllium BioBank: 2. Lymphocyte proliferation testing. J Occup Environ Med. 2014;56:857.

Hines SE, Pacheco K, Maier LA. The role of lymphocyte proliferation tests in assessing occupational sensitization and disease. Curr Opin Allergy Clin Immunol. 2012;12:102.

Honma K, Abraham JL, Chiyotani K, et al. Proposed criteria for mixed-dust pneumoconiosis: definition, descriptions, and guidelines for pathologic diagnosis and clinical correlation. Hum Pathol. 2004;35:1515.

Kelleher PC, Martyny JW, Mroz MM, et al. Beryllium particulate exposure and disease relations in a beryllium machining plant. J Occup Environ Med. 2001;43:238.

Kreiss K, Fechter-Leggett ED, McCanlies EC, Schuler CR, Weston A. Research to practice implications of high-risk genotypes for beryllium sensitization and disease. J Occup Environ Med. 2016;58:855.

Kreiss K, Mroz MM, Zhen B, Martyny JW, Newman LS. Epidemiology of beryllium sensitization and disease in nuclear workers. Am Rev Respir Dis. 1993;148:985.

Li L, Silveira LJ, Hamzeh N, et al. Beryllium-induced lung disease exhibits expression profiles similar to sarcoidosis. Eur Respir J. 2016;47:1797.

Madl AK, Unice K, Brown JL, Kolanz ME, Kent MS. Exposure-response analysis for beryllium sensitization and chronic beryllium disease among workers in a beryllium metal machining plant. J Occup Environ Hyg. 2007;4:448.

Mayer A, Hamzeh N. Beryllium and other metal-induced lung disease. Curr Opin Pulm Med. 2015;21:178.

Newman LS, Bobka C, Schumacher B, et al. Compartmentalized immune response reflects clinical severity of beryllium disease. Am J Respir Crit Care Med. 1994;150:135.

Newman LS, Lloyd J, Daniloff E. The natural history of beryllium sensitization and chronic beryllium disease. Environ Health Perspect. 1996;104:937.

Occupational Safety and Health Administration (OSHA), Department of Labor. Occupational exposure to beryllium. Final rule. Fed Regist. 2017;82:247.

Samuel G, Maier LA. Immunology of chronic beryllium disease. Curr Opin Allergy Clin Immunol. 2008;8:126.

Santo Tomas LH. Beryllium hypersensitivity and chronic beryllium lung disease. Curr Opin Pulm Med. 2009;15:165.

Sharma N, Patel J, Mohammed TL. Chronic beryllium disease: computed tomographic findings. J Comput Assist Tomogr. 2010;34:945.

Sizar O, Talati %. Berylliosis (Chronic Beryllium Disease). StatPearls. https://www.ncbi.nlm.nih.gov/books/NBK470364/. Published Dec 12, 2018. Accessed Jan 3, 2019.

Stoeckle JD, Hardy HL, Weber AL. Chronic beryllium disease. Long-term follow-up of sixty cases and selective review of the literature. Am J Med. 1969;46:545.

Thomas CA, Deubner DC, Stanton ML, Kreiss K, Schuler CR. Long-term efficacy of a program to prevent beryllium disease. Am J Ind Med. 2013;56:733.

Zacharisen MC, Fink JN. Hypersensitivity pneumonitis and related conditions in the work environment. Immunol Allergy Clin North Am. 2011;31:769, vii.

CASE 9

A 44-year-old man presents to your clinic with dyspnea that has been progressively worsening over the last several years but has only recently begun impacting his activities of daily living. Otherwise, the patient has HTN, for which he currently takes amlodipine. He takes no illicit drugs and does not smoke. He noted the gradual onset of symptoms approximately 3 months ago. Initially, he had a nonproductive cough and mild shortness of breath with strenuous exertion and thought he had some allergy issues; however, over-the-counter antihistamines did not help. The symptoms have progressed a bit, and now he is noticing that he is winded after climbing one to two flights of stairs. He works in a manual labor job, and his symptoms have begun to significantly impact his ability to work. His BMI is 22 kg/m². His vitals are T 36.7°C, HR 80, BP 120/80, RR 16, and O_2 saturation 96% on room air. You note that he has some increased work of breathing when asked to walk briskly around the hallway, with a mild drop in his O_2 saturation to 92%, HR 130. The pulmonary examination demonstrates some inspiratory crackles throughout. The patient is sent for a chest radiograph, which is shown in Image 9-1.

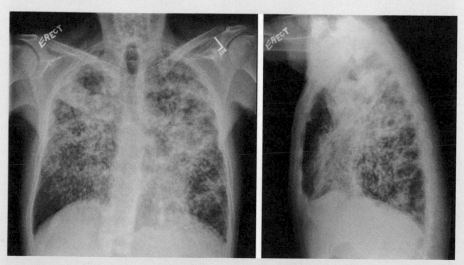

Image 9-1 • PA and lateral chest radiographs for the patient in **Question 9-1**.

QUESTIONS

Q9-1: How would you describe the abnormalities on the chest radiograph in Image 9-1?

A. Lower lobe–predominant linear interstitial opacities
B. Upper lobe–predominant nodular opacities with areas of consolidation
C. Diffuse bilateral alveolar opacities
D. Lower lobe–predominant reticular opacities and volume loss
E. Cystic lung lesions distributed diffusely throughout the lung

Q9-2: How would you describe the abnormalities on the chest CT in Image 9-2?

A. Traction bronchiectasis, interlobular septal thickening, and honeycombing
B. Scattered areas of ground-glass opacification with tree-in-bud opacities
C. Right upper lobe focal consolidation with air bronchograms
D. Linear interstitial opacities with scattered cystic lesions
E. Scattered nodular opacities, with larger areas of consolidation with central necrosis
F. Atelectasis

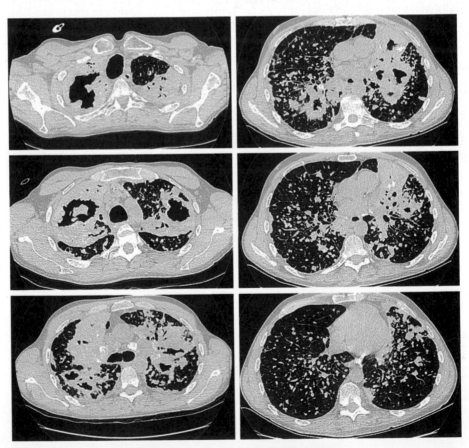

Image 9-2 • Chest CT images for the patient in **Question 9-2.**

Q9-3: Which abnormality is seen on the CT scan from the same patient shown in Image 9-3?

A. Pneumomediastinum
B. Pericardial effusion
C. Anterior mediastinal mass
D. Calcified hilar and mediastinal lymph nodes
E. Patulous esophagus

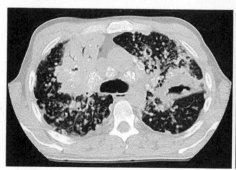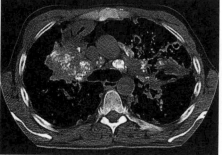

Image 9-3 • Chest CT images (left, lung window; right, mediastinal window) for the patient in **Question 9-3.**

Q9-4: The patient denies any constitutional symptoms. Given the constellation of findings, what would you pursue next in his evaluation?

A. Risk factors for *Mycobacterium tuberculosis* infection
B. Occupational history
C. Family history of malignancy
D. ECG
E. Antinuclear antibody (ANA) testing

Q9-5: The patient provides an occupational history that confirms your suspicion. Which occupation is most likely for this patient?

A. Naval shipyard worker
B. Pilot
C. Coal miner
D. Laboratory researcher
E. Gardener
F. Prison guard

Q9-6: Match the following patient vignettes to the most likely diagnosis.

Conditions:

A. Chronic silicosis
B. Accelerated silicosis
C. Acute silicosis
D. Caplan syndrome
E. Erasmus syndrome

Vignettes:

1. A 28-year-old man presents with fever, pleuritic pain, cough, weight loss, and dyspnea for the last week. He states he has worked in a stone quarry for the last 6 months and rarely wears his personal protective equipment. His chest radiograph shows bilateral, lower-lobe predominant hazy opacities in an alveolar-filling pattern, in addition to a small apical pneumothorax on the right.

2. A 42-year-old woman presents with worsening dyspnea on exertion over the last year. She has worked as a sandblaster for the past 10 years at a quarry. She also notes a dry cough, tightening of the skin on her hands and face, a cyanotic appearance of her bilateral digits in colder weather, bilateral lower extremity edema, and mild weight loss. She denies any fevers, chills, or sweats. An examination demonstrates hypoxemia on room air with some mild digital clubbing. A CXR shows small nodular opacities in the middle and upper lung fields.

3. A 51-year-old man with 22 years of experience as a coal miner presents with worsening dyspnea. He has an intermittently productive cough with black-tinged sputum for years. He does not smoke. He was diagnosed with rheumatoid arthritis 2 years ago with predominantly joint symptoms, including his hands and knees. He has been on immunosuppressive therapy. He denies any fevers, chills, sweats, or weight loss. His chest imaging shows bilateral nodular opacities, predominantly in the periphery. Several of the lesions are calcified, and one shows evidence of cavitation.

Q9-7: Which is NOT a potential complication of silica exposure?

A. Increased risk of lung cancer
B. Increased risk of mycobacterial infection
C. Increased risk of myocardial infarction
D. Increased risk of autoimmune/rheumatologic disease
E. Increased risk of chronic kidney diseases

Q9-8: For patients with either CWP or silicosis, what is the most important intervention?

A. Systemic steroids
B. Inhaled steroids
C. Inhaled bronchodilator
D. Whole lung lavage
E. Prevention of further exposure

Q9-9: What percentage of coal miners with CWP will develop complicated CWP or progressive massive fibrosis?

A. 1%
B. 5%
C. 10%
D. 50%

Q9-10: Which radiographic study is most useful for differentiating the lesions in PMF from lung malignancy?

A. FDG- PET
B. MRI
C. Thoracic ultrasonography.
D. High-resolution CT (HRCT) of the chest

ANSWERS

Q9-1: B
Upper-lobe predominant nodular opacities with areas of consolidation

Rationale: The chest radiograph demonstrates an upper lobe–predominant process, with some sparing of the lower lobes (more notable on the right). There are scattered nodular or reticulonodular opacities throughout, with what appear to be two larger opacities without clear cavitation in the upper lobes bilaterally. The opacity on the right almost has a linear appearance with regular borders, whereas the lesion on the left is more central and seems to have irregular borders. There is no apparent pneumothorax or pleural effusion. The central airways are patent.

Given the abnormalities seen on the chest radiograph, the patient is sent for a CT scan of the chest, which is shown in **Image 9-2**.

Q9-2: E
Scattered nodular opacities, with larger areas of consolidation with central necrosis

Rationale: In this case, there is a diffuse, upper-lobe predominant process with two large upper lobe cavitary lesions. The cavitary lesions are irregular but have well-defined borders. The nodules are opaque rather than ground glass in appearance. There some other scattered cavitary lesions moving inferiorly. The lower lobes and the right middle lobe show less involvement of the disease process overall. The distribution of the smaller nodules is predominantly perilymphatic. There is no evidence of honey-combing in the lower lobes (though images at the bases of the lower lobes are not pro-vided), and there is no significant traction bronchiectasis. Although there are some air bronchograms in the areas of consolidation (B), this does not best describe the diffuse abnormalities. The walls of the cavitary lesions are too thick to be described as cysts.

Q9-3: D
Calcified hilar and mediastinal lymph nodes

Rationale: The images are matched transverse images showing the lung and corre-sponding mediastinal windows at the level of the carina. On the left, an enlarged cal-cified mediastinal node is present (station 4R node). Additionally, there are scattered calcifications throughout the hilum and opacified areas. The esophagus is normal in appearance. There is no apparent area in the mediastinum outside of the airways. The heart is not clearly visible in these images to evaluate for pericardial effusion. There is no apparent anterior mediastinal mass.

Q9-4: B
Occupational history

Rationale: The patient's constellation of chest imaging abnormalities is highly con-cerning for a type of occupational lung disease, often referred to as *pneumoconiosis*.

Therefore, obtaining an occupational history would be the most reasonable next step in his evaluation. Although malignancy is certainly another consideration and a family history of a first-degree relative with lung cancer may increase suspicion, this is less likely to establish the diagnosis. Both *M. tuberculosis* and nontuberculous mycobacterial (NTM) infections may present with similar imaging findings (and often complicate underlying pneumoconiosis), but the lack of any associated symptoms such as cough, fever, weight loss, or hemoptysis makes infection less likely. An ECG could be useful to establish where the patient has evidence of pulmonary HTN; however, this again is less likely to establish the diagnosis for the underlying condition. An ANA test is useful in patients with suspected vasculitis or rheumatologic disease. Although some vasculitides can present with cavitary lung nodules (particularly the antineutrophilic cytoplasmic antibody [ANCA]-positive vasculitides), the lack of any other associated symptoms makes this less likely. Sarcoidosis would also be in the differential diagnosis.

Q9-5: C
Coal miner

Rationale: Again, the abnormalities on the patient's chest imaging are most concerning for pneumoconiosis, marked by the presence of diffuse, upper-lobe predominant nodular opacities, calcified hilar and mediastinal adenopathy, and larger mass-like opacities with central cavitation. In simple cases, the nodules are typically less than 1 cm in diameter. The larger opacifications arise from a conglomeration of smaller lesions and are generally lentiform or "sausage"-like in shape. Once these lesions reach approximately 4 to 5 cm in size, central cavitation becomes more likely. These areas may contain air bronchograms and can be calcified, as is seen above. The presence of these larger, bilateral lesions (typically more than 1 cm in diameter) is classically termed *progressive massive fibrosis* (PMF). A number of occupational exposures can lead to very similar radiographic findings, but of the options provided, only coal mining is associated with such changes. Naval shipyard workers are at increased risk for asbestos-related lung disease, which generally does not consist of diffuse nodular disease, even in asbestosis. Coal miners who develop such changes after exposure to washed coal have coal workers' pneumoconiosis (CWP). Coal workers may also develop silicosis if exposed to unwashed coal. A prison guard may have an increased risk of *M. tuberculosis* exposure. Gardeners may have an increased risk of exposure to endemic fungi as well as NTM species. Laboratory researchers are more likely to experience acute inhalational exposures, though long-term exposure to any of a number of metals, dusts, or fibers during research could also lead to a similar condition.

Patients with simple CWP have a limited form of the disease, with lesions generally less than 1 cm in diameter. The presence of these larger bilateral lesions heralds the development of complicated CWP, also termed PMF. Additionally, patients can develop a more diffuse picture of pulmonary fibrosis that will also involve the lower lobes and is associated with severe hypoxemia. The risk of developing CWP is related to the duration, severity, and type of coal dust exposure. It has been estimated that up to 20% to 30% of coal miners have CWP. The usual exposure period before the onset of disease is 25 to 30 years. Exposure to coal that is high in silica content significantly increases the risk of developing CWP. Aside from exposure-related risk factors, smoking also increases the risk of CWP in exposed workers. The Internal Labor Organization (ILO) developed a diagnostic classification system based on chest radiography that has long been used for screening.

Nearly all coal miners will have evidence of carbon dust deposition in the lung (termed *anthracosis* when there is no associated lung pathology). In the terminal bronchioles, carbon dust is phagocytosed by macrophages. The macrophages transport the dust to the lymphatics, or dust-laden macrophages are expelled from the airway by coughing. When the ability to clear the dust particles via the lymphatics is overwhelmed, dust-laden macrophages accumulate, and dust itself may be retained in the alveoli. Eventually, the coal dust will lead to an inflammatory or immune response that ultimately results in fibroblast activation, collagen deposition, and focal interstitial fibrosis. This tends to occur in perilymphatic areas. The finding of coal dust-laden macrophages (coal macules) in areas of focal fibrosis is diagnostic, though lung biopsy is rarely necessary because the diagnosis can often be made clinically. These focal areas may then coalesce as more dust is deposited and fibroblasts activate. These larger, coalescent areas will appear as black lesions in the lung on gross pathology. This latter finding of larger coalescing lesions is PMF. The architectural distortion in these areas can lead to surrounding emphysematous changes and strangulation of blood supply. The latter may be responsible for the cavitation seen in larger lesions. Some patients may also go on to develop changes of diffuse pulmonary fibrosis, with more irregular opacities at the lung bases.

Numerous occupational exposures may lead to chronic lung disease similar to CWP. Silica exposure and the development of silicosis may occur in mining (including exposure to unwashed coal or metals), sand-blasting, brick-laying or other masonry work, and stone-cutting. Talcosis can result from exposure to talc powder, which is found in the rubber and cosmetic industries. Hard metal pneumoconiosis results from exposure during sintering of cobalt. Berylliosis results from exposures to beryllium used in ceramics, dental laboratories, and aerospace applications. Byssinosis results from the inhalation of textile fibers during manufacturing. All can have a very similar appearance on CT to CWP, and therefore a detailed occupational history is necessary to aid in differentiating these conditions.

For nearly all forms of pneumoconiosis, there is increased risk of tuberculosis and NTM infections. Other prominent considerations in the differential for this patient would include lung cancer (likely bronchoalveolar or bronchogenic carcinoma), sarcoidosis, rheumatoid arthritis–associated interstitial lung disease, Langerhans cell histiocytosis (LCH), and vasculitis or other autoimmune diseases.

Q9-6-1: C
Acute silicosis

Rationale: Acute silicosis is a rare condition occurring typically after a high concentration exposure to silica-containing dust. The presentation may be similar to that of viral pneumonitis. Imaging typically demonstrates a lower-lobe predominant process with fluffy alveolar infiltrates or ground-glass opacities. Patients with acute silicosis are at increased risk for chronic silicosis. Pneumothorax is seen more commonly in acute silicosis as well.

Q9-6-2: E
Erasmus syndrome

Rationale: Erasmus syndrome is silica-induced scleroderma that is indistinguishable from system sclerosis.

Q9-6-3: D
Caplan syndrome

Rationale: Caplan syndrome is the development of CWP or silicosis in patients with manifestations of rheumatoid arthritis. The nodules likely represent a mix of rheumatoid lung nodules and coal macules. However, these lesions tend to evolve more rapidly than in simple or complicated CWP, and they have a greater tendency to cavitate.

Chronic silicosis closely parallels CWP, including simple silicosis and complicated silicosis (PMF). A classic finding that is highly suggestive of silicosis is the presence of "eggshell" calcifications in the hilar nodes, in which just the outer edges of the lymph node are calcified. The radiographic findings otherwise mirror CWP. The time from first exposure to the development of disease is typically 20 to 30 years. Accelerated silicosis has the same clinical presentation as chronic silicosis, though it occurs over a very rapid period from the time of initial exposure (less than 10 years).

Q9-7: C
Increased risk of myocardial infarction

Rationale: All the other answers have been associated with silica exposure.

Q9-8: E
Prevention of further exposure

Rationale: For patients with pneumoconiosis, it is imperative to limit any and all future exposures to the inciting substance for fear of disease progression. Unfortunately, as the symptoms and radiographic findings of many of the pneumoconioses lag significantly from the time of last exposure, this intervention may be of little help. However, for patients with accelerated silicosis, immediate removal from exposure is associated with a reduced risk of progression to PMF. Treatment otherwise is largely supportive, with only anecdotal evidence for the use of glucocorticoids in cases of accelerated silicosis. For patients with rapidly progressive disease, lung transplantation is typically the only viable option.

Q9-9: C
10%

Rationale: Approximately 10% of patients with CWP will develop PMF (about 2%-3% overall). However, up to 30% of patients with CWP may go on to develop diffuse pulmonary fibrosis.

Q9-10: B
MRI

Rationale: The lesions seen in PMF (complicated silicosis or CWP) are difficult to differentiate from malignancy on HRCT or ultrasound. Unfortunately, the majority of the lesions are FDG-avid on PET-CT. There is some evidence that MRI can be useful to differentiate these conditions. On T2-weighted images, PMF lesions will appear dark, and malignant lesions will appear white. Additionally, PMF lesions may show rim enhancement.

References

Ajlani H, Meddeb N, Sahli H, Sellami S. [Erasmus syndrome: case report]. Rev Pneumol Clin. 2009; 65:16.

Antao VC, Pinheiro GA, Terra-Filho M, et al. High-resolution CT in silicosis: correlation with radiographic findings and functional impairment. J Comput Assist Tomogr. 2005;29:350.

Bégin R, Bergeron D, Samson L, et al. CT assessment of silicosis in exposed workers. AJR Am J Roentgenol. 1987;148:509.

Blackley DJ, Reynolds LE, Short C, et al. Progressive massive fibrosis in coal miners from 3 clinics in Virginia. JAMA. 2018;319:500.

Chong S, Lee KS, Chung MJ, et al. Pneumoconiosis: comparison of imaging and pathologic findings. Radiographics. 2006;26:59.

Cox CW, Rose CS, Lynch DA. State of the art: imaging of occupational lung disease. Radiology. 2014;270:681.

Dee P, Suratt P, Winn W. The radiographic findings in acute silicosis. Radiology. 1978;126:359.

Garg K, Lynch DA. Imaging of thoracic occupational and environmental malignancies. J Thorac Imaging. 2002:198.

International Labour Office. Guidelines for the use of the ILO international classification of radiographs of pneumoconioses. Geneva, Switzerland: International Labour Office, 2011.

Karam M, Roberts-Klein S, Shet N, Chang J, Feustel P. Bilateral hilar foci on 18F-FDG PET scan in patients without lung cancer: variables associated with benign and malignant etiology. J Nucl Med. 2008;49:1429.

Kim KI, Kim CW, Lee MK, et al. Imaging of occupational lung disease. Radiographics. 2001;21:1371.

Kuempel ED, Wheeler MW, Smith RJ, Vallyathan V, Green FH. Contributions of dust exposure and cigarette smoking to emphysema severity in coal miners in the United States. Am J Respir Crit Care Med. 2009;180:257.

Laney AS, Weissman DN. Respiratory diseases caused by coal mine dust. J Occup Environ Med. 2014;56:S18.

Marchiori E, Ferreira A, Müller NL. Silicoproteinosis: high-resolution CT and histologic findings. J Thorac Imaging. 2001;16:127.

McCunney RJ, Morfeld P, Payne S. What component of coal causes coal workers' pneumoconiosis? J Occup Environ Med. 2009;51:462.

Rapidly progressive coal workers' pneumoconiosis in the United States: geographic clustering and other factors. Occup Environ Med. 2005;62:670.

Seaman DM, Meyer CA, Kanne JP. Occupational and environmental lung disease. Clin Chest Med. 2015;36:249.

Wade WA, Petsonk EL, Young B, Mogri I. Severe occupational pneumoconiosis among West Virginian coal miners: one hundred thirty-eight cases of progressive massive fibrosis compensated between 2000 and 2009. Chest. 2011;139:1458.

CASE 10

A 56-year-old man presents with several acute episodes of dyspnea over the last few weeks. He has a history of HTN and GERD. He takes an angiotensin-converting enzyme (ACE) inhibitor and omeprazole. He has never smoked. He exercises three to four times a week, though he has not been able to recently because of fatigue. He has no family history of cardiac, pulmonary, or rheumatologic history and no history of malignancy. He works as a consultant for an engineering firm. He initially experienced intermittent episodes of fever, myalgia, dyspnea, and dry cough, which started in the middle of the night about 3 weeks ago. This coincided with starting a new project at work, which the patient attributed to a likely viral infection. After 2 days of these symptoms, the patient presented to the ED with the aforementioned symptoms because of some lightheadedness and tachycardia.

The ED notes show that on examination he was tachycardic to 105, regular. He was saturating 92% on room air at rest, and 88% on room air with activity, improving to 94% on 2 L NC. He had no adenopathy. He had some bibasilar inspiratory crackles. He had no clubbing, cyanosis, or edema. There was no murmur. His abdominal examination was benign. He had no musculoskeletal or joint findings of note. He was diagnosed as having some type of viral infection and treated supportively.

He was sent home from his assignment and started feeling better upon returning home. After another week, he returned to complete his consulting assignment, and after 2 nights, the symptoms returned. He presented to urgent care, where his CXR appeared abnormal. Due to the recurrence of his symptoms, he was referred to the pulmonary clinic for evaluation. He returned home, and since then his symptoms have improved significantly.

His CXRs at the time of the urgent care evaluation (Images 10-1 and 10-2) and on his follow-up visit to the pulmonary clinic 10 days later (Image 10-3) are shown below.

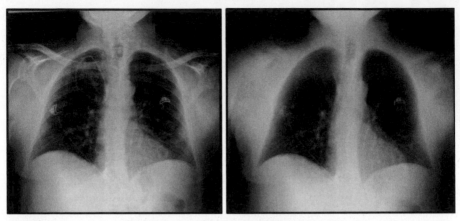

Image 10-1 • Chest radiographs for the patient in **Question 10-1** at time of presentation (febrile) (left image, standard AP CXR; right, clear view image with bone images suppressed).

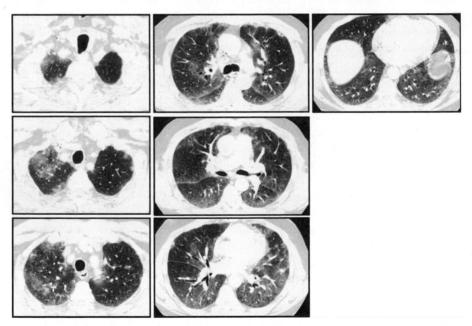

Image 10-2 • Chest CT imaging for the patient in **Question 10-1** from time of presentation (febrile).

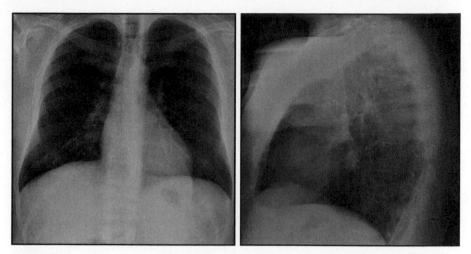

Image 10-3 • Chest radiographs (PA and lateral) for the patient in **Question 10-1** approximately 10 days later while on leave from work.

QUESTIONS

Q10-1: Which is the most appropriate description of the findings?

A. Bilateral pleural effusions on CXR with ground-glass opacities on CT, which resolved on follow-up

B. Bilateral upper lobe cavitary lesions, with nodules, cavitary nodules, and cysts on CT, which resolved on follow-up

C. Bilateral diffuse reticulonodular interstitial opacities, with ground glass and septal thickening on CT, which resolved on follow-up

D. Miliary nodular pattern with diffuse nodules on CT, which has persisted in the interval

Q10-2: Given the patient's recurrent symptoms, which question would be most appropriate to determine the etiology of the CXR abnormalities?

A. Do you have any pets at home?

B. Did you start any new medications recently?

C. Did you have any sick contacts/encounters recently?

D. Did you have any new exposures at works recently?

Q10-3: You inquire further about the patient's current job assignment. He reports that he was recently assigned to help design a new manufacturing plant that had flooded recently and is being demolished soon because of mold. What is the most likely diagnosis?

A. Sarcoidosis

B. Asthma

C. Acute/subacute hypersensitivity pneumonitis (HP)

D. Noncardiogenic pulmonary edema

E. Cryptogenic organizing pneumonia (COP)

Q10-4: Which exposure history is not consistent with acute/subacute HP? Assume the same general clinical presentation as in this case.

A. A farmer who just completed harvesting and baling hay

B. A carpenter who just completed a job where welding was performed and who was not wearing personal protective equipment (PPE)

C. An employee in a chemical manufacturing plant that produces isocyanates who did not wear any PPE at work while cleaning equipment

D. An employee who worked in a grain mill for years and who recently had exposure to a large plume of grain dust

E. A chicken farmer whose ventilation system malfunctioned the day prior

Q10-5: Which of the following is most useful to establish a diagnosis of acute/subacute HP in patients with the above imaging abnormalities?

A. Elevated serum LDH
B. Peripheral eosinophilia
C. Bronchoalveolar lavage with lymphocyte percentage 10%
D. Pulmonary function testing with expiratory airflow obstruction present
E. Serum precipitins (IgG) against thermophilic actinomyces
F. Exposure history
G. Skin testing (IgE) against environmental antigens

Q10-6: What is the most common abnormality on PFT in acute/subacute HP?

A. Restrictive findings (reduced TLC and FVC)
B. Air-trapping/hyperinflation
C. Isolated reduced RV
D. Reduced DLCO
E. Elevated DLCO

Q10-7: What abnormality on histopathology is most consistent with acute/subacute HP?

A. Organizing pneumonia
B. Poorly formed, noncaseating granulomatous inflammation
C. Usual interstitial pneumonia
D. Fibrotic nonspecific interstitial pneumonia
E. Well-formed granulomas around respiratory bronchioles with numerous CD1a+ cells

Q10-8: What is the primary treatment for patients with acute/subacute hypersensitivity pneumonitis?

A. Systemic glucocorticoids
B. Methotrexate
C. Mycophenolate
D. Rituximab
E. Plasmapheresis
F. Antigen avoidance
G. Azathioprine
H. Start smoking tobacco
I. Antifibrotics (eg, pirfenidone)

ANSWERS

Q10-1: C
Bilateral diffuse reticulonodular interstitial opacities, with ground glass and septal thickening on CT, which resolved on follow-up

Rationale: These appear to have resolved on follow-up. Although somewhat difficult to see, diffuse reticulonodular interstitial opacities are shown in **Image 10-1**, and they appear to have improved on follow-up in **Image 10-3**. On CT, there are upper-lobe predominant but relatively diffuse patchy areas of ground-glass opacities and some septal thickening. These findings are largely nonspecific.

Q10-2: D
Did you have any new exposures at work recently?

Rationale: This patient had the development of symptoms (fevers, myalgias, dyspnea, cough) starting shortly after traveling to a new consulting assignment a few weeks prior. The symptoms persisted while at that job site and then resolved upon the patient's return home. Although this could certainly be due to a viral/atypical pulmonary infection (answer C), the constellation of symptoms recurred after the patient returned to the worksite a few weeks later, suggesting that there may be some type of exposure at work causing the symptoms. Question (A) would be appropriate if the symptoms occurred when at home but resolved when the patient travels. Question (B) is an alternative choice, but the temporal relationship favors question (D) rather than (B).

Q10-3: C
Acute/subacute hypersensitivity pneumonitis (HP)

Rationale: The patient's symptoms started with exposure to a moldy environment, resolved with removal of the antigen, and then recurred with antigen reexposure, suggesting a diagnosis of HP. Mold is a very common antigen in cases of HP. Although asthma can have a similar temporal course, the constitutional symptoms and CXR abnormalities are much less likely to occur. COP can have a similar temporal pattern of symptoms, but the CXR abnormalities are typically more focal. Noncardiogenic edema is a nonspecific term and can be related to infections, inflammation, etc, and HP is a more specific diagnosis here. Sarcoidosis does not typically have such a relapsing/remitting pattern without immunosuppressive intervention (eg, steroids), though this is possible. Heart failure with pulmonary edema may also have a similar appearance; however, the presence of constitutional symptoms and the lack of any evidence on heart failure on examination makes this less likely.

Hypersensitivity pneumonitis (also referred to as *extrinsic allergic alveolitis*) is an immune response to an organic allergen and may be seen in acute, subacute, and chronic forms. However, it should be noted that not all presentations of HP fit nicely into this schema. Some clinicians have suggested using a different classification system similar to nonspecific interstitial pneumonia (NSIP), with an acute/inflammatory/cellular form of the disease and a chronic/fibrotic subtype. The subacute subtype may fall into either a more acute or a more chronic pattern. HP is believed to be a two-hit pathogenic mechanism, with a genetic predisposition to developing the disorder coupled with some prior, typically lower-level, exposure to a specific antigen that leads to the development of a hypersensitivity reaction. In acute HP, there is a high-level antigen exposure to which the patient is sensitized, while the chronic form is associated with a more indolent, likely lower level antigen exposure over a long period of time.

Q10-4: B
A carpenter who just completed a job where welding was performed and who was not wearing personal protective equipment (PPE)

Rationale: This is a difficult question. To identify a case of acute HP in this instance, one needs to identify if the patient had a large acute exposure to an antigen to which the patient has previously been sensitized. In answer (B), the patient, a carpenter, likely does not have significant prior exposure to welding fumes. This is actually a different disease process termed "metal fume" or inhalation fever, which does not require prior sensitization. All the other exposure histories would be consistent with possible acute/subacute HP, as the patients in these cases had prior exposure to antigens and recently had a high-level exposure. However, it is important to note that in patients with no prior sensitization, high-level exposure to grain dust (silo filer disease), organic dust (organic dust toxic syndrome or pulmonary mycotoxicosis), or chemical compounds (chemical inhalation fever) can cause acute febrile respiratory illnesses. Animal dander, aerosolized molds/fungi, organic chemical compounds, and many other compounds have been implicated as antigens in HP. There have been reported outbreaks of HP as well, typically associated with contaminated water supply systems or water damage leading to the development of mold. Isocyanates have most commonly been associated with asthma and HP in chemical manufacturing or other industrial processing. Infection or colonization with *Mycobacterium avium* complex has also been associated with the development in HP in patients with prolonged hot water exposure, often termed "hot tub lung." Patients with suspected HP should be questioned about their occupational and environmental exposures, with particular interest to the following:

1. Presence of mold or water damage in the house or place of employment: This may arise from multiple sources, including heat and air conditioning systems, swimming pools, hot tubs, and humidifiers. Often, patients may not be aware of water damage in the house, and it should be recommended to have crawl and attic spaces inspected as well as an inspection of the ventilation system.

2. Exposure to farms or farm animals, as well as exposure to bird droppings or bird dander: Essentially any prolonged exposure to animal dander or droppings may lead to the development of HP, including household pets. Note, there is a condition known as *organic dust toxic syndrome* that is similar to acute berylliosis in that it requires a high antigen exposure load over a short period of time (1 day), whereas

farmer lung disease (HP) results from a more subacute or prolonged exposure to the antigen.

3. Exposure to any processing of organic materials that are associated with the development of aerosolized particles, including woodworking/lumber processing, granaries, flour mills, and tobacco processing plants.

4. Exposure to any organic chemical vapors, with particular attention to isocyanates or plastics: It is important to differentiate HP from inhalation fever ("metal fume fever") as well.

5. Exposure to textile manufacturing: This is controversial, and some clinicians consider textile-related lung injury to be a process separate from HP. However, this aspect of the patient's exposure history must also be addressed.

6. Of course, it is important to address exposures more commonly associated with other types of lung disease (coal dust, beryllium in aerospace or electronics manufacturing, silica) to aid in narrowing the differential diagnosis.

Q10-5: F
Exposure history

Rationale: The diagnosis of acute/subacute HP is often difficult to establish because it mimics community-acquired pneumonia and resolves rapidly. In combination with the appropriate imaging findings, an appropriate exposure history would be most helpful to establish a diagnosis of acute/subacute HP. Serum precipitins are the most useful laboratory test for HP; however, there are several drawbacks to the serum precipitins testing: (1) these antibodies are often found in asymptomatic subjects with prior exposure to the antigens, who have no evidence of lung disease; (2) there is a significant risk of false-negative testing; and (3) there is an infinite number of potential antigens, but currently testing is limited to around 100 to 200 antigens through the National Jewish Hospital, and some *a priori* knowledge of the antigen must be known to narrow the search. PFT findings of expiratory airflow obstruction would be nonspecific and could represent asthma or chronic bronchitis. It is possible to obtain environmental samples and test them against a patient's blood to determine if an immune complex forms; however, this is limited to specific reference laboratories and likely also depends on the purity of the environmental samples obtained. For subacute and chronic HP, there are no widely available lymphocyte proliferation tests, which, again, would require a significant number of antigens. Skin testing is not useful because this is a test of antigen-specific IgE antibodies, representing a different hypersensitivity mechanism (type 1). Other acute phase or inflammatory marker testing (erythrocyte sedimentation rate [ESR], C-reactive protein [CRP], LDH, procalcitonin) is generally not useful in the diagnosis of HP. Peripheral eosinophilia is more commonly seen in acute eosinophilic pneumonia (AEP). Bronchoalveolar lavage with a lymphocyte population of 10% is nonspecific; a lymphocyte count above 20% would help support the diagnosis, but it is not as useful as a clear exposure history.

Q10-6: D
Reduced DLCO

Rationale: In acute HP, following resolution, most patients' PFTs are normal, though during acute events, PFTs are likely to demonstrate a reduced DLCO. In subacute and chronic HP, the most common abnormality is a reduced DLCO. Most patients have some degree of restrictive lung disease, but patients with more evidence of air-trapping may have a predominant obstructive pattern with an elevated RV and RV/TLC ratio. For the most part, patients have a mixed restrictive and obstructive pattern. It is important to look at the shape of the flow-volume curve on expiration and not just the spirometric indices because significant restriction can cause pseudonormalization of the FEV1/FVC ratio (the percent reduction in FVC is typically more significant than the FEV1 in restriction) and the presence of underlying obstruction can be missed and untreated.

Q10-7: B
Poorly formed, noncaseating granulomatous inflammation

Rationale: This abnormality is typically accompanied by cellular interstitial pneumonitis. The pathology in acute and subacute HP generally shows noncaseating granulomatous inflammation in the respiratory bronchioles with lymphocytes and monocytes in the peribronchiolar regions (ie, cellular bronchiolitis and pneumonitis). In the end-stages of the disease, the pathology may show usual interstitial pneumonia, fibrotic NSIP, or areas of organizing pneumonia. Well-formed granulomas staining positive for CD1a+ cells would be more consistent with pulmonary Langerhans cell histiocytosis (PLCH).

Q10-8: F
Antigen avoidance

Rationale: The primary treatment for patients with all forms of HP is antigen avoidance. As acute HP typically resolves quickly with antigen avoidance (within hours), this typically the only treatment needed. In patients with persistent symptoms or imaging/PFT abnormalities despite antigen avoidance, consideration can be given to the use of glucocorticoids. Rituximab, mycophenolate, and azathioprine can be used in patients with disease refractory to glucocorticoids. Antifibrotic medications could also be considered in patients with a chronic/fibrotic disease subtype. Plasmapheresis has not been used in the treatment of HP. Although a history of smoking tobacco is associated with a reduced risk of developing HP, starting smoking tobacco after a diagnosis is not associated with an attenuated or stable disease course and is more likely to lead to further reductions in pulmonary function with time.

Here is a brief summary of acute and subacute HP (**Table 10-1**). Chronic HP will be covered in an additional case in this text.

TABLE 10-1 • Characteristics of Acute and Subacute Hypersensitivity Pneumonitis				
	Time to Onset From Antigen Exposure	Symptoms	Radiographic Findings	Progression/ Recurrence	Treatment
Acute	Several hours (4-8 hours)	Resembles community-acquired pneumonia, with fevers, chills, malaise, dyspnea, and dry cough. Patients may have inspiratory crackles on examination.	Often normal, though patients may have reticulonodular opacities with a lower lobe predominance. Alveolar opacities can be seen in a similar pattern in severe cases. CT may demonstrate ground-glass opacities and micronodules.	Typically resolves rapidly in the absence of the antigen (1-2 days) but may recur with antigen reexposure. Not thought to be a significant risk for progression to chronic disease, assuming the antigen is avoided.	Antigen avoidance; if symptoms persist, search for an alternative antigen. A course of glucocorticoids may be necessary for patients with persistent abnormalities on imaging or pulmonary function testing or in those with continued symptoms.
Subacute	Days-weeks (typically less than 6 months)	Subacute (4-6 weeks) onset and progression of dyspnea and cough, without fever, chills, or night sweats.	As opposed to acute HP, subacute HP displays an upper lung predominance, typically with a reticulonodular pattern. CT may demonstrate ground-glass opacities and micronodules. On CT, patients may have evidence of interlobular thickening, and if expiratory imaging is performed, there may be evidence of air-trapping in a mosaic pattern.	Increased risk of progression to chronic HP.	Same as above. Prednisone is typically dosed at 0.5 mg/kg/day with an unspecified period of time and tapered during follow-up based on symptoms and objective testing.

CASE 11

A 33-year-old White woman with no medical history presents to a primary care clinic with a painful rash on her legs. She had a low-grade fever and arthralgia recently as well. The symptoms began approximately 3 days ago. She takes no medications, does not smoke, and does not use illicit drugs. She works as a chef at a local restaurant and has no new occupational or environmental exposures. She denies any dyspnea but does endorse a dry cough intermittently that she attributes to postnasal drip.

Her BMI is 30 kg/m^2. Her vitals are HR 67, BP 150/100, RR 10, and O$_2$ saturation 96% on room air. Her oxygen saturation does not drop with ambulation.

Her examination is unremarkable aside from the following abnormalities:

1. There are moderate effusions of the ankles bilaterally, associated with warmth and tenderness, and somewhat limited range of motion; and
2. These lesions on the leg are palpable, nonblanching, warm, erythematous, and painful on palpation.

Image 11-1 depicts these findings.

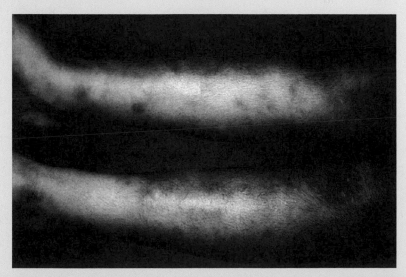

Image 11-1 • Dermatologic abnormalities discovered on examination of the patient in **Question 11-1.** (*Reproduced with permission from Mana J, Marcoval J. Erythema nodosum, Clin Dermatol May-Jun 2007;25(3):288-294.*)

The patient's CXR is shown in **Image 11-2**.

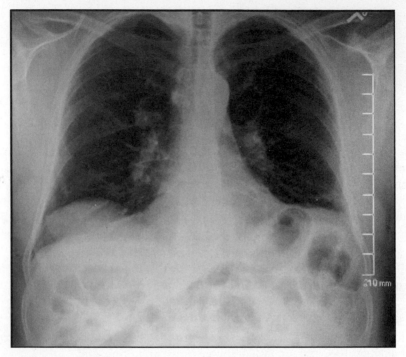

Image 11-2 • Chest radiograph (AP) for the patient in **Question 11-1**.

QUESTIONS

Q11-1: What is the likely diagnosis?

A. Reactive (postinfectious arthritis)
B. Rheumatoid arthritis (RA)
C. Systemic lupus erythematosus (SLE)
D. Lofgren syndrome
E. Acute leukemia
F. Loeffler syndrome

Q11-2: What percentage of patients with sarcoidosis have lung involvement?

A. 5%
B. 20%
C. 40%
D. 70%
E. 90%

Q11-3: Match the following chest images to the appropriate radiographic disease stage of sarcoidosis.

A. Stage I
B. Stage II
C. Stage III
D. Stage IV

Note: The rationale for the answers will follow the last of the image sets.

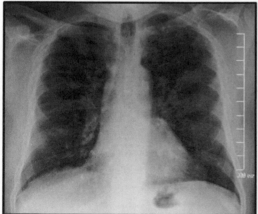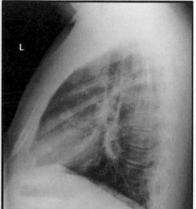

Image 11-3 • Chest radiographs (PA and lateral) for **Question 11-3-A**.

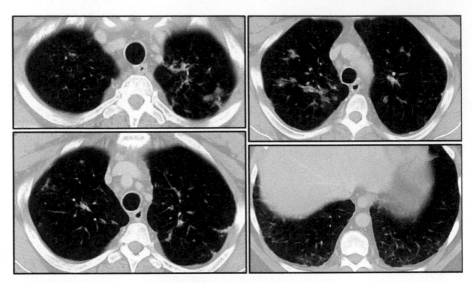

Image 11-4 • Chest CT images for **Question 11-3-A**.

Q11-3-A: Answer: _____

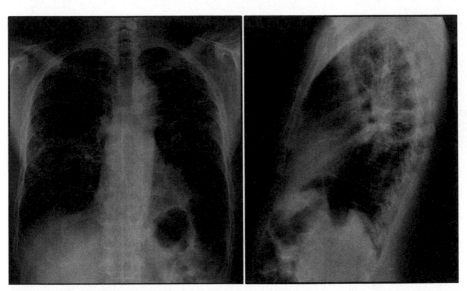

Image 11-5 • Chest radiographs (PA and lateral) for **Question 11-3-B**.

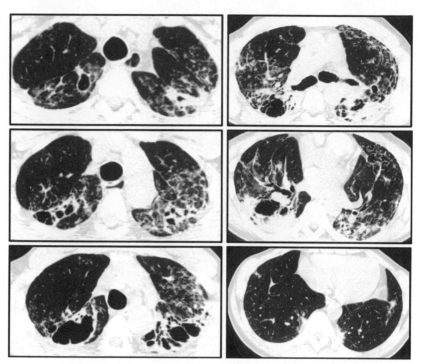

Image 11-6 • Chest CT images for **Question 11-3-B**.

Q11-3-B: Answer: _____

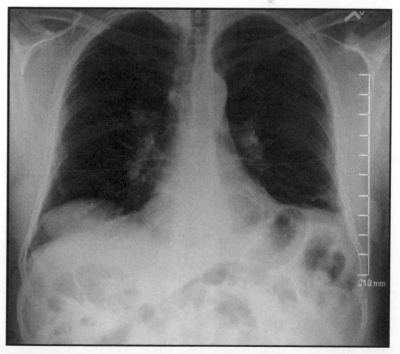

Image 11-7 • Chest Radiograph (AP) for the **Question 11-3-C**.

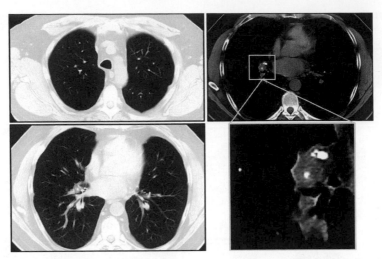

Image 11-8 • Chest CT images (left images, lung window; right images, mediastinal window) for **Question 11-3-C**.

Q11-3-C: Answer: _____

Q11-4: Match the following cutaneous manifestations of sarcoidosis to the images below.

A. Lupus pernio
B. Plaque sarcoidosis
C. Papular sarcoidosis
D. Ulcerated sarcoidosis

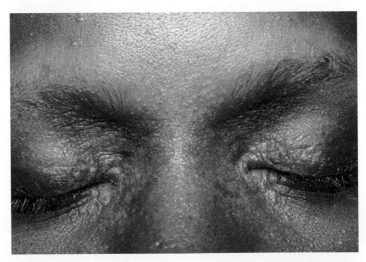

Image 11-9 • Dermatologic abnormalities noted during examination of the patient in **Question 11-4-A**. (*Reproduced with permission from Marchell RM, Judson MA. Chronic cutaneous lesions of sarcoidosis, Clin Dermatol May-Jun 2007;25(3):295-302.*)

Q11-4-A: Answer: _____

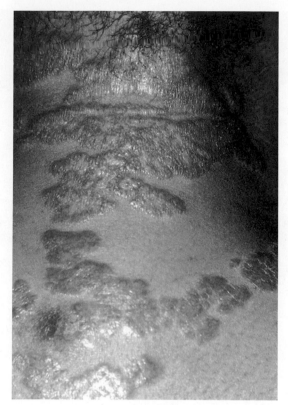

Image 11-10 • Dermatologic abnormalities noted during examination of the patient in **Question 11-4-B**. *(Reproduced with permission from Marchell RM, Judson MA. Chronic cutaneous lesions of sarcoidosis, Clin Dermatol May-Jun 2007;25(3):295-302.)*

Q11-4-B: Answer: _____

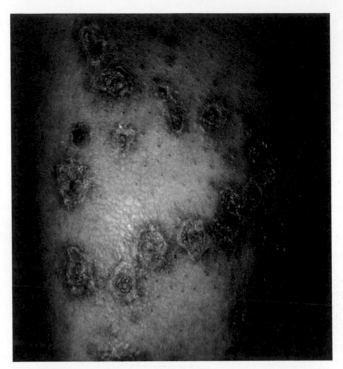

Image 11-11 • Dermatologic abnormalities noted during examination of the patient in **Question 11-4-C.** (*Reproduced with permission from Marchell RM, Judson MA. Chronic cutaneous lesions of sarcoidosis, Clin Dermatol May-Jun 2007;25(3):295-302.*)

Q11-4-C: Answer: _____

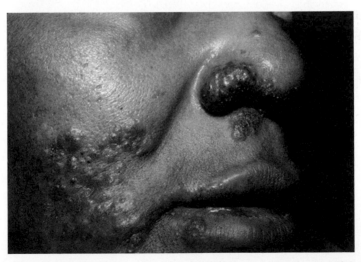

Image 11-12 • Dermatologic abnormalities noted during examination of the patient in **Question 11-4-D**. (*Reproduced with permission from Marchell RM, Judson MA. Chronic cutaneous lesions of sarcoidosis, Clin Dermatol May-Jun 2007;25(3):295-302.*)

Q11-4-D: Answer: _____

Q11-5: Which test is NOT recommended for the initial screening of asymptomatic patients with sarcoidosis?

A. Echocardiogram
B. ECG
C. Ophthalmologic examination
D. Serum ACE level
E. Pulmonary function testing
F. B and D
G. A and D
H. C and D

Q11-6: A 44-year-old White man presents to your office with an intermittent dry cough for the last 4 months, mild dyspnea on exertion, and new bilateral hilar adenopathy on chest radiography performed for a workup for a chronic cough. He has been afebrile, there is no evidence of parenchymal lung disease on chest radiography, and he takes no medications at baseline. He has an EKG that shows sinus rhythm with normal intervals and no conduction abnormalities. He denies any chest pain or syncope. He has no ocular or neurologic symptoms. His serum calcium level is 9.0 mg/dL with an ionized calcium level of 1.12 mmol/L. PFTs are performed and show the following:

FVC   93%

FEV1   79%

Ratio: 72% predicted

DLCO   84%

He requires no oxygen at rest, with an oxygen saturation of 97% on room air at rest and 96% with activity. He had a biopsy of his hilar adenopathy that returned with noncaseating granulomas and no evidence of infection. Treatment options are discussed, and the patient elects not to start on glucocorticoid therapy given the potential complications. He returns 6 months later with interval improvement in his cough but slightly worsened dyspnea on exertion that he attributes to an interval weight gain of 5 lb. His CXR appears stable with continued hilar adenopathy but no apparent parenchymal disease. His PFTs are as follows:

FVC   78%

FEV1   72%

Ratio: 86% predicted

DLCO: 70%

He again does not require oxygen at rest or with activity. What is the best option for the patient?

A. Inhaled glucocorticoids
B. Systemic glucocorticoids
C. Methotrexate
D. Antitumor necrosis factor (TNF)-α therapy
E. No change in therapy; have the patient return in 3 months for repeat PFTs and chest imaging
F. Leflunomide

Q11-7: **Which bronchoscopic modality is considered to have the highest diagnostic yield for sarcoidosis in suspected patients with hilar adenopathy but no or minimal parenchymal abnormalities?**

A. Airway examination only
B. Bronchoalveolar lavage (BAL) with flow cytometry demonstrating a CD4-to-CD8 ratio
C. Endobronchial biopsy (EBB)
D. Transbronchial biopsy (TBB)
E. Endobronchial ultrasound (EBUS)-guided transbronchial needle aspiration (TBNA)

ANSWERS

Q11-1: D
Lofgren syndrome

Rationale: This is Lofgren syndrome, in which patients present with erythema nodosum (EN; skin lesion shown in **Image 11-1**), arthralgia, and bilateral hilar adenopathy (shown on CXR in **Image 11-2**). Lofgren syndrome is an acute form of sarcoidosis, which occurs in only a small percentage of patients with sarcoidosis (less than 10%). The other manifestations of Lofgren syndrome may include fever and uveitis. This form of sarcoidosis is often self-resolving over a few weeks' time, though more persistent cases may require initiation of oral corticosteroid therapy. Although the diagnosis is often made clinically, a tissue biopsy is generally recommended, particularly when cutaneous lesions are a potential target.

EN is a nonspecific dermatologic finding, and it is the most common form of panniculitis. It is characterized by raised, nonulcerative, painful lesions most commonly found on the anterior tibia, though other portions of the lower extremities and the upper extremities may also be involved. Again, EN is nonspecific; the presence of bilateral hilar adenopathy helps to narrow the differential diagnosis, as the combination of fever, arthralgia, and EN may be seen in drug toxicity, infections, inflammatory bowel disease, Behçet syndrome, and other rheumatologic conditions. EN lesions are generally not biopsied because the findings rarely demonstrate evidence of sarcoidosis.

Loeffler syndrome is an eosinophilic pulmonary response to a parasitic infection. Reactive arthritis can be associated with polyarthritis and uveitis, and EN can be associated with infections; however, bilateral hilar adenopathy is not typical or reactive arthritis. RA is not typically associated with EN. Acute leukemia can cause skin lesions such as EN, but it is usually accompanied by other findings such as fatigue. EN is far less frequently associated with SLE.

Q11-2: E
90%

Rationale: Sarcoidosis is a multisystem granulomatous disorder that is characterized by the presence of noncaseating granulomas in involved organ systems. The etiology of sarcoidosis is not clearly understood. Sarcoidosis most commonly presents in patients 30 to 50 years of age, though it may also be seen in younger and older patients. Although data on prevalence and incidence vary by geography, the disease is thought to be more common in Black people than White people. It is estimated that more than half of cases are asymptomatic and found incidentally as abnormalities on chest radiographs obtained for other reasons. Sarcoidosis most commonly involves the lymph nodes of the thoracic cavity, with up to 90% of patients having lung involvement. Up to 40% of patients may have extrapulmonary organ involvement of any organ system. More commonly, extrapulmonary sarcoidosis involves the cutaneous, neurologic, cardiac, renal, GI, bone marrow, and ocular organ systems. As the saying goes, "sarcoidosis can do anything."

The finding of noncaseating granulomas on tissue biopsy is the gold standard for the diagnosis of sarcoidosis. However, there is a number of granulomatous lung diseases that need to be excluded before a diagnosis of sarcoidosis can be confirmed. This includes infection (mycobacterial, fungal, with the latter including *Pneumocystis jirovecii*), hypersensitivity pneumonitis (including drug-induced), foreign body granulomatosis, antineutrophil cytoplasmic antibodies (ANCA)-associated pulmonary vascular disease (granulomatosis with polyangiitis, eosinophilic granulomatosis with polyangiitis), the pneumoconioses, and pulmonary Langerhans cell histiocytosis (PLCH).

Q11-3-A: B
Stage II

Q11-3-B: D
Stage IV (Fibrocavitary disease)

Q11-3-C: A
Stage I

Rationale: Sarcoidosis has most often been staged according to radiographic findings (Scadding staging); however, this does not necessarily have any prognostic value.

Stage I disease is defined by the presence of bilateral hilar adenopathy, as is seen in **Images 11-7** and **11-8**, without evidence of parenchymal involvement. Approximately 50% of patients present with bilateral hilar adenopathy, while some patients with stage I disease present with dyspnea and cough. Most patients presenting with stage I disease will not develop disease beyond stage I, and the bilateral hilar adenopathy will typically resolve within 2 years with or without treatment. These hilar nodes often develop calcifications as the disease process resolves, as can be seen in the mediastinal window of **Image 11-8**, highlighted in red. Here, one can see calcifications within the right hilar nodes. This process of acute inflammation being replaced with calcification in the lymph nodes is often referred to as sarcoidosis "burning out."

Stage II disease is defined by the presence of hilar adenopathy and reticular opacities without volume loss or scarring. In **Image 11-3**, one can see bilateral hilar adenopathy and faint linear or reticulonodular opacities on the CXR. The reticulonodular opacities and ground glass are more easily seen on the accompanying CT scan in **Image 11-4**. Although the reticular opacities are more commonly located in the upper lung zones, they may be widely distributed, as seen here. A common finding in sarcoidosis is the presence of micronodules ("beading") along the bronchovascular bundles/central airways and also along the lymphatics seen on high-resolution CT. Patients may also have nodular consolidations or predominantly ground-glass opacities rather than reticular changes. Approximately 25% of patients present with stage II disease, of which only 25% typically have progressive disease.

Stage III disease is defined by the presence of reticular changes in the lung parenchyma (again without volume loss) but with resolving/resolved hilar adenopathy. Again, the reticular changes in the lung are predominantly seen in the upper lobes but, again, may involve any lung segment.

Stage IV disease is defined by the presence of parenchymal volume loss. This may be due to cysts, cavitation, honeycombing changes/fibrosis, traction bronchiectasis, or conglomerated nodules/masses (sometimes referred to as the "galaxy" sign). Examples are shown in **Images 11-5** and **11-6**. In **Image 11-5**, the chest radiograph shows perhaps some mild hilar adenopathy but is dominated by the reticular opacities in both lung fields with an upper-lobe predominance, which is more apparent on the lateral film. On chest CT (**Image 11-6**), one can see extensive parenchymal volume loss/scarring with the presence of large cavities, nodules and ground glass changes, septal thickening, and traction bronchiectasis in the upper lobes, with relative sparing of the lung bases bilaterally.

Q11-4-A: C
Papular sarcoidosis

Q11-4-B: B
Plaque sarcoidosis

Q11-4-C: D
Ulcerative sarcoidosis

Q11-4-D: A
Lupus pernio

Rationale: Although cutaneous manifestations may only arise in 10% to 30% of patients with sarcoidosis, it is often present at disease onset, and recognizing these changes may aid in forming a differential diagnosis. Lupus pernio (**Image 11-12**) is the presence of symmetric, violaceous, plaque-like lesions that involve the node, face, ear lobes, and, occasionally, the digits. This should raise concern for possible mucosal involvement. Papular sarcoidosis (**Image 11-9**) is likely the most common form of cutaneous sarcoidosis. These small papules are commonly found in the periorbital areas and around the scalp. The lesions have a yellowish-brown color that is termed "apple jelly" when the erythematous background is blanched with a glass slide. The papules may eventually develop into plaques, such as those seen in **Image 11-10**. Papules are less likely to cause scarring when compared with plaque lesions, while plaque lesions may also be associated with more chronic disease. These plaques may also eventually ulcerate (**Image 11-11**), which is more commonly seen in patients with systemic disease than isolated cutaneous involvement.

Q11-5: G
A (Echocardiogram) and D (Serum ACE level)

Rationale: Initial screening for an asymptomatic patient with sarcoidosis includes a chest radiograph, complete pulmonary function testing, ophthalmologic examination, complete laboratory testing (electrolytes, renal function, liver function, blood counts with differential), ECG, and screening for tuberculosis (TB). An echocardiogram or more advanced testing for cardiac involvement (cardiac MRI or PET) is indicated for patients with palpitations, syncope, or conduction abnormalities on electrocardiography. Serum ACE levels, while often elevated in patients with active TB, are highly nonspecific for sarcoidosis. There is some evidence of the use of serum soluble IL-2 receptor alpha (sIL2Ra) as a biomarker to determine if patients have extrapulmonary involvement of sarcoidosis; however, this is nonspecific and may be elevated in a number of conditions, including other rheumatologic conditions, malignancy, and infection.

Q11-6: B
Systemic glucocorticoids

Rationale: Most patients with sarcoidosis do not require initiation of glucocorticoids because they are either asymptomatic or mildly symptomatic and the risks of systemic corticosteroid use will often outweigh the potential benefits. Typical indications for glucocorticoid therapy at the initial visit are shown below.

Initial indications for glucocorticoid therapy in sarcoidosis:

(A) Symptoms that impact function or quality of life to such a degree that the risks of systemic glucocorticoid therapy are outweighed by the potential benefits;

(B) The presence of significant lung disease at initial presentation, including the need for supplemental oxygen, or the presence of significant abnormalities on pulmonary function testing (FEV1, FVC, or TLC less than 70%, DLCO less than 60% predicted);

(C) The presence of extrapulmonary sarcoidosis that would necessitate systemic glucocorticoid therapy, including, but not limited to, cardiac, renal, endocrine, and neurologic involvement.

In this case, as the patient did not meet the aforementioned criteria, it was reasonable to adopt a conservative treatment approach and monitor at 3- to 6-month intervals. The patient's PFTs demonstrate a significant drop in FVC and DLCO, and the patient has had a worsening of his dyspnea.

Indications of disease progression that indicate systemic glucocorticoid therapy in sarcoidosis:

(A) Development of any extrapulmonary organ involvement that would necessitate system glucocorticoids;

(B) Progressive imaging abnormalities or clinical symptoms, including the development of signs of pulmonary HTN or the need for supplemental oxygen;

(C) Reductions in lung function testing, including a fall in FEV1, FVC, or TLC by 10% to 15% and a reduction in DLCO by 20%.

As such, it would be reasonable to initiate therapy with glucocorticoids. Although there is some marginal evidence for the use of inhaled glucocorticoids for symptom management, the mainstay of initial therapy for sarcoidosis is systemic glucocorticoids. For pulmonary sarcoidosis, systemic steroids are generally started at 0.5 mg/kg/day of prednisone (or equivalent) and tapered gradually over several months while monitoring for improvement. Relapse is not uncommon and is marked by worsening symptoms, thoracic imaging, or PFT findings and may necessitate an increase in steroid dosing and a slower tapering period. Patients with disease that is refractory to glucocorticoids or who are unable to be tapered to a reasonable dose of steroids (eg, 10 mg or less of prednisone daily) may require initiation of a steroid-sparing agent to further taper the steroid dose. Methotrexate is the preferred steroid-sparing agent because there is the most data for its efficacy. Leflunomide is an antimetabolite similar to methotrexate that may also be considered as a second-line agent in patients unable to tolerate methotrexate. Azathioprine and mycophenolate are other options, but they are associated with limited data as well. Anti-TNF therapy is reserved for disease that is refractory to these steroid-sparing agents, though is not currently approved for the treatment of sarcoidosis by the FDA. The treatment of extrapulmonary sarcoidosis often involves more prolonged tapers or even lifelong therapy depending on the organ system, and it is outside the scope of this discussion.

Q11-7: E
Endobronchial ultrasound (EBUS)-guided transbronchial needle aspiration (TBNA)

Rationale: Results have been somewhat mixed and likely are dependent on both patient factors (eg, the size of the hilar/mediastinal adenopathy, degree of calcification of the adenopathy, the severity of parenchymal abnormalities) and technique (eg, experience, number of biopsies performed, on-site or frozen pathology). The literature has generally demonstrated that BAL with an elevated CD4-to-CD8 ratio (usually greater than 3.5 to 4:1) has a diagnostic yield between 20% and 50%. BAL is typically more useful to rule out an infectious or eosinophilic process. Endobronchial biopsies have a diagnostic yield between 20% and 60%; this is higher in patients with evidence of airway mucosal involvement. Transbronchial biopsies have a diagnostic yield ranging from 60% to 90%, depending on the severity of abnormalities in the lung parenchyma (increasing from 60% in stage I to nearly 85% in stage III disease). Although the diagnostic yield of traditional/conventional transbronchial needle aspiration of mediastinal lymph nodes is around 50%, the use of endobronchial ultrasound to guide the biopsy site has greatly increased the yield of this procedure, reported to be between 70% and 90% in much of the literature and is thus the modality with the highest yield. Therefore, in this patient with hilar adenopathy but with minimal parenchymal changes, this is likely the most useful procedure. However, in reality, combining various modalities provides the highest yield. In general, most procedures would include BAL, EBUS-TBNA, and TBB, with EBB usually limited to patients with evidence of possible mucosal involvement (ie, cobblestoning, nodules). The recent introduction of transbronchial lung cryobiopsy (TBLC) may also increase the diagnostic yield in these patients; however, this procedure does have some increased risk that should be considered.

References

Baughman RP, Grutters JC. New treatment strategies for pulmonary sarcoidosis: antimetabolites, biological drugs, and other treatment approaches. Lancet Respir Med. 2015;3:813.

Baughman RP, Lower EE, Drent M. Inhibitors of tumor necrosis factor (TNF) in sarcoidosis: who, what, and how to use them. Sarcoidosis Vasc Diffuse Lung Dis. 2008;25:76.

Baughman RP, Lower EE. Leflunomide for chronic sarcoidosis. Sarcoidosis Vasc Diffuse Lung Dis. 2004;21:43.

Broos CE, Poell LHC, Looman CWN, et al. No evidence found for an association between predni- sone dose and FVC change in newly-treated pulmonary sarcoidosis. Respir Med. 2018;138S:S31.

Cremers JP, Drent M, Bast A, et al. Multinational evidence-based World Association of Sarcoidosis and Other Granulomatous Disorders recommendations for the use of methotrexate in sarcoidosis: integrating systematic literature research and expert opinion of sarcoidologists worldwide. Curr Opin Pulm Med. 2013;19:545.

Dziedzic DA, Peryt A, Orlowski T. The role of EBUS-TBNA and standard bronchoscopic modali- ties in the diagnosis of sarcoidosis. Clin Respir J. 2017;11:58.

Ferrer G, Khosla R. Endobronchial ultrasonography vs conventional transbronchial needle aspira- tion in the diagnosis of sarcoidosis. Chest. 2010;137:235.

Gupta D, Dadhwal DS, Agarwal R, Gupta N, Bal A, Aggarwal AN. Endobronchial ultra- sound-guided transbronchial needle aspiration vs conventional transbronchial needle aspiration in the diagnosis of sarcoidosis. Chest. 2014;146:547.

Hamzeh N, Voelker A, Forssén A, et al. Efficacy of mycophenolate mofetil in sarcoidosis. Respir Med. 2014;108:1663.

Hamzeh NY, Wamboldt FS, Weinberger HD. Management of cardiac sarcoidosis in the United States: a Delphi study. Chest. 2012;141:154.

Iannuzzi MC, Rybicki BA, Teirstein AS. Sarcoidosis. N Engl J Med. 2007;357:2153.

Judson MA, Baughman RP, Costabel U, et al. Efficacy of infliximab in extrapulmonary sarcoidosis: results from a randomised trial. Eur Respir J. 2008;31:1189.

Judson MA. The diagnosis of sarcoidosis. Clin Chest Med. 2008;29:415.

Korsten P, Strohmayer K, Baughman RP, Sweiss NJ. Refractory pulmonary sarcoidosis - proposal of a definition and recommendations for the diagnostic and therapeutic approach. Clin Pulm Med. 2016;23:67.

Kouba DJ, Mimouni D, Rencic A, Nousari HC. Mycophenolate mofetil may serve as a steroid-spar- ing agent for sarcoidosis. Br J Dermatol. 2003;148:147.

Lewis SJ, Ainslie GM, Bateman ED. Efficacy of azathioprine as second-line treatment in pulmonary sarcoidosis. Sarcoidosis Vasc Diffuse Lung Dis. 1999;16:87.

Mana J, Marcoval J. Erythema nodosum. Clin Dermatol. 2007;25:288.

Marchell RM, Judson MA. Chronic cutaneous lesions of sarcoidosis. Clin Dermatol. 2007;25:295.

Pedro C, Melo N, Novais E, et al. Role of bronchoscopic techniques in the diagnosis of thoracic sarcoidosis. J Clin Med. 2019;8:1327.

Rahaghi FF, Baughman RP, Saketkoo LA, et al. Delphi consensus recommendations for a treatment algorithm in pulmonary sarcoidosis. Eur Respir Rev. 2020;29.

Terushkin V, Stern BJ, Judson MA, et al. Neurosarcoidosis: presentations and management. Neurologist. 2010;16:2.

Thomas KW, Hunninghake GW. Sarcoidosis. JAMA. 2003;289:3300.

Ungprasert P, Carmona EM, Utz JP, et al. Epidemiology of sarcoidosis 1946-2013: a population-based study. Mayo Clin Proc. 2016;91183.

von Bartheld MB, Dekkers OM, Szlubowski A, et al. Endosonography vs conventional bronchoscopy for the diagnosis of sarcoidosis: the GRANULOMA randomized clinical trial. JAMA. 2013;309:2457.

Wijsenbeek MS, Culver DA. Treatment of sarcoidosis. Clin Chest Med. 2015;36:751.

CASE 12

A 28-year-old White woman with a history of an ovarian cyst presents to the clinic following a recent pneumothorax. She experienced the sudden onset of chest pain and some diaphoresis and mild dyspnea 2 weeks ago while exercising. She did not experience any known trauma. She presented to a local hospital where she was found to have a pneumothorax on CXR, along with other abnormalities. She had a chest tube placed with resolution of the pneumothorax over the next 2 days and was discharged with follow-up in the pulmonary clinic.

On examination, she is a tall (5 feet 10 inches) female with a BMI of 20 kg/m². Her vitals are HR 65, BP 110/70, and O₂ saturation of 95% on room air. She has a healing wound in the right hemithorax from prior chest tube placement. She has a normal cardiopulmonary examination. She has no clubbing, and her musculoskeletal and joint examination is normal as well. She has no peripheral edema.

She does report some dyspnea in the recent months, as well as a dry, nonproductive cough and some unexpected weight loss, though she has been trying to exercise. She has no family history of lung disease, rheumatologist disease, or malignancy. She has smoked two to three packs per day for the last 8 years.

The CXR and CT scan are shown below.

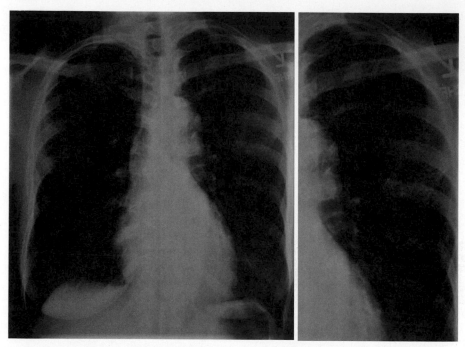

Image 12-1 • Chest radiograph (AP film) for the patient in **Question 12-1**. The image on the left is the full view, and the image on the right is a magnified view of the left airspace.

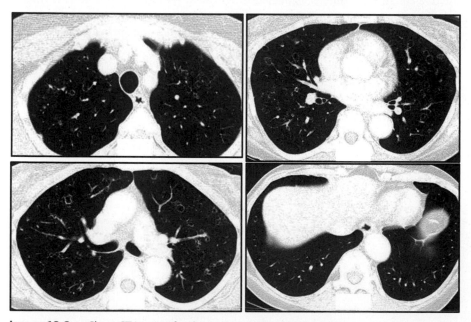

Image 12-2 • Chest CT images for the patient in **Question 12-1**.

QUESTIONS

Q12-1: What best describes the changes seen on the chest radiograph in Image 12-1 and the CT scan in Image 12-2?

A. Upper lobe–predominant cavitary lesions with air-fluid levels
B. Lower lobe–predominant linear interstitial opacities with honeycombing and traction bronchiectasis
C. Bilateral, upper lobe–predominant reticulonodular opacities with possible cysts
D. Bilateral alveolar infiltrates
E. Miliary nodular pattern

Q12-2: The patient is scheduled for bronchoscopy with a transbronchial biopsy, but this procedure will not be performed for several days. The patient requests counseling regarding her imaging. Based on the history and imaging provided, what is the most likely diagnosis?

A. Idiopathic pulmonary fibrosis (IPF)
B. Pulmonary Langerhans cell histiocytosis (PLCH)
C. Respiratory bronchiolitis interstitial lung disease (RB-ILD)
D. Cystic fibrosis (CF)
E. Nonspecific interstitial pneumonia (NSIP)
F. Pulmonary tuberculosis (TB)

Q12-3: What is the predominant abnormality identified on PFTs?

A. Reduced FEV1/FVC ratio
B. Reduced VC
C. Reduced DLCO
D. Increased RV/TLC ratio

Q12-4: What finding on electron microscopy identifies Langerhans cells?

A. Birbeck granules
B. Sulfur granules
C. Cytoplasmic inclusion bodies
D. Giant cells (fused macrophages)

Q12-5: Which special stain on histopathology is specific for identifying Langerhans cells?

A. S100
B. Cytokeratin (CK) 7
C. CD1a
D. CD19
E. CD3
F. Bcl-2

Q12-6: Which organ system is not usually involved in LCH?

A. Central nervous system
B. Skeletal system
C. Skin
D. Bone marrow
E. Heart

Q12-7: What is the most important treatment for patients with PLCH?

A. Lung transplantation
B. Cytotoxic chemotherapy
C. Glucocorticoids
D. Smoking cessation
E. Pulmonary rehabilitation
F. Sirolimus

Q12-8: Which genetic mutation has recently been associated with PLCH?

A. ΔF508
B. BRCA
C. BCR-ABL
D. BRAF V600E
E. TSC1/2

ANSWERS

Q12-1: C
Bilateral, upper-lobe predominant reticular opacities with cysts

Rationale: There are diffuse bilateral reticulonodular opacities on the CXR more prominent in the lower lobes. However, on the CT images (mid-lung zones based on the appearance of the right and left mainstem bronchi), the volume loss is due to the presence of numerous thin-walled cysts and possibly some small nodules with central cavitation without air-fluid levels. Additionally, there a number of ill-defined nodules (also termed *stellate nodules*), all less than 1 cm in diameter, associated with reticular interstitial opacities/thickening. Note that the cysts are highly variable in size and irregularly shaped. Additionally, they are positioned close to vascular structures. Note the preservation of the costophrenic angles and the relative sparing of the basilar segments on the chest radiograph and the CT images.

Q12-2: B
Pulmonary Langerhans cell histiocytosis (PLCH)

Rationale: Here, the patient is presenting with cystic and nodule lung lesions, with some of the nodules potentially cavitating. The other primary differential diagnoses would include lymphangioleiomyomatosis (LAM) and lymphocytic interstitial pneumonia, changes from *Pneumocystis jiroveci* pneumonia, and centrilobular emphysema. Earlier in the disease process, when nodules are the predominant finding, the differential would include sarcoidosis and miliary TB, metastatic cancer (eg, renal cell carcinoma), and other causes of granulomatous lung disease, such as hypersensitivity pneumonitis or coal worker pneumoconiosis. In cases where fibrosis is the primary finding, it can mimic the end stages of pulmonary fibrosis.

PLCH is a proliferation of monoclonal Langerhans cells in the pulmonary interstitium and extending to the alveolar space. The primary risk factor for PLCH is smoking tobacco use. The disease primarily affects patients between the ages of 20 and 45, with a strong predilection for those of European descent. PLCH is distributed equally between men and women, though women are often diagnosed later in life. There is some association with acute lymphoblastic and myeloid leukemias. Patients often present with cough, dyspnea, and reduced exercise tolerance, but patients may also experience constitutional symptoms (fever, night sweats, weight loss), pleuritic chest pain, and fatigue. Up to 25% of patients will experience spontaneous pneumothorax.

It is believed that PLCH results from the recruitment and abnormal proliferation of histiocytes, and this process is driven through cytokine and growth factor secretion from type I alveolar macrophages in response to tobacco smoke particles deposited in the alveoli and respiratory bronchioles. This is supported by the fact that the disease has a slight upper lobe predominance on imaging and pathology as well. These monoclonal Langerhans cells proliferate along the epithelium, forming granulomas. These granulomas initially appear as nodules on CT imaging. Over time, they may cavitate, leaving first thick-walled cavitary lesions, which will eventually lead to cystic lesions.

Early in the disease course, the chest radiograph will often demonstrate bilateral, symmetric nodular opacities evenly distributed throughout the upper lobes, with relative sparing of the bases. These may start off small in a reticulonodular or miliary pattern. With time, these nodules may grow, coalesce, and cavitate, leading to thick-walled cysts with irregular shapes. Eventually, these may completely cavitate leaving only a thin-walled cyst. Imaging typically demonstrates significant temporal variation. Similarly, CT will show a similar pattern of irregularly shaped nodules (1-10 mm in diameter) progressing to thick-walled cavitary lesions and eventually to cysts. These cysts may coalesce, yielding unusual shapes. In more severe cases, evidence of fibrosis (traction bronchiectasis, interlobular thickening, honeycombing) may be seen.

Q12-3: C
Reduced DLCO

Rationale: PFTs generally demonstrate obstructive expiratory airflow pattern with air trapping (elevated RV and RV/TLC), with a reduced DLCO. Restriction is present only in patients with more severe disease or in patients with extrathoracic restriction (eg, obesity).

Q12-4: A
Birbeck granules

Rationale: Langerhans cells are the only cells known to contain Birbeck granules, which are rod-shaped organelles believed to be involved in antigen processing and presentation.

Q12-5: C
CD1a

Rationale: Special stains for CD1a and CD207 are commonly used to identify Langerhans cells in cytologic or histopathologic specimens. CD1a staining can be performed in bronchoalveolar lavage specimens. While Langerhans cells stain positive for S100, other macrophages and neuroendocrine cells are also S100+. CD19 is a stain for B cells, while CD3 is a stain for T cells. Bcl-2 staining is used in the diagnosis of specific hematologic malignancies. CK7 staining is used to differentiate thoracic and abdominal adenocarcinomas, along with CK20.

Diagnosis can often be made from an appropriate history, typical radiologic findings, and PFT. However, when a definitive diagnosis is desired, bronchoscopy with bronchoalveolar lavage and transbronchial biopsies can be performed. BAL findings include CD1a+ cells. A biopsy will show Langerhans cells that stain positive for CD1a and S100 (**Images 12-3** and **12-4**).

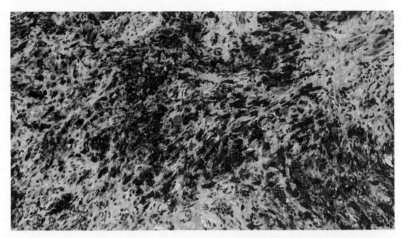

Image 12-3 • CD1a staining in a histopathologic specimen from a patient with pulmonary Langerhans cell histiocytosis (the black staining is positive). Note the organization of the cells into granulomas.

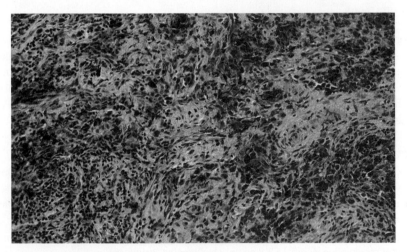

Image 12-4 • S100 staining in a histopathologic specimen from a patient with pulmonary Langerhans cell histiocytosis (the black staining is positive).

Q12-6: E
Heart

Rationale: Although pulmonary manifestations are the most common, LCH is a systemic disease that can affect other organ systems as well, most notably the skin, long bones, lymph nodes, bone marrow, and pituitary gland). Isolated PLCH accounts for more than 80% of all LCH cases. The most common extrapulmonary manifestations are bone pain (20%), dermatologic manifestations (predominantly macular rash) (10%), and central diabetes insipidus (less than 5% of cases).

Q12-7: D
Smoking cessation

Rationale: The primary treatment for all patients is smoking cessation, as more than 95% of patients with PLCH have a smoking history. In patients who experience disease progression, corticosteroids or other cytotoxic or immunosuppressive drugs have been used, but evidence of their effectiveness is lacking. Glucocorticoids are typically reserved for patients early in the disease course (ie, with predominantly micronodular disease). Cytotoxic chemotherapeutics, namely cladribine and cytarabine, have been used in patients with PLCH that is refractory to smoking cessation and glucocorticoids. Lung transplantation can be considered, but there is a risk of disease recurrence in the allograft if the patient resumes smoking following transplantation. Pulmonary rehabilitation is an important component of treatment for PLCH, but it does not stop disease progression if patients continue to smoke tobacco. Sirolimus is the treatment for patients with progressive LAM.

Q12-8: D
BRAF V600E

Rationale: Recent evidence suggests that the V600E mutation in the *BRAF* gene may be associated with PLCH. Targeted small molecule inhibitors are under investigation to treat this kinase mutation. A related disease process, termed *Erdheim-Chester disease*, involved the BRAF V600E mutation, and there is currently an approved treatment (vemurafenib). Erdheim-Chester disease is clinically very similar to PLCH but does not involve Langerhans cells.

References

Aricò M, Girschikofsky M, Généreau T, et al. Langerhans cell histiocytosis in adults. Report from the International Registry of the Histiocyte Society. Eur J Cancer. 2003;39:2341.

Auerswald U, Barth J, Magnussen H. Value of CD-1-positive cells in bronchoalveolar lavage fluid for the diagnosis of pulmonary histiocytosis X. Lung. 1991;169:305.

Castoldi MC, Verrioli A, De Juli E, Vanzulli A. Pulmonary Langerhans cell histiocytosis: the many faces of presentation at initial CT scan. Insights Imaging. 2014;5:483.

Dauriat G, Mal H, Thabut G, et al. Lung transplantation for pulmonary langerhans' cell histiocytosis: a multicenter analysis. Transplantation. 2006;81:746.

Gupta N, Langenderfer D, McCormack FX, et al. Chest computed tomographic image screening for cystic lung diseases in patients with spontaneous pneumothorax is cost effective. Ann Am Thorac Soc. 2017;14:17.

Harari S, Torre O, Cassandro R, et al. Bronchoscopic diagnosis of Langerhans cell histiocytosis and lymphangioleiomyomatosis. Respir Med. 2012;106:1286.

Hyman DM, Puzanov I, Subbiah V, et al. Vemurafenib in multiple nonmelanoma cancers with BRAF V600 mutations. N Engl J Med. 2015;373:726.

Nasser M, Traclet J, Cottin V. Effect of cladribine therapy on lung cysts in pulmonary Langerhans cell histiocytosis. ERJ Open Res. 2018;4.

Néel A, Artifoni M, Fontenoy AM, et al. Long-term efficacy and safety of 2CdA (cladribine) in extra-pulmonary adult-onset Langerhans cell histiocytosis: analysis of 23 cases from the French Histiocytosis Group and systematic literature review. Br J Haematol. 2020;189:869.

Radzikowska E, Błasińska-Przerwa K, Wiatr E, et al. Pneumothorax in patients with pulmonary Langerhans cell histiocytosis. Lung. 2018;196:715.

Sundar KM, Gosselin MV, Chung HL, Cahill BC. Pulmonary Langerhans cell histiocytosis: emerging concepts in pathobiology, radiology, and clinical evolution of disease. Chest. 2003;123:1673.

Tazi A. Adult pulmonary Langerhans' cell histiocytosis. Eur Respir J. 2006;27:1272.

Vassallo R, Ryu JH. Pulmonary Langerhans' cell histiocytosis. Clin Chest Med. 2004;25:561.

CASE 13

A 27-year-old White woman is referred to the clinic for evaluation following the development of a spontaneous left-sided pneumothorax. She has no significant medical history. She is adopted and has no information on her biological family. She reports that she had about 3 to 4 months of progressively worsening dyspnea on exertion, with an intermittent nonproductive cough. However, she did have one episode of blood-tinged sputum a few days prior that resolved spontaneously. She takes no medications. She has smoked two to three cigarettes a day for the last 2 years but has intermittently quit. She takes no illicit drugs. She drinks alcohol socially.

The pneumothorax developed while she was out of the country. She works as a business accountant and was recently in Chile for a conference when the episode occurred. She was never in a nonurbanized area on the trip, and she did not travel from the hotel other than to a hospital in the capital city. She has not experienced fever or diarrhea but has had some pleuritic chest pain on the left side. She notes the chest tube was in place for 3 days and then removed. She was forced to remain in Chile for 1 week before flying back to the United States.

On examination, she is well appearing and well nourished. Her oxygen saturation is 93% on room air. Her RR is 14. She does not become dyspneic with walking, though she does not desaturate with walking. She has a BMI of 22 kg/m². She has some diminished breath sounds throughout. The remainder of the examination is unremarkable.

Her CXR is shown below.

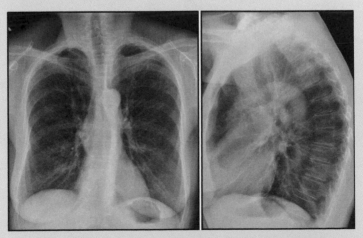

Image 13-1 • Chest radiographs (PA and lateral) for the patient in **Question 13-1**.

QUESTIONS

Q13-1: How would one describe the abnormalities in the chest film in Image 13-1?

A. Atelectasis
B. Lung mass in the left upper lobe
C. Focal consolidative opacity in the left lower lobe
D. Hyperinflation
E. Pneumothorax
F. Unilateral pleural effusion

Q13-2: Given the patient's reported history, you obtain a high-resolution CT scan of the chest, which is shown in Image 13-2.

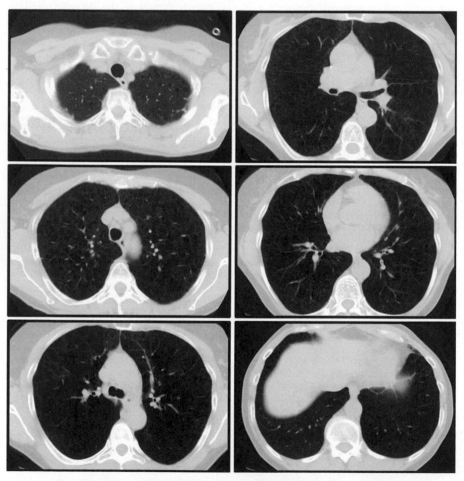

Image 13-2 • Chest CT images for the patient in **Question 13-2**.

Q13-2: How would you describe the changes?

A. Nodular interstitial opacities and centrilobular cystic lesions
B. Scattered centrilobular cystic lesions
C. Cavitary lesions with air-fluid levels
D. Bilateral reticulonodular opacities with honeycombing
E. Pneumothorax
F. Both A and E
G. Both B and E
H. Both C and D
I. Both D and E

Q13-3: The patient reports that approximately 4 months ago she also was diagnosed as having a pleural effusion after presenting to an ED with shortness of breath. She had a thoracentesis at the facility, which completely relieved her symptoms. She reports that the physician that performed the procedure reported its appearance as "milky." What is the most likely diagnosis?

A. Alpha-1-antitrypsin (A1AT)
B. Cystic fibrosis (CF)
C. Pulmonary Langerhans cell histiocytosis (PLCH)
D. Pulmonary lymphangioleiomyomatosis (PLAM)
E. Lymphocytic interstitial pneumonia (LIP)

Q13-4: What genetic disorder is associated with pulmonary lymphangioleiomyomatosis (LAM)?

A. *BRCA* mutation
B. Down syndrome
C. Klinefelter syndrome
D. Short telomere syndrome
E. Hermansky-Pudlak syndrome
F. Tuberous sclerosis complex (TSC)
G. Neurofibromatosis

Q13-5: What extrapulmonary manifestation is much more commonly seen in patients with TSC-LAM and patients with sporadic LAM?

A. Chylothorax (chylous pleural effusion)
B. Chlyoperitoneum (chylous ascites)
C. Renal angiolipoma
D. Lymphadenopathy

Q13-6: Which is NOT a common finding on PFT in patients with PLAM?

A. Reduced DLCO
B. Reduced FEV1
C. Reduced FEV1/FVC
D. Reduced RV/TLC

Q13-7: What treatment is indicated for patients with PLAM with progressive disease?

A. Tacrolimus
B. Sirolimus
C. Methotrexate
D. Azathioprine
E. Mycophenolate (CellCept)
F. Rituximab

Q13-8: What laboratory value may aid in distinguishing patients with LAM from those with other cystic lung diseases?

A. D-dimer
B. Serum ACE level
C. Serum cortisol level
D. Serum VEGF-D (vascular endothelial growth factor-D) level
E. Serum brain natriuretic peptide (BNP) level

ANSWERS

Q13-1: D
Hyperinflation

Rationale: This plain film has a relatively normal appearance of the lung fields, with the exception of perhaps some hyperinflation with some mild flattening of the diaphragm. Additionally, one could say that there are some increased faint reticular opacities bilaterally, but this is subtle.

Q13-2: B
Scattered centrilobular cystic lesions

Rationale: The CT scan demonstrates the presence of scattered centrilobular cystic lesions without evidence of nodular, reticulonodular, or cavitary lesions. Note the important difference between cysts (thin-walled structures) and cavitary lesions (thick-walled structures) (**Images 13-3** and **13-4**).

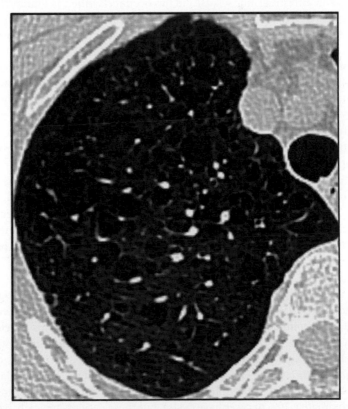

Image 13-3 • Example of cystic lesions on chest CT imaging.

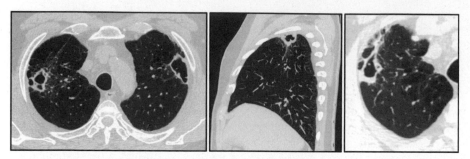

Image 13-4 • Examples of cavitary (thick-walled) lesions on chest CT imaging.

Q13-3: D
Pulmonary lymphangioleiomyomatosis (PLAM)

Rationale: PLAM is a disease that predominantly affects premenopausal women, but it can occur in postmenopausal women and in men as well. PLAM was previously referred to as an interstitial lung disease but has been reclassified as a tumor/low-grade neoplasm of perivascular epithelioid cell origin (PEComa). The etiology of PLAM will be discussed below. The primary pulmonary manifestation of PLAM is progressive cystic lung lesions with continued volume loss over time. Patients with PLAM most often present with dyspnea on exertion, though patients may also be asymptomatic and identified by chest imaging obtained for other purposes. Patients can also present with spontaneous pneumothoraces (up to 30%) or the development of pleural effusions (10%-30%), often chylous in nature. The pneumothoraces result from the coalescence of these cystic structures and eventual rupture of the thin-walled structures. The chylous effusions develop as a result of these LAM cells accumulating and proliferating in the lymphatic system, causing obstruction of the lymphatic drainage to the venous system. The chyle then backs up and overwhelms local lymphatics in the lungs, as well as in other organs. These effusions will have high levels of cholesterol, triglycerides, and chylomicrons. Patients may also develop chylous effusions in other potential spaces, including chylous ascites. LAM should be suspected in any premenopausal female with spontaneous pneumothorax or chylous effusion and no other reasonable explanation (eg, evidence of another interstitial lung disease).

LIP is an interstitial pneumonitis that is commonly associated with Sjogren syndrome, end-stage HIV/AIDs, rheumatoid arthritis (RA), systemic lupus erythematosus (SLE), and common variable immune deficiency (CVID). This develops most commonly in middle age, between the ages of 40 and 60. Chest imaging is notable for bilateral lower-lobe predominant reticular opacities and airspace opacities, with variable features on CT that may include cystic changes, ground-glass opacities, interstitial thickening, and micronodules. PLCH is another cystic lung disease (only approximately 20% of cases have cysts), but these patients typically have upper lobe-predominant reticulonodular opacities present. This disease is often associated with smoking and may also be associated with spontaneous pneumothorax. Chylothorax is not a common finding of either of these processes. There is no evidence of bronchiectasis to suggest CF. A1AT is associated with panlobular emphysema.

In LAM, the classic HRCT findings include thin-walled cysts of variable sizes that are surrounded by normal lung parenchyma. There may also be interlobular septal thickening. Patients may also have a dilated thoracic duct, thoracic or abdominal chylous effusions, renal angiolipomas, lymphadenopathy, or lymphatic malformations. The 2011 European Respiratory Society and 2016 American Thoracic Society guidelines provide diagnostic criteria of LAM based on history, laboratory, fluid cytology, and radiographic findings without the absolute need for tissue biopsy.

Q13-4: F
Tuberous sclerosis (TSC)

Rationale: LAM is classified as either sporadic or TSC-associated; however, in both instances, the primary etiology is the loss of function of the tuberous sclerosis complex, which is composed of two proteins, TSC1 (hamartin) and TSC2 (tuberin). Patients with TSC-LAM have germline mutations in either TSC1 or TSC2, while patients with sporadic LAM develop somatic mutations in the *TSC2* gene. The TSC complex is a tumor suppressor that regulates the activity of the mTOR complex, which is a key signal integrator in cells that controls cellular metabolism, cell survival, and proliferation. The loss of function of the TSC leads to unchecked mTOR activity, which drives the proliferation of LAM cells. However, estrogen and other growth factors (eg, VEGF-D) may also drive the proliferation of these LAM cells.

Q13-5: C
Renal angiolipoma

Rationale: Renal angiolipomas are more common in patients with TSC-LAM (about 80%) compared with sporadic LAM (10%-30%). Alternatively, the lymphatic complications in sporadic LAM are much more frequent than those encountered in patients with TSC-LAM. The reason for the latter finding is unclear. Patients with TSC-LAM also may have other symptoms of TSC, including angiofibromas, cortical tubers, cognitive dysfunction, and seizures. Uterine LAM lesions may also be seen more frequently in patients with TSC-LAM.

Q13-6: D
Reduced RV/TLC

Rationale: The ratio of the residual volume (the residual volume of air in the lung following forced expiration) over the TLC (total lung capacity at maximum or forced inspiration) is a measure of air trapping or dynamic hyperinflation. As lung tissue is destroyed with disease progression, patients will begin to lose some elastic recoil in the lung, resulting in increased residual volume at the end of forced expiration. This increase in RV is larger than the increase in TLC, so the ratio of RV to TLC will increase rather than decrease. The remaining abnormalities (reduced DLCO, reduced FEV1, and reduced FEV1/FVC) may all occur. Pulmonary function testing is also a noninvasive way to monitor disease severity without additional radiation exposure.

Q13-7: B
Sirolimus

Rationale: Patients with pulmonary LAM should undergo initial testing with high-resolution chest CT, PFT (with spirometry, lung volumes, and DLCO), and evaluation of the need for supplemental oxygenation. Patients with clinical evidence of pulmonary HTN should be evaluated using either echo or right heart catheterization. For patients with mild disease (FEV1 greater than 70%, DLCO greater than 80%), no supplemental O_2 requirement, and no evidence of pulmonary HTN, conservative management can be considered with close follow-up at 3- to 4-month intervals with repeat spirometry and full pulmonary function testing at least once a year. For patients with more severe disease at presentation or with evidence of disease progression during monitoring (eg, worsening gas exchanges as marked by 20% reduction in DLCO, need for supplemental oxygen with exercise or at rest, symptoms of pulmonary HTN; worsening hyperinflation as marked by increasing RV and RV/TLC ratio; worsening FEV1) initiation of therapy with sirolimus is appropriate. Recall from Question 4 that TSC1/2 is a tumor suppressor that regulates the function of the mTOR complex. Sirolimus (rapamycin) is an mTOR inhibitor. This is the first-line treatment option for patients with PLAM. This is generally effective in stopping the decline in lung function and reversing the lymphatic complications associated with sporadic LAM. Everolimus is a second-line option, though it is not FDA-approved at this time. Lung transplantation is an option for patients with refractory or severe disease. Patients with evidence of expiratory airflow obstruction on spirometry often will respond to bronchodilators or inhaled glucocorticoids, so these should be considered even in patients with mild disease. Patients should be counseled about the potential increased risk of using estrogen-based birth control and against the use of any smoking tobacco.

Q13-8: D
Serum VEGF-D (vascular endothelial growth factor-D) level

Rationale: Recent evidence suggests that a serum VEGF-D level above 800 pg/dL has a specificity approaching 100% for a diagnosis of LAM, though it does not necessarily differentiate TSC-LAM from sporadic LAM. The presence of renal angiolipomas or lymphatic complications may help differentiate the germline versus somatic mutations forms of this disease.

References

Ando K, Kurihara M, Kataoka H, et al. Efficacy and safety of low-dose sirolimus for treatment of lymphangioleiomyomatosis. Respir Investig. 2013;51:175.

Carsillo T, Astrinidis A, Henske EP. Mutations in the tuberous sclerosis complex gene TSC2 are a cause of sporadic pulmonary lymphangioleiomyomatosis. Proc Natl Acad Sci U S A. 2000;97:6085.

Glasgow CG, Avila NA, Lin JP, et al. Serum vascular endothelial growth factor-D levels in patients with lymphangioleiomyomatosis reflect lymphatic involvement. Chest. 2009;135:1293.

Goncharova EA, Goncharov DA, Lim PN, et al. Modulation of cell migration and invasiveness by tumor suppressor TSC2 in lymphangioleiomyomatosis. Am J Respir Cell Mol Biol. 2006;34:473.

Gu X, Yu JJ, Ilter D, et al. Integration of mTOR and estrogen-ERK2 signaling in lymphangioleiomyomatosis pathogenesis. Proc Natl Acad Sci U S A. 2013;110:14960.

Gupta N, Lee HS, Ryu JH, et al. The NHLBI LAM registry: prognostic physiologic and radiologic biomarkers emerge from a 15-year prospective longitudinal analysis. Chest. 2019;155:288.

Gupta N, Lee HS, Young LR, et al. Analysis of the MILES cohort reveals determinants of disease progression and treatment response in lymphangioleiomyomatosis. Eur Respir J. 2019;53.

Harari S, Torre O, Cassandro R, Moss J. The changing face of a rare disease: lymphangioleiomyomatosis. Eur Respir J. 2015;46:1471.

Henske EP, McCormack FX. Lymphangioleiomyomatosis – a wolf in sheep's clothing. J Clin Invest. 2012;122:3807.

Johnson SR, Cordier JF, Lazor R, et al. European Respiratory Society guidelines for the diagnosis and management of lymphangioleiomyomatosis. Eur Respir J. 2010;35:14.

McCormack FX, Gupta N, Finlay GR, et al. Official American Thoracic Society/Japanese Respiratory Society clinical practice guidelines: lymphangioleiomyomatosis diagnosis and management. Am J Respir Crit Care Med. 2016;194:748.

McCormack FX, Inoue Y, Moss J, et al. Efficacy and safety of sirolimus in lymphangioleiomyomatosis. N Engl J Med. 2011;364:1595.

McCormack FX, Travis WD, Colby TV, et al. Lymphangioleiomyomatosis: calling it what it is: a low-grade, destructive, metastasizing neoplasm. Am J Respir Crit Care Med. 2012;186:1210.

McCormack FX. Lymphangioleiomyomatosis: a clinical update. Chest. 2008;133:507.

Muzykewicz DA, Sharma A, Muse V, et al. TSC1 and TSC2 mutations in patients with lymphangioleiomyomatosis and tuberous sclerosis complex. J Med Genet. 2009;46:465.

Ogórek B, Hamieh L, Lasseter K, et al. Generalised mosaicism for TSC2 mutation in isolated lymphangioleiomyomatosis. Eur Respir J. 2019;54.

Ryu JH, Moss J, Beck GJ, et al. The NHLBI lymphangioleiomyomatosis registry: characteristics of 230 patients at enrollment. Am J Respir Crit Care Med. 2006;173:105.

Taveira-DaSilva AM, Hathaway O, Stylianou M, Moss J. Changes in lung function and chylous effusions in patients with lymphangioleiomyomatosis treated with sirolimus. Ann Intern Med. 2011;154:797.

Xu KF, Zhang P, Tian X, et al. The role of vascular endothelial growth factor-D in diagnosis of lymphangioleiomyomatosis (LAM). Respir Med. 2013;107:263.

Yano S. Exacerbation of pulmonary lymphangioleiomyomatosis by exogenous oestrogen used for infertility treatment. Thorax. 2002;57:1085.

Yao J, Taveira-DaSilva AM, Jones AM, et al. Sustained effects of sirolimus on lung function and cystic lung lesions in lymphangioleiomyomatosis. Am J Respir Crit Care Med. 2014;190:1273.

Young L, Lee HS, Inoue Y, et al. Serum VEGF-D a concentration as a biomarker of lymphangioleiomyomatosis severity and treatment response: a prospective analysis of the Multicenter International Lymphangioleiomyomatosis Efficacy of Sirolimus (MILES) trial. Lancet Respir Med. 2013;1:445.

Young LR, Inoue Y, McCormack FX. Diagnostic potential of serum VEGF-D for lymphangioleiomyomatosis. N Engl J Med. 2008;358:199.

CASE 14

A 51-year-old White woman presents to the clinic with 18 months of progressive dyspnea and cough. She reports no other medical problems and takes no prescribed medications. She reports that she was in a good state of health approximately 2 years ago when she noticed some mild dyspnea on excrtion that she thought might be related to some mild weight gain or deconditioning. However, over the last 18 months, she has developed a dry cough, and her dyspnea has progressed to the point she can only tolerate household distances (about 50-100 feet) before needing to rest. She reports no history of smoking tobacco use or drug use. She denies any significant occupational or environmental exposures. She has lost approximately 10 lb over this time, with her BMI now 23 kg/m² from 25 kg/m² 18 months ago. She reports no family history of lung disease. She does not follow-up regularly with any physicians.

On examination, her vital signs are within normal limits: HR 89, BP 110/80, RR 12, and O_2 saturation of 96% on room air at rest, 93% with activity. There are some faint inspiratory crackles. She has a normal cardiac examination. There is no clubbing, cyanosis, or edema.

Her CXR is shown in **Image 14-1**.

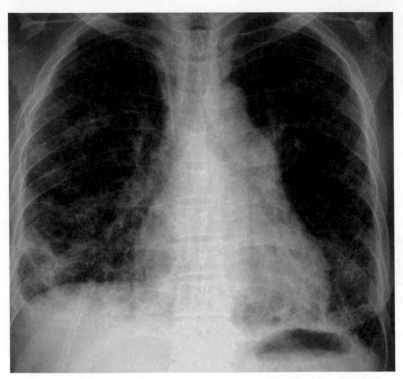

Image 14-1 • Chest Radiograph (AP) for the patient in **Question 14-1**. (*Reproduced with permission from Filipek MS, Thompson ME, Wang PL, et al: Lymphocytic interstitial pneumonitis in a patient with systemic lupus erythematosus: radiographic and high-resolution CT findings, J Thorac Imaging 2004 Jul;19(3):200-203.*)

QUESTIONS

Q14-1: How would one best describe the abnormalities on the chest radiograph?

A. Diffuse, hazy, alveolar opacities

B. Focal infiltrate in the left and right lower lobes, with linear opacities in the upper lobes

C. Reticulonodular opacities and cysts in a lower lobe-predominant pattern.

D. Pleural effusion on the left

E. Deep sulcus sign on the left

E. Nodular opacities in a miliary pattern

Q14-2: The patient's high-resolution CT scan of the chest is shown in Image 14-2A and 14-2B.

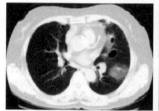 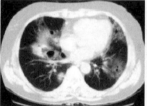 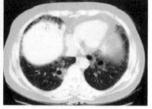

Image 14-2A • Chest CT images for the patient in **Question 14-2**. (*Reproduced with permission from Dong X, Gao YL, Lu Y, et al: Characteristics of primary Sjögren's syndrome related lymphocytic interstitial pneumonia, Clin Rheumatol 2021 Feb;40(2):601-612.*)

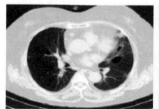 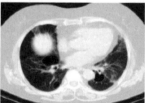 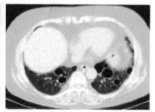

Image 14-2B • Chest CT images for the patient in **Question 14-2**. (*Reproduced with permission from Dong X, Gao YL, Lu Y, et al: Characteristics of primary Sjögren's syndrome related lymphocytic interstitial pneumonia, Clin Rheumatol 2021 Feb;40(2):601-612.*)

Which is the best description of the abnormalities seen in the patient's CT scan of the chest?

A. Honeycombing, traction bronchiectasis, and reticular interstitial opacities

B. Diffusely distributed ground-glass opacities with linear interstitial opacities

C. Scattered areas of ground-glass opacities with nodular interstitial opacities

D. Diffuse cystic lesions, ground-glass opacities, nodules, and septal thickening with areas of normal lung tissue

E. Nodular opacities along bronchovascular and lymphatic structures with hilar adenopathy

Q14-3: The patient's review of symptoms reveals the following affirmatives: fatigue, mild pleuritic chest pain, weight loss of 10 lb over 12 to 18 months, xerostomia, intermittent episodes of diarrhea (limited to 1-2 times a month), arthralgia without joint deformities but with mild effusions occasionally. She denies any constitutional symptoms otherwise.

Based on these findings, the patient is referred for a surgical lung biopsy. The biopsy is shown in Image 14-3. The pathology reports is as follows:

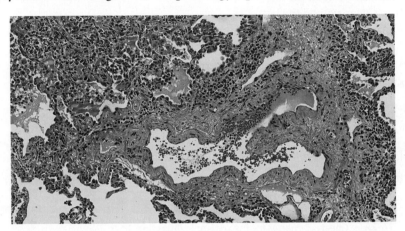

Image 14-3 • Representative image of the lung histopathology for the patient in **Question 14-3**.

"There is diffuse infiltration of mononuclear cells into the interlobular and alveolar septa. There is a polyclonal inflammatory infiltrate that consists predominantly of T cells, with pre-B cells, plasma cells, and scattered multinucleated giant cells also seen. There are scattered germinal centers identified predominantly along the bronchovascular bundles. There is no involvement of the pleura."

What is the likely diagnosis?

A. Pulmonary Langerhans cell histiocytosis (PLCH)
B. Lymphocytic interstitial pneumonia (LIP)
C. Sarcoidosis
D. Desquamative interstitial pneumonia (DIP)
E. Usual interstitial pneumonia (UIP)

Q14-4: Which of the following comorbid disease processes is NOT commonly associated with the form of interstitial lung disease in this case

A. Sjogren syndrome (SS)
B. Rheumatoid arthritis (RA)
C. Human immunodeficiency virus (HIV)
D. Hypogammaglobulinemia
E. Type 2 diabetes mellitus
F. Human T cell lymphotropic virus type I (HTLV-1)
G. Pernicious anemia

Q14-5: Given the patient's symptoms of xerostomia and some mild parotid gland swelling on examination, you suspect the patient has SS. Which laboratory test would you expect to be positive in a patient with SS?

A. Rheumatoid factor (Rf)
B. Anticitrullinated peptide (anti-CCP) antibodies
C. Anti-Ro/anti-La antibodies
D. Anti-Scl70 antibodies
E. Elevated serum beta-galactomannan

Q14-6: For patients with LIP not caused by immunodeficiency, what is the primary treatment?

A. Smoking cessation
B. Immunoglobulin (IgG) supplementation
C. Systemic glucocorticoids
D. Sirolimus
E. Transplantation

ANSWERS

Q14-1: C
Reticulonodular opacities and cysts in the lower > upper lobes.

Rationale: The patient's chest radiograph shows multiple cysts throughout the lung fields, perhaps more prominently in the lower lobes. Additionally, there is a "net-like" or reticular pattern of interstitial opacities throughout the bilateral lungs, again more prominently in the lower lobes. There is no focal infiltrate present. There is no apparent pleural effusion on the left, but there is a deepened costophrenic angle on the left that could be concerning for deep sulcus sign in the appropriate context. To make this call, the patient is usually placed supine, and the image needs to capture the entire diaphragm. The air in the costophrenic angle will classically maintain a clear separation between the diaphragm and the parietal pleura as seen in **Image 14-4** below.

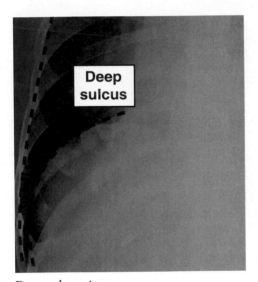

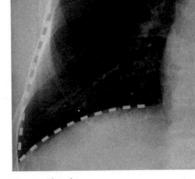

Deep sulcus sign.   Normal sulcus.

Image 14-4 • Example of "Deep Sulcus" sign on chest radiograph (left), consistent with presence of a pneumothorax. Note the exaggerated separation of the diaphragm and the chest wall in the image on the left (black), compared to the normal anatomy on the right (gray) where there is a clear costophrenic angle.

Q14-2: D
Diffuse cystic lesions and ground glass opacities scattered in areas of normal lung tissue

Rationale: The CT scan of the chest shows cystic lung lesions in the upper and lower lobes, with the presence of ground-glass opacities, nodules, and interstitial thickening, more marked in the lower than in the upper lobes. Note particularly how the cysts are predominantly located along the bronchovascular structures as well. Here, there is no overt evidence of honeycombing or traction bronchiectasis. Also, there is no significant adenopathy seen in the hilum. Although options B and C could be considered here, these do not mention the cystic lung lesions, which significantly helps to narrow the differential diagnosis.

Q14-3: B
Lymphocytic interstitial pneumonia (LIP)

Rationale: The findings of a polyclonal infiltrate, consisting predominantly of T cells, into the alveolar septa is a classic finding in LIP. This is consistent with the patient's chest imaging as well, which demonstrates cystic lung disease with scattered ground-glass opacities and a lower-lobe predominance. As the disease progresses, the cysts may coalesce. **Image 14-2B** shows a follow-up CT scan for the patient in **Image 14-2A**, where some of areas of ground-glass opacities on the initial image have transitioned to cysts and some of the cysts have coalesced. Similar to patients with LAM, these patients are at an increased risk of spontaneous pneumothorax.

LIP is an interstitial pneumonitis that consists of a benign (polyclonal) expansion of T cells, pre-B cells, and plasma cells into the alveolar and interlobular septa. There is some evidence for a role for aberrant Bcl-6 expression as a driver for this process, which may suggest the involvement of T follicular helper cells. Although it may arise without a clear etiology (ie, idiopathic), patients commonly present with dyspnea, cough, and fatigue, and constitutional symptoms are rare. The polyclonal infiltrate is important to differentiate the condition from malignant conditions, including extranodal marginal zone lymphoma, angioimmunoblastic T cell lymphoma and pulmonary lymphoma. CT imaging classically demonstrates loose centrilobular nodules (ie, not well defined), cysts, peribronchovascular thickening, septal thickening, lymphadenopathy, and possibly areas of consolidation. This is different from follicular bronchiolitis, a B-cell–driven process that affects the airways with sparing of the alveoli. Unlike LAM, there is typically a basilar predominance of abnormalities on CT.

Sarcoidosis is identified on pathology by the presence of tight, well-formed noncaseating granulomas composed of multinucleated cells, with mild inflammatory cell infiltrate present. Asteroid bodies may be seen in the giant cells. There may be areas of fibrosis and vascular involvement. The CT findings are highly variable but typically include hilar or mediastinal adenopathy. Sarcoidosis is a diagnosis of exclusion.

PLCH is also a cystic lung disease that affects predominantly smokers and can involve other sites, primarily bone. Similar to LIP and LAM, patients can be predisposed to develop pneumothoraces. CT generally demonstrates centrilobular nodules scattered in the upper and lower lung fields, with the presence of cysts typically evolving out of these nodular areas. The pathology demonstrates the presence of Langerhans cells (staining positive for S100, CD1a) in the nodules, in addition to eosinophils. Lymphocytes, plasma cells, and histiocytes may also be present.

DIP is a interstitial pneumonia that occurs almost exclusively in smokers. The CT findings are generally lower-lobe predominant ground-glass opacities, though nodules can be seen. On pathology, one would see a diffuse filling of alveoli and terminal bronchioles with "smokers' macrophages," which contain a golden-brown pigment and stain positive for iron. These patients often also have evidence of chronic bronchitis or emphysema.

UIP is a progressive interstitial pneumonia marked by temporal and geographic heterogeneity. The classic findings on pathology include areas of fibrosis and inflammation alternating with normal lung, with both temporal and geographic heterogeneity in terms of the degree of fibrosis. In areas of more severe fibrosis, there is architectural distortion and traction bronchiectasis; these changes are typically most severe in the subpleural or paraseptal regions. On CT, the findings include, in a basal and peripheral predominance, reticular interstitial opacities, traction bronchiectasis, and honeycomb changes.

Q14-4: E
Type 2 diabetes mellitus

Rationale: LIP most commonly occurs in patients with rheumatologic disease, and immunodeficiencies. Although often associated with HIV/AIDS, LIP is quite rare in HIV-positive patients, particularly those receiving antiretroviral therapy. Of the rheumatologic disorders, LIP has been most closely associated with Sjogren syndrome, though may be seen in RA, systemic lupus erythematosus (SLE), autoimmune thyroid disease, pernicious anemia, Castleman disease, and myasthenia gravis. For patients with immunodeficiencies (eg, CVID), a form of LIP termed *granulomatous and lymphocytic interstitial pneumonia* (or lung disease; G-LIP or GLILD) may also be seen. Infections such as Epstein-Barr virus (EBV) or HTLV-1 have also been proposed to cause LIP. Therefore, of the options available, type 2 diabetes mellitus is the only condition not associated with LIP.

Q14-5: C
Anti-Ro/anti-La antibodies (anti-SSA/anti-SSB)

Rationale: Up to 80% of patients with SS will have antibodies against either Ro (SSA) or La (SSB) antigen, in addition to a positive anti-nuclear antibody (ANA) titer. Patients with SS may also have a positive Rf or anti-CCP, but this much less common. Rf and anti-CCP antibodies are used to screen for seropositive rheumatoid arthritis. Anti-Scl70 (topoisomerase 1) antibodies are serologic markers for systemic scleroderma (SSc). Beta-galactomannan and 1,3-beta-D-glucan are non–culture-based tools used for diagnosis of fungal infections.

Q14-6: C
Systemic glucocorticoids

Rationale: As with most interstitial lung diseases, the decision to initiate treatment is dependent on the severity of the patient's symptoms, the degree of lung/physiologic impairment at the time of diagnosis, and the disease progression. Most patients with

LIP are initiated on therapy with glucocorticoids; however, definitive clinical trials demonstrating the utility of glucocorticoids are lacking. The typical dosing is 0.5 mg/kg/day prednisone or its equivalent, which is tapered slowly over the course of several months while monitoring for improvement. Patient with rheumatologic disease–associated LIP may also require a second immunosuppressive medication to control extrapulmonary symptoms. For patients who fail to respond to systemic glucocorticoids, there is no clear evidence to guide the choice of second-line therapy, with the reported use of azathioprine, mycophenolate, cyclosporine, and rituximab, among others. All patients, and particularly those with interstitial lung disease, should be counselled against the use of smoking tobacco, but this is not the primary driver. Immunoglobulin supplementation should be used for patients with immunoglobulin deficiencies, but again, this is not the primary treatment for LIP. Median survival from the time of diagnosis if approximately 10 to 13 years. LIP has the potential for malignant transformation, most commonly into mucosa-associated lymphoid tissue (MALT) lymphomas. Lung transplantation has been performed for end-stage disease.

References

Cha SI, Fessler MB, Cool CD, et al. Lymphoid interstitial pneumonia: clinical features, associations and prognosis. Eur Respir J. 2006;28:364.

Dong X, Gao YL, Lu Y, Zheng Y. Characteristics of primary Sjögren's syndrome related lymphocytic interstitial pneumonia. Clin Rheumatol. 2020:1.

Dufour V, Wislez M, Bergot E, et al. Improvement of symptomatic human immunodeficiency virus-related lymphoid interstitial pneumonia in patients receiving highly active antiretroviral therapy. Clin Infect Dis. 2003;36:e127.

Filipek MS, Thompson ME, Wang PL, Gosselin MV, Primack SL. Lymphocytic interstitial pneumonitis in a patient with systemic lupus erythematosus: radiographic and high-resolution CT findings. J Thorac Imaging. 2004;19:200.

Fishback N, Koss M. Update on lymphoid interstitial pneumonitis. Curr Opin Pulm Med. 1996;2:429.

Hare SS, Souza CA, Bain G, et al. The radiological spectrum of pulmonary lymphoproliferative disease. Br J Radiol. 2012;85:848.

Hatron PY, Tillie-Leblond I, Launay D, et al. Pulmonary manifestations of Sjögren's syndrome. Presse Med. 2011;40:e49.

Johkoh T, Fukuoka J, Tanaka T. Rare idiopathic intestinal pneumonias (IIPs) and histologic patterns in new ATS/ERS multidiciplinary classification of the IIPs. Eur J Radiol. 2015;84:542.

Kramer MR, Saldana MJ, Ramos M, Pitchenik AE. High titers of Epstein-Barr virus antibodies in adult patients with lymphocytic interstitial pneumonitis associated with AIDS. Respir Med. 1992;86:49.

Kurosu K, Weiden MD, Takiguchi Y, et al. BCL-6 mutations in pulmonary lymphoproliferative disorders: demonstration of an aberrant immunological reaction in HIV-related lymphoid interstitial pneumonia. J Immunol. 2004;172:7116.

Rao N, Mackinnon AC, Routes JM. Granulomatous and lymphocytic interstitial lung disease: a spectrum of pulmonary histopathologic lesions in common variable immunodeficiency—histologic and immunohistochemical analyses of 16 cases. Hum Pathol. 2015;46:1306.

Seaman DM, Meyer CA, Gilman MD, McCormack FX. Diffuse cystic lung disease at high-resolution CT. AJR Am J Roentgenol. 2011;196:1305.

Setoguchi Y, Takahashi S, Nukiwa T, Kira S. Detection of human T-cell lymphotropic virus type I-related antibodies in patients with lymphocytic interstitial pneumonia. Am Rev Respir Dis. 1991;144:1361.

Swigris JJ, Berry GJ, Raffin TA, Kuschner WG. Lymphoid interstitial pneumonia: a narrative review. Chest. 2002;122:2150.

Teirstein AS, Rosen MJ. Lymphocytic interstitial pneumonia. Clin Chest Med. 1988;9:467.

Travis WD, Costabel U, Hansell DM, et al. An official American Thoracic Society/European Respiratory Society statement: update of the international multidisciplinary classification of the idiopathic interstitial pneumonias. Am J Respir Crit Care Med. 2013;188:733.

CASE 15

A 44-year-old White man presents with complaints of dyspnea on exertion. The symptoms have been gradually worsening over the past 1 to 2 years. He also notes a nonproductive cough that has worsened over the last 6 months. He notes no pleuritic chest pain, hemoptysis, lower-extremity edema, or palpitations. He denies any fevers, chills, sweats, or abdominal symptoms. He has no family history of pulmonary disease, malignancy, or rheumatologic disease. He has smoked cigarettes since the age of 18, between one and two packs per day on average. He has attempted quitting multiple times unsuccessfully. He smokes marijuana approximately one to two times a month. He denies illicit drug use. He works as a paralegal and has no known occupational exposures. On examination, he is saturating 93% on room air at rest but requires 2 L NC to maintain his saturations above 88% when walking. His 6-minute walk distance is 60% predicted. His vitals otherwise are T 98.2°F, HR 87, BP 151/67. He has inspiratory crackles at the bases and some moderate clubbing. The patient had a chest radiograph with his primary care physician that was reported as "normal."

QUESTIONS

Q15-1: The patient undergoes pulmonary function testing at your clinic prior to the appointment. The following results are reported in Image 15-1:

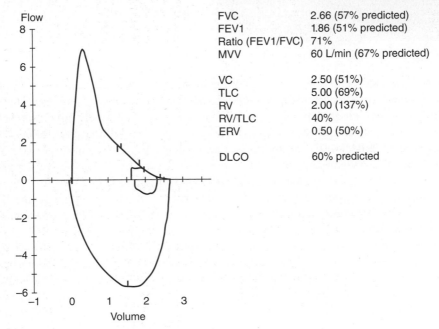

FVC	2.66 (57% predicted)
FEV1	1.86 (51% predicted)
Ratio (FEV1/FVC)	71%
MVV	60 L/min (67% predicted)
VC	2.50 (51%)
TLC	5.00 (69%)
RV	2.00 (137%)
RV/TLC	40%
ERV	0.50 (50%)
DLCO	60% predicted

Image 15-1 • Pulmonary function testing for the patient in **Question 15-1**.

How would you interpret the PFT results?

A. Mixed restrictive and obstruction with evidence of air trapping and a reduced DLCO
B. Restrictive defect with a reduced DLCO
C. Obstructive defect with air trapping and a normal DLCO
D. Normal spirometry, lung volumes, and a reduced DLCO
E. An elevated DLCO concerning for alveolar hemorrhage or polycythemia

Q15-2: Given the patient's PFT abnormalities and clinical symptoms (both subject and objective), what is the next test you would like to order?

A. MRI of the C-spine and brain, EMG and NCS studies including the diaphragm, a neck CT scan, and anticholinesterase antibodies studies
B. Echocardiogram, VQ scan, and right heart catheterization
C. Noncontrasted CT scan of the chest with rheumatologic antibody, serum precipitins studies
D. No further testing is indicated; discharge the patient from the clinic
E. A cardiac MRI and angiotensin enzyme levels

Q15-3: The patient's rheumatologic antibody panel test results are negative or normal. The serum precipitins testing results are negative. The patient undergoes high-resolution CT scanning, which demonstrated the following in Image 15-2:

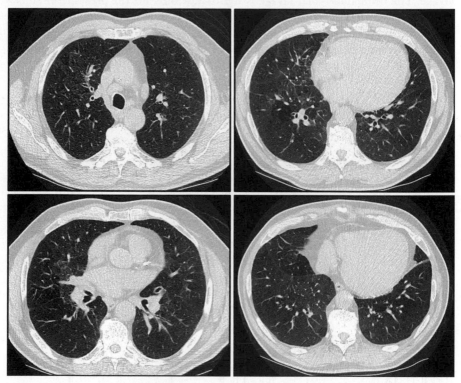

Image 15-2 • CT imaging of the patient in **Case 15**.

How would you describe the abnormalities on the CT scan?

A. Septal thickening, traction bronchiectasis, and honeycomb changes
B. Ground-glass and micronodular interstitial opacities
C. Centrilobular emphysematous changes
D. Tree-in-bud opacities
E. Consolidation with air bronchograms

Q15-4: The patient completes a comprehensive environmental and occupational exposure history without a clear precipitating or instigating factor. The patient undergoes a bronchoscopy with a transbronchial biopsy and bronchoalveolar lavage. The bronchoalveolar lavage is significant only for the presence of smokers' macrophages. The transbronchial biopsy shows only scant alveolar tissue and is nondiagnostic. The patient undergoes a video-assisted thoracoscopic thoracotomy with a lung biopsy. The result is shown in Image 15-3. The staining is negative for CD1a. What is the likely diagnosis?

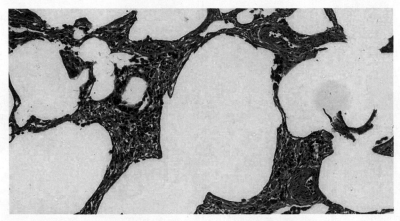

Image 15-3 • Pathology specimen from the patient in **Case 15**.

A. Hypersensitivity pneumonitis (HP)
B. Respiratory bronchiolitis–associated interstitial lung disease (RB-ILD)
C. Pulmonary Langerhans cell histiocytosis (PLCH)
D. Idiopathic pulmonary fibrosis (IPF)
E. Sarcoidosis

Q15-5: The pathology is consistent with RB. Why is the diagnosis RB-ILD and not simply RB?

A. The patient has less than a 100–pack-year history of smoking.
B. The patient has clinical evidence of interstitial lung disease.
C. The patient has a family history of emphysema in a grandfather who smoked tobacco for years.
D. The patient is under the age of 50.

Q15-6: What is the primary risk factor for RB-ILD?

A. Lipid exposure from chronic aspiration
B. Silica exposure
C. Chewing tobacco exposure
D. Smoking tobacco exposure
E. Isocyanate exposure
F. Grain dust exposure
G. Heavy metal exposure

Q15-7: What is the primary treatment for patients with RB-ILD?

A. Systemic glucocorticoids
B. Azathioprine
C. Pulmonary rehabilitation
D. Smoking cessation
E. Age-appropriate vaccination

ANSWERS

Q15-1: A
Mixed restrictive and obstruction with evidence of air trapping and a reduced DLCO

Rationale: An examination of the spirometric indices and the flow-volume loop reveals evidence of both restrictive and obstructive defects. The FVC is low, suggesting possible restriction, and while the FEV1/FVC ratio is borderline normal (71%), the flow-volume loop clearly has a concave shape, suggesting worsening airflow obstruction at lower lung volumes, which is consistent with an obstructive defect. This is an example of pseudonormalization of the FEV1/FVC ratio. This is encountered mostly in restrictive lung disease, where the FVC is reduced out of proportion to the FEV1. The lung volumes show a reduced TLC (69%) consistent with at least moderate restriction of the lung volume excursion. The patient's RV is elevated (137%), and the RV/TLC ratio is elevated at 40%, both suggesting air trapping is present. The ERV is low, but the reduction in the ERV is consistent with the severity of the reduction in VC. The MVV, while low at 60 L/min, is appropriate for the patient's reduced FEV1 (30 * FEV1 = 55.8 L/min expected), so there is no evidence of neuromuscular disease. The DLCO is substantially reduced. Therefore, the appropriate answer is option (A).

Q15-2: C
Noncontrasted CT scan of the chest with rheumatologic antibody studies

Rationale: The patient's PFT abnormalities, with a large restrictive component and reduced DLCO, raise concern for interstitial lung disease, despite the "normal" chest radiograph. The presence of concomitant obstruction may be related to the patient's smoking history or the presence of airway-centric interstitial lung disease (ie, sarcoidosis, chronic HP). Therefore, a high-resolution CT scan of the chest coupled with appropriate rheumatologic antibody testing would be an appropriate next step. High-resolution CT of the chest is much more specific for identifying interstitial lung disease than chest radiographs alone. Option (A) would be a good option in a patient with concern for neuromuscular disease–associated dyspnea (restriction with reduced MVV, but normal DLCO). Option (B) would be a good option for patients with primary concern for pulmonary vascular disease (eg, pulmonary HTN, chronic thromboembolic pulmonary hypertension [CTEPH], acute pulmonary embolism). In isolated pulmonary vascular disease (PVD), the PFTs are generally normal, with a reduction in DLCO. While these PVDs may also occur as a result of interstitial lung disease, vasculitis, or emphysema, identifying the underlying cause in these nonidiopathic cases is most important. Option (D) is clearly inappropriate as the patient has not only subjective but objective evidence of interstitial lung disease. Cardiac MRI in Option (E) would be a viable choice for a patient with sarcoidosis or pulmonary amyloidosis who is experiencing increased dyspnea without changes in lung volumes or spirometry, and it may indicate infiltrative heart disease. The use of angiotensin enzyme level testing has no general utility.

Q15-3: B
Ground-glass and micronodular interstitial opacities

Rationale: The arrows are pointing to centrilobular areas of the lung parenchyma, with hazy opacities that do not completely obscure the underlying lung architecture, consistent with ground-glass opacities. Although somewhat difficult to see in this image, micronodules are present as well. There is no evidence of significant septal thickening or consolidation. There are no cysts or cavitary lesions. There is no evidence of traction bronchiectasis or honeycombing, as can be seen in fibrotic processes.

Q15-4: B
Respiratory bronchiolitis–associated interstitial lung disease (RB-ILD)

Rationale: The pathology shows an accumulation of tan/brown pigmented macrophages. Note here these cells, along with some lymphocytes (gray), are infiltrating into the peribronchiolar spaces, but the alveoli are generally spared. Note the preservation of the general alveolar architecture with some respiratory bronchiole thickening that is due to the inflammatory cell infiltrate. Importantly, note the lack of any significant fibrosis or granulomas. There is preservation of the vascular structures as well. This pathology is consistent with respiratory bronchiolitis (RB).

Q15-5: B
The patient has clinical evidence of interstitial lung disease.

Rationale: An explanation will be provided following the next question.

Q15-6: D
Smoking tobacco exposure

Rationale: RB is marked by the presence of smokers' macrophages in respiratory bronchioles, with patchy infiltration of lymphocytes and dendritic cells (histiocytes) in the peribronchiolar areas. This inflammation can lead to areas of mild focal peribronchiolar fibrosis that extends into the interstitium of adjacent alveoli. RB-ILD is typically a clinical diagnosis with the same pathologic abnormalities, but patients have clinical evidence of interstitial lung disease, including radiographic abnormalities not associated with emphysema and a reduced DLCO.

RB and RB-ILD are most identified in current smokers who undergo lung biopsies for other reasons, such as sampling a suspicious lung nodule during lung cancer screening or in patients with clinical evidence of ILD without a clear diagnosis otherwise.

Nearly all cases of RB-ILD are associated with current or recent smoking tobacco use. Rarely, patients with significant second-hand exposure have been diagnosed with RB-ILD. There is some evidence that vaping may also lead to the development of RB-ILD.

Patients with RB-ILD often present in the third to fifth decade of life. The primary presenting symptoms include dyspnea with exertion, dry or productive cough, intermittent expiratory wheezing, and occasional pleuritic chest pain. Hemoptysis is relatively uncommon. Patients may have a normal examination, or they may have dry bibasilar expiratory crackles. Clubbing and cyanosis are atypical. Patients may have exercise- or rest-related hypoxia as well.

Chest radiographs are often normal in patients with RB-ILD, though those patients with more severe disease may have fine reticulonodular opacities as well as evidence of hyperinflation (diaphragmatic flattening) and emphysema (increased translucency in the upper lobes). High-resolution CT is more revealing in this disease process and often shows patchy, diffuse ground-glass opacities and centrilobular nodules. RB-ILD more commonly has an upper-lobe predominance, but it may be relatively diffuse as well. Patients may also have bronchial wall thickening. A diagnosis of RB-ILD requires clinical features of ILD to accompany such changes.

Bronchoscopy is typically of limited utility and primarily used to rule out infection or granulomatous disease processes (HP, sarcoidosis). Video-assisted thoracoscopic surgery/open lung biopsy is often required for a formal diagnosis in patients in whom the diagnosis is questionable, particularly in those with a more severe presentation. This is typically necessary to rule out other forms of interstitial pneumonia.

Q15-7: D
Smoking cessation

Rationale: The primary treatment in RB-ILD is smoking cessation (or stopping tobacco or other smoke inhalation). Approximately 70% of patients have clinical improvement with abstinence alone. However, 30% to 50% of patients may have persistent abnormalities on PFT, particularly obstructive expiratory airflow obstruction and hyperinflation. Continued tobacco use is associated with a progression of the lung disease process. Some patients with progressive disease despite tobacco cessation have been treated with glucocorticoids, and those with an initial response to glucocorticoid who are unable to be weaned have been placed on immunosuppressive medications (mycophenolate, azathioprine). However, the data for such interventions are lacking, and a response to these therapies should raise concern for an alternative diagnosis. Otherwise, treatment is primarily supportive, including pulmonary rehabilitation, age- and comorbidity-appropriate vaccination, treatment of underlying or existing obstructive lung disease, and, in appropriate clinical settings, supplemental oxygen. In patients with more severe disease, the role of antifibrotic agents has not been explored. Lung transplantation would be a reasonable option for patients with severe disease who demonstrate the ability to refrain from further smoking tobacco use. However, this is unlikely to be necessary. Lung cancer screening should be considered in patients who meet the appropriate screening criteria.

A final note: the diagnosis of RB-ILD requires the finding of smokers' macrophages in respiratory bronchioles with evidence of focal, patchy peribronchiolar and alveolar wall fibrosis, an appropriate smoking-tobacco exposure history, the exclusion of an infectious, granulomatous, or other interstitial pneumonia process, and clinical evidence of interstitial lung disease (most objectively by abnormalities in PFTs that are not solely attributable to COPD/emphysema). A clinical diagnosis, without the need for a lung biopsy, can often suffice if the radiographic and clinical manifestations fit and the patient experiences clinical improvement with abstinence from smoking tobacco use or exposure.

References

American Thoracic Society, European Respiratory Society. American Thoracic Society/European Respiratory Society International Multidisciplinary Consensus Classification of the Idiopathic Interstitial Pneumonias. This joint statement of the American Thoracic Society (ATS), and the European Respiratory Society (ERS) was adopted by the ATS board of directors, June 2001 and by the ERS Executive Committee, June 2001. Am J Respir Crit Care Med. 2002;165:277.

Bradley B, Branley HM, Egan JJ, et al. Interstitial lung disease guideline: the British Thoracic Society in collaboration with the Thoracic Society of Australia and New Zealand and the Irish Thoracic Society. Thorax. 2008;63 Suppl 5:v1.

Caminati A, Cavazza A, Sverzellati N, Harari S. An integrated approach in the diagnosis of smoking-related interstitial lung diseases. Eur Respir Rev. 2012;21:207.

Colby TV. Bronchiolitis. Pathologic considerations. Am J Clin Pathol. 1998;109:101.

Fraig M, Shreesha U, Savici D, Katzenstein AL. Respiratory bronchiolitis: a clinicopathologic study in current smokers, ex-smokers, and never-smokers. Am J Surg Pathol. 2002;26:647.

English C, Churg A, Lam S, Bilawich AM. Respiratory bronchiolitis with fibrosis: prevalence and progression. Ann Am Thorac Soc. 2014;11:1665.

Holt RM, Schmidt RA, Godwin JD, Raghu G. High resolution CT in respiratory bronchiolitis-associated interstitial lung disease. J Comput Assist Tomogr. 1993;17:46.

Mavridou D, Laws D. Respiratory bronchiolitis associated interstitial lung disease (RB-ILD): a case of an acute presentation. Thorax. 2004;59:910.

Nakanishi M, Demura Y, Mizuno S, et al. Changes in HRCT findings in patients with respiratory bronchiolitis-associated interstitial lung disease after smoking cessation. Eur Respir J. 2007;29:453.

Portnoy J, Veraldi KL, Schwarz MI, et al. Respiratory bronchiolitis-interstitial lung disease: long-term outcome. Chest. 2007;131:664.

Ryu JH, Myers JL, Capizzi SA, et al. Desquamative interstitial pneumonia and respiratory bronchiolitis-associated interstitial lung disease. Chest. 2005;127:178.

Travis WD, Costabel U, Hansell DM, et al. An official American Thoracic Society/European Respiratory Society statement: update of the international multidisciplinary classification of the idiopathic interstitial pneumonias. Am J Respir Crit Care Med. 2013;188:733.

Wells AU, Nicholson AG, Hansell DM. Challenges in pulmonary fibrosis . 4: smoking-induced diffuse interstitial lung diseases. Thorax. 2007;62:904.

CASE 16

A 51-year-old woman presents with symptoms of dry cough and dyspnea on exertion that have progressively worsened over the last 5 months. She reports a history of 5 years of smoking between the ages of 8 and 23 but says she has not smoked since. She works as a sales associate at a local furniture store, but therc is no furniture repaired, manufactured, painted, or stained there. She has no apparent occupational exposures. There was no apparent prodrome prior to the development of the symptoms, which was insidious at best. She was on an ACE inhibitor for HTN (her only other known medical problem), which was stopped 3 months ago without effect. She has also been given two short courses of antibiotics, a nasal steroid spray, and a proton pump inhibitor, but none have been effective in reducing her symptoms. She had one chest radiograph at an urgent care center a few weeks ago, and she has never had PFTs performed. She reports no abdominal pain, nausea, emesis, chest pain, pleuritic pain, diaphoresis, or hemoptysis, and the cough is nonproductive. She reports no stridor. She notes her exercise tolerance has dropped from walking 3 miles a day to barely being able to get to her mailbox and back without stopping (approximately 200 feet). She has difficulty with stairs but no evidence of focal neuromuscular weakness or neuropathy. She saw a cardiologist a few weeks ago who noted she was hypoxic at rest on room air, and she was started on supplemental O_2. Her vitals are T 99.1°F, HR 89, BP 123/66, RR 18, and O_2 saturation 93% on 2 L/min supplemental O_2. On echocardiogram, she had a mild tricuspid regurgitation jet identified, with an estimated right ventricular systolic pressure (RVSP) of 30 mm Hg. The LV is normal in size and functional, and the RV is normal in size and functional with a normal tricuspid annular plane systolic excursion (TAPSE) of 2.1 cm. A chest radiograph is shown in Image 16-1.

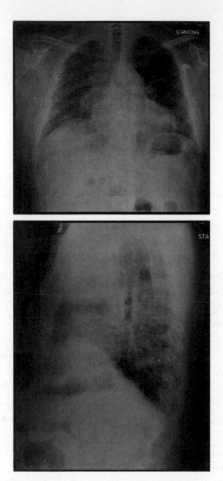

Image 16-1 • Chest radiograph for the patient in **Question 16-1**.

QUESTIONS

Q16-1: How would you describe the abnormalities in the chest radiograph shown in Image 16-1?

A. Reticular interstitial opacities
B. Linear interstitial opacities
C. Diffuse alveolar/airspace opacities
D. Focal consolidative opacities
E. Diffuse cavitary lesions

Q16-2: The patient's CT scan is shown in Image 16-2.

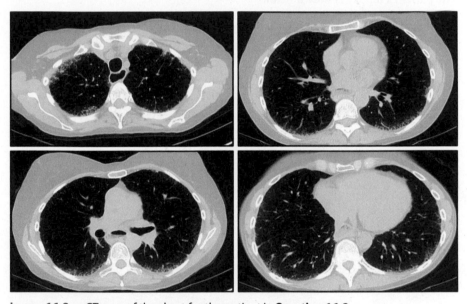

Image 16-2 • CT scan of the chest for the patient in **Question 16-2**.

Which findings are in the CT scan shown in Image 16-2? Select all that apply.

A. Subpleural interlobular and septal thickening
B. Honeycomb changes
C. Bronchial wall thickening
D. Ground-glass opacities
E. Focal consolidations

Q16-3: The patient undergoes an extensive evaluation in the clinic, including a completely negative evaluation for rheumatologic disease. There are no abnormalities on any of the patient's laboratory studies otherwise. What is the most appropriate next step in evaluation?

A. Right heart catheterization (RHC)
B. Left heart catheterization (LHC)
C. Cardiac MRI with stress test
D. Ventilation–perfusion (VQ) scan
E. Bronchoscopy with bronchoalveolar lavage and cryobiopsy

Q16-4: The patient undergoes a biopsy. All stains for organisms are negative. The patient's biopsy is shown below.

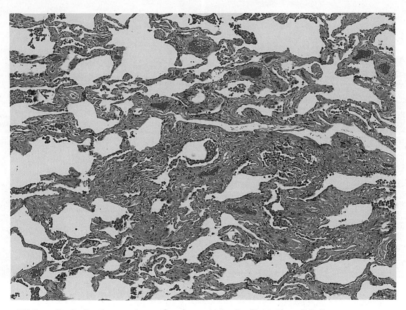

Image 16-3 • Pathologic specimen for the patient in **Question 16-4**.

What is the likely diagnosis?

A. Idiopathic pulmonary fibrosis (IPF)
B. Nonspecific interstitial pneumonia (NSIP)
C. Lymphocytic interstitial pneumonia (LIP)
D. Cryptogenic organizing pneumonia (COP)
E. Silicosis
E. Pulmonary tuberculosis

Q16-5: Which subtype of NSIP is shown in Image 16-3?

A. Cellular
B. Fibrotic

Q16-6: Which abnormalities on PFTs are not associated with NSIP? Select all that apply.

A. Reduced FEV1-to-FVC ratio, below 70% predicted
B. Reduced FVC, less than 70% predicted
C. Increased RV, greater than 130% predicted
D. Reduced DLCO, less than 70% predicted
E. A and B
F. A and C
G. A and D
H. B and C
I. B and D
J. C and D

Q16-7: A patient with severe NSIP is admitted to the inpatient service with worsening disease. He is requiring 4 L NC at rest and greater than 10 L/min O_2 with activity. The patient has received supplemental O_2, and all other causes of NSIP have been evaluated and ruled out, including rheumatologic disease. He is 44 years old and has not responded to several days of high-dose steroids. He has no signs of infection. What is the most appropriate next therapeutic option in the short term?

A. Lung transplantation
B. Extracorporeal membrane oxygenation (ECMO)
C. Plasmapheresis
D. Photopheresis
E. Cyclophosphamide therapy
F. Antibiotics

Q16-8: A 48-year-old man with no prior pulmonary history presents to the clinic for evaluation of an unresolved infiltrate. He has a history of HTN, for which he takes amlodipine and carvedilol. He initially presented to his primary care provider approximately 2 months ago, during the summer, with fevers to 101.3°F, nonproductive cough, and dyspnea. He had an abnormal chest radiograph and was treated with a course of azithromycin (5 days) for community-acquired pneumonia. However, the patient's symptoms have persisted, with intermittently low-grade fevers and progressive dyspnea. He denies any productive cough, but the dry cough persists. About a week after completing the azithromycin, he was treated with an additional course of moxifloxacin for 7 days, but again his symptoms persisted. A repeat CXR demonstrated persistent abnormalities, so he was referred to the pulmonary clinic for evaluation. He is otherwise known to be immunocompetent and to have never smoked, and he has no exposure history, including occupational or travel exposures. He denies any hemoptysis, chest pain, abdominal pain, lower-extremity edema, or weight loss, but he does endorse occasional night sweats. He had a purified protein derivative (PPD) skin test 1 month ago at his primary care office that was negative (0 mm in duration). His examination demonstrates only some dry crackles that are scattered throughout the lung fields but more prominent at the bases. The CT scan of his chest is shown in Image 16-4.

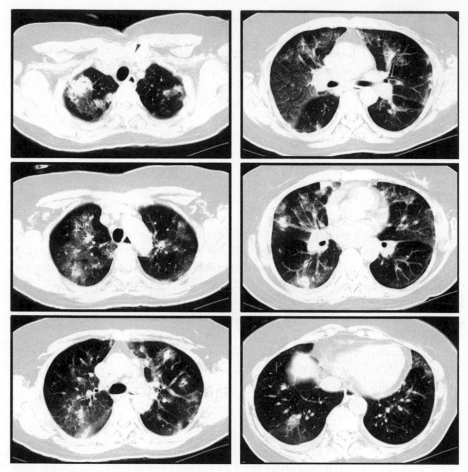

Image 16-4 • Chest CT images for the patient in **Question 16-8**.

How would you describe the primary CT scan abnormalities?

A. Reticulonodular interstitial opacities
B. Centrilobular ground-glass opacities
C. Scattered areas of consolidation and ground-glass opacities
D. Scattered cavitary lung lesions
E. Fibrocystic scarring

Q16-9: The patient has a negative rheumatologic evaluation and undergoes a bronchoscopy with bronchoalveolar lavage and cryobiopsy of the lung. The BAL returns with the following differential: 30% lymphocytes, 20% neutrophils, 5% eosinophils, and 45% macrophages. The stains for fungus and mycobacterium are negative. All bacterial cultures are negative, including the Gram stain. All other cultures are reported as "no growth to date." The pathology returns with the following report:

"The abnormal portion of the lung is characterized by the presence and proliferation of granulation tissue (fibroblasts, myofibroblasts, loose collagen fibers) in alveoli with extension into the terminal bronchioles. There is temporal homogeneity with affected areas, but there is geographic heterogeneity."

What is the most likely diagnosis?

A. Lymphocytic interstitial pneumonia (LIP)
B. Asbestosis
C. Respiratory bronchiolitis–associated interstitial lung disease (RB-ILD)
D. Sarcoidosis
E. Cryptogenic organizing pneumonia (COP)
F. Silicosis

Q16-10: Which condition or exposure is NOT commonly associated with the development of organizing pneumonia (OP) on lung pathology?

A. RA
B. Amiodarone
C. Ulcerative colitis (UC)
D. Radiation
E. Lung transplantation
F. GVHD
G. Lymphoma
H. All of the above
I. None of the above

Q16-11: What is the primary treatment for COP?

A. Supplement oxygen and supportive care
C. Corticosteroids
C. Rituximab
D. Anti–TNF-α therapy
E. Lung transplantation
F. Hyperbaric oxygen therapy (HBOT)

ANSWERS

Q16-1: A
reticular interstitial opacities

Rationale: This is a PA and lateral film. The costophrenic angles are clear. There are fine, net-like interstitial opacities present in both lower lobes as well as some notable in the upper lobes, particularly on the right. Although there may be some linear interstitial opacities, the predominant finding here is that of reticular opacities. There are no overt cavitary lesions, nor are there hazy alveolar opacities.

Q16-2: A; C; D
Subpleural interlobular and septal thickening; Bronchial wall thickening; Ground-glass opacities

Rationale: The CT scan is a standard inspiratory study. The patient has a slightly patulous esophagus more proximally. There are relatively diffuse subpleural reticular opacities (interlobular), and septal thickening is present, with some areas of bronchial wall thickening bordering perhaps on traction bronchiectasis. There are no overt honeycomb changes seen (note that there are some thickened bronchioles present at the lung bases which can give the appearance of possible early honeycombing). There are also some ground-glass opacities in a peripheral distribution.

Q16-3: E
Bronchoscopy with bronchoalveolar lavage and cryobiopsy

Rationale: The patient's CT scan is concerning for interstitial lung disease. The pattern seen on the scan could be an early fibrotic process, but it may be caused by a number of different underlying conditions. Additionally, this may be an idiopathic process. The patient's echocardiogram demonstrated only mild evidence of pulmonary HTN but no evidence of left ventricular (LV) dysfunction and no RV dysfunction to suggest a need for RHC or LHC currently. As the patient has evidence of parenchymal lung disease, there is a plausible reason for the hypoxemia and elevated pulmonary artery pressures, so an evaluation for pulmonary embolism is not needed at this point. Additionally, the patient's chest radiograph is abnormal, and a VQ scan is not an ideal study. A cardiac MRI would be useful if the primary concern was for cardiac sarcoidosis, but it would not provide a definitive diagnosis. Bronchoscopy with BAL and cryobiopsy will serve multiple purposes. Cryobiopsy can provide tissue samples large enough for a diagnosis of usual interstitial pneumonia (UIP), granulomatous disease, drug toxicity, and infectious causes. Therefore, this would be the most reasonable next step.

Q16-4: B
Nonspecific interstitial pneumonia (NSIP)

Rationale: Here, the biopsy shows a relatively uniform appearance of collagen deposition with a light mononuclear cell infiltrate within the interstitium and alveolar walls with general preservation of the overall lung architecture. There are no overt granulomas or granulomatous inflammatory lesions, and there is no evidence of organizing pneumonia. This is most consistent with a diagnosis of NSIP.

Q16-5: B
Fibrotic

Rationale: NSIP, along with UIP, is a chronic fibrosing interstitial pneumonia that may be idiopathic or may be associated with a number of other conditions, including connective tissue diseases (dermatomyositis [DM], polymyositis [PM], systemic sclerosis [SSc], systemic lupus erythematosus [SLE], Sjogren syndrome [SS], antisynthetase syndrome), rheumatoid arthritis [RA], HIV, drug toxicity (including chemotherapeutics such as the taxanes), IgG4-related sclerosing lung disease, and graft-versus-host disease (GVHD). Additionally, patients with a classic appearance of chronic hypersensitivity pneumonitis, including the presence of mosaic attenuation on CT scan, may lack the necessary findings of poorly formed granulomas on biopsy and receive a diagnosis of NSIP. It is the second most common form of IIP, following UIP, and accounts for between 15% and 30% of all IIPs.

The clinical presentation is in the fourth to fifth decade of life, with a female predominance due primarily to an increased incidence of connective tissue/rheumatologic disorders. Idiopathic NSIP shows a female predominance and is more common in patients of Eastern European descent. It is more common in patients who have never smoked, similar to chronic HP. Up to 20% of patients with NSIP eventually are diagnosed with a connective tissue disorder. Patients most commonly present with dyspnea, dry cough, and exercise intolerance with a more subacute than insidious onset. NSIP may also be the presenting symptoms of any of the connective tissue, rheumatologic, or collagen vascular disorders, and therefore patients may present with any signs or symptoms associated with those etiologies. Patients will commonly have basilar inspiratory crackles, and some patients may have clubbing. Patients with chronic hypoxemia related to their lung disease may present with signs and symptoms of right heart failure and pulmonary HTN.

The evaluation for a patient with suspected NSIP includes a thorough medical, family, occupational, and environmental exposure history. A thorough review of all prior medication use, including any prior chemotherapy or radiation therapy treatments, should be included. Laboratory testing is necessary to rule out rheumatologic disorders and HIV. Pulmonary function testing most commonly demonstrates a restrictive lung disease with reduced TLC and VC, in addition to a reduced DLCO. Bronchoscopy is generally not recommended unless cryobiopsy is performed because transbronchial biopsy has a low diagnostic yield. BAL findings are nonspecific, but they do help rule out other causes, particularly if the chest imaging findings are atypical. A definitive diagnosis requires histopathologic analysis of lung tissue, preferably from multiple lobes. The decision to pursue a surgical lung biopsy depends on the pretest probability that the patient has NSIP. Patients with a very high likelihood of NSIP (known underlying connective tissue disorder, prior known drug exposure with an appropriate temporal relationship to the development of symptoms) can defer biopsy begin treatment. Patients with an atypical course or in whom a biopsy would change the management plan significantly are more appropriate candidates for surgical biopsy if their clinical condition permits the procedure.

The radiographic findings of cellular and fibrotic NSIP may overlap considerably (**Images 16-5** and **16-6**), with the presence of both subpleural fibrosis and diffuse ground glass, and may represent episodes of acute exacerbations of an underlying fibrotic NSIP phenotype.

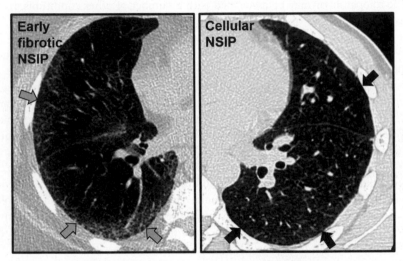

Image 16-5 • Comparison of the findings of fibrotic and cellular NSIP.

A. Cellular NSIP: Findings include ground-glass opacities, possibly in basilar predominance but may be heterogeneously or diffusely dispersed, with fine, but not coarse, reticular opacities. All the ground glass may exist in subpleural areas; there is typically immediate subpleural sparing (ie, a clear border between the lung and parietal pleura).

B. Early fibrotic NSIP: findings include reticular interstitial opacities, particularly in the subpleural areas, thickening of the bronchovascular bundles, associated ground-glass opacities, evolving traction bronchiectasis.

C. Late fibrotic NSIP: Findings include subpleural and septal thickening, traction bronchiectasis, generally with a lack of honeycomb changes, though they may also be seen. The distribution may be lower-lobe predominant, but it may also be diffuse. Overall, there is a loss of lung volume (**Image 16-7**).

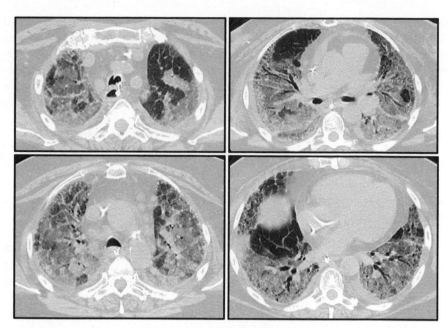

Image 16-6 • Example of a patient with NSIP with both cellular and fibrotic elements.

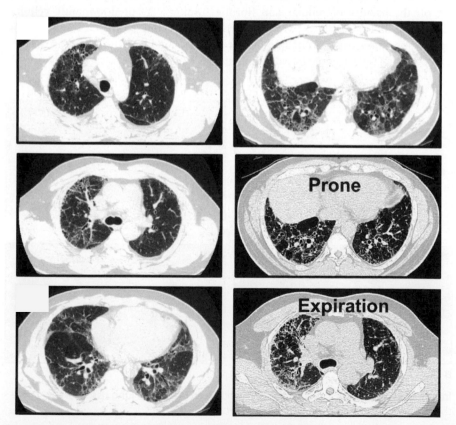

Image 16-7 • Example of a patient with advanced Fibrotic NSIP.

Similar to the radiographic findings, the pathology associated with cellular and fibrotic NSIP often overlaps as well. Additionally, patients with NSIP often have areas of the biopsy consistent with UIP. Unfortunately, patients with mixed UIP/NSIP findings have outcomes more consistent with UIP. There may also be areas of focal organizing pneumonia; however, these areas may not account for more than 10% of the cross-sectional area of the abnormal tissue.

The pathology of cellular NSIP is characterized by interstitial inflammation with a predominance of lymphocytes but without hyaline membrane deposition, overt fibrosis, or type II alveolar cell hyperplasia and with overall preservation of the lung architecture. There is also a lack of fibroblastic foci, viral inclusions, infectious organisms, eosinophils, granulomas, and granulomatous inflammation and significant areas of organizing pneumonia.

The pathology of fibrotic NSIP is characterized by mild inflammation with diffuse alveolar wall thickening due to collagen deposition. Unlike UIP, the natural lung architecture is maintained, and there is temporal and spatial homogeneity rather than heterogeneity. Recall that in UIP, there are areas of normal lung interspersed with areas of dense fibrosis.

NSIP had previously been classified into three different pathologic groups depending on the balance of cellular and fibrotic findings: (1) predominantly cellular; (2) cellular and fibrosis; (3) predominantly fibrosis (rare). However, there were no significant differences in outcomes between the second and third groups, so now the pathology is considered based on the presence or absence of a significant fibrotic component.

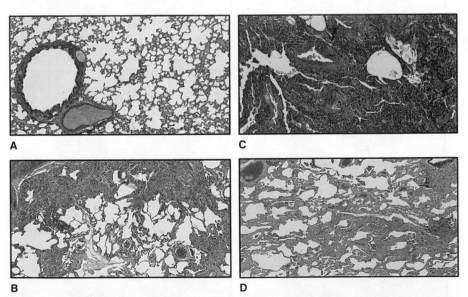

Image 16-8 • Comparison of pathology specimens: (A) normal lung tissue; (B) UIP (note the heterogeneity and dense fibrosis); (C) chronic HP; (D) NSIP.

Q16-6: C

(A) Reduced FEV1-to-FVC ratio, less than 70%, and (C) Increased RV, greater than 130% predicted

Rationale: A reduced FEV1/FVC is associated with airflow obstruction, such as in COPD. An increased RV is associated with hyperinflation, such as may be seen in the emphysematous subtype of COPD. NSIP is a restrictive lung disease associated with reductions in lung volumes, namely the vital capacity and reduced DLCO.

Q16-7: E

Cyclophosphamide

Rationale: For nonidiopathic NSIP, the treatment must first address the underlying cause. For the lung disease itself, the treatment is dependent on the severity of disease and the response to prior treatment. Patients with mild abnormalities on chest imaging and pulmonary function testing can possibly be monitored initially with close follow-up. Most patients will require treatment with systemic glucocorticoids (0.5-1 mg/kg/day), which may be tapered slowly over several months to observe for stability or improvement. If there is improvement, this can eventually be tapered off. If patients are unable to be tapered off glucocorticoids, initiation of a steroid-sparing agent is often required, possibly mycophenolate or azathioprine. For patients with more severe disease presentations, pulse-dose steroids (500-1000 mg/day for 3-5 days) can be attempted. For refractory disease, which is the case here, the cyclophosphamide has the most evidence, though there are reports of patients responding to rituximab therapy as well. Lung transplantation is an option, and the patient should be referred, but this should be reserved as a last option. Plasmapheresis has a role for certain rheumatologic diseases, but not in idiopathic disease. Antibiotics have no role in this patient. ECMO would be reserved for patients with acute respiratory failure who were awaiting a lung transplant. For further information regarding cyclophosphamide use in NSIP (as well as other immunosuppressives) and prognosis, please refer to the following section.

Q16-8: C

Scattered areas of consolidation and ground-glass opacities

Rationale: Note that all the areas of consolidation and ground glass are localized to the lung periphery. There are no reticulonodular opacities. Although there may be some areas of centrilobular ground glass, the predominant lesions here are consolidative. There are no obvious cavitary lesions or evidence of cystic changes present.

Q16-9: E

Cryptogenic organizing pneumonia

Rationale: This is a classic presentation of COP. COP is a diagnosis that falls under the category of the IIPs and is a diagnosis of exclusion. This will be discussed further below.

Q16-10: I
None of the above

Rationale: All the above conditions or exposures have been associated with the development of organizing pneumonia on lung pathology. This will be discussed further below.

Q16-11: B
Corticosteroids

Rationale: Cryptogenic organizing pneumonia is an idiopathic form of organizing pneumonia. Organizing pneumonia may also be seen as a result of a number of other conditions, including connective tissue disease, drug toxicity, pulmonary edema, infection, and malignancy. Additionally, organizing pneumonia is a common finding on histopathology in patients with other interstitial pneumonias, including NSIP.

The classic pathologic finding in COP is areas of organizing pneumonia, characterized by the presence and proliferation of granulation tissue (fibroblasts, myofibroblasts, loose collagen fibers) in alveoli with possible involvement of the terminal bronchioles. There is temporal homogeneity with affected areas, but there is geographic heterogeneity. Although COP may be seen in other IIPs such as NSIP, the areas of affected tissue should contain less organizing pneumonia (ie, less than 10% of the cross-sectional area).

COP presents most commonly in the fifth through sixth decades of life, with no sexpredilection. There is some evidence that smoking may be associated with an increased risk, but this is not confirmed. Patients often present with a subacute onset (4-8 weeks) of a flu-like illness, often with fever, malaise, fatigue, and cough. Night sweats and weight loss are relatively uncommon. Many patients have previously been treated for bronchitis, sinusitis, or community-acquired pneumonia without success. The physical examination findings are nonspecific, but patients may present with inspiratory crackles. Again, as this can be associated with any of the connective tissue disorders/rheumatologic conditions, patients may present with symptoms consistent with these as well.

Laboratory studies often demonstrate leukocytosis, but this is clearly nonspecific. Patients often have a very elevated ESR and CRP, but again, these are nonspecific. Testing for infectious and rheumatologic causes is necessary.

Chest radiographs often demonstrate patchy or hazy alveolar opacities, which may migrate with time. CT of the chest often demonstrates more extensive disease than expected from the plain chest radiographs, with patchy areas of consolidation, ground-glass opacities, and possible nodules. Cavitation is a rare finding but has been reported. It may have a peripheral distribution, as is seen in chronic eosinophilic pneumonia.

On BAL, there is traditionally a mixed cellular pattern, with lymphocytes, neutrophils, and eosinophils, but overall, it is nonspecific. BAL and transbronchial lung biopsy are primarily useful to rule out infection, hemorrhage, and malignancy as a cause of the abnormalities. Transbronchial biopsy has a moderate diagnostic yield for a diagnosis of organizing pneumonia, but cryobiopsy or surgical lung biopsy is often required for a definitive diagnosis.

A diagnosis of COP requires the predominant presence of organizing pneumonia on histopathology with the absence of findings suggestive of granulomatous disease, fibrosis, infection, or eosinophils. Additionally, one must rule out the multitude of potential causes of secondary organizing pneumonia.

The differential diagnoses for COP include community-acquired pneumonia, NSIP, subacute presentations of HP or eosinophilic pneumonia, chronic eosinophilic pneumonia, and granulomatous disease.

The treatment for COP is dependent on the severity of the patient's clinical presentation.

A. Mild-moderate disease (ie, no O_2 requirement): Consideration for monitoring for 4 to 8 weeks for improvement. Consideration can also be given to macrolide therapy for the anti-inflammatory effects, but this is less effective than glucocorticoids. Most patients will require treatment with glucocorticoids, initially at a dose of 1 mg/kg/day of oral equivalents of prednisone for 1 to 2 months, followed by a reduction to 0.5 mg/kg/day for another 1 to 2 months, then a gradual taper over approximately 6 months while monitoring for improvement/relapse. Overall, the evidence for steroid-sparing agents is lacking.

B. Glucocorticoid-refractory disease: An attempt can be made to add a macrolide to glucocorticoid therapy, but the patient may require oral cyclophosphamide (typically 150 mg daily) for a period of at least 3 months. Rituximab is also an option.

C. Fulminant disease (ie, respiratory failure on admission): Patients presenting with advanced respiratory failure or requiring mechanical ventilation should receive pulse-dose steroids (1000 mg/day of methylprednisolone) for 3 to 5 days, followed by oral prednisone (60 mg daily), followed by a taper. Cyclophosphamide or rituximab could also be considered.

References

American Thoracic Society, European Respiratory Society. American Thoracic Society/European Respiratory Society International Multidisciplinary Consensus Classification of the Idiopathic Interstitial Pneumonias. This joint statement of the American Thoracic Society (ATS), and the European Respiratory Society (ERS) was adopted by the ATS board of directors, June 2001 and by the ERS Executive Committee, June 2001. Am J Respir Crit Care Med. 2002;165:277.

Belloli EA, Beckford R, Hadley R, Flaherty KR. Idiopathic non-specific interstitial pneumonia. Respirology. 2016;21:259.

Bradley B, Branley HM, Egan JJ, et al. Interstitial lung disease guideline: the British Thoracic Society in collaboration with the Thoracic Society of Australia and New Zealand and the Irish Thoracic Society. Thorax. 2008;63 Suppl 5:v1.

Cho YH, Chae EJ, Song JW, et al. Chest CT imaging features for prediction of treatment response in cryptogenic and connective tissue disease-related organizing pneumonia. Eur Radiol. 2020;30:2722.

Cordier JF. Cryptogenic organising pneumonia. Eur Respir J. 2006;28:422.

Corte TJ, Ellis R, Renzoni EA, et al. Use of intravenous cyclophosphamide in known or suspected, advanced non-specific interstitial pneumonia. Sarcoidosis Vasc Diffuse Lung Dis. 2009;26:132.

Dina R, Sheppard MN. The histological diagnosis of clinically documented cases of cryptogenic organizing pneumonia: diagnostic features in transbronchial biopsies. Histopathology. 1993;23:541.

Fischer A, Antoniou KM, Brown KK, et al. An official European Respiratory Society/American Thoracic Society research statement: interstitial pneumonia with autoimmune features. Eur Respir J. 2015;46:976.

Flaherty KR, Travis WD, Colby TV, et al. Histopathologic variability in usual and nonspecific interstitial pneumonias. Am J Respir Crit Care Med. 2001;164:1722.

Fujita J, Yamadori I, Suemitsu I, et al. Clinical features of non-specific interstitial pneumonia. Respir Med. 1999;93:113.

Grinblat J, Mechlis S, Lewitus Z. Organizing pneumonia-like process: an unusual observation in steroid responsive cases with features of chronic interstitial pneumonia. Chest. 1981;80:259.

Hartman TE, Swensen SJ, Hansell DM, et al. Nonspecific interstitial pneumonia: variable appearance at high-resolution chest CT. Radiology. 2000;217:701.

Jegal Y, Kim DS, Shim TS, et al. Physiology is a stronger predictor of survival than pathology in fibrotic interstitial pneumonia. Am J Respir Crit Care Med. 2005;171:639.

Kim HC, Ji W, Kim MY, et al. Interstitial pneumonia related to undifferentiated connective tissue disease: pathologic pattern and prognosis. Chest. 2015;147:165.

Katzenstein AL, Fiorelli RF. Nonspecific interstitial pneumonia/fibrosis. Histologic features and clinical significance. Am J Surg Pathol. 1994;18:136.

Monaghan H, Wells AU, Colby TV, et al. Prognostic implications of histologic patterns in multiple surgical lung biopsies from patients with idiopathic interstitial pneumonias. Chest. 2004;125:522.

Nizami IY, Kissner DG, Visscher DW, Dubaybo BA. Idiopathic bronchiolitis obliterans with organizing pneumonia. An acute and life-threatening syndrome. Chest. 1995;108:271.

Oymak FS, Demirbaş HM, Mavili E, et al. Bronchiolitis obliterans organizing pneumonia. Clinical and roentgenological features in 26 cases. Respiration. 2005;72:254.

Purcell IF, Bourke SJ, Marshall SM. Cyclophosphamide in severe steroid-resistant bronchiolitis obliterans organizing pneumonia. Respir Med. 1997;91:175.

Radzikowska E, Wiatr E, Langfort R, et al. Cryptogenic organizing pneumonia-Results of treatment with clarithromycin versus corticosteroids-Observational study. PLoS One. 2017;12:e0184739.

Travis WD, Costabel U, Hansell DM, et al. An official American Thoracic Society/European Respiratory Society statement: Update of the international multidisciplinary classification of the idiopathic interstitial pneumonias. Am J Respir Crit Care Med. 2013;188:733.

Travis WD, Hunninghake G, King TE Jr, et al. Idiopathic nonspecific interstitial pneumonia: report of an American Thoracic Society project. Am J Respir Crit Care Med. 2008;177:1338.

Ujita M, Renzoni EA, Veeraraghavan S, et al. Organizing pneumonia: perilobular pattern at thin-section CT. Radiology. 2004;232:757.

Weill D, Benden C, Corris PA, et al. A consensus document for the selection of lung transplant candidates: 2014—an update from the Pulmonary Transplantation Council of the International Society for Heart and Lung Transplantation. J Heart Lung Transplant. 2015;34:1.

Xu W, Xiao Y, Liu H, et al. Nonspecific interstitial pneumonia: clinical associations and outcomes. BMC Pulm Med. 2014;14:175.

CASE 17

A 53-year-old man presents with a 1½-week course of progressive shortness of breath associated with a dry cough and moderate fevers to 101.1°F. He has a history of gout and HTN. His only medications are over-the-counter vitamin D supplements and amlodipine 10 mg daily. He reports no recent sick contacts. The symptoms initially started with a low-grade fever, a nonproductive cough, and some general malaise. The dyspnea started a few days later, and the dyspnea and cough have progressively worsened. He notes no chest pain, pleuritic pain, hemoptysis, or lower-extremity edema. He has a 10–pack-year smoking history (quit 15 years prior). He takes no medications. He has no known occupational or environmental exposures. He decided to go to an urgent care center, where he was noted to be tachypneic with a respiratory rate in the high 20s and an O_2 saturation of 93% on 6 L/min supplemental O_2 via NC (75% on room air on presentation). He was sent directly to the ED. He is afebrile, normotensive, mildly tachycardic to 110, and has inspiratory crackles bilaterally. The patient has a negative influenza A/B test and a negative SARS2-COVID19 rapid test. Additionally, the results of an extended respiratory viral panel are negative. The patient has blood cultures drawn and is started on community-acquired pneumonia coverage, including ceftriaxone 1 g IV every 24 hours and azithromycin 500 mg IV every 24 hours. He is admitted to the medical ICU. The patient's chest imaging will be reviewed below.

The patient's chest radiography is shown in Image 17-1.

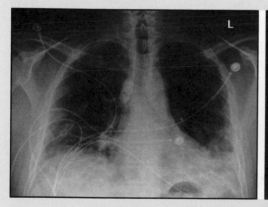
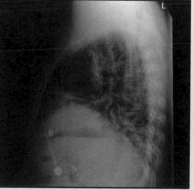

Image 17-1 • Chest radiograph for the patient in **Case 17**.

QUESTIONS

Q17-1: How would you describe the abnormalities in the chest radiograph?

A. Normal chest radiograph
B. Upper-lobe predominant linear interstitial opacities
C. Bilateral diffuse reticular and airspace opacities
D. Focal consolidative opacities at the bilateral bases
E. Scattered diffuse cavitary lesions

Q17-2: The patient undergoes a CT scan of the chest, which is shown in Image 17-2.

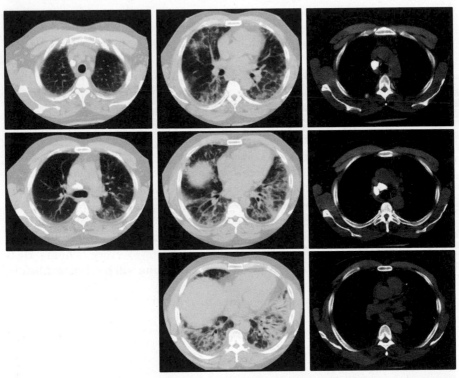

Image 17-2 • Chest CT imaging for the patient in **Case 17** (left two panels, lung windows; right panel, mediastinal windows).

Which abnormalities are present in the chest CT imaging shown in Image 17-2? Select all that apply.

A. Cavitary lung lesions
B. Mosaic pattern of air trapping
C. Diffuse consolidative opacities
D. Ground-glass opacities
E. Traction bronchiectasis
F. Septal thickening
G. Calcified mediastinal adenopathy
H. Noncalcified mediastinal adenopathy

Q17-3: The patient is admitted to the ICU, and over the next several hours the patient's condition deteriorates, necessitating intubation. The patient is on pressure-assist control with inspiratory pressure of 10 mm Hg, positive end-expiratory pressure (PEEP) of 14 cm H_2O, RR 12, and the fraction of inspired oxygen (FIO_2) is 0.70. The patient has the following laboratory testing return:

Laboratory Test	Value	Normal
Brain (B-type) natriuretic peptide (BNP)	31 pg/mL	1-100 pg/mL
C-reactive protein, high-sensitivity (hsCRP)	15.2 mg/L	<1.1 mg/L
Erythrocyte sedimentation rate (ESR)	67 mm/h	0-15 mm/h
Rheumatoid factor (Rf)	2 U/mL	<40 U/mL
Procalcitonin	0.02 ng/mL	<0.15 ng/mL
Arterial Blood Gas		
pH	7.48	7.35-7.45
$PaCO_2$	27	35-45 mm Hg
PaO_2	65	80-120 mm Hg

The patient undergoes a point-of-care ultrasound by a cardiac anesthesia critical care colleague who reports the following: "A hyperdynamic LV, evidence of LVH, normal wall motion, normal size of LA, normal RV function with normal size of the RA, inferior vena cava (IVC) 1.4 cm with normal respiratory variation." The patient also underwent a contrasted pulmonary embolism (PE) protocol CT scan that is negative for PE to subsegmental pulmonary arteries.

What is the most appropriate diagnosis at this point?

A. Diffuse alveolar hemorrhage (DAH)
B. Mild acute respiratory distress syndrome (ARDS)
C. Moderate acute respiratory distress syndrome (ARDS)
D. Severe acute respiratory distress syndrome (ARDS)
E. Very severe acute respiratory distress syndrome (ARDS)
F. Acute hypercarbic respiratory failure

Q17-4: The patient makes no improvement with broad-spectrum antibiotics and lung-protective ventilation, including a trial of prone positioning and paralysis. He remains on 60% FIO_2. The patient undergoes an extensive evaluation over the next 3 days, including the following studies: negative cardiac markers (troponin, CK-MB) × 3; normal creatine kinase (CK) and negative or normal values for the following: ANA, Scl70, ANCA, Rf, CCP antibodies, Smith/Ro/La antibodies, Jo-1 antibody; normal thyroid function; normal liver function; negative respiratory viral panel; and negative sputum culture from admission in the ED. Which treatment would you pursue next to evaluate the source of the patient's respiratory demise?

A. Bronchoscopy with bronchoalveolar lavage, transbronchial biopsy, and cell count
B. Barium swallow study to evaluate for aspiration
C. Serum precipitin studies to evaluate for possible hypersensitivity pneumonitis
D. Serum immunoglobulin levels to rule out IgA deficiency
E. Serum galactomannan level

Q17-5: The patient undergoes a bronchoscopy with BAL, transbronchial biopsies, and cell counts. The results of all fungal, mycobacterial, bacterial, and viral studies are negative, with no evidence of infection on histopathology. The serial lavage is negative for DAH. All rheumatologic testing has returned negative. The histopathology report demonstrates no evidence of organizing pneumonia, granulomatous disease (caseating or noncaseating), or malignancy, though there is mention of squamous metaplasia. The BAL had a normal cell count with an abundance of macrophages and no eosinophilia (less than 1%). The patient has made minimal progress thus far and is on 14 cm H_2O PEEP and 55% FIO_2 with marginal oxygenation; however, he remains within the limits of lung-protective mechanical ventilation. What is the most appropriate next step?

A. Consideration for extra-corporeal membrane oxygenation (ECMO) support
B. Lung transplant evaluation
C. Surgical lung biopsy
D. Empiric plasmapheresis and rituximab therapy
E. Salvage therapy with cyclophosphamide

Q17-6: The patient's respiratory status remains tenuous. Given the findings on the CT scan and the laboratory testing, the patient is scheduled for a video-assisted thoracoscopic surgery (VATS) lung biopsy. The result is shown in Image 17-3.

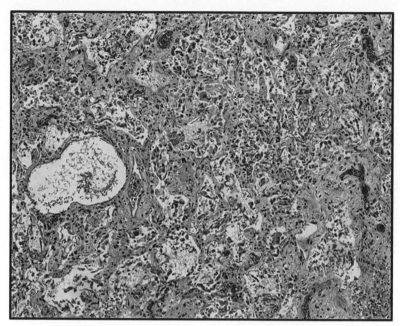

Image 17-3 • Histopathology from patient's lung biopsy in **Case 17**.

What is the most likely diagnosis?

A. Cardiogenic pulmonary edema
B. Lymphangitic spread of an unknown primary malignancy
C. Pulmonary alveolar proteinosis (PAP)
D. Acute interstitial pneumonia (AIP)
E. Cryptogenic organizing pneumonia (COP)
F. Scleroderma-associated interstitial lung disease

Q17-7: What is the primary treatment for patients with AIP?

A. Corticosteroids
B. Cyclophosphamide
C. Vincristine
D. Doxorubicin
E. Anti-TNF-α therapy
F. Supportive care
G. Methotrexate

Q17-8: What percentage of patients with AIP survive beyond the first 3 to 6 months?

A. More than 70%

B. 60%

C. 50%

D. 40%

E. Less than 30%

ANSWERS

Q17-1: C
Bilateral, diffuse reticular and airspace opacities

Rationale: Here, the pattern of abnormalities is diffuse and bilateral, though there may be some lower-lobe predominance present. The abnormalities could be considered reticular or "interstitial" in some areas, while others appear a bit more organized with a question of faint air bronchograms. These latter areas are better characterized as alveolar or airspace opacities. There is no focal consolidation. There may be some linear interstitial opacities present at higher magnification, but the overall pattern is not that of predominant linear opacities. There are no cavitary lesions. Note the prominence of the paratracheal/mediastinal lymph nodes.

Q17-2: C; D; F; G
Diffuse consolidative opacities; Ground-glass opacities; Septal thickening; and Calcified mediastinal adenopathy

Rationale: The distribution of abnormalities is lower-lobe predominant, though there are some ground-glass opacities in the upper lobes. These are peripheral and in dependent areas of the lung. In the lower lobes, the opacities are more organized and opaque, obscuring the underlying lung architecture. There are some air bronchograms (better visualized on sagittal images). There is septal thickening as well. Finally, on the mediastinal windows, one can see completely calcified mediastinal lymph nodes, representing prior granulomatous disease (likely histoplasmosis based on the patient's splenic calcifications).

Q17-3: D
Severe acute respiratory distress syndrome (ARDS)

Rationale: The patient meets the Berlin criteria for a diagnosis of ARDS with the following manifestations: (1) respiratory symptoms resulting from a known insult in the last week *or* new or worsening symptoms in the last week; (2) bilateral opacities on chest imaging not better explained by pleural effusions, atelectasis, or pulmonary nodules/masses; (3) respiratory failure not explained by cardiogenic causes (ie, cardiogenic pulmonary edema); and (4) a PaO_2/FIO_2 ratio (measure of impairment in oxygenation) or less than 300 mm Hg (while on a PEEP of 5 cm H_2O or greater). The laboratory and examination values suggest that cardiogenic pulmonary edema is not the source of the patient's respiratory failure, with a normal echocardiogram aside from LVH, normal IVC collapse, hyperdynamic LV and normal RV function, and a normal BNP value. The PaO_2/FIO_2 value of 65 mm Hg/0.70 is less than 100 mm Hg; this places the patient in the severe category because the patient is on greater than 5 cm H_2O. Mild ARDS is classified as values between 200 and 300 mm Hg, while moderate is between 100 and 200. There is no category termed "very severe" (do not get this confused with the severity of expiratory airflow obstruction on pulmonary function testing). The patient does not have hypercarbic respiratory failure as the $PaCO_2$ is low; rather, this patient has a primary respiratory alkalosis, which is the most common acid-base disorder in ARDS. The CT scan is not entirely consistent with diffuse alveolar hemorrhage (typically more fluffy alveolar infiltrates), and the patient has no risk factors for DAH (stem cell transplantation, use of anticoagulation, vasculitis) or evidence of hemoptysis. Serial lavage during bronchoscopy is most commonly used to confirm this diagnosis.

Q17-4: A
Bronchoscopy with bronchoalveolar lavage and cell count

Rationale: This would be next highest yield study to perform in this patient to discern the cause of his respiratory failure/acute respiratory distress syndrome. Some potential causes of ARDS are infection, drug toxicity, connective tissue disease, transfusion reactions and aspiration; however, a number of other conditions may cause or mimic ARDS and include acute eosinophilic pneumonia, acute hypersensitivity pneumonitis, acute inhalation syndromes, lymphangitic carcinomatosis, diffuse alveolar hemorrhage, atypical presentation of sarcoidosis, and radiation pneumonitis. Bronchoscopy is most useful in ARDS when the etiology remains unclear, which is the case here. The patient's initial testing indicates no bacterial pneumonia, and this is supported by the lack of improvement on broad-spectrum antibiotics. A bronchoscopy with biopsies and lavage would help eliminate several of the aforementioned potential causes, including fungal or viral infection, tuberculosis, diffuse alveolar hemorrhage (serial lavage), acute eosinophilic pneumonia (BAL cell count), aspiration (lack of lipid-laden macrophages), granulomatous disease (sarcoidosis), lymphangitic carcinomatosis (biopsy), drug toxicity, and organizing pneumonia. A barium swallow is not possible because this patient is currently intubated. The serum precipitin study is unfortunately not specific for hypersensitivity pneumonitis, only for prior exposure to an antigen, and in this case, there is no particular antigen to consider. A serum immunoglobulin level would potentially be helpful to rule out common variable immune deficiency (CVID) or an immunocompromised state as well as to evaluate for possible IgG-4 disease; however, IgA deficiency would be unlikely to cause these manifestations. A serum galactomannan level is helpful to make a diagnosis of disseminated aspergillus infection, but it would not be as useful as a bronchoscopy with the aforementioned studies.

Q17-5: C
Surgical lung biopsy

Rationale: This is a difficult situation, and the risk of undergoing a surgical lung biopsy is obviously very high in this patient, with a significant risk of further exacerbating the inflammatory condition. However, of the options available, this would be most appropriate next choice. The patient is currently stable on invasive mechanical ventilation with lung-protective settings, and the use of ECMO in a patient with an unclear etiology for respiratory failure and therefore an unclear trajectory would require a multiteam discussion. Similarly, referral for lung transplant evaluation could be considered, but generally some attempt to obtain a diagnosis would be preferred because some conditions can recur in lung allografts. A case could certainly be made for an empiric course of immunosuppression; however, the first-line immuno-suppressive therapy would more likely be systemic corticosteroids/glucocorticoids. However, it is often advantageous to perform a biopsy before initiation of immuno-suppression because therapy can alter the histopathology and obscure the original diagnosis.

Q17-6: D
Acute interstitial pneumonia (AIP)

Rationale: The pathology demonstrates the classic findings of diffuse alveolar dam-age (DAD). Note the lack of any alveolar space in the specimen, with infiltrating inflammatory cells (predominantly macrophages but also including lymphocytes) and hyaline membrane deposition (gray material) in the interstitial spaces. Hyaline membrane is composed of dead cell debris, protein, and surfactant. The hyaline membranes collect in the interstitium and in alveolar spaces, leading to alveolar col-lapse and interstitial thickening and ultimately to reduced oxygen diffusion. Diffuse alveolar damage is a nonspecific pathologic finding that may be seen in a number of conditions, including ARDS, AIP, acute exacerbations of UIP/IPF, primary graft dysfunction following lung transplantation, and O_2 toxicity. AIP (Hamman-Rich syn-drome) is an idiopathic interstitial pneumonia (IIP) characterized by an acute onset (1-2 weeks) and rapid progression, and it is almost indistinguishable from ARDS. In fact, AIP is essentially idiopathic ARDS (ie, ARDS in which no discernable cause may be identified). Therefore, AIP is a diagnosis of exclusion that requires: (1) a diagnosis of ARDS that is not caused by infection, rheumatologic condition, vasculitis, or other clear pulmonary pathology and (2) a lung biopsy demonstrating diffuse alveolar damage. Here, we have effectively ruled out all other potential causes of the patient's ARDS, and AIP would be an appropriate diagnosis.

Similar to ARDS, AIP likely progresses through an acute inflammatory (exudative) phase, followed by a proliferative phase and, potentially, a fibrotic phase. Unlike patients with ARDS, most patients with AIP progress to the fibrotic phase. During the exudative phase, the histopathology will show massive neutrophil, macrophage, and lymphocyte recruitment to the alveolar space, with the development of leaky alveoli and edema. Additionally, there is deposition of hyaline membranes in the alveolar spaces and in the interstitium. During the proliferative phase, there is dif-fuse fibroblastic proliferation in both the interstitium and alveoli, type II alveolar cell hyperplasia, and the presence of thrombi in pulmonary arterioles. The hyaline mem-brane material can become trapped. AIP tends to show a more significant fibroblastic proliferation that that seen in ARDS. The fibroblast proliferation leads to architec-tural distortion, traction bronchiolectasis, and septal thickening; however, unlike UIP, there is very minimal collagen deposition/fibrosis. This finding helps differenti-ate AIP from UIP. Additionally, pathologically, AIP appears as a single injury event, with a diffuse presentation across the biopsy specimen and a temporal uniformity to the fibrosis; UIP is defined by the scattered areas of disease interspersed with areas of normal lung tissue, and the disease areas shows considerable temporal heterogene-ity, indicating ongoing or repeated insults over time. Acute exacerbation of UIP may appear as AIP on a background of UIP.

There is no clear sex or ethnic predisposition to developing AIP. Similar to the other IIPs, AIP is encountered most commonly in the fourth through sixth decades of life. The clinical presentation is acute to subacute in onset, typically with a 1- to 2-week illness with dyspnea, dry cough, hypoxemia, fatigue, malaise, and fever. As stated previously, the disease progresses rapidly, and patients often require invasive mechanical ventilation. Depending on the disease process stage, the patient may have a normal examination, inspiratory crackles particularly at the bilateral bases, tachypnea, and increased work of breathing. Patients may also present in extremis and require emergency intubation.

On chest radiographs, AIP presents similar to ARDS, with diffuse bilateral airspace opacities and possibly reticulonodular opacities (**Image 17-1**). As the disease progresses and patients develop more chronic changes, there may be a shift toward a more reticular appearance of the chest radiograph (**Image 17-4**). Early in the disease process, CT of the chest shows bilateral, diffuse ground-glass opacities and possible areas of consolidation and septal thickening (**Image 17-2**). Later stages of the disease demonstrate reduced ground glass, which is replaced by areas of consolidation, interstitial/septal thickening, and architectural distortion with traction bronchiectasis (**Image 17-5**). Honeycombing changes in a subpleural distribution may be seen but are generally much more limited than that seen in UIP.

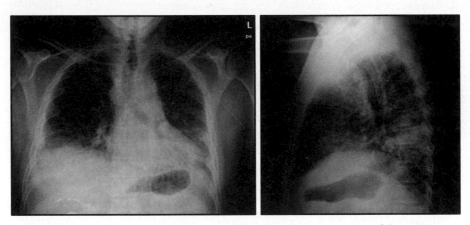

Image 17-4 • Radiograph of the chest 3 weeks after the presentation of the patient in **Case 17.**

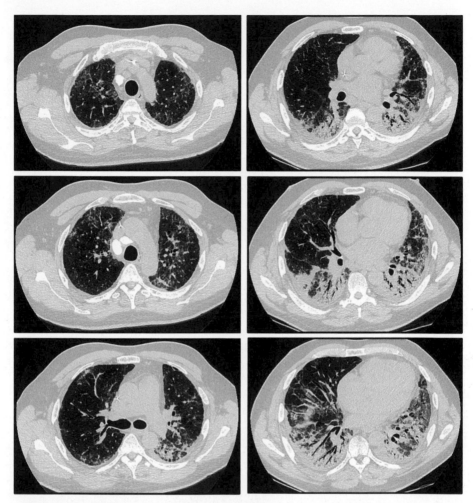

Image 17-5 • CT of the chest 3 weeks after the presentation of the patient in **Case 17**.

Q17-7: F
Supportive care

Rationale: Unfortunately, there is very limited evidence for the use of any immunosuppressive medications in the treatment of AIP. The primary treatment for these patients is supportive care, including broad-spectrum antibiotics, supplemental O_2, and positive-pressure ventilation when necessary. Although high doses of corticosteroids are often used (and are generally recommended by consensus groups such as the American Thoracic Society and the European Respiratory Society), evidence is lacking for their clinical efficacy. Data from small case series suggest a good response to glucocorticoids; however, there are no randomized trials, and comparison to older cohorts does not take into account advances in mechanical ventilation over the last several decades. There are case reports and small series that describe the use of cyclophosphamide and vincristine for treatment as well; however, this is typically salvage therapy, and again, evidence is lacking. A recent case report suggested a role for polymyxin-B-immobilized hemofilter as a possible treatment. Any consideration for advanced immunosuppression beyond a trial of glucocorticoids should be discussed with an advanced lung disease or transplantation specialist. Lung transplantation has been used in patients who survive the initial process.

Q17-8: E
Less than 30%

Rationale: More than 70% to 80% of patients with AIP succumb to illness within the first 3 to 6 months of presentation. The prognosis is very poor overall, and patients who survive the initial process are often left with significantly reduced pulmonary reserve and are at risk for recurrence.

References

Acute Respiratory Distress Syndrome Network; Brower RG, Matthay MA, Morris A, Schoenfeld D, Thompson BT, Wheeler A. Ventilation with lower tidal volumes as compared with traditional tidal volumes for acute lung injury and the acute respiratory distress syndrome. N Engl J Med. 2000;342:1301.

ARDS Definition Task Force. Ranieri VM, Rubenfeld GD, Thompson BT, et al. Acute respiratory distress syndrome: the Berlin Definition. JAMA. 2012;307:2526.

Avnon LS, Pikovsky O, Sion-Vardy N, Almog Y. Acute interstitial pneumonia-Hamman-Rich syndrome: clinical characteristics and diagnostic and therapeutic considerations. Anesth Analg. 2009;108:232.

Bonaccorsi A, Cancellieri A, Chilosi M, et al. Acute interstitial pneumonia: report of a series. Eur Respir J. 2003;21:187.

Bouros D, Nicholson AC, Polychronopoulos V, du Bois RM. Acute interstitial pneumonia. Eur Respir J. 2000;15(2):412.

Hamman L, Rich AR. Fulminating diffuse interstitial fibrosis of the lungs. Trans Am Clin Climatol Assoc. 1935;51:154.

Ichikado K, Johkoh T, Ikezoe J, et al. Acute interstitial pneumonia: high-resolution CT findings correlated with pathology. AJR Am J Roentgenol. 1997;168:333.

Ichikado K. High-resolution computed tomography findings of acute respiratory distress syndrome, acute interstitial pneumonia, and acute exacerbation of idiopathic pulmonary fibrosis. Semin Ultrasound CT MR. 2014;35:39.

Johkoh T, Müller NL, Taniguchi H, et al. Acute interstitial pneumonia: thin-section CT findings in 36 patients. Radiology. 1999;211:859.

Katzenstein AL, Myers JL, Mazur MT. Acute interstitial pneumonia. A clinicopathologic, ultrastructural, and cell kinetic study. Am J Surg Pathol. 1986;10:256.

Katzenstein AL, Myers JL. Idiopathic pulmonary fibrosis: clinical relevance of pathologic classification. Am J Respir Crit Care Med. 1998;157:1301.

Olson J, Colby TV, Elliott CG. Hamman-Rich syndrome revisited. Mayo Clin Proc. 1990;65:1538.

Primack SL, Hartman TE, Ikezoe J, Akira M, Sakatani M, Müller NL. Acute interstitial pneumonia: radiographic and CT findings in nine patients. Radiology. 1993;188:817.

Robinson DS, Geddes DM, Hansell DM, Shee CD, Corbishley C, Murday A, Madden BP. Partial resolution of acute interstitial pneumonia in native lung after single lung transplantation. Thorax. 1996;51:1158.

Suda T, Kaida Y, Nakamura Y, et al. Acute exacerbation of interstitial pneumonia associated with collagen vascular diseases. Respir Med. 2009;103:846.

Travis WD, Costabel U, Hansell DM, et al; ATS/ERS Committee on Idiopathic Interstitial Pneumonias. An official American Thoracic Society/European Respiratory Society statement: update of the international multidisciplinary classification of the idiopathic interstitial pneumonias. Am J Respir Crit Care Med. 2013;188:733.

Vourlekis JS, Brown KK, Cool CD, et al. Acute interstitial pneumonitis. Case series and review of the literature. Medicine (Baltimore). 2000;79:369.

Vourlekis JS. Acute interstitial pneumonia. Clin Chest Med. 2004;25:739.

CASE 18

A 40-year-old man presents with progressive symptoms of dyspnea and an abnormal CXR, referred from his primary care physician. He is former smoker (0.25 packs per day for 15 years, though he quit 9 months ago at onset of symptoms) and exercises regularly. He reports the gradual onset of dyspnca on exertion over the last 6 to 9 months, which has been impacting his exercise tolerance. He was running 5 miles three to four times a week but now feels like he has difficulty completing more than 1 to 2 miles twice a week. He does not use illicit drugs or drink alcohol. He has no other associated symptoms except a dry cough and some mild fatigue. He specifically denies any fevers, chills, sweats, or hemoptysis. He has no other significant medical history and takes no other medications. He denies any environmental or occupational exposures and is currently working as a teacher in a local high school. He has no recent sick contacts. The patient's vital signs are T 36.4°C, HR 78, BP 123/56, RR 18, oxygen saturation 93% on room air. The results of a full set of laboratory studies from his primary physician, including a CBC, chemistry panel, cardiac biomarkers, BNP, and d-Dimer, were within normal limits. An ECG demonstrated no abnormalities, and an ECG showed no evidence of right- or left-sided heart failure or valvular disease. His examination demonstrates scattered inspiratory crackles throughout on both the left and right.

His CXR is shown in Image 18-1.

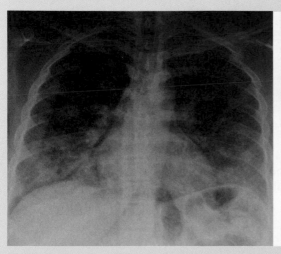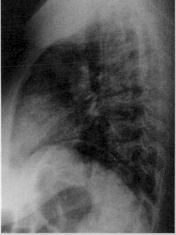

Image 18-1 • Chest Radiographs (PA and lateral) for the patient in **Question 18-1**.

QUESTIONS

Q18-1: **How would you described the abnormalities on the CXR?**

A. Reticular opacities most prominent in bilateral lower lobes
B. Focal consolidation in the right lower and middle lobes
C. Linear interstitial opacities
D. Diffuse alveolar opacities
E. Numerous cavitary lung lesions

Q18-2: **The patient undergoes a CT scan of the chest because of the abnormalities, which is shown in Image 18-2. How would you describe the abnormalities?**

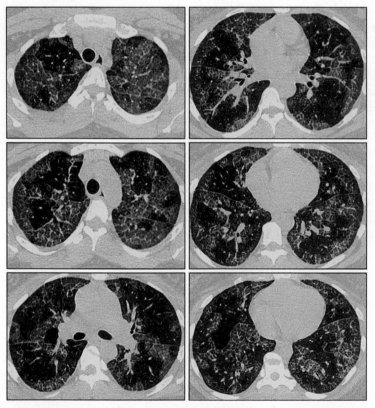

Image 18-2 • Chest CT images for the patient in **Question 18-2**.

A. Diffuse ground-glass opacities
B. Honeycombing and traction bronchiectasis
C. Smooth interlobular and intralobular septal thickening
D. Cystic lung lesions
E. A and B
F. A and C
G. B and C
H. B and D

Q18-3: How is the patient's constellation of findings on CT generally described?

A. Mosaic pattern
B. Miliary pattern
C. Crazy paving
D. Usual interstitial pneumonia (UIP)

Q18-4: Based on this patient's presentation, what is the most likely diagnosis?

A. Acute respiratory distress syndrome (ARDS)
B. Radiation pneumonitis
C. Cardiogenic pulmonary edema
D. Idiopathic pulmonary fibrosis (IPF)
E. Pulmonary alveolar proteinosis (PAP)
F. Emphysema

Q18-5: The patient has a normal CBC, and there is no evidence of a monoclonal gammopathy on protein electrophoresis. The patient denies any occupational history in which he was exposed to dusts, aerosols, or vapors. Which test would you recommend next to confirm the diagnosis of PAP?

A. Bronchoscopy with transbronchial biopsy and bronchoalveolar lavage
B. Open lung biopsy
C. Right and left heart catheterization
D. Induced sputum cultures for bacteria, AFB, and fungal cultures
E. Cryptococcal serum antigen test
F. Ventilation–perfusion (VQ) scan

Q18-6: Antibodies against which of the following is commonly associated the autoimmune form of PAP?

A. Colony stimulating factor (CSF)
B. Granulocyte-Monocyte colony stimulating factor (GM-CSF)
C. Interleukin-6 (IL-6)
D. CFTR
E. Surfactant protein A (SP-A)

Q18-7: What is the primary treatment for patient with PAP who develop symptoms of respiratory impairment?

A. Corticosteroids
B. Antibiotics
C. Immunosuppression
D. Whole lung lavage (WLL)
E. Lung transplantation

ANSWERS

Q18-1: A
Reticular opacities most prominent in the bilateral lower lobes

Rationale: There is the appearance of reticular (net-like) opacities versus a miliary pattern in the bilateral lower lobes. There is no evidence of cavitary lung lesions or focal consolidations on the chest imaging. The appearance of the opacities is more reticular in appearance, and the opacities are not consistent with a diffuse alveolar filling process. There is no evidence of pleural effusions, pneumothorax, hilar adenopathy, or cardiomegaly.

Q18-2: F
Options (A) Diffuse ground-glass opacities and (C) Smooth interlobular and intralobular septal thickening

Rationale: There are no cysts present, and there is no evidence of traction bronchiectasis or honeycombing throughout the lung fields. This will be further clarified in the question.

Q18-3: C
Crazy paving

Rationale: The combination of (1) diffuse ground-glass opacities and (2) associated, smooth interlobular and intralobular septal thickening is often referred to as "crazy paving" because it gives the appearance of a nonlinear city road pattern if viewed from far above (such as a satellite image). This is a nonspecific finding overall and can be associated with a number of different conditions. A miliary pattern generally refers a diffuse micronodular pattern. UIP is a radiographic finding that, in the appropriate clinical context, can confirm a diagnosis of IPF. The Fleischner Society recently updated the diagnostic criteria for UIP, which includes definitions for typical UIP, probable UIP, indeterminate for UIP, and most consistent with non-IPF diagnosis. The most common features in UIP are subpleural (occurring less than 1 cm from the pleural surface) reticular opacities (interlobular and intralobular septal thickening in a net-like pattern) and honeycombing, usually in a basal-predominant pattern.

Q18-4: F
Pulmonary alveolar proteinosis (PAP)

Rationale: The patient presents with a slowly progressive process with worsening dyspnea on exertion, a mild nonproductive cough, and findings of crazy paving on a CT scan. Although crazy paving can be associated with a wide variety of conditions (ARDS, eosinophilic pneumonia, pulmonary edema, cryptogenic organizing pneumonia, sarcoidosis), none of the other diagnoses provided seem to fit here.

PAP is caused by the abnormal accumulation of lipoproteinaceous material (predominantly surfactant phospholipids) in distal airways and the alveoli. This material will stain positive on PAS (periodic acid-Schiff) staining. The pathogenesis will be discussed further below. Although there are congenital or hereditary forms of PAP that may present in childhood, cases of acquired PAP that present in adulthood typically present between the ages of 30 and 50, with a male predominance. Overall, the severity of changes in chest imaging in PAP far outweigh the severity of the clinical presentation. On CXR, PAP can present with a number of different findings, including batwing pulmonary edema, a miliary pattern of nodular opacities, and reticular or reticulonodular opacities. Patients with a long-standing history of poorly-controlled PAP may also have evidence of scarring or fibrosis. Although PAP most commonly presents with crazy paving on CT, it can also present with focal consolidation. Scarring in the form of fibrosis is rare, but it can be seen in patients with long-standing disease and those who have gone for long periods without appropriate therapy. PFT typically shows a reduced DLCO and, occasionally, some degree of restriction. Patients generally have an elevated A-a gradient as well. Patients may be asymptomatic at the time of presentation (due to abnormalities on chest imaging), but many patients present with progressive dyspnea over a period of months to years. Patients may also note a dry or productive cough and, more rarely, weight loss and fever. The latter symptoms may herald a bacterial (mycoplasma, legionella, nocardia), mycobacterial (either tuberculous or nontuberculous), or fungal (aspergillus, *Pneumocystis jiroveci* pneumonia [PCP]PCP) superinfection, which can accelerate the accumulation of surfactant. On examination, the presence of inspiratory crackles generally correlates with the severity of abnormalities on chest imaging.

With regard to the other diagnoses, there is no evidence of cardiogenic edema on any other study or on examination, and the patient has a normal BNP. The patient has no history of radiation exposure or prior cancer history to suggest such. To consider a diagnosis of IPF here, one would need to consider whether a UIP pattern is found on CT. Although there is smooth interlobar interlobular septal thickening (reticulations), the lack of traction bronchiectasis suggests no significant fibrosis, and the predominant ground-glass opacifications seen would be atypical (unless the patient were in the midst of an acute exacerbation of IPF). This would likely be classified as a CT with features most consistent with non-IPF diagnosis. Additionally, there is no evidence of either centrilobular or panlobular emphysema on the CT imaging to suggest emphysema. Other conditions that could be considered here would include an atypical infection (viral, mycoplasma), *P. jirovecii* infection, nontuberculous mycobacterial infection, sarcoidosis (atypical alveolar sarcoidosis), pulmonary veno-occlusive disease (PVOD), lipoid pneumonia, diffuse alveolar hemorrhage, drug-induced pneumonitis, cryptogenic organizing pneumonia, and chronic eosinophilic pneumonia.

Q18-5: A
Bronchoscopy with transbronchial biopsies and bronchoalveolar lavage

Rationale: In this patient, we have a general suspicion for PAP as the primary cause of his dyspnea and chest imaging abnormalities.

Q18-6: B
GM-CSF

Rationale:. GM-CSF regulates the ability of type II alveolar cells to turnover pulmonary surfactant. In terms of causes, PAP may be hereditary or congenital (mutations in surfactant protein and GM-CSF receptors), auto-immune (antibodies against GM-CSF), secondary to hematologic malignancies, HIV, PCP, or other autoimmune disorders, or secondary to environmental or occupational exposures. A diagnosis of PAP can be obtained by bronchoscopy, but the critical factor is determining the underlying cause.

Q18-7: D
Whole lung lavage (WLL)

Rationale: Patients with PAP should undergo routine surveillance for evidence of disease progression, including clinical assessment, evaluation for hypoxemia with exercise and at rest, pulmonary function testing, and thoracic imaging. Patients who remain asymptomatic and are without other objective evidence of accelerated pulmonary function decline do not require intervention, although avoidance of pulmonary infections or use of systemic steroids should be encouraged. If the patient has what is presumed to be PAP secondary to an occupational exposure, avoidance of the known precipitant or use of appropriate personal protective equipment is appropriate. When patients with PAP develop respiratory symptoms or demonstrate evidence of accelerated pulmonary function decline or hypoxemia, the primary treatment option is whole lung lavage (WLL). This is not without risk. The procedure requires the patient to undergo general anesthesia during which a double lumen endotracheal tube is placed to allow for individual lung ventilation. One lung is then lavage with approximately 10-20 times with 1-1.5 liters volumes of warmed normal saline. After instillation of the saline, chest percussion and/or bag-mask ventilation of the lavaged lung, and after approximately 5 minutes the saline is removed by using both postural drainage techniques and a flexible bronchoscope. Initially, the lavage fluid will appear milky, but by the end of the procedure the drained saline should appear clear. The same procedure is then performed on the opposite lung, typically in one to two weeks time. Clearly, the patient must be able to appropriately oxygenate and ventilate with single lung ventilation to allow for the first lung to be lavaged. In some centers, hyperbaric oxygen chambers or even extracorporeal membrane oxygenation (ECMO) have been used to allow for lavage of both lungs on the same encounter, or to allow for more unstable patients to tolerate the procedure. Some patient's may only require one treatment during their lifetime, while others may require multiple WLL sessions. Antibiotics are not the first line therapy for symptomatic PAP, however, pulmonary infections increase secretion of pulmonary surfactant and can worsening PAP, so antibiotics should be administered quickly if there are signs or symptoms of infection. Similarly, corticosteroids increase surfactant production, and should be avoided. As some cases of PAP are caused by an autoimmune disorder, yielding anti-GM-CSF antibodies, immunosuppression is appropriate thought. There is some initial evidence that rituximab (anti-CD20 antibody) has some efficacy in the treatment of PAP, but this has not been substantiated in further studies and rituximab is not indicated for the treatment of PAP at this time. No other immunosuppressive has been shown to improve outcomes in PAP. Lung transplantation is reserved for patients who develop significant, irreversible lung damage resulting from PAP, although the disease may recur in the allograft.

More recently, there have been studies examining the use of recombinant GM-CSF, utilizing either a subcutaneous or inhaled route of administration. These studies have generally shown some improvement in pulmonary function and some reduction in ant-GM-CSF antibody levels. While this therapy has not yet been approved for use in PAP at the time of publication of this case, clinicians should continue to monitor developments in this area.

References

Beccaria M, Luisetti M, Rodi G, et al. Long-term durable benefit after whole lung lavage in pulmonary alveolar proteinosis. Eur Respir J. 2004;23:526.

Bonfield TL, Kavuru MS, Thomassen MJ. Anti-GM-CSF titer predicts response to GM-CSF therapy in pulmonary alveolar proteinosis. Clin Immunol. 2002;105:342.

Borie R, Debray MP, Laine C, et al. Rituximab therapy in autoimmune pulmonary alveolar proteinosis. Eur Respir J. 2009;33:1503.

Chew R, Nigam S, Sivakumaran P. Alveolar proteinosis associated with aluminium dust inhalation. Occup Med (Lond). 2016;66:492.

Cummings KJ, Donat WE, Ettensohn DB, et al. Pulmonary alveolar proteinosis in workers at an indium processing facility. Am J Respir Crit Care Med. 2010;181:458.

Gaine SP, O'Marcaigh AS. Pulmonary alveolar proteinosis: lung transplant or bone marrow transplant? Chest. 1998;113:563.

Gay P, Wallaert B, Nowak S, et al. Efficacy of Whole-Lung Lavage in Pulmonary Alveolar Proteinosis: A Multicenter International Study of GELF. Respiration. 2017;93:198.

Kavuru MS, Sullivan EJ, Piccin R, et al. Exogenous granulocyte-macrophage colony-stimulating factor administration for pulmonary alveolar proteinosis. Am J Respir Crit Care Med. 2000;161:1143.

Khan A, Agarwal R, Aggarwal AN. Effectiveness of granulocyte-macrophage colony-stimulating factor therapy in autoimmune pulmonary alveolar proteinosis: a meta-analysis of observational studies. Chest. 2012;141:1273.

Kumar A, Abdelmalak B, Inoue Y, Culver DA. Pulmonary alveolar proteinosis in adults: pathophysiology and clinical approach. Lancet Respir Med. 2018;6:554.

Latzin P, Tredano M, Wüst Y, et al. Anti-GM-CSF antibodies in paediatric pulmonary alveolar proteinosis. Thorax. 2005;60:39.

Malur A, Kavuru MS, Marshall I, et al. Rituximab therapy in pulmonary alveolar proteinosis improves alveolar macrophage lipid homeostasis. Respir Res. 2012;13:46.

Robinson TE, Trapnell BC, Goris ML, et al. Quantitative analysis of longitudinal response to aerosolized granulocyte-macrophage colony-stimulating factor in two adolescents with autoimmune pulmonary alveolar proteinosis. Chest. 2009;135:842.

Shah PL, Hansell D, Lawson PR, et al. Pulmonary alveolar proteinosis: clinical aspects and current concepts on pathogenesis. Thorax. 2000;55:67.

Soyez B, Borie R, Menard C, et al. Rituximab for auto-immune alveolar proteinosis, a real life cohort study. Respir Res. 2018;19:74.

Sui X, Du Q, Xu KF, et al. Quantitative assessment of Pulmonary Alveolar Proteinosis (PAP) with ultra-dose CT and correlation with Pulmonary Function Tests (PFTs). PLoS One. 2017;12:e0172958.

Suzuki T, Trapnell BC. Pulmonary Alveolar Proteinosis Syndrome. Clin Chest Med. 2016;37:431.

Takaki M, Tanaka T, Komohara Y, et al. Recurrence of pulmonary alveolar proteinosis after bilateral lung transplantation in a patient with a nonsense mutation in CSF2RB. Respir Med Case Rep. 2016;19:89.

Tazawa R, Ueda T, Abe M, et al. Inhaled GM-CSF for Pulmonary Alveolar Proteinosis. N Engl J Med. 2019;381:923.

Venkateshiah SB, Yan TD, Bonfield TL, et al. An open-label trial of granulocyte macrophage colony stimulating factor therapy for moderate symptomatic pulmonary alveolar proteinosis. Chest. 2006;130:227.

CASE 19

A 44-year-old Black man presents to the clinic for evaluation after being referred by his primary care provider. He had an abnormal chest radiograph and hence was referred to the pulmonary clinic for evaluation. He has noted some progressively worsening dyspnea on exertion and a productive cough, which is usually clear, but he has been treated multiple times in the past 3 to 4 years for episodes of "pneumonia" by various urgent care centers. He has no other associated symptoms aside from generalized fatigue and a possible 3- to 4-lb weight loss over the last year, though he states his weight waxes and wanes. He has no significant medical history, and he has never smoked or used illicit drugs. He served in the military for approximately 3 years but was never overseas or on a navy vessel, and he has no known exposures. He reports no family history of pulmonary disease, malignancy, or rheumatologic disease. His BMI is 19 kg/m². He is tall and thin. He requires no O_2 at rest or with activity. His vitals are T 36.7 °C, HR 67, BP 119/71. He has no tachypnea. His cardiac examination is normal, and his pulmonary examination demonstrates bronchovesicular and vesicular crackles. He has slight clubbing as well. His CXR is shown in Image 19-1.

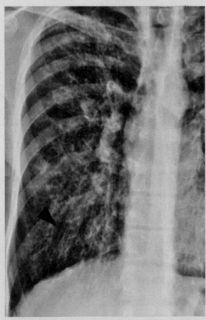

Image 19-1 • Chest radiograph (PA, magnified view of right airspace) for the patient in **Question 19-1**. (*Reproduced with permission from Chiarenza A, Ultimo LE, Falsaperla D, et al: Chest imaging using signs, symbols, and naturalistic images: a practical guide for radiologists and non-radiologists, Insights Imaging 2019 Dec 4;10(1):114.*)

QUESTIONS

Q19-1: How would you describe the abnormality indicated by the black arrow-head in Image 19-1?

A. Reticulonodular opacity
B. Alveolar infiltrate
C. Pleural thickening
D. Hyperinflation
E. Bronchial thickening
F. Atelectasis

Q19-2: The patient was sent for a CT scan, shown in Image 19-2.

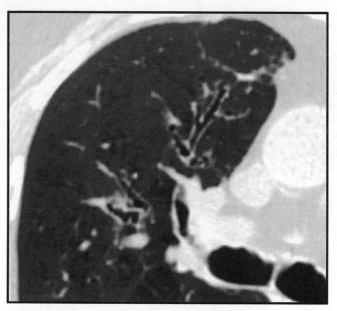

Image 19-2 • Chest CT images for the patient in **Question 19-2**.

What abnormalities are present on the CT scan?

A. Cystic lung lesions
B. Lobar atelectasis
C. Cavitary lung lesions with air-fluid levels
D. Cylindrical bronchiectasis
E. Empyema

Q19-3: Which flow-volume loop is most consistent with a patient with bronchiectasis (Image 19-3)?

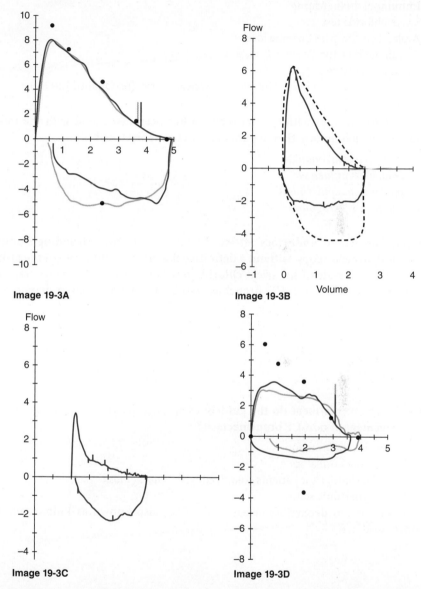

Image 19-3A

Image 19-3B

Image 19-3C

Image 19-3D

Image 19-3 • A and D, (*Reproduced with permission from McKean S, Ross JJ, Dressler DD, et al: Principles and Practice of Hospital Medicine, 2nd ed. New York NY: McGraw Hill; 2017.*)

Q19-4: Which test would be the most appropriate to obtain next to determine the etiology of the pulmonary disease?

A. Immunoglobulin testing
B. Sweat chloride test
C. Alpha-1-antitrypsin enzyme level
D. Rheumatoid factor
E. Nasal nitric oxide
F. *Mycobacterium tuberculosis* interferon-γ release assay (ie, QuantiFERON)

Q19-5: Colonization with which organism has been associated with the most rapid decline in lung function in patients with bronchiectasis?

A. *Streptococcus pneumoniae*
B. *Haemophilus influenzae*
C. *Staphylococcus epidermidis*
D. *Pseudomonas aeruginosa*

Q19-6: The patient undergoes extensive laboratory testing, including sputum testing and bronchoscopy, without a definitive diagnosis as the cause of the bronchiectasis. The result of his sweat chloride test is normal. What percentage of cases of non-cystic fibrosis (CF) bronchiectasis fail to have an etiology diagnosed?

A. 0% to 5%
B. 5% to 10%
C. 25% to 50%
D. 75% to 100%
E. 80% to 90%

Q19-7: Which treatment do the guidelines specifically recommend against in the management of non-CF bronchiectasis?

A. Pulmonary rehabilitation
B. Inhaled bronchodilators
C. Inhaled antibiotics for patients colonized with *P. aeruginosa*
D. Inhaled hypertonic saline
E. Inhaled human deoxyribonuclease (rhDNase, also known as Pulmozyme or dornase alfa)

ANSWERS

Q19-1: E
Bronchial thickening

Rationale: The black arrowhead denotes the appearance of "tram-tracks," which represent bronchial and bronchiolar wall thickening.

Q19-2: D
Cylindrical bronchiectasis

Rationale: To evaluate for bronchiectasis, one must compare the luminal diameter of the airway with the diameter of the adjacent vessel on high-resolution CT of the chest. Bronchiectasis is defined as a luminal airway diameter of 1½ times the diameter of the adjacent vessel. There are multiple types of bronchiectasis, including varicose, cylindrical, and cystic or saccular, with examples shown in **Image 19-4** and **19-5**. Another imaging finding in bronchiectasis is the "signet ring" finding, also shown in **Image 19-6.** Bronchiectasis and bronchial wall thickening may also produce a tram-track appearance on chest radiography, as is seen in **Image 19-1**.

Patients with bronchiectasis often have a history of recurrent respiratory infections and report a chronic cough that produces sputum. Dyspnea is also common, but it is not universal. A high-resolution CT scan of the chest that reveals abnormal dilatation of the airways in this clinical context confirms a diagnosis of bronchiectasis. Bronchiectasis is more commonly seen in women and in patients of advanced age.

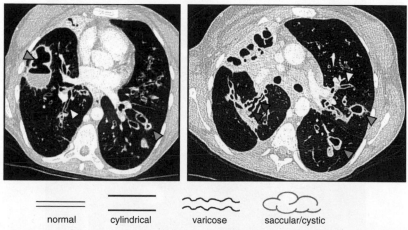

Image 19-4 • Examples of different morphologies of bronchiectasis: cyclindrical bronchiectasis (white arrows), varicose bronchiectasis (dark blue arrows); and saccular or cystic bronchiectasis (light blue arrows). All three morphologies may be present in the same patient, as is seen here. In cylindrical bronchiectasis, there is bronchial wall thickening, with an increased airway diameter; however, the airways appear relatively linear. In varicose bronchiectasis, the airways have an irregular and tortuous course, and there may be a heterogeneous distribution of dilitation along the tract of the airway. In cystic or saccular bronchiectasis, the bronchi appear as clusters of cystic or saccular structures.

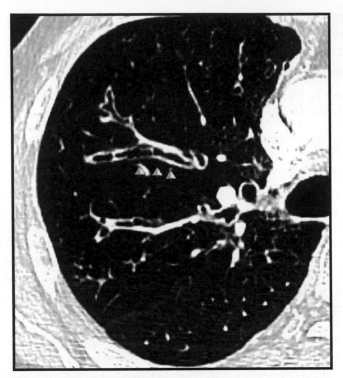

Image 19-5 • Cylindrical bronchiectasis.

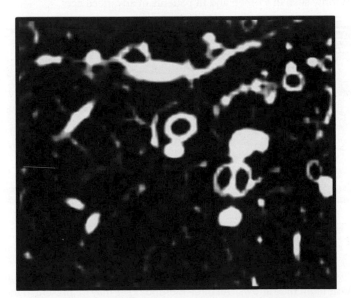

Image 19-6 • The signet ring finding often seen in bronchiectasis.

Q19-3:
Image 19-3C

Rationale: The flow-volume loop depicted in **Image 19-3A** is a normal flow-volume loop with a nearly linear decrease in flow as the lung volume decreases during expiration and with a normal inspiratory flow pattern. The flow-volume loop depicted in **Image 19-3B** has a nearly normal expiratory portion with an abnormal inspiratory portion, consistent with an extrathoracic obstruction, likely a lesion in the upper airway (or at least outside of the thoracic cavity). **Image 19-3C** shows a typical obstructive flow volume loop, where the airflow reduces nonlinearly with reducing lung volumes during expiration ("scooping" of the flow-volume curve), similar to someone with an airway-centric disease process such as COPD or bronchiectasis. **Image 19-3D** has variable obstruction during expiration (note that the line oscillates, with some portions increasing with reducing lung volumes), which is consistent with a variable intrathoracic obstruction, such as an intraluminal mass with ball-valve action. This is a possible finding in a patient with focal bronchiectasis due to a bronchial obstruction, but this patient has a more diffuse process. Bronchiectasis may present with a normal flow-volume loop initially, though many patients will have flow-volume loops consistent with obstruction. Patients with severe disease will usually develop restrictive disease as the disease progresses and the patient develops scarring. A reduced DLCO is common as the disease progresses as well.

Q19-4: B
Sweat chloride test

Rationale: Cystic fibrosis remains the most common cause of bronchiectasis in the United States. Although the presentation is atypical, patients can present later in life with more mild mutations that result in residual *CFTR* activity, and therefore a sweat chloride test should be sent for this patient. The remainder of the testing is also appropriate. Bronchiectasis can result from prior infections or exposures, current indolent infections such as nontuberculous mycobacteria (NTM), congenital disorders such as primary ciliary dyskinesia (nasal nitric oxide testing), autoimmune disorders (particularly rheumatoid arthritis or inflammatory bowel disease), A1AT, immunodeficiency (immunoglobulin deficiencies, particularly IgG_2; HIV), COPD, or a complication of aspergillus sensitivity in a process called *allergic bronchopulmonary aspergillosis* (ABPA). At a minimum, in the evaluation of bronchiectasis, patients should have a CBC with differential and serum immunoglobulins checked, as well as an evaluation for ABPA. Sputum cultures may also be of value.

Q19-5: D
Pseudomonas aeruginosa

Rationale: *P. aeruginosa* colonization is associated with the greatest reduction in lung function and more severe chronic lung damage than in patients without colonization. Although *H. influenzae* and *S. pneumoniae* colonization can occur, they are often less virulent. And while *S. aureus* colonization can be associated with significant lung damage, *S. epidermidis* is an uncommon colonizer of the airway.

Q19-6: C
25% to 50%

Rationale: Between 25% and 50% of cases of non-CF bronchiectasis fail to have an etiology established and are termed "idiopathic."

Q19-7: E
Inhaled human deoxyribonuclease (rhDNase, also known as Pulmozyme or dornase alfa)

Rationale: Pulmonary rehabilitation is recommended for all patients with bronchiectasis who have dyspnea that interferes with their ability to perform their activities of daily living. Inhaled bronchodilators are recommended in patients with dyspnea and evidence of airflow obstruction. Inhaled corticosteroids are not recommended except in those patients with asthma or COPD, where inhaled corticosteroids may be indicated. In patients colonized with *P. aeruginosa* who have three or more bronchiectasis exacerbations per year, long-term inhaled antibiotics are recommended. Airway clearance techniques, including the use of hypertonic saline, are recommended. These therapies are designed to prevent exacerbations of bronchiectasis, which are associated with an accelerated decline in lung function, increased mortality, and a lower quality of life. Inhaled rhDNase is associated with a higher rate of exacerbations in patients with non-CF bronchiectasis and with a decrease in FEV1 and is therefore not recommended in the management of patients with non-CF bronchiectasis.

References

Chiarenza A, Ultimo LE, Falsaperla D, et al. Chest imaging using signs, symbols, and naturalistic images: a practical guide for radiologists and non-radiologists. Insights Imaging. 2019;10:114.

Contarini M, Finch S, Chalmers JD. Bronchiectasis: a case-based approach to investigation and management. Eur Respir Rev. 2018;27:180016.

Miaskiewicz JJ. Pulmonary function testing. In: Principles and Practice of Hospital Medicine, 2nd ed, McKean SC, Ross JJ, Dressler DD, Scheurer DB (Eds), McGraw-Hill, 2017.

O'Donnell AE, Barker AF, Ilowite JS, et al. Treatment of idiopathic bronchiectasis with aerosolized recombinant human DNase I. Chest. 1998;113:1329.

Pasteur MC, Bilton D, Hill AT. British Thoracic Society guideline for non-CF bronchiectasis. Thorax. 2010;65:i1.

Polverino E, Goeminne PC, McDonnell MJ, et al. European Respiratory Society guidelines for the management of adult bronchiectasis. Eur Respir J. 2017;50:1700629.

CASE 20

A 45-year-old man presents to the ED reporting fever, productive cough, dyspnea, and some mild chest pain on the right. He has a history of right lower lobe lung adenocarcinoma, stage Ib. The patient recently completed concurrent chemotherapy and radiation therapy; the chemotherapy regimen included platinum- and taxane-based drugs in addition to pembrolizumab immunotherapy. He completed his radiation treatments (6 weeks in duration, a total of 70 Gy to the primary target) 6 weeks ago. He completed four cycles of chemotherapy as well. He denies any sick contacts recently and has no constitutional symptoms currently. He denies any hemoptysis, abdominal pain, skin changes, nausea, emesis, or diarrhea. He notes the onset of symptoms just about a week before presentation. He is not currently working, and he has no known occupational or environmental exposures. He denies any tobacco or drug use and denies any aspiration events at home. On examination, he requires 4 L NC at rest and 6 L NC with activity; at baseline, the patient has no O_2 requirement either at rest or with activity. He has a normal cardiovascular examination and has some moderate crackles and bronchial breath sounds on the right. The patient's vital signs are T 101.3°F, HR 122, BP 108/55, RR 23, and saturation 93% on 4 L/min supplemental O_2 at rest, which drops to 85% with activity, requiring 6 L/min supplemental O_2.

The patient's chest radiograph is shown in Image 20-1.

QUESTIONS

Q20-1: How would you describe the abnormalities seen on the CXR?

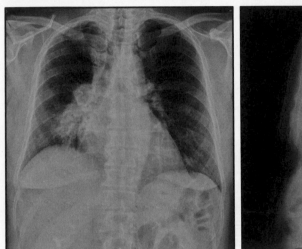 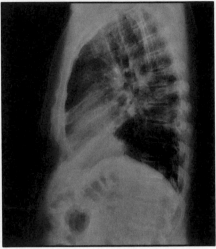

Image 20-1 • Chest radiograph for the patient in **Case 20**.

A. Reticulonodular interstitial opacities
B. Linear interstitial opacities
C. Hilar adenopathy
D. Opacification or consolidation
E. Alveolar infiltrates
F. Atelectasis

Q20-2: The patient undergoes a CTA, which shows no evidence of a pulmonary embolism, though it does reveal the abnormality shown in Image 20-2.

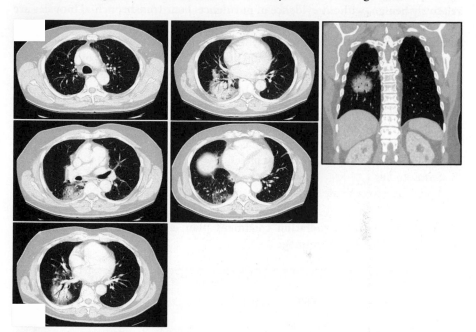

Image 20-2 • Chest CT for the patient in **Case 20**.

How would you describe the abnormalities in the CT scan in Image 20-2?

A. Cavitary lung lesion
B. Consolidation surrounded by ground-glass opacities (reverse-halo sign)
C. Ground-glass opacities surrounded by an area of consolidation (halo sign)
D. Rounded atelectasis in the right lower lobe
E. Tree-in-dub opacities in the right lower lobe
F. Crazy paving

20-3: Which diagnosis would be an appropriate differential diagnosis for the patient?

A. Idiopathic pulmonary fibrosis (IPF), nonspecific interstitial pneumonia (NSIP), cryptogenic organizing pneumonia (COP), and infection
B. Drug-induced toxicity, radiation pneumonitis, cryptogenic organizing pneumonia (COP), and infection
C. Radiation fibrosis, drug toxicity, infection, and anterior mediastinal mass (thymoma)
D. Sarcoidosis, radiation fibrosis, infection, drug toxicity, and nonspecific interstitial pneumonia

Q20-4: The patient is admitted to the inpatient service and is started on broad-spectrum antibiotics. He undergoes a bronchoscopy with lavage, which appears relatively benign, without evidence of purulence. Four transbronchial biopsies are performed, which show no evidence of organizing pneumonia or granulomatous inflammation. There is also no evidence of lymphangitic spread of adenocarcinoma. He is started on broad-spectrum antibiotics, and a number of cultures are currently pending. Special stains for fungal and acid fast bacilli (AFB) elements are negative. In the meantime, what would be the next step in his evaluation?

A. Echocardiogram
B. CT scan of the abdomen and pelvis to evaluate for other sources of infection
C. MRI of the brain to evaluate for metastatic disease
D. Review of the radiation treatment plan
E. Stool studies
F. Endoscopy to evaluate for a tracheoesophageal fistula (TEF)

Q20-5: The patient's radiation treatment plan is provided by the radiation oncologist and is shown in Image 20-3.

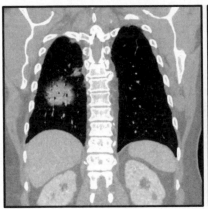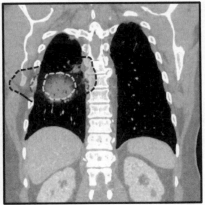

Image 20-3 • Isodose mapping from the patient's lung cancer radiation therapy using image-guided radiation therapy. The gray outline represents the volume of tissue receiving 20 Gy, the black circle 30 Gy, and the white circle 70 Gy.

The results of the patient's silver stain, KOH stain, and Gram stain are negative. A *Pneumocystis jirovecii* pneumonia (PCP) polymerase chain reaction (PCR) is also negative. A beta-D-glucan test returns within normal limits.

What is the most likely diagnosis?

A. Radiation pneumonitis
B. Cytomegalovirus (CMV) pneumonia
C. Radiation fibrosis
D. Fungal pneumonia
E. Radiation pleuritis
F. Pneumocystis pneumonia
G. Radiation-induced bronchial stenosis

Q20-6: What would be the next course of action?

A. Captopril
B. Weight-based glucocorticoids (0.5 to 1 mg/kg prednisone or equivalent daily)
C. Methotrexate
D. Cyclophosphamide
E. *N*-acetylcysteine (NAC)

Q20-7: What is the relationship between mean lung radiation dose (in Gy) and the probability of developing radiation pneumonitis?

A. There is no relationship between the total mean lung dose and the risk of radiation pneumonitis.
B. There is an inverse relationship between the total mean lung dose and the risk of radiation pneumonitis.
C. There is a positive relationship between the total mean lung dose and the risk of radiation pneumonitis.
D. The risk of radiation pneumonitis is more dependent on the administration of concurrent chemotherapy than on total mean lung radiation dose.
E. The risk of radiation pneumonitis is more dependent on the administration of concurrent immunotherapy than on the total mean lung radiation dose.

Q20-8: What are risk factors for the development of RILI? Select all that apply.

A. Concurrent treatment with chemotherapy
B. Smoking tobacco use
C. Underlying structural lung disease, including interstitial lung disease (ILD) or COPD
D. Concurrent treatment with immunotherapy
E. Male genetic sex
F. Radiation dose fractionation
G. Use of conformal radiation therapy (eg, intensity-modulated radiotherapy [IMRT], image-guided radiotherapy [IGRT], stereotactic body radiation therapy [SBRT]) as compared with single-beam/single-field radiation therapy

Q20-9: What is the severity of this patient's radiation pneumonitis?

A. Grade 1
B. Grade 2
C. Grade 3
D. Grade 4
E. Grade 5

Q20-10: The patient is started on prednisone 40 mg daily with a plan for a slow taper over several months. What additional medication should be prescribed?

A. Metformin
B. Albuterol inhaler PRN
C. Trazadone
D. Bactrim
E. Calcium carbonate
F. Escitalopram

ANSWERS

Q20-1: D
Opacification or consolidation

Rationale: This chest radiograph demonstrates a large right-sided infiltrate (opacity or consolidation) that does not appear to conform to normal anatomic barriers. There is no evidence of reticulonodular opacities, linear opacities, or hilar adenopathy. Alveolar infiltrates do not appear in this manner (see **Case 48** for an example). The important distinction is between choices D and F. Atelectasis refers to collapse of the lung resulting in the appearance of consolidation on chest films. As this pattern does not fit any particular pattern consistent with a lobe, segment, or subsegment of the right lung, it is less likely atelectasis and is best described as an opacity or infiltrate.

Q20-2: B
Consolidation surrounded by ground-glass opacities (reverse-halo sign)

Rationale: In this CT scan, there is an ill-defined area of consolidation with air bronchograms that is surrounded by a sphere of ground-glass opacities. This is termed the *reverse-halo sign*, as opposed to the halo sign, where an area of ground-glass is surrounded by consolidative opacities. The lesions are not cavitary, but there are air bronchograms present. The pattern is not consistent with simple rounded atelectasis, a common pulmonary complication of asbestos exposure. Rounded atelectasis classically has a comet-tail appearance and lacks ground glass as well as such extensive air bronchograms. There is also more evidence of volume loss in rounded atelectasis than is seen here. Although there may be some tree-in-bud opacities, this is not the predominant abnormality. There is no evidence of crazy paving.

Q20-3: B
Drug-induced toxicity, radiation pneumonitis, cryptogenic organizing pneumonia (COP), and infection

Rationale: Drug-induced toxicity, radiation pneumonitis, cryptogenic organizing pneumonia (COP), and infection would be the most appropriate differential diagnosis for this patient. The patient was on several drugs that may cause pulmonary drug toxicity, including taxane-based chemotherapy, platinum-based chemotherapy, and immunotherapy, so drug toxicity is certainly possible. Radiation pneumonitis is an acute reaction (6 weeks to 6 months) following radiation therapy that presents similarly to pneumonia; radiation fibrosis, on the other hand, would present with evidence of fibrosis and is a late complication (years) after radiation and is not necessarily preceded by radiation pneumonitis. Cryptogenic organizing pneumonia can also present with a focal infiltrate or consolidation and symptoms of pneumonia. Given that the patient was recently on chemotherapy, he is at increased risk for opportunistic infections as well as community-acquired pneumonia. IPF and NSIP do not typically present as focal consolidations, nor does sarcoidosis (though remember, sarcoidosis can present in nearly any fashion). On the lateral film, the consolidation does not appear to be in the anterior mediastinum.

Q20-4: D
A review of the radiation treatment plan

Rationale: A review of the radiation treatment plan would be an appropriate next step. The patient has undergone appropriate evaluation for an infectious cause and is on appropriate antibiotic therapy. There is no evidence of organizing pneumonia to suggest COP, and there is no granulomatous disease. Before initiation of any additional treatment, reviewing the radiation treatment plan may shed light on the cause of the patient's consolidation. An echocardiogram would be helpful if there was concern for a cardiac issue. CT of the abdomen and pelvis would be appropriate if there was not a likely cause of the patient's fever; however, with a clear process ongoing in the lung and no localizing symptoms, this would not be the next step. Similarly, the patient has no diarrhea, and the lack of abdominal symptoms indicates that a stool specimen would not be terribly helpful. An endoscopy to evaluate for a TEF is an interesting thought; however, this patient has no symptoms consistent with TEF, there was no evidence of TEF on bronchoscopy or CT scan, and the bronchoscopy showed no evidence of purulence.

Q20-5: A
Radiation pneumonitis

Rationale: The patient's radiation treatment field replicates the distribution of the patient's abnormalities on chest radiography. CMV pneumonia, fungal pneumonia, and pneumocystis pneumonia are unlikely as the bronchoscopy BAL and biopsy results do not suggest an infectious process. Again, radiation fibrosis is a chronic finding occurring years after radiation therapy and is usually associated with reticulonodular interstitial opacities associated with areas of consolidation, traction bronchiectasis, honeycomb changes, and septal thickening in the same distribution as the radiation field. Radiation pleuritis is an acute complication that can be seen in a similar time frame to radiation pneumonitis and usually presents with severe pleuritic chest pain, dyspnea, a pleural effusion (exudative), and, occasionally, a rub audible on examination. Radiation-induced bronchial stenosis usually results from the treatment of perihilar tumors and can lead to complications, including necrosis and fistulas.

There are two forms of radiation-induced lung injury (RILI). The subacute form of injury is termed *radiation pneumonitis*, while the chronic form of injury is termed *radiation fibrosis*. This is determined primarily by the dose of radiation delivered to the lung tissue and surrounding pleura, though it may be modulated by concurrent or subsequent chemotherapy or immunotherapy. Radiation pneumonitis can be difficult to differentiate from pure drug toxicity, atypical/viral infection, or edema. Radiation fibrosis is generally more easily identified if dose mapping is available from the patient's treatment planning/report.

An example of radiation fibrosis is shown in **Image 20-4**.

Before treatment   **1 year after treatment**

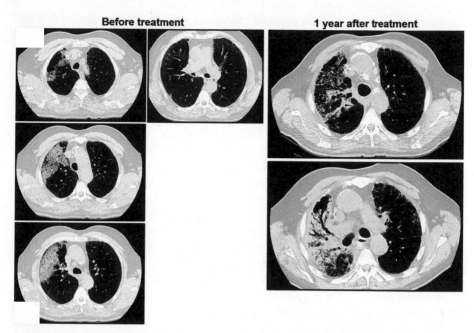

Image 20-4 • An example of radiation fibrosis in a patient with adenocarcinoma of the lung. On the left, the chest CT scan of the patient before radiation therapy is shown, with a classic appearance of primary lung adenocarcinoma. On the right is the CT scan for the same patient 1 year after treatment. Here, there is clear evidence of fibrotic changes, with architectural distortion, traction bronchiectasis, volume loss, areas of consolidation, and septal thickening. Some of this is localized to the primary tumor and is often termed "treatment effect" on radiology reports because these changes are beneficial and anticipated. However, there is also fibrosis in the surrounding lung parenchyma. These bystander areas of lung parenchyma that develop damage are considered to have experienced radiation fibrosis.

Radiation pneumonitis is an acute inflammatory illness occurring most commonly within the first 12 weeks after treatment (but may occur as late as 6 months after treatment ends), while radiation fibrosis represents an organized, fibrotic phase and occurs more than 6 months after therapy completion.

The symptoms of radiation pneumonitis include fever, dyspnea, nonproductive cough, pleuritic chest pain, hemoptysis, fatigue, and other constitutional symptoms, including night sweats and weight loss. Patients most commonly have inspiratory crackles or a pleural rub, and there may be evidence of skin erythema overlying the areas with these crackles. Patients with more severe cases may present with hypoxemia, tachypnea, tachycardia, and increased work of breathing. Patients may also develop inflammatory pleural effusions (exudative) that are typically small to moderate in size.

Radiation fibrosis is more likely to present gradually, with the development of dyspnea and reduced exercise tolerance and perhaps a dry cough. The examination findings are likely to demonstrate inspiratory crackles over the affected area, and effusions are less likely. PFT may demonstrate restriction and a reduced DLCO. Chest imaging is highly useful to aid in making a diagnosis. In radiation pneumonitis, chest radiographs may show patchy airspace disease (alveolar consolidations), typically surrounding the target lesions (most commonly seen as a mass or consolidation on chest imaging). Chest radiographs in radiation fibrosis may demonstrate dense consolidations or reticular interstitial opacities in the affected areas. Before the introduction of 3-dimensional confirmational radiation therapy (CRT), the "straight-line" sign—affected tissue limited to that between the lines representing the treatment area and ignoring anatomic boundaries (fissures)—was diagnostic of radiation pneumonitis and particular fibrosis. Now that modern treatment methods feature multiple low-dose beams at multiple angles in a three-dimensional space, this effect is not commonly seen. However, it may still be seen in cases where the primary lesions allow for only one or two beam paths without causing significant damage to bystander organs or tissue. This may yield any number of topographic dosimetry maps. This is why obtaining dosimetric information in the form of isodose or dose delivery maps overlayed on CT imaging before treatment is essential for diagnosis; it allows one to compare the current and pretreatment scans to determine if the pattern of lung injury observed matches the treatment on delivery-dose maps. CT imaging typically shows ground-glass opacities surrounding the lesion. As the disease shifts from inflammatory/exudative to organizing/proliferative, consolidations may form. This may occur in a patchy pattern, from an inside-out pattern (halo sign—a halo of consolidation around a center of ground-glass opacities) or from inside-out (reverse-halo sign—a halo of ground-glass opacities around a center of consolidation). Patients may also have nodules, tree-in-bud opacities, or septal thickening (the latter, in combination with ground-glass opacities, can lead to a crazy paving pattern). Pulmonary effusions are almost exclusively ipsilateral. As the disease progresses to a fibrotic phase, septal thickening, architectural distortion, traction bronchiectasis, consolidation, and volume loss may be seen. Honeycomb changes may also be seen. Patients may also have small linear opacities that conform to individual beam paths but ignore anatomic boundaries, depending on the radiation delivery technique.

PFT most commonly demonstrates a reduced DLCO and evidence of restriction (reduced TLC or FVC).

The differential diagnosis includes infection (particularly viral or atypical causes, though if the patient is immunocompromised, opportunistic infections must also be considered), drug toxicity/pneumonitis, disease progression/lymphangitic carcinomatosis, organizing pneumonia, acute exacerbations of underlying lung disease (particular interstitial pneumonias), and cardiogenic pulmonary edema.

Laboratory testing and bronchoscopy are most useful to rule out infection, drug toxicity, and lymphangitic spread/disease progression (particularly in adenocarcinoma). The BAL is typically lymphocyte predominant. Biopsies can identify cancer progression, infection, drug toxicity, and organizing pneumonia (radiation can induce organizing pneumonia in addition to the above).

Q20-6: B
Weight-based glucocorticoids (0.5 to 1 mg/kg prednisone or equivalent daily)

Rationale: Weight-based glucocorticoids are an appropriate choice in this case because dramatic improvement can often be observed and a failure to respond to therapy can be associated a worse overall prognosis. Other immunosuppressive medications such as methotrexate (which can have lung toxicity) or cyclophosphamide are not currently indicated. There is no evidence that NAC has an effect on radiation pneumonitis. Interestingly, captopril has been studied as potential therapeutic for the prevention of radiation pneumonitis, but it has not been examined for the treatment of pneumonitis itself.

Q20-7: C
There is a positive relationship between the total mean lung dose and the risk of radiation pneumonitis

Rationale: This will be discussed further in the following question.

Q20-8: A, C, D, F
Aside from the mean dose of radiation to the lung, all of the following are associated with an increased risked risk of RILI: concurrent use of chemotherapy or immunotherapy, the presence of underlying structural lung disease (particularly ILD), and radiation dose fractionation. The evidence for smoking tobacco use increasing the risk of RILI is limited. There is no sex predilection in radiation pneumonitis. The use of conformal radiation therapy is associated with a reduced risk of RILI compared with prior single-beam/single-field techniques.

Although the dose of ionizing radiation is critical, there are a number of other factors to consider: the volume of lung parenchyma exposed, the method of irradiation, concurrent chemotherapy or immunotherapy, the dose fractionation (time-dose factor), underlying/existing parenchymal lung disease at the time of treatment initiation, and smoking tobacco use.

In terms of volume, the true risk is likely related to the volume-mean dose product. In treatment planning, dose/isodose mapping will show color-coded distributions, wherein tissue denoted with a particular color is expected to be (or have been, if after treatment) exposed to same mean dose of radiation. The product of the mean dose by the volume of tissue exposed is a primary predictor for RILI. For lung parenchyma, the risk of RILI increases as the volume of lung exposed to more than 20 Gy per day increases. In terms of fractionation and the "time-dose" factor, this refers to the time (or here, the number of sessions) over which a dose is given. Given the constraints on medical equipment and personnel, most radiation therapy is performed in fractions of one or two doses a day. The method of delivery of the ionizing radiation is also a significant factor. Over the past 50 years, much progress has been made to optimize radiation delivery to the target lesion while minimizing radiation to other tissues (broadly termed "conformal radiation therapy"). This includes a number of different methods that involve using multiple low-dose beam paths at different angles to maximize delivery to one point of intersection of these beams while minimizing the radiation dose delivered to the tissue on the individual beam paths outside the area of intersection. The most common forms of CRT are IGRT, IMRT, and SBRT. These likely carry a risk of approximately 5% to 10% for the development of clinically significant radiation pneumonitis (grade 3 or above). An alternative form of radiation that uses protons rather than photons is also beginning to be used in breast and lung cancer and has shown promising results with a very low incidence of radiation pneumonitis (less than 5%). The presence of underlying structural lung disease of any kind (COPD, interstitial pneumonia) is likely to increase the risk of radiation fibrosis, though the presence of interstitial pneumonia (eg, IPF, chronic HP, NSIP, sarcoidosis) is associated with a significantly increased risk of severe or very severe radiation pneumonitis.

The use of concurrent chemotherapy or immunotherapy is also a significant risk factor. This is particularly true for gemcitabine as well as taxanes, anthracyclines, and cyclophosphamide. Additionally, immunotherapy drugs (immune checkpoint inhibitors targeting PD-1/PD-L1 or CTLA-4) may be associated with an increased risk of developing pneumonitis. The complicating factor is that many of these drugs may directly cause pneumonitis themselves, even in the absence of radiation. Additionally, in patients who have previously received radiation to the lung parenchyma, either as a target or indirectly as a result of radiation to other surrounding tissue, may also experience what is called "recall pneumonitis" if they are exposed to these chemotherapeutic or immunotherapy drugs after radiation treatment.

It should be noted that there is an entity termed *radiation hypersensitivity pneumonitis* that occurs bilaterally and typically also involves lung tissue not exposed to pathologic doses of ionizing radiation. This can be difficult to differentiate from combined radiation and drug-induced pneumonitis or drug-induced pneumonitis.

Q20-9: C
Grade 3

Rationale: The severity of radiation pneumonitis is graded using the following scale:
- Grade 1 – increase in pulmonary symptoms not requiring initiation or increase of corticosteroids
- Grade 2 – increase in pulmonary symptoms requiring initiation or increase of corticosteroids
- Grade 3 – requiring initiation or increase of supplemental O_2 therapy
- Grade 4 – requiring ventilatory support or causing life-threatening illness
- Grade 5 – causing death

As this patient has pulmonary symptoms and a new O_2 requirement, he is at least grade 3. He has not progressed to need ventilatory support, so he is not at grade 4. However, patients can progress at any point, necessitating a personalized, slow taper with frequent follow-up to evaluate for new or worsening symptoms.

Q20-10: D
Bactrim

Rationale: The patient is being initiated on prednisone therapy for a prolonged period. Prednisone at such doses is associated with a number of potential complications, including mood swings/aggression, sleep disturbances and vivid nightmares, cataracts, GERD and the development of gastric ulcers, increased blood glucose levels, increased bone resorption and risk of osteoporosis, and increased risk of infection due to immunosuppression. This patient should be initiated on *Pneumocystis* pneumonia (PCP) PCPprophylaxis with trimethoprim/sulfamethoxazole (or alternative). Although the patient should be informed to monitor his blood glucose once a daily, empiric initiation of metformin is not called for at this point. Similarly, sleep aids and mood stabilizers are not empirically initiated, so trazadone or escitalopram would not be required here. Calcium carbonate may aid in the treatment of GERD, but the use of a preventive medication (proton pump inhibitor [PPI] or H2-blocker) would be preferential. Patients initiated on long-term prednisone therapy often receive PCP prophylaxis, a PPI or an H2-blocker, and calcium/vitamin D supplementation (not calcium alone). Patients are instructed to monitor their blood glucose typically once daily or three times a week and to monitor for the development of vision issues (cataracts).

References

Arbetter KR, Prakash UB, Tazelaar HD, Douglas WW. Radiation-induced pneumonitis in the "nonirradiated" lung. Mayo Clin Proc. 1999;74:27.

Abratt RP, Morgan GW, Silvestri G, Willcox P. Pulmonary complications of radiation therapy. Clin Chest Med. 2004;25:167.

Abratt RP, Morgan GW. Lung toxicity following chest irradiation in patients with lung cancer. Lung Cancer. 2002;35:103.

Arroyo-Hernández M, Maldonado F, Lozano-Ruiz F, Muñoz-Montaño W, Nuñez-Baez M, Arrieta O. Radiation-induced lung injury: current evidence. BMC Pulm Med. 2021;21:9.

Choi YW, Munden RF, Erasmus JJ, et al. Effects of radiation therapy on the lung: radiologic appearances and differential diagnosis. Radiographics. 2004;24:985.

Graham MV, Purdy JA, Emami B, et al. Clinical dose-volume histogram analysis for pneumonitis after 3D treatment for non-small cell lung cancer (NSCLC). Int J Radiat Oncol Biol Phys. 1999;45:323.

Giridhar P, Mallick S, Rath GK, Julka PK. Radiation induced lung injury: prediction, assessment and management. Asian Pac J Cancer Prev. 2015;16:2613.

Giuranno L, Ient J, De Ruysscher D, Vooijs MA. Radiation-induced lung injury (RILI). Front Oncol. 2019;9:877.

Kimsey FC, Mendenhall NP, Ewald LM, et al. Is radiation treatment volume a predictor for acute or late effect on pulmonary function? A prospective study of patients treated with breast-conserving surgery and postoperative irradiation. Cancer. 1994;73:2549.

Kouloulias V, Zygogianni A, Efstathopoulos E, et al. Suggestion for a new grading scale for radiation induced pneumonitis based on radiological findings of computerized tomography: correlation with clinical and radiotherapeutic parameters in lung cancer patients. Asian Pac J Cancer Prev. 2013;14:2717.

Linda A, Trovo M, Bradley JD. Radiation injury of the lung after stereotactic body radiation therapy (SBRT) for lung cancer: a timeline and pattern of CT changes. Eur J Radiol. 2011;79:147.

Ma LD, Taylor GA, Wharam MD, Wiley JM. "Recall" pneumonitis: adriamycin potentiation of radiation pneumonitis in two children. Radiology. 1993;187:465.

Marks LB, Bentzen SM, Deasy JO, et al. Radiation dose-volume effects in the lung. Int J Radiat Oncol Biol Phys. 2010;76:S70.

Mazeron R, Etienne-Mastroianni B, Pérol D, et al. Predictive factors of late radiation fibrosis: a prospective study in non-small cell lung cancer. Int J Radiat Oncol Biol Phys. 2010;77:38.

Movsas B, Raffin TA, Epstein AH, Link CJ Jr. Pulmonary radiation injury. Chest. 1997;111:1061.

Park KJ, Chung JY, Chun MS, Suh JH. Radiation-induced lung disease and the impact of radiation methods on imaging features. Radiographics. 2000;20:83.

Poletti V, Costabel U, Semenzato G. Pulmonary complications in patients with hematological disorders: pathobiological bases and practical approach. Semin Respir Crit Care Med. 2005;26:439.

Rosiello RA, Merrill WW, Rockwell S, et al. Radiation pneumonitis. Bronchoalveolar lavage assessment and modulation by a recombinant cytokine. Am Rev Respir Dis. 1993;148:1671.

Roy S, Salerno KE, Citrin DE. Biology of Radiation-induced lung injury. Semin Radiat Oncol. 2021;31:161.

Seidensticker M, Seidensticker R, Damm R, et al. Prospective randomized trial of enoxaparin, pentoxifylline and ursodeoxycholic acid for prevention of radiation-induced liver toxicity. PLoS One. 2014;9:e112731.

Spiro SG, Douse J, Read C, Janes S. Complications of lung cancer treatment. Semin Respir Crit Care Med. 2008;29:302.

Suresh K, Voong KR, Shankar B, et al. Pneumonitis in non-small cell lung cancer patients receiving immune checkpoint immunotherapy: Incidence and risk factors. J Thorac Oncol. 2018;13:1930.

Tian S, Switchenko JM, Buchwald ZS, et al. Lung stereotactic body radiation therapy and concurrent immunotherapy: A multicenter safety and toxicity analysis. Int J Radiat Oncol Biol Phys. 2020;108:304.

Venkatramani R, Kamath S, Wong K, et al. Correlation of clinical and dosimetric factors with adverse pulmonary outcomes in children after lung irradiation. Int J Radiat Oncol Biol Phys. 2013;86:942.

Verma V, Shostrom VK, Zhen W, et al. Influence of fractionation scheme and tumor location on toxicities after stereotactic body radiation therapy for large (≥5 cm) non-small cell lung cancer: A multi-institutional analysis. Int J Radiat Oncol Biol Phys. 2017;97:778.

Voong KR, Hazell SZ, Fu W, et al. Relationship between prior radiotherapy and checkpoint-inhibitor pneumonitis in patients with advanced non-small-cell lung cancer. Clin Lung Cancer. 2019;20:e470.

Yamashita H, Takahashi W, Haga A, Nakagawa K. Radiation pneumonitis after stereotactic radiation therapy for lung cancer. World J Radiol. 2014;6:708.

Yirmibesoglu E, Higginson DS, Fayda M, et al. Challenges scoring radiation pneumonitis in patients irradiated for lung cancer. Lung Cancer. 2012;76:350.

CASE 21

A 33-year-old White man is referred to your office with asthma refractory to standard management. He has no other medical history except asthma that developed approximately 5 years ago. He is currently on a high-dose inhaled corticosteroid, a long-acting beta-agonist, a long-acting muscarinic antagonist, a leukotriene inhibitor, and a low dose of systemic corticosteroids (5 mg prednisone) daily, yet he has persistent symptoms. He reports that he had some allergy testing about 4 years ago but only recalls that he has allergies to "something in the environment." He reports dyspnea with exertion, significant wheezing multiple times a day, frequent use of nebulized albuterol with minimal effect, a frequent and intermittently productive cough, and fatigue. He recently became more concerned as he had developed some scant blood in his sputum, and he requested a referral to a specialist. He endorses some low-grade fevers at times but no weight loss. His examination demonstrates wheezing diffusely and rhonchi that partially clear with a productive deep cough. He does not require O_2 at rest or with activity. His vital signs are T 37.5°C, HR 88, BP 132/78, RR 15, oxygen saturation 95% on room air. Some values from his spirometry are shown below.

	Pre bronchodilator	Post bronchodilator
FEV1	61%	68% predicted
FVC	91%	92% predicted
Ratio	60%	67% predicted

His CXR is shown in Image 21-1.

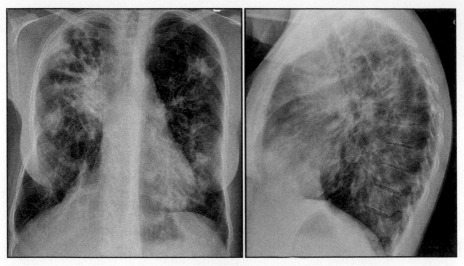

Image 21-1 • Representative chest radiographs (PA and lateral) for the patient in **Case 21**.

QUESTIONS

Q21-1: How would you describe the patient's chest radiograph?

A. Normal
B. Linear interstitial opacities
C. Bronchial wall thickening and focal opacity
D. Hilar adenopathy
E. Pulmonary arterial enlargement
F. Right middle lobe lung mass

Q21-2: A representative CT scan is shown in Image 21-2.

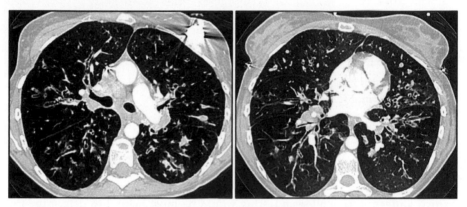

Image 21-2 • CT chest image for the patient in **Question 21-2**.

How would you describe the abnormalities on the CT scan?

A. Lobar infiltrate with air bronchograms
B. Mosaic pattern of air trapping and crazy paving
C. Tree-in-bud opacification
D. Cylindrical bronchiectasis
E. A and B
F. B and C
G. C and D
H. B and D

Q21-3: You receive some additional testing for the patient that was performed recently. The results of a tuberculosis skin test and an HIV test are negative. He has no risk factors for tuberculosis. He reports working in an office and states that the company for whom he works has twice had the air conditioning and heating system checked for mold contamination because of his symptoms, without any findings. Which test would you send to further evaluate the patient's condition?

A. ESR, CRP, CBC with differential, ANA, ANCA, dsDNA, Jo-1, Scl70
B. Peripheral blood smear for thick-and-thin analysis
C. Neutrophil function and oxidative burst test and cystic fibrosis (CF) gene mutation study
D. Sweat chloride test, immunoglobulin panel, CBC with differential, and a quantitative IgE study

Q21-4: The patient's studies return as follows:

Sweat chloride: 40 (normal)

Immunoglobulin panel: total IgG (predominantly IgG$_2$) is elevated at 2300 IU/mL. Otherwise, normal IgA and IgM levels.

Peripheral blood count with differential: 7% eosinophils, WBC count is 14,000/mm^3 with a neutrophilic predominance.

IgE: 9450 IU/mL.

Which antigen during allergen testing would be most helpful to determine the etiology of the patient's condition?

A. *Aspergillus versicolor*
B. *Aspergillus fumigatus*
C. Cat epithelium
D. Ragweed
E. *Dermatophagoides farinae*

Q21-5: The patient in the above vignette is diagnosed with ABPA. Given the presence of central bronchiectasis on the CT scan, he is diagnosed with ABPA-central bronchiectasis (CB) as opposed to ABPA-S (seropositive without evidence of bronchiectasis). Which is not a criterion for the diagnosis of ABPA?

A. IgE level greater than 1000 U/mL
B. IgE level greater than 417 IU/mL
C. Severe uncontrolled asthma
D. Positive skin hypersensitivity test to *A. fumigatus* (or equivalent serum precipitins IgG or IgE level specific for *A. fumigatus*)

Q21-6: Which clinical stage of ABPA does this patient have?

A. Stage I
B. Stage II
C. Stage III
D. Stage IV
E. Stage V

Q21-7: In addition to corticosteroids, what treatment is recommended for patients with ABPA by the Infectious Disease Society of America (IDSA)?

A. Omalizumab (anti-IgE antibody)
B. Rapamycin
C. Methotrexate
D. Itraconazole
E. Fluconazole

ANSWERS

Q21-1: C
Bronchial wall thickening with focal opacity

Rationale: The PA and lateral chest radiographs are certainly not normal. There is relatively diffuse bronchial wall thickening with cystic changes seen as well. The right upper lobe appears heterogenously opacified and there may be some endobronchial mucoid impaction. There is also a right upper or middle lobe opacity present near the fissure. There is no clear evidence of pulmonary artery enlargement or hilar adenopathy. While there may well be some linear interstitial opacities, this is not the predominant abnormality.

Q21-2: G
C and D

Rationale: There are areas of cylindrical bronchiectasis bilaterally, though they are more predominant on the right. There are also some areas of tree-in-bud opacification, particularly noticeable on the right. There is no lobar infiltrate, and there are no air bronchograms. There is no evidence of a mosaic pattern of ground-glass opacities that is seen in some conditions associated with hyperinflation and air trapping or evidence of crazy paving, as can be seen in pulmonary alveolar proteinosis (PAP).

Q21-3: D
Sweat chloride test, immunoglobulin panel, CBC with differential, and a quantitative IgE study

Rationale: The patient has evidence of bronchiectasis on CT and refractory asthma symptoms, including recurrent bronchitis symptoms. The panel of tests indicated in choice D would best evaluate the patient, including a sweat chloride test for CF, an immunoglobulin panel for immunodeficiency, a CBC with differential to evaluate for peripheral eosinophilia, and a quantitative IgE study to help determine the asthma phenotype. Choice A is a good choice for the evaluation of a patient with restrictive lung disease and suspected interstitial lung disease (ILD). A peripheral blood smear for thick-and-thin analysis is used to evaluate for parasitic diseases. Choice C would be appropriate for a child with recurrent bacterial infections, as the neutrophil function test would evaluate for the presence of chronic granulomatous disease (CGD).

Q21-4: B
Aspergillus fumigatus

Rationale: The primary concern in this patient at this point in the evaluation is for allergic bronchopulmonary aspergillosis (ABPA), a severe inflammatory disease of the lung often associated with bronchiectasis and refractory asthma that can lead to fibrosis and permanent lung scarring if not treated appropriately. The disease is closely associated with sensitization to colonization of the lung with *A. fumigatus*, though it may be associated with other fungi, including *Candida*, *Alternaria*, *Cladosporium*, and *Fusarium*, among others. *A. versicolor* is generally not associated with this condition. Cat epithelium tests for cat allergy, ragweed is a seasonal weed allergen, and *D. farinae* is the test for allergies to common house dust mites.

Q21-5: B
IgE level greater than 417 IU/mL

Rationale: An IgE level of greater than 1000 U/mL is required for a diagnosis of ABPA. However, a separate clinical term describing a very similar clinical entity (termed *severe asthma with fungal sensitivity* [SAFS]) is used to describe patients meeting criteria B, C, and D but with IgE levels less than 1000 U/mL.

Serum IgE level is always elevated in ABPA unless the patient is already on corticosteroids. Checking an IgE level is helpful for both diagnosing ABPA and monitoring a patient's response to steroids. A decrease in the serum IgE level by 35% to 50% constitutes remission. On the contrary, relapse of ABPA is indicated by a doubling of the patient's baseline IgE level.

Patients with ABPA generally present with fevers, wheezing, and a productive cough. Cough is typically productive of brownish-black mucus plugs. PFTs generally show an obstructive ventilatory defect.

Diagnostic criteria for ABPA include: a diagnosis of asthma, a positive skin test for *A. fumigatus* or elevated serum precipitins IgG or IgE to *A. fumigatus*, and serum IgE greater than 1000 IU/mL. Other supporting evidence includes pulmonary infiltrates and bronchiectasis on imaging, peripheral eosinophilia, cough productive of mucus plugs, and positive sputum culture for *A. fumigatus*.

Q21-6: D
Stage IV

Rationale: This patient has stage IV disease, with refractory steroid-dependent asthma, elevated levels of serum IgE, and likely elevated serum precipitins to *A. fumigatus*, but without evidence of fibrotic lung disease, which would push him into stage V (example shown in **Image 21-3**).

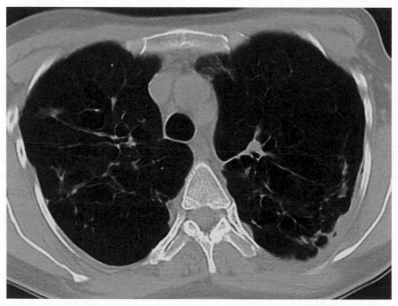

Image 21-3 • Representative chest CT image for the patient in **Question 21-6**. (*Reproduced with permission from Grippi MA, Elias JA, Fishman JA, et al: Fishman's Pulmonary Diseases and Disorders, 5th ed. New York, NY: McGraw Hill; 2015.*)

There are five stages of ABPA. Stage I is acute, active ABPA. Stage II is remission. Stage III is relapsed disease. Stage IV is refractory, steroid-dependent asthma with ABPA, and stage V is fibrotic lung disease.

Typical chest radiographic findings in ABPA include pulmonary opacities, which may be fleeting in nature or persistent, finger-in-glove opacities, bronchiectasis, and lobar collapse (related to mucus impaction). On CT imaging, typical findings include centrilobular nodules, tree-in-bud opacities, central bronchiectasis, air trapping, and mucus plugging.

Image 21-4 shows images taken from a patient with ABPA demonstrating the finger-in-glove sign on the chest radiograph with the corresponding CT scan of the chest.

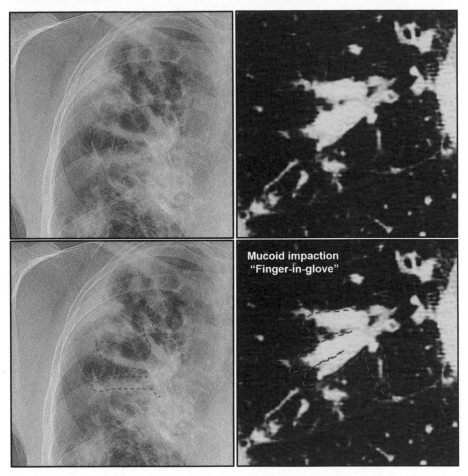

Mucoid impaction
"Finger-in-glove"

Image 21-4 • Chest radiograph (left) and CT chest image (right) demonstrating "finger-in-glove" sign as discussed in **Question 21-6**.

Q21-7: D
Itraconazole

Rationale: In addition to systemic glucocorticoids, itraconazole is recommended by the IDSA for initial treatment of ABPA in patients who are on chronic steroids, those with frequent exacerbations, and those with advanced disease felt to be at high risk for developing chronic lung scarring. Airway clearance, exercise, and allergen avoidance are also recommended, as they are for all patients with bronchiectasis.

Corticosteroids are generally tapered over the course of 6 to 12 months. There are no data on the ideal dosing or duration of corticosteroid therapy in ABPA. Duration and dosing are guided by disease severity and the patient's clinical response. As the steroid dose is tapered, the IgE level is followed, and repeat chest imaging is obtained. IgE level should drop by 35% to 50% to mark remission, and pulmonary infiltrates should resolve. Pulmonary function testing can also be monitored and should improve over the course of therapy. A rise in IgE level of greater than 100% indicates that the steroid dose should be increased.

References

Agarwal R. Allergic bronchopulmonary aspergillosis. Chest. 2009;135:805.

Chupp GL. Allergic bronchopulmonary aspergillosis (mycosis) and severe asthma with fungal sensitivity. In: Grippi MA, Elias JA, Fishman JA, Kotloff RM, Pack AI, Senior RM, Siegel MD, eds. *Fishman's Pulmonary Diseases and Disorders.* 5th ed. McGraw-Hill; 2015.

Nussbaumer-Ochsner Y, Kohler M. Finger-in-glove sign in bronchial atresia. Thorax. 2011;66:182.

Panchabhai TS, Mukhopadhyay S, Sehgal S, Bandyopadhyay D, Erzurum SC, Mehta AC. Plugs of the air passages: a clinicopathologic review. Chest. 2016;150:1141.

Patterson K, Strek ME. Allergic bronchopulmonary aspergillosis. Proc Am Thorac Soc. 2010;7:237-244.

Shah A, Panjabi C. Allergic aspergillosis of the respiratory tract. Eur Respir Rev. 2014;23:8.

CASE 22

A 54-year-old man presents to an urgent care clinic with a cough, fever, and dyspnea. He has a CXR that shows possible pneumonia, and he is prescribed a course of azithromycin. His symptoms do not improve, so he is scheduled for evaluation at the clinic. He has never smoked, and he does not use drugs or drink alcohol. He is a computer engineer who recently returned from a business trip to the Philippines where he was installing new software at a local factory. The factory produces some type of plastic bottles, and none of the other engineers that he traveled with has developed any issues. He reports no issues while away from home and states he returned about 4 months ago. He notes perhaps 2 to 3 weeks of worsening fatigue, some low-grade fevers, and a persistent cough that is largely nonproductive. He notes no improvement on the antibiotics given to him 2 weeks ago. He has no family history of pulmonary disease, no malignancy history, and no rheumatologic disease. He did have Hodgkin lymphoma as a young adult (25 years ago), for which he received chemotherapy and mantle radiation. The mantle radiation was complicated by mitral and aortic valve replacements approximately 10 years ago. He takes an oral anticoagulant but denies any bleeding complications or hemoptysis. On examination, he has decreased breath sounds over the right base, with dullness to percussion. His vitals are T 99.9°F, HR 85, BP 120/70, RR 14, and O₂ saturating 97% on room air. His chest radiograph is shown in Image 22-1.

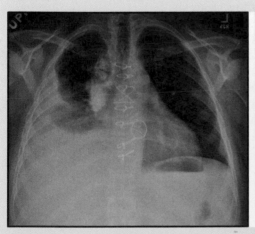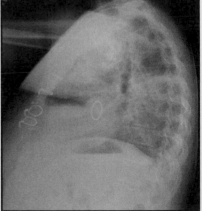

Image 22-1 • Chest radiograph for the patient in **Case 22**.

QUESTIONS

Q22-1: Which findings are identifiable on this patient's chest radiograph? Select all that apply.

A. Reticulonodular interstitial opacities
B. Left-sided pneumothorax
C. Right-sided pleural effusion
D. Right-sided thoracostomy (chest) tube
E. Valve replacement rings
F. Sternal wires
G. Hilar adenopathy/fullness
H. Left upper lobe lung mass

Q22-2: The patient is sent to the hospital ED from urgent care because of the abnormalities, and a sputum sample and blood cultures are obtained. The patient's brain (B-type) natriuretic peptide (BNP) level is within normal limits. The patient stopped his warfarin 2 days ago, and his current INR is 1.3. The patient's platelets are 245 ×10⁹/L. The patient is started on antibiotics for community-acquired pneumonia, including ceftriaxone and doxycycline. What is the next step in management?

A. CT scan of the chest
B. Thoracentesis
C. Lumbar puncture
D. Repeat sputum culture in 8 hours
E. Echocardiogram

Q22-3: The patient undergoes a thoracentesis with the following results:

Volume	600 mL
Color	Yellow/straw
pH	7.30
Glucose	44 mg/dL (serum 133)
Protein	3.4 g/dL
Lactate dehydrogenase (LDH)	544 IU/L
Nucleated cell count	3000 cells/mm³
Differential	94% lymphocytes
Triglycerides	40 mg/dL
Adenosine deaminase	48 units/L

The sputum gram stain is negative, and the sputum KOH stain and acid-fast bacillus (AFB) smear are both negative. An HIV study is also negative. What is the likely diagnosis?

A. Yellow fever
B. Dengue fever
C. Tuberculous pleuritis, possibly with primary pulmonary *Mycobacterium tuberculosis* infection
D. Miliary tuberculosis
E. Histoplasmosis
F. Sarcoidosis

Q22-4: The patient undergoes a CT scan of the chest that demonstrates no obvious parenchymal opacities. The cytology returns negative. He has had three consecutive induced AFB cultures return negative for AFB on smear. The patient is anxious to start treatment and be discharged home.

What is the gold standard diagnostic method for confirming a diagnosis of tuberculous pleurisy?

A. Standard sputum culture
B. Induced sputum culture
C. Pleural fluid microscopy/cytology and culture
D. *M. tuberculosis* IGRA from pleural fluid
E. Elevated ADA
F. Pleural biopsy

Q22-5: The patient undergoes a pleural biopsy that confirms the diagnosis of tuberculous pleurisy. The patient has three induced sputum cultures that return negative after 6 weeks. What is the likelihood of the patient developing active TB in the future if the patient foregoes treatment?

A. Less than 10%
B. 10% to 25%
C. 25% to 60%
D. 80% to 100%

Q22-6: What is the most appropriate treatment regimen for tuberculous pleurisy to prevent the development of active MTB infection when sensitivity data are not yet available?

A. Ethambutol monotherapy
B. INH monotherapy
C. INH and rifampin
D. INH, rifampin, and pyrazinamide
E. INH, rifampin, pyrazinamide, and ethambutol
F. INH, rifampin, pyrazinamide, ethambutol, and streptomycin

ANSWERS

Q23-1: D
Focal bronchiectasis, ground-glass opacities, and tree-in-bud opacities

Rationale: In the right middle lobe, there is evidence of ground-glass opacities as well as tree-in-bud opacities (seen best in **Image 23-2**), which represent distal filling of the terminal bronchioles into the alveolar sac, with the opacified appearance of a tree branch leading into a tree bud at the end. Additionally, there is evidence of bronchiolar wall thickening (bronchiectasis). There is no evidence of atelectasis or bronchial obstruction, reticulonodular opacities, honeycombing, or cavitation. Further examples of tree-in-bud opacities are shown in **Image 23-3**.

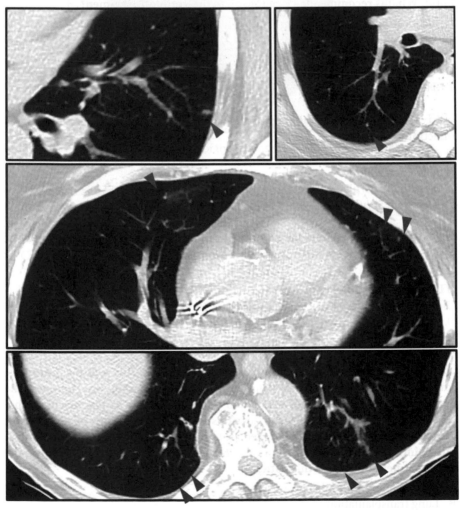

Image 23-3 • Examples of tree-in-bud opacities.

Q23-2: A
Sputum cultures

Rationale: This patient has structural abnormalities on CT and has failed a prior course of antibiotics. Although the structural changes (bronchiectasis) may be the result of scarring from prior infection or insult, the presence of ground-glass and tree-in-bud opacities suggests an active process of inflammation or infection. Given this patient's abnormalities on CT, a sputum culture would be an appropriate next step to determine the etiology of the patient's symptoms, and if the patient is not able to produce sputum, an induced sputum test could be performed in the clinic. Alternatively, if this is not successful, bronchoscopy would be the next step with bronchoalveolar lavage and perhaps a transbronchial biopsy. An open lung biopsy would be a last step. Bronchial artery embolization would be of use in a patient with active hemoptysis. An echocardiogram would not be particularly helpful at this point in the evaluation. However, if the patient did not have any focal findings in the lung parenchyma, consideration could be given to mitral stenosis (again, there is no evidence of murmur on examination).

Q23-3: B
Mycobacterium avium complex (MAC)

Rationale: MAC infection is the most likely diagnosis. The negative cultures at 7 days are not significant for AFB cultures, as these will not become final until 6 weeks, and many NTM species will not grow for at least 14 days in culture. Infection with MTB (eg, MAC) is broadly referred to as NTM. This is a classic presentation of "Lady Windermere" syndrome, an "atypical" or environmental, nontuberculous mycobacterial infection that has been classically associated with middle-aged women, older adult patients, or immunocompromised hosts (HIV, organ transplantation). The patient failed an outpatient course of antibiotics that would have covered most atypical bacteria and community-acquired organisms, including mycoplasma. The patient has no TB risk factors and has a negative TB skin test (PPD), so TB is unlikely. Sarcoidosis is a "great mimicker" and could potentially present in this fashion; however, there is no adenopathy, so this seems unlikely. PAP typically presents with a crazy-paving pattern marked by substantial ground-glass opacities, while NSIP is usually marked by septal thickening, ground-glass opacities, and interstitial opacities. Diagnosis requires (1) pulmonary symptoms; (2) radiographic abnormalities (nodular opacities, bronchiectasis, cavitations, tree-in-bud opacities); and (3) a positive culture on at least two sputum cultures or a positive culture from one BAL or a transbronchial biopsy with evidence of NTM infection.

There are a number of species of NTM that can cause lung pathology. While MAC is a very common cause, other common species include *M. abscessus*, *M. fortuitum*, and *M. kansasii*, with the latter more likely to cause cavitary lung lesions. On chest radiographs, NTM commonly presents in the mid-lung fields (right middle lobe, lingula) with tree-in-bud opacities, ground glass, micronodular disease, and bronchiectasis. Resolved or resolving infections may present with calcifications as well. In severe cases (particularly in patients with underlying structural lung disease such as cystic fibrosis (CF) or COPD, patients may have large cavitations that mimic primary TB infection. An example of a patient with severe MAC infection with cavitation (termed *fibrocavitary disease*) is shown in **Image 23-4**.

NTM are ubiquitous in the environment, and it is believed that NTM infections occur primarily through direct inoculation from soil; however, there is growing evidence that NTM infections may also be spread through the water supply. In fact, several lung transplant centers require patients to only use bottled or boiled water for bathing for the first year after the transplant to prevent such infection. In immunocompetent hosts, NTM infections primarily involve the lung. This is most seen in patients with underlying structural lung disease, particularly in patients with underlying COPD/emphysema and CF or non-CF bronchiectasis. These patients are particularly at risk for the development of fibrocavitary disease. In patients with no structural lung disease, NTM most commonly affects nonsmoking women between the ages of 50 and 70. Soft tissue, skin infections, and lymphadenitis may occur in some immunocompetent hosts, though the predominance of disseminated disease occurs in immunocompromised hosts.

In immunocompetent hosts, patients may be asymptomatic, with abnormalities only seen incidentally. Alternatively, patients may have a cough (productive or nonproductive), pleuritic chest pain, and dyspnea or shortness of breath. Patients with more severe disease may present with constitutional symptoms that closely mimic mycobacterium tuberculosis infection, including night sweats, weight loss, fatigue, and fevers. Disseminated MAC occurs in patients who are severely immunocompromised (eg, AIDS), with fever, night sweats, weight loss, and fatigue. Disseminated MAC may involve any other organ system as well, particularly the reticuloendothelial system, bone marrow, and the GI tract.

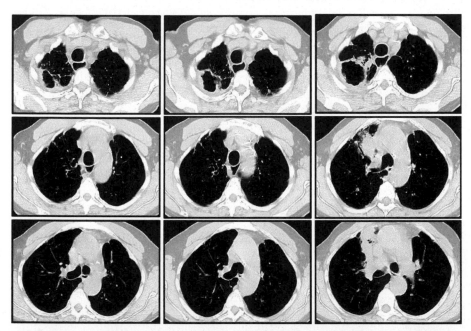

Image 23-4 • *Mycobacterium avium* complex infection over time (left panel, initial imaging; center panel, 3 months follow-up; right panel, 1 year follow-up) with progression of the cavitary lesion (thick-walled).

Q23-4: D
Ophthalmology consultation

Rationale: Due to the potential toxicities associated with ethambutol, the patient should be referred to an ophthalmologist for visual acuity and color vision testing. A hearing test is recommended for patients with evidence of fibrocavitary disease because the regimen often involves the use of amikacin or streptomycin.

Q23-5: D
Less than 50/μL

Rationale: Note that some resources will cite less than 100/μL. Azithromycin (1200 mg once weekly or 600 mg PO twice a week; alternatives: clarithromycin 500 mg PO twice daily, or rifabutin) is commonly prescribed for prophylaxis at CD4 counts below 50 to prevent disseminated disease. Patients with HIV are at increased risk for bacterial infections, MTB, herpes simplex and zoster, Kaposi sarcoma, and hairy cell leukemia, even with normal CD4 counts. At CD4 counts below 200/μL, there is an increased risk of *Pneumocystis jirovecii* pneumonia (PCP), toxoplasmosis, cryptosporidium, and opportunistic fungal infections, such as cryptococcosis or coccidioidomycosis. At CD4 counts below 50, patients are at increased risk for disseminated MAC infection, histoplasmosis, cytomegalovirus retinitis, and CNS lymphoma.

Q23-6: C
Hot tub use

Rationale: There are case reports of patients developing hypersensitivity pneumonitis in the setting of positive MAC cultures from BAL specimens. There is a close association with hot tub use in this cohort of patients, and the process has been termed "hot tub lung."

Q23-7: C
Lung resection following several weeks of a revised, three-drug antibiotic course

Rationale: The patient has focal bronchiectasis and is unlikely to clear this infection without antibiotics. As her disease is focal and limited to the right middle lobe, she would be an appropriate candidate for a minimally invasive lung resection. Monotherapy with amikacin or linezolid would not be effective, and lung transplantation is certainly not indicated in a patient with suspected active infection. A three-drug regimen has been strongly supported by literature to date. A bronchoscopy may be helpful in ruling out other etiologies; however, her imaging has not changed, and the symptoms are consistent with her prior presentation. As she can produce sputum, BAL is not necessary. Continued observation could be undertaken, but the patient has clearly expressed a desire to avoid this route. Once the patient has been counseled regarding the risks and benefits of lung resection, she can make an educated and informed decision. If the patient elects for surgical intervention, it is typically done only after a period of antibiotic therapy (here with a revised three-drug regimen that does not include ethambutol). This is prescribed for a period of 6 to 12 weeks with repeat sputum cultures to ensure clearance prior to resection, with the hopes of reducing the risk of colonizing other portions of the lung. A case could also be made to refer the patient for bronchial artery embolization in the region where the bronchiectasis is present or when her next episode of active bleeding occurs.

References

Daley CL, Iaccarino JM, Lange C, et al. Treatment of nontuberculous mycobacterial pulmonary disease: an official ATS/ERS/ESCMID/IDSA clinical practice guideline: executive summary. Clin Infect Dis. 2020;71:e1.

Griffith DE, Aksamit T, Brown-Elliott BA, et al. An official ATS/IDSA statement: diagnosis, treatment, and prevention of nontuberculous mycobacterial diseases. Am J Respir Crit Care Med. 2007;175:367.

Griffith DE, Brown BA, Girard WM, et al. Azithromycin-containing regimens for treatment of *Mycobacterium avium* complex lung disease. Clin Infect Dis. 2001;32:1547.

Haworth CS, Banks J, Capstick T, et al. British Thoracic Society guidelines for the management of nontuberculous mycobacterial pulmonary disease (NTM-PD). Thorax. 2017;72:ii1.

Hwang JA, Kim S, Jo KW, Shim TS. Natural history of *Mycobacterium avium* complex lung disease in untreated patients with stable course. Eur Respir J. 2017;49.

Jarand J, Davis JP, Cowie RL, et al. Long-term follow-up of *Mycobacterium avium* complex lung disease in patients treated with regimens including clofazimine and/or rifampin. Chest. 2016;149:1285.

Koh WJ, Jeong BH, Jeon K, et al. Clinical significance of the differentiation between *Mycobacterium avium* and *Mycobacterium intracellulare* in *M avium* complex lung disease. Chest. 2012;142:1482.

Kotilainen H, Valtonen V, Tukiainen P, et al. Prognostic value of American Thoracic Society criteria for nontuberculous mycobacterial disease: a retrospective analysis of 120 cases with four years of follow-up. Scand J Infect Dis. 2013;45:194.

Lee G, Lee KS, Moon JW, et al. Nodular bronchiectatic *Mycobacterium avium* complex pulmonary disease. Natural course on serial computed tomographic scans. Ann Am Thorac Soc. 2013;10:299.

Levin DL. Radiology of pulmonary *Mycobacterium avium-intracellulare* complex. Clin Chest Med. 2002;23:603.

Mitchell JD, Bishop A, Cafaro A, et al. Anatomic lung resection for nontuberculous mycobacterial disease. Ann Thorac Surg. 2008;85:1887.

Miwa S, Shirai M, Toyoshima M, et al. Efficacy of clarithromycin and ethambutol for *Mycobacterium avium* complex pulmonary disease. A preliminary study. Ann Am Thorac Soc. 2014;11:23.

Mullis SN, Falkinham JO 3rd. Adherence and biofilm formation of *Mycobacterium avium*, *Mycobacterium intracellulare* and *Mycobacterium abscessus* to household plumbing materials. J Appl Microbiol. 2013;115:908.

Olivier KN, Shaw PA, Glaser TS, et al. Inhaled amikacin for treatment of refractory pulmonary nontuberculous mycobacterial disease. Ann Am Thorac Soc. 2014;11:30.

Shiraishi Y, Fukushima K, Komatsu H, Kurashima A. Early pulmonary resection for localized *Mycobacterium avium* complex disease. Ann Thorac Surg. 1998;66:183.

Shiraishi Y, Nakajima Y, Katsuragi N, et al. Pneumonectomy for nontuberculous mycobacterial infections. Ann Thorac Surg. 2004;78:399.

Shiraishi Y, Nakajima Y, Takasuna K, et al. Surgery for *Mycobacterium avium* complex lung disease in the clarithromycin era. Eur J Cardiothorac Surg. 2002;21:314.

Winthrop KL, Ku JH, Marras TK, et al. The tolerability of linezolid in the treatment of nontuberculous mycobacterial disease. Eur Respir J. 2015;45:1177.

Yu JA, Pomerantz M, Bishop A, et al. Lady Windermere revisited: treatment with thoracoscopic lobectomy/segmentectomy for right middle lobe and lingular bronchiectasis associated with nontuberculous mycobacterial disease. Eur J Cardiothorac Surg. 2011;40:671.

CASE 24

You are called to the ED to examine a 44-year-old man with hypoxemia and cyanosis who requires admission to the ICU. He was diagnosed with sarcoidosis approximately 5 months ago. He reports that he was started on prednisone 60 mg daily and has continued on that medication after missing two follow-up appointments in the clinic. He has been experiencing 2 to 3 weeks of worsening fatigue, cough, and dyspnea and is now requiring 10 L/min supplement O_2 via high-flow nasal cannula to maintain his oxygen saturations. A review of his CXR at the time of his diagnosis of sarcoidosis reveals stage I disease, involving only hilar adenopathy without parenchymal findings. His primary complaint at the time of diagnosis was a persistent cough, which resolved after a month of steroids, and he was well until about 3 weeks ago. He reports no sick contacts, no travel, and no environmental or occupational exposures. His vital signs are T 100.9°F, HR 122, BP 110/65, RR 21, and saturation 94% on 10 L/min supplemental O_2. He does not smoke or use drugs. A CT scan of the chest is negative for acute pulmonary embolism. His CXRs from admission and approximately 24 hours later are shown below in Images 24-1A and 24-1B, respectively.

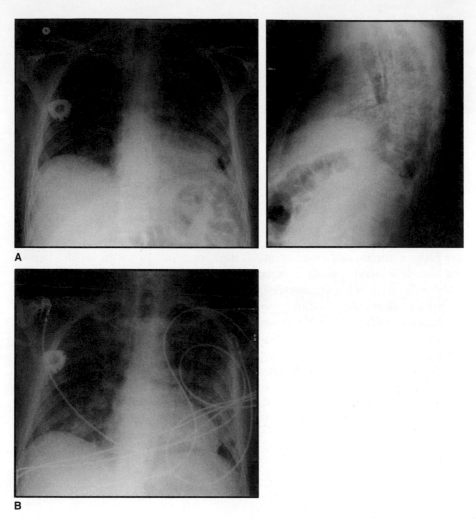

Image 24-1A and B • Chest radiographs for the patient in **Question 24-1**. (A) PA and lateral chest radiographs from admission. (B) AP chest radiograph approximately 24 hours following admission.

QUESTIONS

Q24-1: How would you describe the abnormalities on the chest radiographs?

A. Diffuse bilateral linear/reticular and alveolar opacities
B. Focal lobar consolidative opacity
C. Pneumomediastinum and hilar adenopathy
D. Cavitary lung lesions with air-fluid levels
E. Hyperinflation

Q24-2: The patient's condition deteriorates quickly after you examine the patient, and he requires endotracheal intubation. The patient's CT scans from admission are shown in Image 24-2. The patient's CT scan was negative for pulmonary embolism.

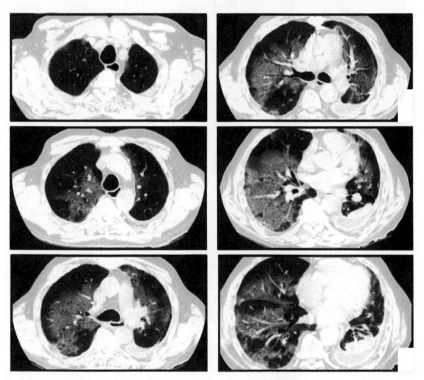

Image 24-2 • Chest CT images for the patient in **Question 24-2**.

How would you describe the abnormalities shown on CT in Image 24-2?

A. Diffuse ground-glass opacities and interlobular septal thickening consistent with crazy paving
B. Diffuse cystic lung disease with surrounding ground glass
C. Lower-lobe predominant interstitial thickening, honeycombing, and traction bronchiectasis
D. Focal opacification of the right lower and middle lobes
E. Pneumothorax on the left side

Q24-3: The patient is admitted to the medical ICU, and blood cultures are drawn. The patient is placed on broad-spectrum antibiotics (vancomycin and ceftazidime). Given the patient's immunocompromised state, you recommend the patient undergo bronchoscopy for BAL. The Gram stain is negative. The results of a silver stain are similar and shown in Image 24-3.

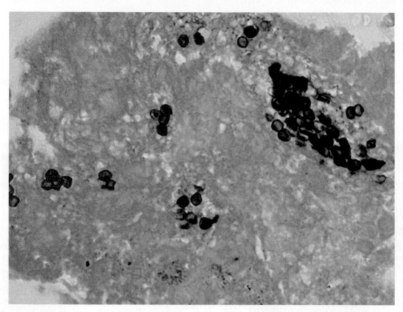

Image 24-3 • Representative silver stain results for the patient in **Question 24-3**. (*Used with permission from Dr. K. Volmar.*)

What is the likely diagnosis?

A. *Streptococcus pneumoniae* pneumonia
B. *Staphylococcus aureus* pneumonia
C. *Pneumocystis jiroveci* pneumonia (PJP or PCP)
D. *Pseudomonas aeruginosa* pneumonia
E. *Mycobacterium avium* complex (MAC) pneumonia

Q24-4: Which is not a risk factor for PCP?

A. Solid-organ transplantation
B. Hematologic malignancy
C. HIV
D. Diabetes mellitus
E. Corticosteroid use

Q24-5: Which medication is not an option for prophylaxis against PCP?

A. Bactrim
B. Atovaquone
C. Azithromycin
D. Dapsone
E. Pentamidine

Q24-6: What is the first-line therapy for patients with PCP?

A. Intravenous pentamidine
B. Intravenous trimethoprim/sulfamethoxazole
C. Dapsone
D. Atovaquone
E. Clindamycin and primaquine

Q24-7: You have a patient with severe acute respiratory distress syndrome (ARDS) resulting from PCP who is allergic to trimethoprim/sulfamethoxazole, with the allergy listed as anaphylaxis. What is the next treatment option?

A. Intravenous pentamidine
B. Intravenous clindamycin and dapsone
C. Intravenous clindamycin and PO primaquine
D. Atovaquone
E. Intravenous colistin

Q24-8: In addition to antibiotics, what adjunctive therapy may be useful in the treatment of PCP?

A. Corticosteroids
B. *N*-acetylcysteine (NAC)
C. Ribavirin
D. Oseltamivir
E. Montelukast

Q24-9: What is a potential complication of dapsone use NOT related to G6PDH deficiency?

A. Hemolytic anemia
B. Carboxyhemoglobinemia
C. Methemoglobinemia
D. Hypoglycemia
E. Pancreatitis

Q24-10: The gold standard for the diagnosis of PCP is the direct visualization of cystic or trophic forms of the organism in specimens obtained from the respiratory tract (from highest to lowest sensitivity: biopsy [either video-assisted thoracic surgery or transbronchial], BAL, endotracheal aspirate, or induced sputum). Of the following tests that do not meet the above criteria of direct visualization, which is the most specific to aid in the diagnosis of PCP?

A. Serum lactate dehydrogenase (LDH)
B. Serum galactomannan
C. Serum β-1,3-d-glucan (βGD)
D. *P. jiroveci* PCR performed using induced sputum
E. Serum lactate

ANSWERS

Q24-1: A
Diffuse bilateral linear and alveolar opacities

Rationale: In the PA image in **Image 24-1A**, the patient's CXR shows a more linear or reticular pattern with a lower lobe predominance, though the opacities are more diffusely distributed on the lateral film. In **Image 24-1B**, there is a clear progression on the AP image, with diffuse linear/reticular opacities but also some opacities that could be characterized as alveolar opacities. There is no evidence of cavitary lesions, cysts, pneumomediastinum, adenopathy, consolidation, or bronchiectasis. This pattern also is not consistent with an alveolar infiltrate or consolidation.

Q24-2: A
Diffuse ground-glass opacities and interlobular septal thickening consistent with crazy paving

Rationale: The CT scan demonstrates bilateral, relatively diffuse ground-glass opacities associated with interlobular septal thickening. This is a pattern commonly referred to as "crazy paving." Unfortunately, crazy paving can be seen in a number of conditions and therefore is nonspecific. There is no pneumothorax seen, but there are likely bilateral small pleural effusions. There is no apparent pericardial effusion. Additionally, there are no cystic changes. There is no lower-lobe predominant honeycombing or traction bronchiectasis either. There are no focal consolidations or opacifications to suggest bronchopneumonia or a mass or nodule.

Q24-3: C
Pneumocystis jiroveci pneumonia (PCP)

Rationale: The silver stain is used to identify fungal elements by staining carbohydrate structures in the cell membrane. On the Gomori methenamine silver stain, *P. jiroveci* appears as variations of a crushed sphere or ping-pong ball, ranging from slightly malformed to flattened. The GMS stain can also identify a number of other conditions (microsporidia, *Entamoeba histolytica*, intracytoplasmic inclusions bodies in cytomegalovirus [CMV], *Nocardia*, and *Mycobacterium* species), and gram-positive organisms can also stain with GMS (however, since the Gram stain is negative, the positive results on the GMS stain are not *Staphylococcus aureus*, *Streptococcus pneumoniae*, or *Pseudomonas pneumonia*). The primary differential here is between PCP and MAC infection. The appearance of the organisms on silver stain is very distinctive for PCP, as the stain attaches to the cyst wall yielding the dark shell around a lighter center, with some containing comma-shaped spores in the center. Recall that *Pneumocystis* cannot be cultured in the laboratory. Silver stain is not used in isolation to diagnose PCP, and it is usually accompanied by an immunofluorescence study using monoclonal antibodies against specific surface antigens. Diff-Quick stains (a modified form of the Wright stain that can be performed at the bedside) can identify the presence of trophozoites, which are missed on silver stain (which only stains the cyst wall). If a diagnosis cannot be made by sputum samples, bronchoscopy with

BAL, tissue biopsy, needle aspiration (can be transthoracic), or open lung biopsy may be necessary. Co-infection with bacteria, other fungal species, or CMV (or other viruses) and superinfection during treatment for PCP are exceedingly common, so all specimens should be sent for broad evaluation, particularly because patients are immunocompromised.

Now, a quick word on taxonomy. *P. jiroveci* was previously termed *P. carinii*, and the pulmonary infection caused by the organism was abbreviated PCP (*P. carinii* pneumonia). However, it was determined that the species of Pneumocystis that causes disease in humans is not the same as that the which causes disease in other species, and the human pathogen was renamed *P. jiroveci* to provide distinction. To avoid confusion, the abbreviation "PCP" is still commonly used, but is now stands for *Pneumocystis* pneumonia and is used interchangeable with the abbreviation PJP (*P. jiroveci* pneumonia). We will the abbreviation PCP in this case, although the reader should be aware that PJP and PCP may be used in the literature and refer to the same infectious disease.

The appearance of PCP on radiographic studies can vary widely. Chest radiographs are highly nonspecific and may show evidence of a diffuse focal process. Early in the disease course, such as in this case, the patient may present with a fine linear or reticular interstitial pattern that can progress to an alveolar filling pattern. Some patients may then go on to develop cysts and cavitations, areas of consolidation with air bronchograms, and fibrosis or scarring. The more classic board questions present a similar patient with cystic changes on chest imaging; however, the lack of cystic changes does not rule out PCP. Additionally, patients are at increased risk for pneumothoraces and pleural effusions.

Q24-4: D
Diabetes mellitus

Rationale: The primary risk factor for PCP before the introduction of modern highly active antiretroviral therapy (HAART) and the use of prophylaxis was HIV, followed by organ transplantation and patients receiving immunosuppression for rheumatologic disease. Although these therapies have reduced the risk of PCP, the patients at highest risk are those with HIV with a CD4 count less than 200, following by organ transplantation patients, patients with hematologic malignancy, and those receiving corticosteroids (usually greater than 20-30 mg prednisone daily for at least 3 months or multiple other immunosuppressive medications used in conjunction). Diabetes mellitus is a potentially immunosuppressive state, but it is not associated with the development of PCP.

Q24-5: C
Azithromycin

Rationale: All the remaining answers are potential therapies that may be used for prophylaxis against PCP, including nebulized or inhaled pentamidine.

Q24-6: B
Intravenous trimethoprim/sulfamethoxazole

Rationale: Trimethoprim/sulfamethoxazole remains the first-line antibiotic for the treatment of PCP when tolerated, including for all degrees of severity and for extrapulmonary disease. The dosing is 15 to 20 mg/kg of the trimethoprim component per day, every 8 hours. In addition to the other potential adverse events associated with trimethoprim/sulfamethoxazole use, the PCP dosing of trimethoprim/sulfamethoxazole can lead to issues with volume overload, as it often requires 1.5 to 2 L of carrier fluid per day. For patients with less severe disease, oral trimethoprim/sulfamethoxazole would be an appropriate choice.

Q24-7: C
Intravenous clindamycin and PO primaquine

Rationale: While either option A or C would be appropriate for patients with severe disease, clindamycin and primaquine are generally preferred to IV pentamidine as the latter is associated with significant adverse events, most notably hypoglycemia, hypotension, and nephrotoxicity. Atovaquone can be used as monotherapy in patients with mild disease. As most patients with an allergy to trimethoprim/sulfamethoxazole are primarily allergic to the sulfa component (sulfamethoxazole), trimethoprim with dapsone has also been used in mild-to-moderate disease. Disease severity in PCP is typically defined by the A-a gradient or the patient's PaO_2: mild, PaO_2 greater than 70 mm Hg with A-a gradient less than 35 mm Hg; moderate, PaO_2 between 60 and 70 mm Hg or A-a gradient between 35 and 50 mm Hg; severe, anything outside these ranges *or* a patient with impending respiratory failure related to work of breath or respiratory muscle fatigue.

Q24-8: A
Corticosteroids

Rationale: Initial studies in patients with HIV/AIDS demonstrated a significant benefit in the use of corticosteroids for the first 3 to 4 days of treatment in patients with severe disease presentations, thought to be by reducing inflammation during treatment. No formal studies have been performed to demonstrate that this benefit extends to the non–AIDS community, anecdotal evidence does suggest a similar benefit, and this is the standard of care.

Q24-9: C
Methemoglobinemia

Rationale: Methemoglobinemia is a potential complication of dapsone therapy. This is a significant complication that can occur in more than 10% of patients on PCP prophylaxis. Hemolytic anemia is a potential complication of dapsone therapy as well, though this is related to G6PDH activity. Primaquine also shares this potential adverse effect. Hypoglycemia and pancreatitis are more commonly associated with IV pentamidine administration.

Q24-10: D
P. jiroveci PCR performed using induced sputum

Rationale: Often, patients with suspected PCP are too ill to undergo sedation for bronchoscopy but are not so ill as to require endotracheal intubation, which would allow for endotracheal aspirates or bronchoalveolar lavage to be performed safely. In these immunocompromised patients in whom PJP is suspected (based on clinical presentation and imaging), performing PCR for *P. jiroveci* in respiratory specimens is the next most specific test, with a specificity approaching 95% when used on induced sputum samples (ie, induction of deep cough by nebulized hypertonic saline). Although serum LDH and serum βGD are both commonly elevated in patients with PCP and are often used to help determine which patients should receive continued or empiric therapy, they are both nonspecific. Serum LDH may be elevated in hematologic malignancies and hemolytic anemias, while the serum βGD can be elevated in many fungal infections (and these patients are commonly at risk for infection as well). A serum galactomannan is used for the diagnosis of *Aspergillus* infection. A serum lactate level is used to identify tissue ischemia or altered cellular metabolism (ie, glycolysis).

References

Azoulay É, Bergeron A, Chevret S, et al. Polymerase chain reaction for diagnosing pneumocystis pneumonia in non-HIV immunocompromised patients with pulmonary infiltrates. Chest. 2009;135:655.

Catherinot E, Lanternier F, Bougnoux ME, et al. *Pneumocystis jirovecii* pneumonia. Infect Dis Clin North Am. 2010;24:107.

Crans CA Jr, Boiselle PM. Imaging features of *Pneumocystis carinii* pneumonia. Crit Rev Diagn Imaging. 1999;40:251.

DeLorenzo LJ, Huang CT, Maguire GP, Stone DJ. Roentgenographic patterns of *Pneumocystis carinii* pneumonia in 104 patients with AIDS. Chest. 1987;91:323.

Doyle L, Vogel S, Procop GW. Pneumocystis PCR: it is time to make PCR the test of choice. Open Forum Infect Dis. 2017;4:ofx193.

Limper AH. Pneumocystis nomenclature. Clin Infect Dis. 2006;42:1210.

Marty FM, Koo S, Bryar J, Baden LR. (1—>3)beta-D-glucan assay positivity in patients with *Pneumocystis (carinii) jiroveci* pneumonia. Ann Intern Med. 2007;147:70.

Onishi A, Sugiyama D, Kogata Y, et al. Diagnostic accuracy of serum 1,3-β-D-glucan for *Pneumocystis jiroveci* pneumonia, invasive candidiasis, and invasive aspergillosis: systematic review and meta-analysis. *J Clin Microbiol.* 2012;50:7.

Panel on Opportunistic Infections in Adults and Adolescents with HIV. Guidelines for the prevention and treatment of opportunistic infections adults and adolescents with HIV: Recommendations from the Centers for Disease Control and Prevention, the National Institutes of Health, and the HIV Medicine Association of the Infectious Diseases Society of America. https://aidsinfo.nih.gov/contentfiles/lvguidelines/adult_oi.pdf (Accessed on December 18, 2020).

Sepkowitz KA. Opportunistic infections in patients with and patients without acquired immunodeficiency syndrome. Clin Infect Dis. 2002;34:1098.

Tasaka S, Hasegawa N, Kobayashi S, et al. Serum indicators for the diagnosis of *Pneumocystis* pneumonia. Chest. 2007;131:1173.

Theel ES, Jespersen DJ, Iqbal S, et al. Detection of (1, 3)-β-D-glucan in bronchoalveolar lavage and serum samples collected from immunocompromised hosts. Mycopathologia. 2013;175:33.

Thomas CF Jr, Limper AH. Pneumocystis pneumonia. N Engl J Med. 2004;350:2487.

Watanabe T, Yasuoka A, Tanuma J, et al. Serum (1—>3) beta-D-glucan as a noninvasive adjunct marker for the diagnosis of Pneumocystis pneumonia in patients with AIDS. Clin Infect Dis. 2009;49:1128.

CASE 25

A 45-year-old man presents to the ED with nonmassive hemoptysis. He emigrated from sub-Saharan Africa 10 years ago and at that time was treated for latent tuberculosis (TB); otherwise, he has no medical history. He does not smoke or use drugs, and he is HIV negative. He does not regularly see a care provider, so there are no historical chest images available. He states the symptoms started about 2 days ago, and he has been expectorating about 5 to 10 mL of maroon blood two to three times a day. He has had an intermittent chronic cough for years that is nonproductive, but intermittently he has had some blood-tinged sputum over the last few months. He denies any dyspnea with exertion, fevers, chills, sweats, or weight loss. He denies any chest or abdominal pain or any other symptoms. He does not take any nonsteroidal anti-inflammatory drugs (NSAIDs), aspirin, or other blood thinners, and he has never had a propensity towards bleeding. His vital signs are T 37.6°C, HR 121, BP 155/68, RR 20, oxygen saturation 97% on room air.

His chest imaging is shown in Image 25-1.

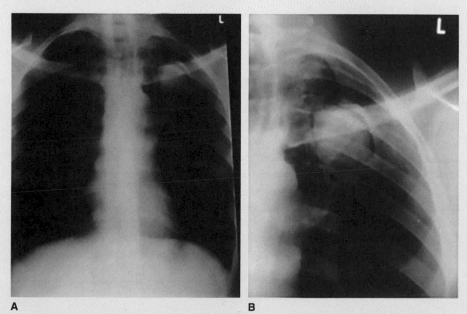

Image 25-1 • Chest radiographs for the patient in **Question 25-1**. (A) AP chest radiograph.
(B) Magnified image of the left upper airspace. (*Reproduced with permission from Ofori A,
Steinmetz AR, Akaasi J, et al: Pulmonary aspergilloma: An evasive disease, Int J Mycobacteriol.
2016 Jun;5(2):235-239.*)

QUESTIONS

Q25-1: Which abnormalities are revealed in the chest imaging?

A. Cystic lung lesion in the left upper lobe
B. Mass in the left upper lobe
C. Mass within a cavitary lesion in the left upper lobe
D. Ranke complex

Q25-2: The patient has a sputum culture sent, which is pending. An anti-nuclear antibody (ANA), antineutrophilic cytoplasmic antibody (ANCA), and rheumatoid factor (RF) are all negative. A serum IgE study for *Aspergillus* returns positive. The serum IgE is normal. What is the likely diagnosis?

A. Invasive aspergillosis
B. Aspergilloma
C. Allergic bronchopulmonary aspergillosis (ABPA)
D. Chronic pulmonary aspergillosis
E. Allergic bronchial asthma

Q25-3: What is the definitive treatment for an aspergilloma?

A. Bronchial artery embolization (BAE)
B. Antifungal therapy
C. Surgical resection
D. Lung transplantation
E. Corticosteroids
F. Intracavitary antifungal instillation

Q25-4: A 33-year-old woman with systemic lupus erythematosus (SLE) on immunosuppression therapy presents with fevers and recurrent cough productive of brownish sputum. The patient is admitted to the medicine service. She presents with dyspnea, hypoxemia (requiring 2 L NC at rest), and mild tachypnea. A rapid HIV study was negative. She does not use illicit drugs. She denies any smoking history. She reports no occupational or environmental exposures. She is a college student studying business. She notes more recently the onset of headaches that have been difficult to control as well. Her WBC count is $2.8/mm^3$, with an absolute neutrophil count of $1200/\mu L$. She takes hydroxychloroquine, mycophenolate, and prednisone for her SLE. She takes trimethoprim-sulfamethoxazole for *Pneumocystis jiroveci* pneumonia (PCP) prophylaxis. She takes pantoprazole for GI protection while on prednisone. She reports night sweats and weight loss over the last 3 weeks. The patient's CT chest images are shown in Image 25-2.

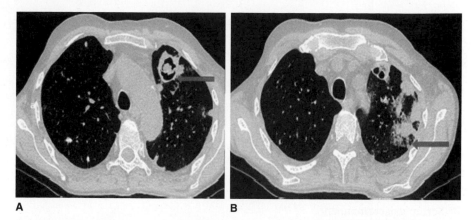

Image 25-2 • Representative chest CT images for the patient in **Question 25-4**. (*Reproduced with permission from Lala H, Manglab IL Prasada R, et al: Imaging features of pulmonary infection in post renal transplantrecipients: A review, Indian J Trans 2017 Jan-Mar;11(1):13-21.*)

On review, she has two prior sputum samples that grew *A. fumigatus*, which was considered colonization as she was asymptomatic at the time. She undergoes bronchoscopy due to the abnormal chest images (shown in Image 25-2). The BAL grew *A. fumigatus*. Biopsies are pending. The patient's laboratory tests show a normal total IgE level, a normal eosinophil count, a positive serum precipitins (IgG) to *A. fumigatus*, and a negative *A. fumigatus*–specific IgE.

What is the most likely diagnosis?

A. Invasive pulmonary aspergillosis
B. Chronic pulmonary aspergillosis
C. Invasive bronchial aspergillosis
D. ABPA
E. Extrinsic allergic alveolitis
F. Pulmonary aspergilloma

Q25-5: What is the name of the abnormality seen in the right CT chest image in Image 25-2?

A. Monod sign
B. Ranke sign
C. Timmon sign
D. Halo sign
E. Ghon sign

Q25-6: What is the name of the abnormality seen in the left CT chest image in Image 25-2?

A. Monod sign
B. Ranke sign
C. Timmon sign
D. Halo sign
E. Air-crescent sign

Q25-7: Which test is most useful in the diagnosis of invasive pulmonary (or bronchial) aspergillosis?

A. Serum beta-D-glucan (BDG)
B. Serum galactomannan
C. Serum procalcitonin
D. *Aspergillus*-specific IgE
E. Examination of sputum specimen

Q25-8: A 55-year-old woman with diabetes mellitus and a prior history of breast cancer who underwent resection and radiation therapy (right-sided) is referred for management. She had breast cancer 22 years ago, and approximately 5 years ago, she developed dyspnea and a cough. She had an abnormal CT scan and underwent an open lung biopsy that showed evidence of fibrosis and scarring consistent with radiation fibrosis. She had a prolonged hospitalization due to a persistent hydropneumothorax, but she was eventually able to be discharged after 2 weeks. Over the last 2 years, she has been experiencing progressively worsening dyspnea on exertion, so she had a repeat CT scan with her primary care physician and was referred to the clinic. She has been treated with steroids numerous times over the last 5 years for "fibrosis." The patient's imaging is shown in Image 25-3.

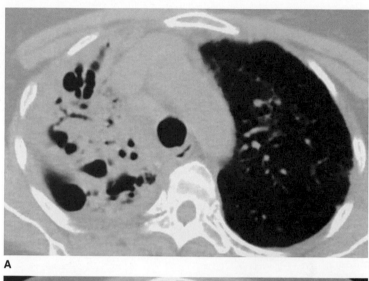

A

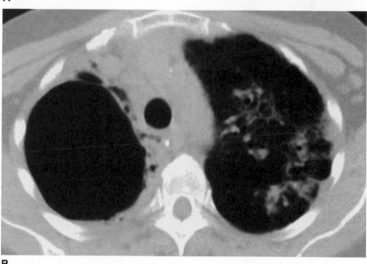

B

Image 25-3 • Chest CT images for the patient in **Question 25-8**. *(Reproduced with permission from Patterson KC, Strek ME: Diagnosis and treatment of pulmonary aspergillosis syndromes, Chest. 2014 Nov;146(5):1358-1368.)*

The patient had a sputum sample that grew *A. fumigatus*. She had some additional laboratory tests, including a positive serum IgG precipitins test for *A. fumigatus*. Bronchoscopy with biopsy is performed that shows "local invasion without dissemination."

What is the likely diagnosis?

A. Invasive pulmonary aspergillosis
B. Invasive bronchial aspergillosis
C. Chronic pulmonary aspergillosis
D. ABPA
E. Extrinsic allergic alveolitis

ANSWERS

Q25-1: C
Mass within a cavitary lesion in the left upper lobe

Rationale: There is a cavitary lesion with an internal mass, and one can barely make out the sliver of air separating the central mass or opacity and the cavity wall. This is called the "Monod sign," in which a solid mass is found within a cavity and the mass and cavity wall are separated by a few thin crests of radiolucent air. This is not always visible on a chest radiograph and is better visualized on CT. The wall is too thick to be a cyst. A Ranke complex is generally more calcified, representing the healed form of a Ghon complex in primary TB. Patients with resolved TB can develop cavitary lesions; however, they are not usually complex lesions containing solids or fluids.

Q25-2: B
Aspergilloma

Rationale: The patient is immunocompetent and previously had primary TB. He likely developed a cavitary lesion in the left upper lobe during resolution, and such structural abnormalities are critical risk factors for the development of an aspergilloma. An aspergilloma represents saprophytic (ie, generates energy from dead or decaying organic matter) colonization of a cavitary lesion in the lung parenchyma, and it is often referred to as a fungal or mycetoma. Although colonization of a post-tuberculous cavity is most common, it may develop from any cavitary lesion arising from any condition. Hemoptysis is the most common presentation. Patients may have positive sputum cultures as well as precipitating antibodies for *Aspergillus* species, and patients with associated hypersensitivity may have eosinophilia or an elevated total IgE level. As this is not an invasive form of *Aspergillus*-associated lung disease, there should be no significant systemic symptoms. Differential diagnoses include sarcoidosis, Wegener granulomatosis, and lung malignancy, as well as other bacterial and fungal infections.

Since the patient has no systemic symptoms, invasive pulmonary aspergillosis and chronic pulmonary aspergillosis are unlikely. The primary differential diagnosis is between an aspergilloma and ABPA. ABPA is a hypersensitivity reaction in response to *Aspergillus fumigatus* colonization of the airways, often presenting as refractory asthma and most often seen in patients with cystic fibrosis (CF). Patients will have sputum production, which may include airway casts or large plugs and possibly hemoptysis. Imaging typically shows central bronchiectasis (discussed separately), debris in the airways (mucous plugs), tree-in-bud opacities, ground-glass opacities, and evidence of air trapping (mosaic attenuation). Patients must have either underlying CF or asthma, with a positive *A. fumigatus*-specific serum IgE test (or positive skin test) and an elevated total serum IgE. Patients must also have two of the following: peripheral total eosinophilia, radiographic findings consistent with ABPA, or a positive serum precipitins study for *A. fumigatus*. Since this patient has a normal serum IgE, there is no diagnosis of ABPA. If there were no evidence of *Aspergillus*-related reactive airway disease, a diagnosis of allergic bronchial asthma could be considered.

An aspergilloma can lead to or overlap with another *Aspergillus*-related lung disease, including all the aforementioned options. As a result, continued observation of such patients is recommended.

Q25-3: C
Surgical resection

Rationale: Surgical resection is the definitive treatment for an aspergilloma. Bronchial artery embolization is an option for recurrent or emergent hemoptysis in patients who are not candidates for surgical resection, as are antifungal therapy (oral) and intracavitary instillation. Antibiotic therapy has been of variable efficacy, in part due to poor blood flow to the cavity. Lung transplantation is not an option for an aspergilloma.

Q25-4: A
Invasive pulmonary aspergillosis

Rationale: Given the systemic symptoms, ABPA and aspergilloma are not likely. Extrinsic allergic alveolitis is a pulmonary disorder that results from high-level or repeated inhalation of organic dust, and symptoms are usually acute in onset and similar to a viral presentation. This patient has significant abnormalities on the CT scan, including nodules with surrounding ground-glass opacities and cavitary lesions with intraluminal debris.

Invasive pulmonary aspergillosis is an aggressive disease process that occurs most commonly in immunocompromised patient populations: patients undergoing stem cell or solid organ transplantation, patients with leukemia or patients receiving chemotherapy, patients with inherited immunodeficiencies (HIV); however, it can also be seen in patients with poorly controlled diabetes mellitus, underlying structural lung disease or COPD, or chronic liver disease. Invasive aspergillosis has high morbidity and mortality, particularly if not recognized early in the disease process. The disease may have a rapid onset in patients with severe neutropenia, though it may also have a subacute presentation over the course of a few weeks to months. Depending on the degree of immunosuppression, patients may present with systemic symptoms, including fever, night sweats, fatigue, and weight loss. Nearly all patients will have cough and dyspnea, and some patients may develop hemoptysis. Any neurologic symptoms should raise suspicion for disseminated disease. A CT scan of the sinuses should be performed in patients with evidence of acute or chronic sinusitis. MRI of the brain is the best modality to examine the possibility of disseminated CNS aspergillosis because CT findings can be nonspecific. MRI can demonstrate evidence of cerebritis or abscess formation (ring-enhancing lesions). Although the gold standard for diagnosis is a tissue biopsy demonstrating septate hyphae with branching at 45-degree angles invading normally sterile tissue (in combination with a positive culture), many patients with invasive disease may not be candidates for biopsy because of thrombocytopenia (hematopoietic stem-cell transplantation [HSCT], leukemia, chemotherapy). In these patients, sputum cultures or BAL specimens may be used for direct imaging and culture; however, treatment should not be held pending these studies because of their poor sensitivity and lengthy time to results. These studies are more sensitive in patients with more severe immunosuppression. In general, a combination of clinical suspicion, serum or BAL galactomannan, and *Aspergillus*-specific PCR studies can provide further evidence of invasive disease. There is no role for serum total IgE, *Aspergillus*-specific serum IgE, or serum precipitins studies in invasive disease. Treatment is with antifungal therapy. Voriconazole, isavuconazole, or a lipid formulation of amphotericin B are the primary treatment options. Recall that amphotericin B has activity against mucormycosis as well, so if the diagnosis of invasive pulmonary aspergillosis is not established and there is evidence for disseminated fungal disease, this is a more appropriate option.

Alternatively, immunocompromised patients can also develop a bronchial- or airway-centric form of invasive aspergillosis, termed *invasive bronchial aspergillosis*. Imaging typically shows tree-in-bud opacities, mucoid impaction of airways, some surrounding ground-glass opacities, and perhaps mild interstitial opacities. Patients will often have progressive symptoms of cough and dyspnea without systemic symptoms. There is no significant hypersensitivity present, but patients may have a positive *Aspergillus* IgE or serum precipitins study. The biopsy demonstrates evidence of A. *fumigatus* invasion in the bronchial epithelium without invasion of the parenchyma. This is most consistent with invasive bronchial aspergillosis. It is most common in lung transplant recipients, occurring within the first 6 months of transplantation and most commonly at the anastomotic sites, but it can be seen in patients undergoing HSCT and patients with rheumatologic disease. Stridor can occur in severe forms. There are three subtypes, including tracheobronchitis/bronchitis, pseudomembranous tracheobronchitis (where pseudomembranes form in the airways), and ulcerative (associated with necrosis and ulceration of the bronchial epithelium). There is also a bronchial stump subtype, which arises at the stump site in patients after lung resection. Antifungal therapy is the mainstay for invasive bronchial aspergillosis. Hyperbaric oxygen therapy has been used as adjuvant therapy in some patients with the pseudomembranous subtype. Stent placement may be necessary for patients who develop complications such as stenosis.

Q25-5: D
Halo sign

Rationale: This is a classic finding of invasive pulmonary aspergillosis, in which a nodule is surrounded by a halo of ground glass and possible micronodules (termed *satellite nodules*). This is believed to be due to hemorrhage or inflammation in the areas surrounding the infectious nodules.

Q25-6: E
Air-crescent sign

Rationale: This should not be confused with the Monod sign, which is a small collection of air separating the internal mass from the wall of a cavitary lesion in an aspergilloma. Rather this is a collection (or crescent) of air that collects around an invasive nodule of aspergillosis. These terms are often confused. As one can see here, there is no well-formed cavity around the nodule, which helps differentiate it from the Monod sign. This is usually seen in late invasive aspergillosis (also termed *angioinvasive disease*) or during the early recovery process, where it may herald clinical improvement.

CT imaging of invasive pulmonary aspergillosis may demonstrate nodules with surrounding ground-glass opacities, larger areas of consolidation with or without cavitation, peribronchial opacities, and pleural effusions.

Q25-7 B
Serum galactomannan

Rationale: While none of the aforementioned tests is 100% specific or sensitive for the diagnosis of invasive pulmonary aspergillosis, a positive serum galactomannan is the most specific test of the options listed, with likely sensitivity and specificity of 70% to 80% in the appropriate patient population. Studies have overall demonstrated variable results for serum as well as BAL fluid galactomannan determinations, though the serum studies tend to be more sensitive overall. There are many potential complications that can lead to a false-positive or false-negative galactomannan study. There is some potential for cross-reactivity with other fungi, namely *Histoplasma capsulatum*. Certain foods may also cause a false positive, which may be due to the presence of *Penicillium* species. More recently developed PCR studies have also been used, with highly variable results, depending on the specific method utilized. The serum BDG is not specific because it is produced by many different bacteria. The examination of sputum samples is generally not specific for *A. fumigatus*. A serum procalcitonin is not useful because it may be positive in any bacterial infection as well.

Q25-8: C
Chronic pulmonary aspergillosis

Rationale: Chronic pulmonary aspergillosis generally presents with a prolonged history of productive cough, fatigue, weight loss, dyspnea, reduced exercise tolerance, chest pain, and possibly hemoptysis. Chronic pulmonary aspergillosis occurs in two subtypes: CFPA (fibrosing) and CCPA (cavitary). The cavitary form usually starts with large areas of consolidation or nodules that eventually cavitate with disease progression. Fibrosing disease is characterized by these findings but with concomitant interstitial fibrosis. Acute or subacute invasive pulmonary aspergillosis used to be termed *chronic necrotizing pulmonary aspergillosis*, but it is now referred to as *invasive pulmonary aspergillosis* (discussed previously). A diagnosis of chronic pulmonary aspergillosis requires one or more cavitary lung lesions (with or without an aspergilloma), systemic symptoms, and evidence of *Aspergillus* as the causative agent (positive sputum culture or positive serum precipitins study). Chronic pulmonary aspergillosis is a chronic, indolent infection with *Aspergillus* that can have local (semi-) invasive disease but is without evidence of dissemination or true invasion. It occurs most commonly in patients with structural lung disease and some mild form immunosuppression (diabetes, chronic steroid use). Morbidity and mortality are high.

Important differential considerations include mycobacterial infections, other endemic functional infections, Wegener granulomatosis, and sarcoidosis, among others. Treatment is prolonged courses of antibiotics, which can lead to regression of disease and shrinkage of the cavities. The primary treatment recommendation is voriconazole, though itraconazole is also an option. Surgery is typically of limited utility in chronic disease.

Spectrum of Pulmonary Disease Caused by *Aspergillus*

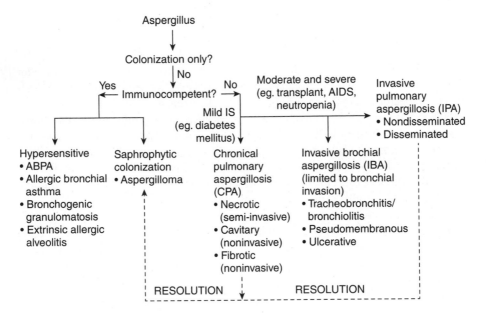

References

Affolter K, Tamm M, Jahn K, et al. Galactomannan in bronchoalveolar lavage for diagnosing invasive fungal disease. Am J Respir Crit Care Med. 2014;190:309.

Aguado JM, Vázquez L, Fernández-Ruiz M, et al. Serum galactomannan versus a combination of galactomannan and polymerase chain reaction-based *Aspergillus* DNA detection for early therapy of invasive aspergillosis in high-risk hematological patients: a randomized controlled trial. Clin Infect Dis. 2015;60:405.

Caillot D, Couaillier JF, Bernard A, et al. Increasing volume and changing characteristics of invasive pulmonary aspergillosis on sequential thoracic computed tomography scans in patients with neutropenia. J Clin Oncol. 2001;19:253.

Cuenca-Estrella M, Bassetti M, Lass-Flörl C, et al. Detection and investigation of invasive mould disease. J Antimicrob Chemother. 2011;i15.

Denning DW, Cadranel J, Beigelman-Aubry C, et al. Chronic pulmonary aspergillosis: rationale and clinical guidelines for diagnosis and management. Eur Respir J. 2016;47:45.

Denning DW, Riniotis K, Dobrashian R, Sambatakou H. Chronic cavitary and fibrosing pulmonary and pleural aspergillosis: case series, proposed nomenclature change, and review. Clin Infect Dis. 2003;37:S265.

Desai SR, Hedayati V, Patel K, Hansell DM. Chronic aspergillosis of the lungs: unravelling the terminology and radiology. Eur Radiol. 2015;25:3100.

Dumollard C, Bailly S, Perriot S, et al. Prospective evaluation of a new *Aspergillus* IgG enzyme immunoassay kit for diagnosis of chronic and allergic pulmonary aspergillosis. J Clin Microbiol. 2016;54:1236.

Fernández-Ruiz M, Silva JT, San-Juan R, et al. *Aspergillus* tracheobronchitis: report of 8 cases and review of the literature. Medicine (Baltimore). 2012;91:261.

Fisher CE, Stevens AM, Leisenring W, et al. The serum galactomannan index predicts mortality in hematopoietic stem cell transplant recipients with invasive aspergillosis. Clin Infect Dis. 2013;57:1001.

Georgiadou SP, Sipsas NV, Marom EM, Kontoyiannis DP. The diagnostic value of halo and reversed halo signs for invasive mold infections in compromised hosts. Clin Infect Dis. 2011;52:1144.

Godet C, Laurent F, Bergeron A, et al. CT imaging assessment of response to treatment in chronic pulmonary aspergillosis. Chest. 2016;150:139.

Herbrecht R, Denning DW, Patterson TF, et al. Voriconazole versus amphotericin B for primary therapy of invasive aspergillosis. N Engl J Med. 2002;347:408.

Judson MA, Stevens DA. The treatment of pulmonary aspergilloma. Curr Opin Investig Drugs. 2001;2:1375.

Lal H, Asmita, Mangla L, Prasad, Gautam M, Nath A. Imaging features of pulmonary infection in post renal transplant recipients: a review. Indian J of Transplant. 2017;11:13.

Leeflang MM, Debets-Ossenkopp YJ, Wang J, et al. Galactomannan detection for invasive aspergillosis in immunocompromised patients. Cochrane Database Syst Rev. 2015;CD007394.

Limper AH, Knox KS, Sarosi GA, et al. An official American Thoracic Society statement: treatment of fungal infections in adult pulmonary and critical care patients. Am J Respir Crit Care Med. 2011;183:96.

McCarthy M, Rosengart A, Schuetz AN, et al. Mold infections of the central nervous system. N Engl J Med. 2014;371:150.

Miceli MH, Grazziutti ML, Woods G, et al. Strong correlation between serum aspergillus galacto-mannan index and outcome of aspergillosis in patients with hematological cancer: clinical and research implications. Clin Infect Dis. 2008;46:1412.

Miceli MH, Maertens J. Role of non-culture-based tests, with an emphasis on galactomannan testing for the diagnosis of invasive aspergillosis. Semin Respir Crit Care Med. 2015;36:650.

Ofori A, Steinmetz AR, Akaasi J, et al. Pulmonary aspergilloma: an evasive disease. Int J Mycobacteriol. 2016;5:235.

Page ID, Richardson MD, Denning DW. Comparison of six *Aspergillus*-specific IgG assays for the diagnosis of chronic pulmonary aspergillosis (CPA). J Infect. 2016;72:240.

Patterson KC, Strek ME. Diagnosis and treatment of pulmonary aspergillosis syndromes. Chest. 2014;146:1358.

Patterson TF, Thompson GR 3rd, Denning DW, et al. Practice guidelines for the diagnosis and management of aspergillosis: 2016 Update by the Infectious Diseases Society of America. Clin Infect Dis. 2016;63:e1.

Pfeiffer CD, Fine JP, Safdar N. Diagnosis of invasive aspergillosis using a galactomannan assay: a meta-analysis. Clin Infect Dis. 2006;42:1417.

Segal BH, Walsh TJ. Current approaches to diagnosis and treatment of invasive aspergillosis. Am J Respir Crit Care Med. 2006;173:707.

Shin B, Koh WJ, Jeong BH, et al. Serum galactomannan antigen test for the diagnosis of chronic pulmonary aspergillosis. J Infect. 2014;68:494.

Stanzani M, Battista G, Sassi C, et al. Computed tomographic pulmonary angiography for diagnosis of invasive mold diseases in patients with hematological malignancies. Clin Infect Dis. 2012;54:610.

White PL, Parr C, Thornton C, Barnes RA. Evaluation of real-time PCR, galactomannan enzyme-linked immunosorbent assay (ELISA), and a novel lateral-flow device for diagnosis of invasive aspergillosis. J Clin Microbiol. 2013;51:1510.

CASE 26

A 23-year-old man is being admitted to the ICU. He was found unconscious at home, and there is limited information regarding his medical history. He was found prone on the floor of his apartment after a neighbor called the police about water leaking into the apartment below. The police found the bathtub overflowing and the patient obtunded and not responsive to sternal rub. The patient's apartment was disheveled, and there was evidence of intravenous drug use. Emergency medical services attempted intranasal naloxone therapy, but this did not reverse his encephalopathy. He is cachectic, with skin lesions on his legs (Image 26-2). No other medications are found in the apartment. The patient is very hypoxemic and was intubated in the field with a King airway. The patient was then intubated with an endotracheal tube on arrival to the ED. He is receiving invasive mechanical ventilation and requires PEEP 12 cm H_2O and 70% FIO_2 to maintain his PaO_2 greater than 55 mm Hg. He has basic laboratory tests sent, pan-cultured, and he is started on broad-spectrum antibiotics. His respiratory acidosis quickly corrects with mechanical ventilation, and a mild metabolic acidosis remains. A drug screen returns positive for opioids but is negative otherwise, including salicylate, acetaminophen, and ethanol levels. There is no osmolar gap. The patient remains unconscious and is requiring no sedation despite being intubated. CT of the brain shows no acute intracranial process, and CT of the cervical spine is negative. The patient is placed in a C-collar. The patient required no sedative, analgesia, anxiolytics, or paralytics for intubation and has not required sedation since that time (approximately 4 hours). On examination, the patient has intact cranial nerve reflexes but does not follow commands, open his eyes, or move his extremities. The patient has severe scars from prior skin-popping and intravenous drug use. He is febrile to 103.1°F, and other vital signs are HR 121 and BP 176/88. He does not withdraw to painful stimuli. The patient's chest radiograph is shown in Image 26-1, and the patient's skin examination abnormalities are shown in Image 26-2.

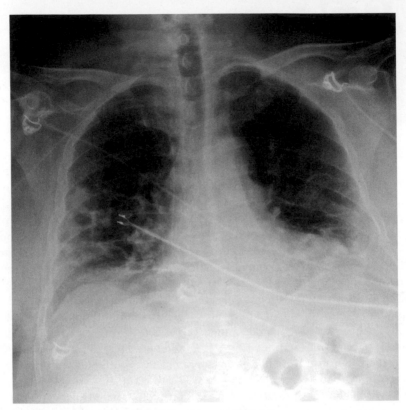

Image 26-1 • Chest radiograph for the patient in **Case 26**.

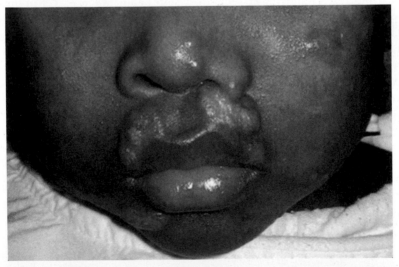

Image 26-2 • Representative images of the skin lesions identified for the patient in **Case 26**, demonstrating pink plaques with crusted erosions on the face. (*Reproduced with permission from Kang S, Amagai M, Bruckner AL, et al: Fitzpatrick's Dermatology, 9th ed. New York, NY: McGraw Hill; 2019.*)

QUESTIONS

Q26-1: How would you best describe the abnormalities on the chest radiograph in Image 26-1?

A. Reticulonodular interstitial pattern
B. Linear interstitial pattern
C. Miliary pattern
D. Focal consolidation
E. Diffuse airspace opacities

Q26-2: The patient's platelet count is within normal limits, and the patient's INR is 1.0 with a normal prothrombin time (PTT) and an elevated fibrinogen level. What would be the next step in your diagnostic evaluation?

A. Bronchoscopy with bronchoalveolar lavage (BAL) and transbronchial biopsy
B. Serum ammonia level
C. Lumbar puncture (LP)
D. Skin biopsy
E. HIV p24 antibody study, HIV RNA PCR, and CD4 count
F. Electroencephalogram (EEG)
G. MRI of the brain

Q26-3: The patient undergoes an LP. The opening pressure was 44 cm H_2O (normal, less than 20). The glucose was 5 mg/dL, the protein 108 mg/dL, and the cell count in tube 4 was 8 nucleated cells/µL with a lymphocyte predominance. The Giemsa stain from the CSF is shown in Image 26-3.

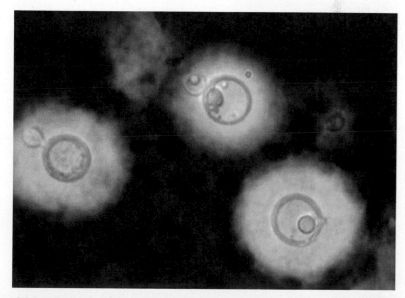

Image 26-3 • Example of the Giemsa stain from cerebral spinal fluid of the patient in **Case 26.** (*Reproduced with permission from Riedel S, Hobden JA, Miller S, et al: Jawetz, Melnick, & Adelberg's Medical Microbiology, 28th ed. New York, NY: McGraw Hill; 2019.*)

What is the likely diagnosis?

A. Disseminated invasive pulmonary aspergillosis (IPA)
B. Disseminated cryptococcal infection
C. Disseminated blastomycosis
D. *Streptococcus pneumoniae* meningitis and pneumonia
E. *Hemophilus influenza* meningitis and pneumonia

Q26-4: The patient's HIV RNA PCR returns positive, as does the patient's anti-body test. Which CD4 count would you anticipate for the patient in this case? Units are number/μL.

A. 300
B. 200
C. 150
D. 75
E. 600

Q26-5: What is the most sensitive test for the diagnosis of disseminated crypto-coccal infection in this patient?

A. India ink study of BAL fluid
B. India ink study of CSF
C. CSF cryptococcal antigen titer
D. Culture of sputum
E. Culture of peripheral blood

Q26-6: What is the first-line antifungal therapy for this patient?

A. Amphotericin-B
B. Voriconazole
C. Fluconazole
D. Posaconazole
E. Amphotericin-B and flucytosine

ANSWERS

Q26-1: E
Diffuse airspace opacities

Rationale: The patient's chest radiograph has components of linear and reticular interstitial opacities coupled with more hazy alveolar opacities (particularly peripherally on the right). Note also the presence of a right-sided peripherally located central venous catheter terminating in the superior vena cava (SVC). There is no apparent pneumothorax, but there is blunting of the left costophrenic angle, which may be due to effusion or consolidation. This mixed pattern with the presence of more alveolar opacities is often termed *diffuse airspace disease*. This pattern is nonspecific and can be seen in a number of different conditions, including multifocal pneumonia, atypical infection, COVID-19 pneumonia, acute interstitial pneumonia (AIP), diffuse alveolar hemorrhage (DAH), and acute respiratory distress syndrome (ARDS). The patient's skin lesions are consistent with acneiform papules and pustules that are characteristic of widespread systemic infections.

Q26-2: C
Lumbar puncture (LP)

Rationale: The overall clinical picture is concerning for possible meningitis given the patient's clinical presentation. He has intact cranial nerve reflexes, but his neurologic examination is poor otherwise, despite not receiving any sedating medications or paralytics. The patient also has an obvious pulmonary process ongoing, and *Streptococcus pneumoniae* infection would be high on the differential in this case. Additionally, the patient has a likely history of intravenous drug use and would be at high risk for HIV infection and the presence of AIDS. An LP would therefore take priority to establish a diagnosis of meningitis or meningoencephalitis because this would alter the patient's treatment. The CT scan of the head did not demonstrate evidence of a mass lesion or hydrocephalus. Although there is a small risk of cerebral herniation if there is elevated intracranial pressure (ICP), the patient is severely ill. The LP will provide immediate clinical information, including anopening pressure, cerebral spinal fluid (CSF) protein, glucose, nucleated and red blood cell counts, differential, Gram stain, KOH/GMS stain, and India ink staining. Bronchoscopy with BAL with or without biopsy would be a bit risky given the patient's current ventilator support settings, and these studies will not help to determine if central nervous system infection is present. An endotracheal aspirate sample should be sent for appropriate culture studies. HIV antibody and RNA PCR are certainly advisable here, but again, they do not rule out meningitis. A serum ammonia level may also be helpful to rule out other causes of encephalitis. An EEG may also be useful to rule out subclinical seizure activity, though the LP would take priority, as the patient's most likely cause of encephalopathy is from infection, cerebrovascular accident (CVA), or drug use. An MRI would be helpful to determine if the patient had a nonhemorrhagic CVA, as this patient would be at risk for an acute embolism if left-sided endocarditis was present. Also, this may identify the presence of active inflammation in the brain or meninges. However, the LP would still be necessary to obtain appropriate cultures. Although most of these tests would be ordered simultaneously, the question is focused on what the most immediate next step should be.

Q26-3: B
Disseminated cryptococcal infection

Rationale: The Giemsa stain demonstrates the classic encapsulated yeast forms as well as budding yeast forms. The presentation with pneumonia and meningo-encephalitis is consistent with likely disseminated disease; however, the diagnosis of cryptococcal pneumonia would still need to be confirmed as the patient may have two separate infectious processes ongoing. In cryptococcal meningoencephalitis, a low nucleated cell count (less than 25-50 cells with a lymphocyte or monocyte predominance), a low glucose level, and very high opening pressure are more classical findings, but they are not specific. Some patients may have completely normal CSF studies aside from a positive CSF cryptococcal antigen. Disease can be disseminated to other sites, notably the liver, spleen, and bone marrow, though any organ system may be affected. *Cryptococcus neoformans* is the species associated with the bulk of cryptococcal infections, though *Cryptococcus gattii* also causes disease in tropical climates as well in the Pacific Northwest of the United States and in British Columbia. The bulk of disseminated cryptococcal disease occurs in immunocompromised hosts, which will be discussed further in this case. Cryptococcal pneumonia rarely presents in isolation in immunocompromised hosts and more often causes a more severe pulmonary presentation and disseminated disease, which may include meningoencephalitis. The acneiform papules or pustules seen in **Image 26-2** are seen in up to 20% of disseminated cases and may progress to warty or vegetating crusted plaques, ulcers, and hard infiltrated plaques or nodules.

Cryptococcal meningitis usually has a subacute pattern of worsening, with symptoms progressively worsening over a 2- to 3-week course. Initial symptoms may include fever, headache, photophobia, stiff neck, nausea, and the development of rash. As the disease progresses and intracranial pressure increases, patients may develop encephalopathy, focal neurologic deficits, and advance to coma or herniation.

Cryptococcal infections in immunocompetent patients may be entirely asymptomatic, or patients with a large exposure or inoculum may have symptoms typical of community-acquired pneumonia. The radiographic findings are variable and may include noncalcified pulmonary nodules, lobar infiltrates, hilar adenopathy, pleural effusions, and cavitary lung nodules or masses (see an example of such findings in **Images 26-4** through **26-7**). The diagnosis of cryptococcal pneumonia in these patients requires either positive culture data from a sputum or bronchoalveolar lavage specimen or a biopsy specimen with subsequent staining. If an effusion is present, these can be samples and are often culture positive as well. The serum antigen and serum serologies are not sensitive in immunocompetent hosts but should still be obtained. Generally, an LP is not necessary for these patients if there are no clinical signs of meningoencephalitis; however, patients with extremely high cryptococcal antigen titers (greater than 1:512) should undergo an empiric LP even if they are asymptomatic. In the absence of severe underlying lung disease and dissemination, the treatment is generally with fluconazole or itraconazole for 6 months or longer.

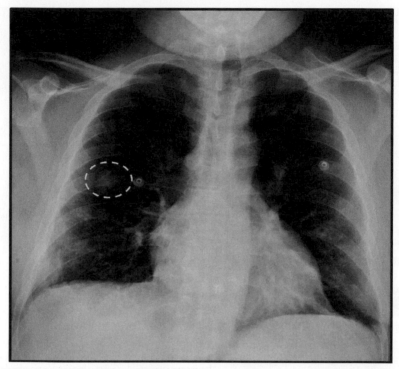

Image 26-4 • An example of isolated pulmonary cryptococcal infection. Note the nodular opacity in the right parenchymal space.

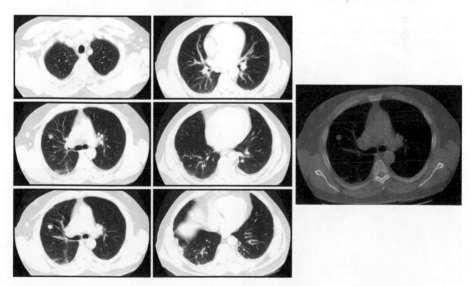

Image 26-5 • CT of the chest demonstrating the nodular appearance of pulmonary cryptococcal infection.

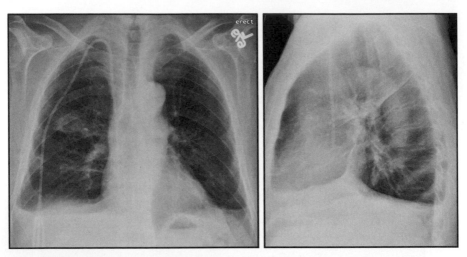

Image 26-6 • Cavitary nodule in a patient with isolated cryptococcal pneumonia.

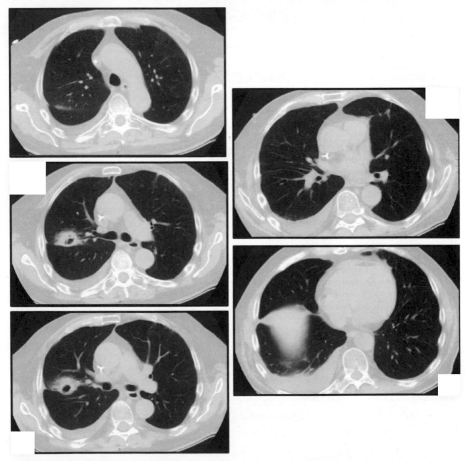

Image 26-7 • Corresponding CT scan for **Image 26-6**, demonstrating cavitation. Note the associated pleural effusion, which was also positive for yeast.

Q26-4: D
75 (/μL)

Patients with HIV are at increased risk of bacterial pneumonia and *Mycobacterium tuberculosis*, independent of CD4 count. At counts below 500, the risk of Kaposi sarcoma increases. At CD4 counts below 300, the risk of *Candida* and parasitic infections increases. Below 200, the risk of PCP pneumonia and toxoplasmosis increases. At counts below 100, the risk of *Mycobacterium avium* complex (MAC) and cryptococcal infection increases, and at counts below 50, the risk of cytomegalovirus (CMV) (particularly retinitis) increases. Therefore, in this case, we would expect the patient's CD4 count to be below 100/μL.

Q26-5: C
CSF cryptococcal antigen titer

Rationale: In immunocompromised patients with disseminated disease, the CSF cryptococcal antigen titer has excellent specificity and sensitivity (approaching 100%), as does the serum antigen test and BAL antigen testing. This is followed by a culture of infected bodily fluid (CSF, BAL). India ink studies have the least sensitivity of the proposed studies. The CSF cryptococcal antigen test is particularly useful as the improvement in antigen titer provides prognostic information, while the serum antigen test is not useful in this manner. PCR tests are currently under investigation.

Q26-6: E
Amphotericin-B and flucytosine

Rationale: Although the duration of each phase of treatment for disseminated cryptococcal infection varies depending on the severity of illness, the presence of neurologic symptoms, and the response to treatment, the induction therapy is liposomal or lipid-based amphotericin B and flucytosine. For patients with meningoencephalitis (with or without HIV), it is given for 4 to 6 weeks for induction, and then fluconazole is administered as "maintenance" or consolidation therapy (8 weeks at 400-800 mg/day) followed by chronic therapy (200-400 mg/day), which is given for at least a year if not longer (potentially life-long in patients requiring ongoing immunosuppression or in HIV-positive patients). The duration of induction therapy can vary depending on follow-up LP testing results, particularly the opening pressure and the reduction in cryptococcal CSF antigen levels. The transition to consolidation is usually hand-tailored by experienced infectious disease physicians. If flucytosine is not available, high-dose fluconazole can be used (800 mg daily) for induction. Patients may also require repeated LP during induction to stabilize intracranial pressures, and patients with elevated levels at the onset of treatment may require shunts or CSF drains. Typically, the CSF is reduced below 20 cm H_2O during each LP (or to a level of 50% of the opening pressure if it is initially greater than approximately 40 cm H_2O). This is usually repeated daily for a few days until the patient is stable. If CSF pressures continually rise despite this approach, a drain or shunt may be necessary. Patients who do not have neurologic symptoms at presentation but have positive CSF antigen titers may be able to transition more rapidly to consolidation; this is usually determined by the clearance of CSF cultures rather than the CSF antigen titers. Glucocorticoids are not indicated for cryptococcal meningitis, but they may be used to prevent immune reconstitution inflammatory syndrome in patients with AIDS who are started on highly active antiretroviral therapy (HAART) during therapy. Typically, HAART is started 4 to 6 weeks after the start of antifungal therapy (or at the time of consolidation or maintenance therapy).

References

Baddley JW, Perfect JR, Oster RA, et al. Pulmonary cryptococcosis in patients without HIV infection: factors associated with disseminated disease. Eur J Clin Microbiol Infect Dis. 2008;27:937.

Cameron ML, Bartlett JA, Gallis HA, Waskin HA. Manifestations of pulmonary cryptococcosis in patients with acquired immunodeficiency syndrome. Rev Infect Dis. 1991;13:64.

Campbell GD. Primary pulmonary cryptococcosis. Am Rev Respir Dis. 1966;94:236.

Chang WC, Tzao C, Hsu HH, et al. Pulmonary cryptococcosis: comparison of clinical and radiographic characteristics in immunocompetent and immunocompromised patients. Chest. 2006;129:333.

Dromer F, Bernede-Bauduin C, Guillemot D, et al. Major role for amphotericin B-flucytosine combination in severe cryptococcosis. PLoS One. 2008;3:e2870.

Dromer F, Mathoulin-Pélissier S, Launay O, et al. Determinants of disease presentation and outcome during cryptococcosis: the CryptoA/D study. PLoS Med. 2007;4:e21.

Ettinger NA, Trulock EP. Pulmonary considerations of organ transplantation. Part I. Am Rev Respir Dis. 1991;143:1386.

Fishman JA, Rubin RH. Infection in organ-transplant recipients. N Engl J Med 1998;338:1741.

Graybill JR, Sobel J, Saag M, et al. Diagnosis and management of increased intracranial pressure in patients with AIDS and cryptococcal meningitis. The NIAID Mycoses Study Group and AIDS Cooperative Treatment Groups. Clin Infect Dis. 2000;30:47.

Ingram PR, Howman R, Leahy MF, Dyer JR. Cryptococcal immune reconstitution inflammatory syndrome following alemtuzumab therapy. Clin Infect Dis. 2007;44:e115.

Larsen RA, Bozzette SA, Jones BE, et al. Fluconazole combined with flucytosine for treatment of cryptococcal meningitis in patients with AIDS. Clin Infect Dis. 1994;19:741.

Mayanja-Kizza H, Oishi K, Mitarai S, et al. Combination therapy with fluconazole and flucytosine for cryptococcal meningitis in Ugandan patients with AIDS. Clin Infect Dis. 1998;26:1362.

Perfect JR, Dismukes WE, Dromer F, et al. Clinical practice guidelines for the management of cryptococcal disease: 2010 update by the infectious diseases society of America. Clin Infect Dis. 2010;50:291.

Perfect JR, Marr KA, Walsh TJ, et al. Voriconazole treatment for less-common, emerging, or refractory fungal infections. Clin Infect Dis. 2003;36:1122.

Shirley RM, Baddley JW. Cryptococcal lung disease. Curr Opin Pulm Med. 2009;15:254.

Singh N, Lortholary O, Alexander BD, et al. Antifungal management practices and evolution of infection in organ transplant recipients with cryptococcus neoformans infection. Transplantation 2005;80:1033.

Sun HY, Singh N. Opportunistic infection-associated immune reconstitution syndrome in transplant recipients. Clin Infect Dis. 2011;53:168.

Sun HY, Wagener MM, Singh N. Cryptococcosis in solid-organ, hematopoietic stem cell, and tissue transplant recipients: evidence-based evolving trends. Clin Infect Dis. 2009;48:1566.

van der Horst CM, Saag MS, Cloud GA, et al. Treatment of cryptococcal meningitis associated with the acquired immunodeficiency syndrome. National Institute of Allergy and Infectious Diseases Mycoses Study Group and AIDS Clinical Trials Group. N Engl J Med. 1997;337:15.

Vilchez RA, Linden P, Lacomis J, et al. Acute respiratory failure associated with pulmonary cryptococcosis in non-aids patients. Chest. 2001;119:1865.

Yang CJ, Hwang JJ, Wang TH, et al. Clinical and radiographic presentations of pulmonary cryptococcosis in immunocompetent patients. Scand J Infect Dis. 2006;38:788.

Young EJ, Hirsh DD, Fainstein V, Williams TW. Pleural effusions due to Cryptococcus neoformans: a review of the literature and report of two cases with cryptococcal antigen determinations. Am Rev Respir Dis. 1980;121:743.

CASE 27

A 28-year-old White woman presents with acute hypoxemic respiratory failure. She has no medical history. She takes no medications, and she does not smoke or use illicit drugs. She gave birth to a healthy child approximately 3 months ago. Her fiancée states she developed a cough, low-grade fevers, and dyspnea about 4 days ago. Two days ago, she was seen at urgent care center and thought to have pneumonia. She was started on azithromycin, but her condition progressively worsened. The patient's vital signs are T 37. 9°C, HR 109, BP 144/81, RR 22, and oxygen saturation 87% on 6 L/min supplemental O_2. She had also noted some myalgia, joint aches, and pleuritic chest pain. On arrival to the ED, the patient required intubation for respiratory distress, and she is now receiving mechanical ventilation. The patient's kidney and liver function are intact and within normal limits. She has a leukocytosis to 17,000/μL with 85% neutrophils and no band forms. The patient's CXR is shown in Image 27-1.

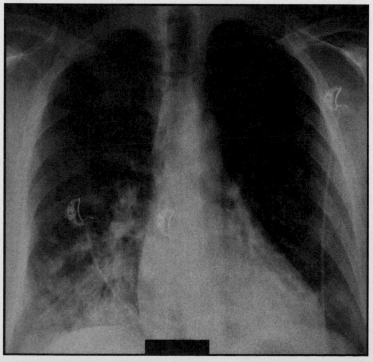

Image 27-1 • Chest radiograph (AP) for the patient in **Question 27-1**.

QUESTIONS

Q27-1: What abnormalities are present on the chest film?

A. Reticulonodular interstitial opacities
B. Diffuse alveolar infiltrates
C. Enlarged cardiac silhouette
D. Left upper lobe cystic lung lesion

Q27-2: The patient's ECG is as shown in Image 27-2:

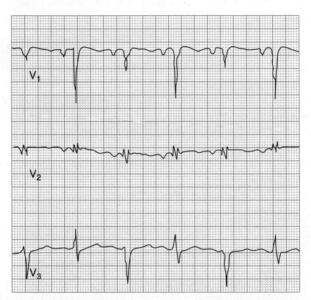

Image 27-2 • Electrocardiogram for the patient in **Question 27-2**. (*Reproduced with permission from McKean S, Ross JJ, Dressler DD, et al: Principles and Practice of Hospital Medicine, 2nd ed. New York NY: McGraw Hill; 2017.*)

Based on the ECG, what would be your primary concern?

A. Dilated cardiomyopathy
B. Hypertrophic cardiomyopathy
C. Acute ST-segment elevation myocardial infarction (STEMI)
D. Pulmonary embolism (PE)
E. Pericardial effusion
F. Pericarditis

Q27-3: You perform a STAT echocardiogram at the bedside that confirms your suspicion as shown in Images 27-3 and 27-4.

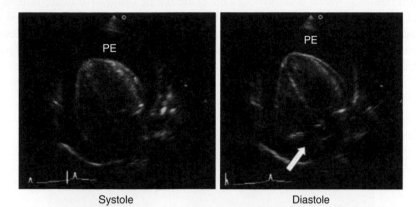

Systole   Diastole

Image 27-3 • Representative ultrasound images for the patient in **Question 27-3**. Large pericardial effusions with tamponade physiology. (*Reproduced with permission from Little WC, Freeman GL. Pericardial disease, Circulation 2006 Mar 28;113(12):1622-1632.*)

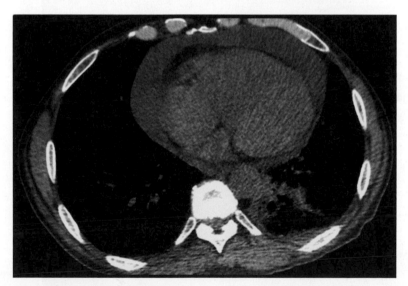

Image 27-4 • Large pericardial effusion on CT.

The patient is rushed to the catheterization laboratory for placement of a pericardial drain. She undergoes a postprocedure echocardiogram and right-heart catheterization, which demonstrates no evidence of congestive heart failure. A STAT CT angiogram of the chest is negative for PE. The patient is started on broad-spectrum antibiotics. You perform a bedside ultrasound and find a pleural effusion as shown in Image 27-5. Additionally, on examination, you identify the following rash shown in Image 27-6:

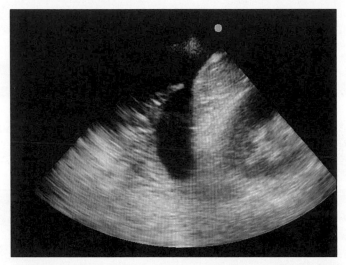

Image 27-5 • Representative thoracic ultrasound image for the patient in **Question 27-3**.

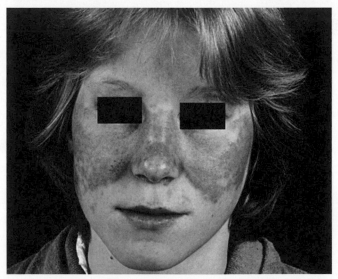

Image 27-6 • Dermatologic abnormalities identified during examination of the patient in **Question 27-3**. (*Reproduced with permission from Wolff K, Johnson RA, Saavedra AP, et al: Fitzpatrick's Color Atlas and Synopsis of Clinical Dermatology, 8th ed. New York, NY: McGraw Hill; 2017.*)

You perform a thoracentesis, and the fluid is serosanguineous. The pH is 7.40, and the glucose level is normal. The Gram stain, KOH, and AFB smear are negative. The cell count is 8,000/µL with a 90% neutrophilic predominance. The fluid is exudative based on the lactate dehydrogenase (LDH) and protein. In addition to the standard laboratory tests sent with the pleural effusion fluid for analysis (cell count, LDH, protein, glucose, and cultures), what additional study should you send from this patient's pleural fluid?

A. Adenosine deaminase
B. Pro-BNP
C. Antinuclear antibody
D. Anti-dsDNA
E. Flow cytometry for leukemia

Q27-4: You send the study, which returns positive at a titer of 1:2560 for the ANA. To rule out an infection, you perform a bronchoscopy with BAL. In addition to the standard studies, what additional study could you perform to help determine the etiology of the patient's respiratory failure?

A. Flow cytometry
B. Serial lavage
C. CD4+/CD8+ cell count
D. Periodic acid-Schiff staining
E. Energy-dispersive electron microscopy

Q27-5: The patient in the above scenario has a no evidence of bloody return on serial lavage and is diagnosed with ALP. What is the primary treatment for this patient?

A. High-dose intravenous steroids (1-2 g/day prednisone equivalent)
B. Mycophenolate
C. Continuous renal replacement therapy
D. Plasmapheresis
E. Weight-based prednisone (0.5 mg/kg per day)

Q27-6: The patient in the above scenario received appropriate therapy, improves clinically, and is lost to follow-up for 5 years. She presents to clinic with complaints of shortness of breath, and her chest imaging is shown in Image 27-7.

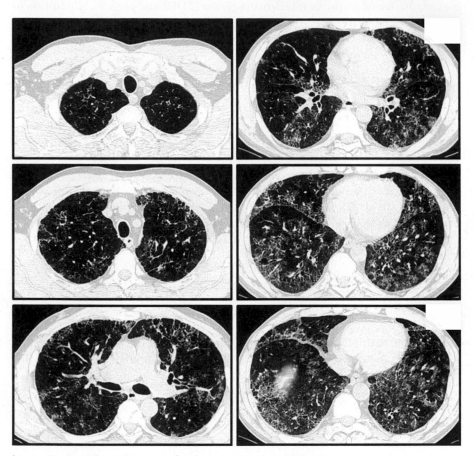

Image 27-7 • Chest CT images for the patient in **Question 27-6**.

How would you describe the abnormalities seen above?

A. Diffuse alveolar infiltrates
B. Reticular interstitial pattern with traction bronchiectasis and honeycombing
C. Mosaic pattern of ground-glass opacities
D. Cavitary lung lesions
E. Centrilobular emphysematous changes
F. Tree-in-bud opacities and scattered ground glass

Q27-7: A patient with known SLE presents to the ED with worsening dyspnea and new-onset hypoxemia. She has no cough, but she has moderate symmetric pitting edema of the lower extremities bilaterally. She is requiring 2 L O$_2$ on NC at rest. She notes that the dyspnea started several months ago and has progressively worsened, with the edema developing over the last month. She has been taking hydroxychloroquine for SLE for the last 6 years. The patient's chest radiograph is shown in Image 27-8.

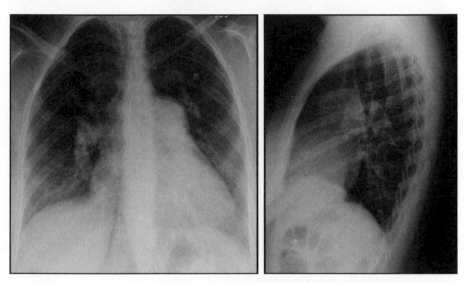

Image 27-8 • Chest radiographs (PA and lateral) for the patient in **Question 27-7**.

What is the likely diagnosis?

A. Acute lupus pneumonitis
B. Acute reversible hypoxia syndrome
C. Diffuse alveolar hemorrhage
D. Pulmonary hypertension
E. Emphysema

Q27-8: Another patient with SLE presents with the following chest radiograph shown in Image 27-9, with worsening dyspnea and intermittent pleuritic chest pain over the last 6 months. She also reports some mild fatigue.

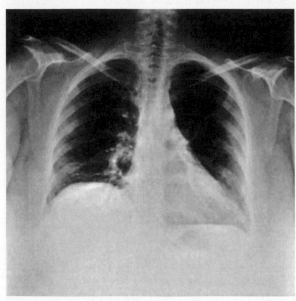

Pulmonary Function Testing:

FEV1	59%
FVC	63%
Ratio	100%
TLC	61%
VC	59%
RV	57%
DLCO	70%

Image 27-9 • Chest radiograph for the patient in **Question 27-8**. (*Reproduced with permission from Warrington KJ, Moder KG, Brutinel WM. The shrinking lungs syndrome in systemic lupus erythematosus. Mayo Clin Proc 2000 May;75(5):467-472.*)

A CT scan demonstrates no evidence of parenchymal disease or pleural disease. What is the likely diagnosis?

A. Pulmonary hypertension
B. SLE-associated ILD
C. Shrinking lung syndrome
D. Chronic obstructive pulmonary disease
E. Trapped lung

ANSWERS

Q27-1: B
Diffuse alveolar infiltrates

Rationale: There is a diffuse alveolar filling pattern present, more prominent on the right. This pattern could be seen in a number of possible pathologies.

Q27-2: E
Pericardial effusion

Rationale: This ECG shows electrical alternans (alternative voltages between beats), a classic finding in patients with large pericardial effusions with tamponade physiology, in which the right ventricular free wall is compressed by the effusion during diastole. This pattern can also be seen in rare cases of Wolf-Parkinson-White (WPW) syndrome and in a pattern of pseudo-alternans that is benign, but when this sign is present, tamponade must be ruled out. There are no ST-segment elevations present to suggest a STEMI. The most common ECG abnormality in PE is sinus tachycardia, which is highly nonspecific. Evidence of right heart strain (S1Q3T3) would be more concerning for an acute PE. Pericarditis can present with PR segment depressions with reciprocal ST elevations (or vice-versa, depending on the lead selected).

Q27-3: C
Antinuclear antibody

Rationale: Although the presence of a pleural effusion in patient with a suspected acute pulmonary process is not uncommon, the finding of an associated pericardial effusion should raise suspicion for a possible autoimmune or rheumatologic condition, and systemic lupus erythematous (SLE) should be high on list given the presence of a pericardial effusion as well as the appearance of the malar rash on the patient's face. Unlike serum studies, the anti-nuclear antibody (ANA) is the most specific test for lupus pleuritis, whereas the dsDNA test can also be positive in tuberculosis and certain types of malignancy. An ANA titer of greater than 1:160 is highly suggestive of lupus pleuritis. Lupus pleuritis is the most common pulmonary manifestation of SLE.

Q27-4: B
Serial lavage

Rationale: The basic studies sent during bronchoscopy will aid in determining if there is an infectious cause of the patient's acute respiratory failure. For patients with SLE, there are two manifestations that may present with acute respiratory failure with chest radiography abnormalities as seen above. The first is acute lupus pneumonitis (ALP), which may be a presenting symptom of SLE. Pleural effusions occur in about 50% of cases overall, and a fulminant form of the disease can occur during or shortly after pregnancy. The second manifestation is diffuse alveolar hemorrhage (DAH), which may be due to pulmonary capillaritis or bland hemorrhage

(**Images 27-10** through **27-13**). DAH more commonly manifests in patients with a known diagnosis of SLE, though it can be the initial presenting symptom. Both conditions are potentially severe and life-threatening. There is significant overlap between ALP and DAH, with a similar radiographic and clinical presentation and potentially similar findings on pathology and immunofluorescence studies. Both may present with hemoptysis as well, though it is more commonly associated with DAH. A diagnosis of DAH may be made by histopathologic examination, but in many patients with DAH biopsy may not be possible because of thrombocytopenia (eg, hematopoietic stem cell transplant recipients). Serial lavage remains an alternative method for diagnosis. In DAH, the return lavage fluid becomes progressively more bloody with sequential lavage. While the treatment for both DAH and ALP is similar, there is clinical value in differentiating between the two etiologies, as they have distinctly different prognosis and risks of recurrence. DAH can also be diagnosed with a DLCO study, if the patient can tolerate this maneuver, as it should be increased. This patient also had lupus pleuritis, which is the most common pulmonary manifestation of SLE. Although pericardial effusions are less common than pericarditis in SLE, they can often occur in concert.

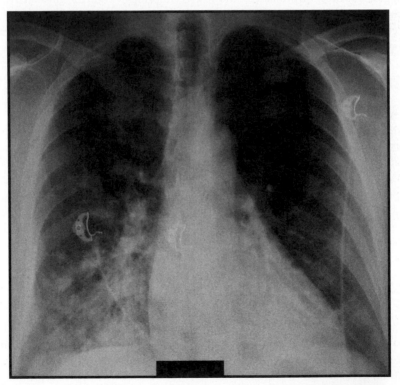

Image 27-10 • Hazy diffuse alveolar infiltrates in a patient with DAH due to SLE.

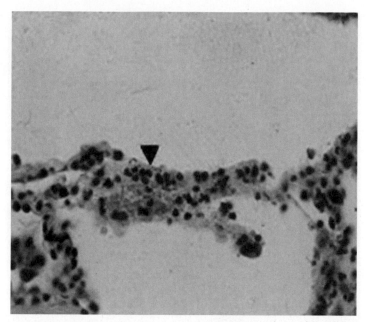

Image 27-11 • Histopathology in DAH consistent with pulmonary capillaritis, with infiltration of the inflammatory cells into and causing expansion of the interstitium. (*Reproduced with permission from Lara AR, Schwarz MI. Diffuse alveolar hemorrhage, Chest 2010 May;137(5):1164-1171.*)

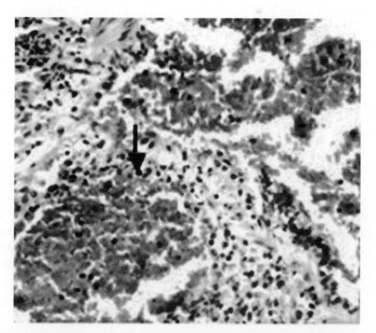

Image 27-12 • Alveolar spaces are filled with red blood cells. (*Reproduced with permission from Lara AR, Schwarz MI. Diffuse alveolar hemorrhage, Chest 2010 May;137(5):1164-1171.*)

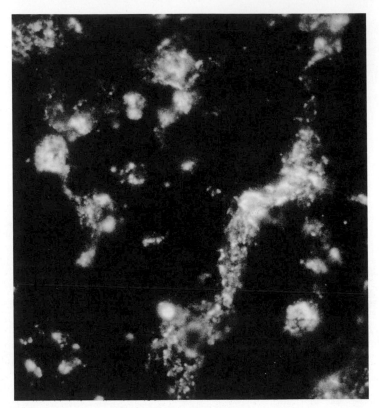

Image 27-13 • Immunofluorescence study of lung tissue in SLE-associated DAH showing a classic "lumpy-bumpy" staining of immune complexes throughout the lung tissue. (*Reproduced with permission from Grippi MA, Elias JA, Fishman JA, et al: Fishman's Pulmonary Diseases and Disorders, 5th ed. New York, NY: McGraw Hill; 2015.*)

Q27-5: A
High-dose intravenous steroids (1-2 g/day prednisone equivalent)

Rationale: Once infection has been ruled out or appropriate antibiotic coverage is provided while awaiting culture data, high-dose intravenous steroids remain the mainstay of treatment for severe/life-threatening pulmonary complications of SLE. This therapy is often supplemented with cyclophosphamide therapy. Plasmapheresis and rituximab or belimumab may be used in patients who failed to respond to therapy. Surgical lung biopsy may also be used in patients who fail to respond to therapy to confirm the diagnosis. Weight-based prednisone may be used for patients with mild or moderate acute symptoms, in conjunction with other oral immunosuppressives such as CellCept mycophenolate or azathioprine.

Q27-6: B
Reticular interstitial pattern with traction bronchiectasis and honeycombing

Rationale: The above CT scan shows subpleural reticulations (reticular interstitial opacities with interlobular/intralobular septal thickening and ground glass), traction bronchiectasis indicating architectural distortion, and honeycombing at the bases. This is consistent with interstitial lung disease (ILD), and more specifically is classic of usual interstitial pneumonia (UIP), the most common type of ILD associated with SLE; however, nonspecific interstitial pneumonia (NSIP), lymphocytic interstitial pneumonia (LIP), and organizing pneumonia are also seen. This is seen more commonly in patients who have had ALP previously. Patients with DAH are more likely to have recurrent DAH, though there is not a clear correlation with the development of ILD. As in other forms of ILD, prognosis depends on the histopathologic findings.

Q27-7: D
Pulmonary hypertension

Rationale: While the lung fields are relatively clear, there is significant enlargement of the right heart and the pulmonary arteries in this patient's chest radiographs. On the PA film, note that the right heart border is quite prominent on the right side of the spine. Additionally, the right pulmonary artery appears enlarged. The enlargement of the pulmonary arteries is better appreciated on the lateral film, directly in the middle of the image. This is primarily concerning for the presence of pulmonary vascular disease, or pulmonary hypertension. SLE is pulmonary vascular disorder than can cause World Health Organization (WHO) group 1 pulmonary hypertension (previously termed *pulmonary arterial hypertension*). Additionally, it may cause pulmonary embolism and with the development of chronic thromboembolic disease lead to WHO group IV pulmonary hypertension (CTEPH). The patient's chest radiograph shows no significant parenchymal or pleural process, but there is prominence of the right heart border, consistent with likely evolving right-sided heart failure from pulmonary hypertension. This supported by the pulmonary function testing, which shows an isolated reduction in the DLCO, consistent with pulmonary hypertension. Acute reversible hypoxia syndrome is an entity unique to patients with SLE that develops with a clear chest radiograph and without signs of right heart failure and is highly responsive to steroids.

Q27-8: C
Shrinking lung syndrome

Rationale: The CXR demonstrates elevation of the right hemidiaphragm, and there are some linear abnormalities likely consistent with atelectasis at the bases. The patient's PFT shows restriction with a reduced DLCO. However, the DLCO is not as significantly reduced as one would expect in ILD necessarily, and there are no parenchymal abnormalities present. Shrinking lung disease is a progressive extrathoracic restrictive disease resulting from reduced inspiratory muscle/diaphragm strength, leading to reductions in lung volumes and atelectasis.

References

Altschul E, Remy-Jardin M, Machnicki S, et al. Imaging of pulmonary hypertension: pictorial essay. Chest. 2019;156:211.

Boyd JS, Melton M, Rupp JD, Ferre RM. Lung ultrasound. In: Knoop KJ, Stack LB, Storrow AB, Thurman R, eds. *The Atlas of Emergency Medicine.* 5th ed. McGraw-Hill, 2021. https://access-medicine.mhmedical.com/content.aspx?bookid=2969&sectionid=250463818

Gupta N, Matta EJ, Oldham SA. Cardiothoracic imaging. In: Elsayes KM, Oldham SA, eds. *Introduction to Diagnostic Radiology.* McGraw-Hill, 2014. https://accessmedicine.mhmed-ical.com/content.aspx?bookid=1562https://accessmedicine.mhmedical.com/content.aspx?bookid=2969&sectionid=250463818sectionid=95876454

Lara AR, Schwarz MI. Diffuse alveolar hemorrhage. Chest. 2010;137:1164.

Little WC, Freeman GL. Pericardial disease. Circulation. 2006;113:1622.

McCann C, Gopalan D, Sheares K, Screaton N. Imaging in pulmonary hypertension, part 1: clinical perspectives, classification, imaging techniques and imaging algorithm. Postgrad Med J. 2012;88:271.

Miranda WR, Imazio M, Greason KL, Stulak JM, Oh JK. Pericardial diseases. In: Fuster V, Harrington RA, Narula J, Eapen ZJ, eds. *Hurst's The Heart.* 14th ed. McGraw-Hill, 2017. https://accessmedicine.mhmedical.com/content.aspx?bookid=2046&sectionid=176561263

Rubin LJ. Pulmonary hypertension. In: Fuster V, Harrington RA, Narula J, Eapen ZJ, eds. *Hurst's The Heart.* 14th ed. McGraw-Hill, 2017. https://accessmedicine.mhmedical.com/content.aspx?bookid=2046&sectionid=176562507

Sorajja P. Pericardial disease. In: Hall JB, Schmidt GA, Kress JP, eds. *Principles of Critical Care.* 4th ed. McGraw-Hill, 2014. https://accessmedicine.mhmedical.com/content.aspx?bookid=1340&sectionid=80031631

The skin in immune, autoimmune, autoinflammatory, and rheumatic disorders. Wolff K, Johnson R, Saavedra AP, Roh EK, eds. *Fitzpatrick's Color Atlas and Synopsis of Clinical Dermatology.* 8th ed. McGraw-Hill, 2017. https://accessmedicine.mhmedical.com/content.aspx?bookid=2043&sectionid=154898980

Warrington KJ, Moder KG, Brutinel WM. The shrinking lung syndrome in systemic lupus erythematosus. Mayo Clin Proc. 2000;75:467.

CASE 28

You are working in an ICU and receive a call to transfer a patient to your facility. The patient is a 52-year-old man who had an orthotopic liver transplant 3 months ago for nonalcoholic fatty liver disease (NAFLD) and who presented 2 days ago to an outside facility with dyspnea and an abnormal chest radiograph. The patient does not smoke, drink alcohol, or use illicit drugs. He experienced a few weeks of fevers, myalgia, malaise, and cough before presenting. His liver function appears at baseline, and a laboratory evaluation of his immunosuppressive medications shows he has been taking his medication. He has progressively worsened over the last 2 days despite initiation of therapy for suspected bacterial pneumonia, which includes ceftriaxone and azithromycin. He had an extended respiratory viral panel that was negative for influenza A/B, respiratory syncytial virus (RSV), metapneumovirus, and adenovirus. He is a long-haul truck driver living in Nashville who resumed his job over the last month. He received alemtuzumab (Campath) for induction therapy for his liver transplant, and he currently takes cyclosporine, prednisone 15 mg daily, and CellCept mycophenolate for maintenance immunosuppression. The outside hospital is planning for urgent intubation and transfer to your facility for further evaluation and management. The patient's vital signs are T 38.3°C, HR 121, BP 100/66, RR 24, and oxygen saturation 88% on 10 L/min supplemental O_2 via high-flow nasal cannula. The patient's chest radiograph is shown in Image 28-1, and an image from the chest CT scan is shown in Image 28-2.

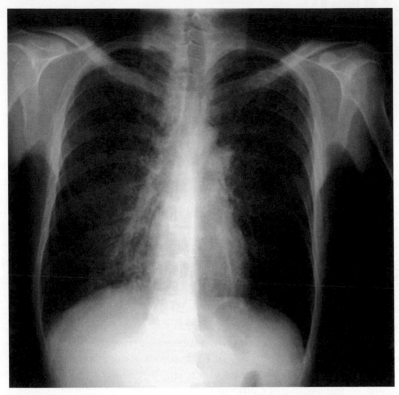

Image 28-1 • Chest radiograph for the patient in **Case 28**. (*Reproduced with permission from Knoop KJ, Stack LB, Storrow AB, et al: The Atlas of Emergency Medicine, 5th ed. New York, NY: McGraw Hill; 2021. Photo contributor: Jake Block, MD.*)

QUESTIONS

Q28-1: How would you describe the abnormalities in the chest radiograph shown in Image 28-1?

A. Miliary pattern with reticulonodular opacities
B. Lower lobe–predominant linear interstitial opacities
C. Upper lobe–predominant cavitary lung lesions
D. Diffuse alveolar consolidations
E. Focal bilateral consolidations with associated pleural effusions

Q28-2: How would you describe the abnormalities in the chest CT shown in Image 28-2?

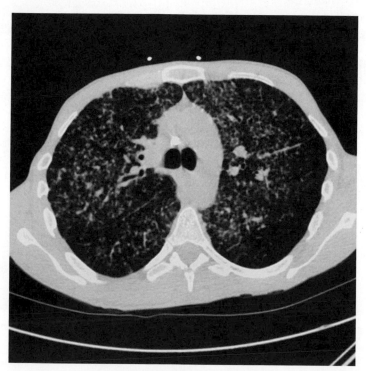

Image 28-2 • Chest CT image for the patient in **Case 28**. (*Reproduced with permission from Knoop KJ, Stack LB, Storrow AB, et al: The Atlas of Emergency Medicine, 5th ed. New York, NY: McGraw Hill; 2021. Photo contributor: Jake Block, MD.*)

A. Nodules and masses with varying stages of cavitation and coalescence
B. Mosaic attenuation
C. Diffuse nodular opacities with interlobular septal thickening
D. Diffuse cavitary lung lesions
E. Centrilobular emphysematous changes

Q28-3: After arrival, the patient undergoes standard admission laboratory testing, and consent is obtained for an immediate bronchoscopy with BAL and biopsy. You also receive a call from the histopathology laboratory that a peripheral blood smear performed for a WBC differential has some abnormalities, as shown in Image 28-3. On examination, the patient is noted to have diffuse erythematous papules and plaques on the upper torso and chest. Before you perform a bronchoscopy, what is the next appropriate step?

A. Interferon-gamma release assay against *Mycobacterium tuberculosis*
B. Three AFB smears from endotracheal aspirates
C. Repeat CT scan to assess for the presence of Ranke complex
D. *Pneumocystis jiroveci* pneumonia (PCP) PCR from endotracheal aspirates
E. *Streptococcus pneumoniae* urine antigen

Q28-4: The patient has three endotracheal aspirate samples sent over the next 24 hours. The patient's blood smear and skin lesions are shown in Image 28-3 below.

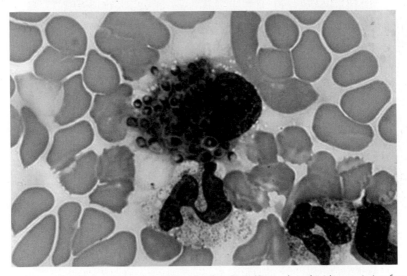

Image 28-3 • Blood smear for the patient in **Case 28**. (*Reproduced with permission from Lichtman MA, Shafer MS, Felgar RE, et al: Lichtman's Atlas of Hematology 2016. New York, NY: McGraw Hill; 2017.*)

What is the next appropriate test to send while waiting for the patient's AFB smears to result negative?

A. *Legionella pneumoniae* urine antigen
B. *S. pneumoniae* urine antigen
C. *Cryptococcus* serum antigen
D. *Pneumocystis jiroveci* PCR
E. *Histoplasma capsulatum* urine antigen

Q28-5: The patient undergoes a lumbar puncture that demonstrates no evidence of meningitis. What is the most appropriate treatment option for the patient?

A. Liposomal amphotericin B for 2 weeks
B. Liposomal amphotericin B for 2 weeks followed by itraconazole
C. Itraconazole monotherapy
D. Fluconazole monotherapy
E. Liposomal amphotericin B for 6 weeks followed by itraconazole

Q28-6: A 56-year-old farmer from western North Carolina with a history of smoking in the distant past is referred to your clinic for an abnormal CT scan. He is asymptomatic. He reports having one prior episode of pneumonia when he was a teenager. He has no fevers, chills, sweats, weight loss, or shortness of breath. His chest radiograph is shown in Image 28-4.

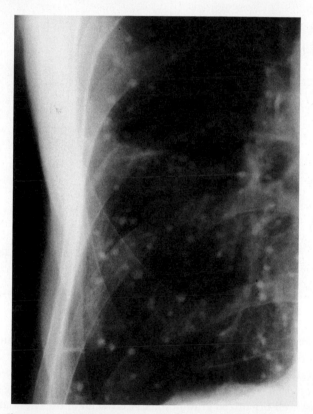

Image 28-4 • Chest radiograph for the patient in **Question 28-6**. (*Reproduced with permission from Schwartz DT, Reisdorff EJ. Emergency Radiology. New York, NY: McGraw Hil; 2000.*)

He had a negative purified protein derivative (PPD) test 2 years ago. He had a PET-CT scan that was negative. He has a positive IgG test to *H. capsulatum* but negative to IgG to *Blastomyces* and *Coccidioides* species. His PET-CT scan also demonstrated some calcifications in the spleen and hilar lymph nodes in addition to the lesions.

What is the likely diagnosis?

A. Acute pulmonary histoplasmosis
B. Chronic pulmonary histoplasmosis
C. Progressive disseminated histoplasmosis
D. Metastatic malignancy
E. Resolved histoplasmosis infection

Q28-7: A 22-year-old marathon runner presents with fevers, dyspnea, and cough. He is otherwise healthy and takes no medications. He has no family history of any medical issues. He completed a marathon 10 days ago in Ohio and felt poorly the next day, but he thought he was simply fatigued from the race, though he never improved. His chest radiograph is shown in Image 28-5.

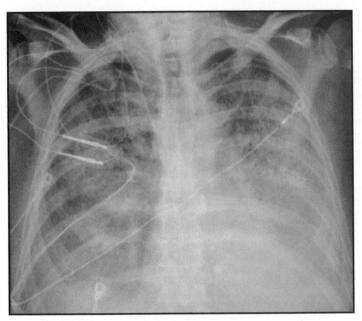

Image 28-5 • Chest radiograph for the patient in **Question 28-7**.

The patient is started on antibiotics for community-acquired pneumonia, but he does not improve. His HIV test is negative. Bacterial and fungal cultures are negative. A respiratory viral panel is negative. A test for serum *Histoplasma* IgG is negative. A *Histoplasma* urine antigen is positive. A transbronchial lung biopsy shows noncaseating, well-organized granulomas. A CT scan of the chest, abdomen, and pelvis shows diffuse micronodules throughout the lung with some ground-glass opacities and mild hilar adenopathy. What is the likely diagnosis in this patient?

A. Acute pulmonary histoplasmosis
B. Fibrosing mediastinitis
C. Chronic pulmonary histoplasmosis
D. Disseminated pulmonary histoplasmosis
E. Sarcoidosis
F. Blastomycosis

Q28-8: A 66-year-old man with COPD presents as a referral from a colleague. He has been experiencing some progressive shortness of breath and an increased cough recently, some of which has been blood-tinged. He reports that he had some abnormalities in this left upper lung on prior chest imaging and has had intermittent episodes similar to this over the last few years that tend to resolve after a few weeks. He is referred for evaluation. His chest radiograph is shown in Image 28-6.

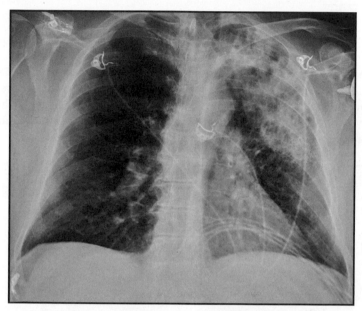

Image 28-6 • Chest radiograph for the patient in **Question 28-8**.

He has a negative interferon-gamma release assay against *M. tuberculosis* antigen. He undergoes a bronchoscopy with biopsies. The biopsies and brushings show no evidence of malignancy but are not diagnostic. Below is the result of all testing.

Gram stain, BAL	Negative
KOH stain, BAL	Positive
AFB smear, BAL	Negative
Histoplasma antigen, urine	Negative
Coccidioides, serum	IgM – negative IgG – negative
Histoplasma, serum	H band – positive M band – positive
Blastomyces, serum	IgM – negative IgG – positive
Aspergillus, serum	IgM – negative IgG – negative
IgE	Normal

What is the likely diagnosis?

A. Acute pulmonary histoplasmosis
B. *Mycobacterium avium* complex (MAC) infection
C. Allergic bronchopulmonary aspergillosis (ABPA)
D. Chronic pulmonary histoplasmosis (CPH)
E. Chronic pulmonary aspergillosis
F. Lung cancer

Q28-9: A 43-year-old man presents to the clinic with fevers, cough, and mild chest pain. He reports no pulmonary or cardiac history and denies any smoking or drug use history. He takes no medications. He spent 6 weeks in rural Tennessee working on a construction site and returned to the West Coast about 6 weeks ago. He has no known tuberculosis risk factors, and his PPD is negative. The symptoms developed slowly over the last few weeks, and they failed to respond to outpatient antibiotics. His chest radiograph is shown below in Image 28-7.

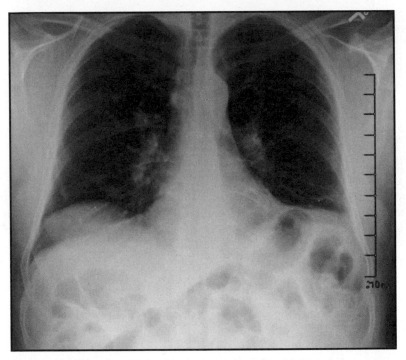

Image 28-7 • Chest radiograph for the patient in **Question 28-9.**

Gram stain, BAL	Negative
KOH stain, BAL	Positive
AFB smear, BAL	Negative
Histoplasma antigen, urine	Negative
Coccidioides, serum	IgM – negative IgG – negative
Histoplasma, serum	H band – negative M band – positive
Blastomyces, serum	IgM – negative IgG – positive
Aspergillus, serum	IgM – negative IgG – negative
IgE	Normal

What is the likely diagnosis?
A. Acute pulmonary histoplasmosis
B. Subacute pulmonary histoplasmosis
C. Blastomycosis
D. Chronic pulmonary histoplasmosis
E. Chronic pulmonary aspergillosis

Q28-10: A 66-year-old woman presents with chest pain, facial and right arm swelling, worsening dyspnea, cough, and lower extremity edema. She notes that the dyspnea and pleuritic chest pain have slowly developed over the last 5 to 6 years, though the remaining symptoms have only developed recently. She presented due to facial swelling and some flushing.

The patient undergoes a CT scan of the chest at an outside facility, and the following image was provided to you (Image 28-8).

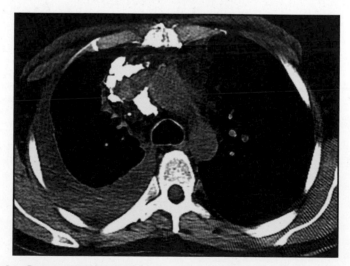

Image 28-8 • Representative image for the patient in **Question 28-10**.

What is the likely diagnosis?

A. Pulmonary embolism
B. Mediastinal granulomas and possible fibrosing mediastinitis
C. Angioinvasive pulmonary aspergillosis
D. Mucormycosis

ANSWERS

Q28-1: A
Miliary pattern with reticulonodular opacities

Rationale: The chest radiograph has relatively diffuse, upper lobe–predominant reticulonodular opacities, almost consistent with miliary pattern of dissemination. This pattern here could also be confused with possible diffuse cystic changes, but there are no obvious cavitary lesions. There are interstitial opacities, but these are more reticular and nodular in appearance. Importantly, this chest radiography shows a slight upper-lobe predominance. There are no apparent effusions or alveolar consolidative opacities.

Q28-2: C
Diffuse nodular opacities with interlobular septal thickening

Rationale: The image shows a coronal view of a CT scan of the chest performed without contrast at the level of the carina. There is diffuse interlobular septal thickening with scattered ground-glass opacities that could be described as "crazy paving" in some areas. There are also scattered micronodular and nodular opacities with some septal thickening. There are no masses or cavitary lesions. There is some mild bronchial wall thickening. There is no apparent mosaic attenuation or hyperinflation (though this would be difficult to call on a single image and without inspiratory–expiratory studies). There are no clear centrilobular emphysematous changes.

Q28-3: B
Three AFB smears from endotracheal aspirates

Rationale: This patient's risk factors for tuberculosis exposure are unknown, but his profession as a long-haul truck driver with considerable recent travel history, his immunosuppressed state, and the miliary pattern on chest imaging should raise suspicion for possible *M. tuberculosis* infection. Bronchoscopy is an aerosol-generating procedure even with the closed circuit of the ventilator because the circuit has to be opened to insert the scope. Therefore, it would be prudent to rule out active tuberculosis infection with three AFB smears prior to performing bronchoscopy. An interferon-gamma release assay would also be appropriate, but this does not differentiate between active and latent infection. A repeat CT scan to assess for Ranke complex (healed primary tuberculosis resulting from Ghon complex) would also not be helpful here, particularly in light of the diffuse abnormalities. Neither PCP nor *S. pneumoniae* infections need to be ruled out before performing bronchoscopy.

Q28-4: E
Histoplasma capsulatum urine antigen

Rationale: The skins described in the question are typical of disseminated histoplasmosis, with multiple erythematous papules and small plaques. These can ulcerate as well. The ears and nose are often involved in patients with severe immunosuppression. **Image 28-3** demonstrates a macrophage containing the yeast forms of *H. capsulatum*. *Histoplasma* tends to have a crescent-shaped nucleus. *Histoplasma* exists in mycelial form in the soil where tuberculate macroconidia grow on septate hyphae. The microconidia are inhaled and persist in phagosomes, yielding encapsulated yeast forms that grow inside the human body (**Image 28-9**).

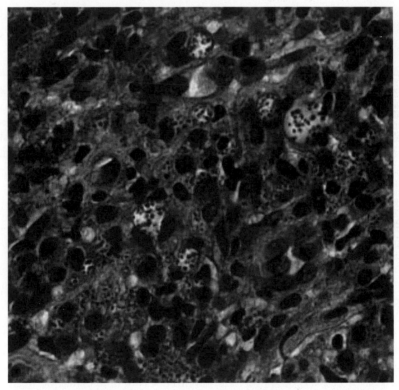

Image 28-9 • Example of yeast forms of *H. capsulatum* in biopsy specimens.

Histoplasma is an endemic fungus most commonly encountered in the southeast United States and the Ohio River valley, where this patient happens to reside. Additionally, the patient is a truck driver and likely has frequent exposure while driving throughout the region. He is significantly immunocompromised from his induction chemotherapy and maintenance immunosuppression. In particular, alemtuzumab is significantly lymphocyte depleting, resulting in CD4+ cell counts that can be very low (less than 100/mm³) for several months. In fact, this patient had a CD4 count less than 50/µL, mimicking AIDS. This patient's presentation is consistent with disseminated disease affecting multiple organ systems outside of the lungs and hilar and mediastinal lymph nodes. This is more common in patients with AIDS than in patients with other immunocompromised states.

The definitive diagnosis is established by antigen testing. Urine antigen testing is very effective in acute pulmonary disease as well as in disseminated disease, but it is less useful in patients with subacute or chronic presentations. The sensitivity of the urine antigen test is approximately 80% to 90% in acute pulmonary histoplasmosis, but generally, it has a less than 35% sensitivity in subacute or chronic cases. Serum serology (IgM and IgG) and culture data are more useful in subacute and chronic cases. Antigen testing (from urine, serum, CNS, ascites, pleural effusion, pericardial effusion) is the most sensitive in disseminated disease, though fungal staining, culture, and serum serology are more effective in disseminated disease than acute pulmonary histoplasmosis.

At body temperature, the fungus grows as an encapsulated yeast, which is the pathogenic form found in human tissue. This patient's presentation is consistent with that of progressive disseminated histoplasmosis (PDH). Disseminated disease can involve the lungs, lymph nodes, liver, skin, oral mucosa, GI tract, adrenal glands, and, most notably, may result in meningitis or focal brain lesions. It is most commonly encountered in patients with AIDS or severe immunosuppression. Abnormalities on chest radiography can vary in PDH and can be similar to the abnormalities seen in this case (diffuse reticulonodular or miliary pattern), areas of consolidation or ground glass, cavitary lesions, and mediastinal and hilar adenopathy. An example of another patient with disseminated histoplasmosis is shown below, with more minimal changes on chest imaging (**Image 28-10**). The patient in the previous vignette should undergo a lumbar puncture to rule out meningitis and MRI of the brain to rule out brain lesions.

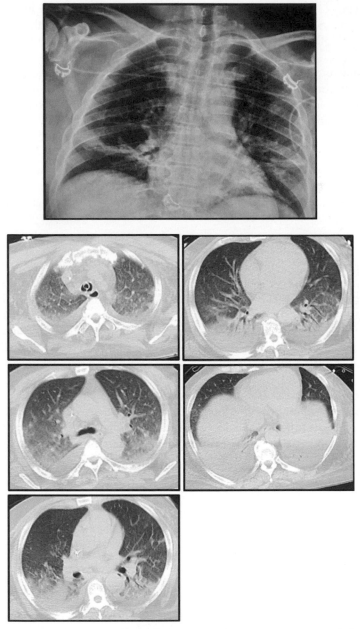

Image 28-10 • Chest radiograph and chest CT scan demonstrating more subtle imaging abnormalities in disseminated histoplasmosis. The initial chest radiograph shows some plate-like atelectasis in the right middle lobe, with some mild basilar opacities. The follow-up CT scan of the chest demonstrates diffuse ground-glass opacities and consolidations with air bronchograms, possible atelectasis, and bilateral pleural effusions.

Q28-5: B
Liposomal amphotericin B for 2 weeks followed by itraconazole

Rationale: When determining treatment for a patient with disseminated histoplasmosis, one first needs to establish disease severity. Patients are classified according to the severity of illness and their immune status. Immunocompromised patients with mild clinical presentations isolated to one organ system and no CNS involvement may be treated with itraconazole therapy alone. Fluconazole is not recommended as first-line therapy. Patients with severe immunocompromised states (such as this case), moderate-to-severe clinical illness, disseminated disease (ie, involving more than one organ system), or with CNS involvement require induction therapy with amphotericin B and maintenance therapy with itraconazole. The duration of induction therapy is typically 2 weeks in patients without CNS involvement but often 4 to 6 weeks in patients with CNS involvement. The treatment for nonimmunocompromised patients differs from these recommendations and is discussed further below.

Q28-6: E
Resolved pulmonary histoplasmosis infection

Rationale: This patient has numerous scattered calcified nodules that are most consistent with the residua of a prior histoplasmosis infection. Calcified granulomas from prior histoplasmosis infection often are found in lymph nodes as well as the spleen. However, this is not specific to resolved histoplasmosis and could be seen in resolved sarcoidosis or other endemic fungal infections, as well as in resolved *M. tuberculosis* infection. The negative result of the PPD test makes this less likely. Malignancy should be excluded as well, but given the number of lesions present in an asymptomatic patient and the calcified nature, histoplasmosis is the most likely diagnosis.

Q28-7: A
Acute pulmonary histoplasmosis

Rationale: The patient recently ran a 26-mile race in an endemic area and likely had a large inoculum. His symptoms developed shortly thereafter, consistent with an acute onset process. The chest radiograph is nonspecific and consistent with diffuse airspace disease. Similarly, the CT scan findings discussed previously are relatively nonspecific and could raise concern for an endemic fungal infection or other noninfectious granulomatous diseases such as sarcoidosis. He is immunocompetent and does not have evidence of disseminated disease, nor does he have symptoms consistent with a chronic disease process. Mediastinal fibrosis is a complication of histoplasmosis that can lead to mediastinal calcification, fibrosis, and extensive vascular scarring, leading to occlusions of airways and invasion of mediastinal structures. The primary differential diagnosis here is between sarcoidosis and acute pulmonary histoplasmosis. Recall that the diagnosis of sarcoidosis is one of exclusion. The negative serum IgG to *Histoplasma* indicates a significant prior exposure resulting in an immune response, whereas the positive urine antigen represents acute infection. A *Histoplasma* IgM may be positive at this point. For this patient, the treatment would depend on the severity of the patient's disease. Patients with mild disease and symptoms lasting less than 4 weeks often require no treatment. If a patient's symptoms progress beyond 4 weeks, oral therapy with itraconazole, fluconazole, or isavuconazole is warranted (posaconazole and voriconazole are also options). Patients with more severe clinical presentations, including acute hypoxemic respiratory failure or acute respiratory distress syndrome (ARDS), should receive induction therapy with itraconazole for 1 to 2 weeks followed by at least 3 months of oral itraconazole. The addition of steroids (prednisone 0.5-1.0 mg/kg/day) can also be considered as adjuvant therapy.

Q28-8: D
Chronic (cavitary) pulmonary histoplasmosis (CPH)

Rationale: For histoplasmosis serologies, an immunodiffusion test is most commonly used, and the results are reported as H and M precipitin bands. This is most useful for the detection of antibodies 4 to 6 weeks from the time of infection. A positive H and M band indicates acute disease *or* chronic progressive disease (such as seen here), while the presence of only the M band represents chronic disease (the anti-H antibodies have reduced in titer to the point they are not detectable, similar to IgM antibodies following acute infection). The M band may present up to 3 to 5 years after infection. Here, the patient has ongoing and progressive symptoms, likely consistent with a more chronic progressive disease. Additionally, there are areas on the chest radiograph that appear cavitary. CPH is characterized by the indolent process of worsening dyspnea, progressive pulmonary infiltrates, cavitary lung lesions, and fibrosis, often mimicking ABPA, chronic pulmonary aspergillosis, and tuberculous. *Aspergillus* superinfection and hemoptysis are common. Malignancy must always be ruled out. The serologies show sensitivity to *Histoplasma* alone (see below). Recall that in chronic pulmonary histoplasmosis, the urine antigen study is only about 40% sensitive. All patients with chronic cavitary pulmonary histoplasmosis require treatment with itraconazole, which may be required for several years, if not life.

Q28-9: B
Subacute pulmonary histoplasmosis

Rationale: This is a similar presentation to acute pulmonary histoplasmosis, but it occurs after a more prolonged exposure to a smaller inoculum. The chest radiograph more commonly shows mediastinal and hilar adenopathy as opposed to the miliary pattern seen in the acute case. The diagnosis is made by serology most commonly; the presence of an M band without an H band may suggest a subacute presentation. H bands are usually seen only in patients with severe acute presentations or in chronic cavitary disease, such as in the case above. The H bands and M bands are part of the immunodiffusion studies, which typically lag slightly behind complement fixation techniques. However, as the M bands may persist for months to years, they can also signal a past resolved infection, so clinical acumen is required. Just as in the other cases, the primary differential diagnoses include TB and sarcoidosis, along with malignancy such as lymphoma.

Q28-10: B
Mediastinal granulomas and possible fibrosing mediastinitis

Rationale: The CT scan demonstrates thickened mediastinum with calcifications, and the mediastinum is compressing local structures, including the airway. This is a condition that is often linked with histoplasmosis or prior *Histoplasma* exposure, though it may be seen in other fungal infections, tuberculosis, sarcoidosis, silicosis, and as a hereditary disorder. Fibrosing mediastinitis and mediastinal granulomas may be caused by *H. capsulatum* infection. Mediastinal granulomas can result from the conglomeration of lymph nodes (seen in the CT in **Image 28-10**) and exaggerated inflammation and fibrosis. As this conglomeration grows, it can begin to compress nearby structures, including the airways (also seen in the image with compression of the right mainstem bronchus), SVC, and esophagus. These are commonly calcified and can erode into the airways, yielding broncholithiasis. This is a benign process that can typically be treated with surgical resection and bronchial or vascular stents. Glucocorticoids and antifungal therapies are not indicated and lack evidence for efficacy. Hemoptysis and bronchopleural fistulas may occur. Fibrosing mediastinitis is more a severe process in which the fibrosis extends beyond the lymph nodes to involve other structures in the mediastinum. Vascular structures can be compressed and completely obstructed. It can often be difficult to differentiate mediastinal fibrosis from granulomas, and the differentiation depends on the identification of a more diffuse process in the mediastinum on contrasted CT imaging. The patient also has a sizable right-sided pleural effusion.

References

Assi M, Martin S, Wheat LJ, et al. Histoplasmosis after solid organ transplant. Clin Infect Dis. 2013;57:1542.

Goodwin RA, Nickell JA, Des Prez RM. Mediastinal fibrosis complicating healed primary histoplasmosis and tuberculosis. Medicine (Baltimore). 1972;51:227.

Goodwin RA Jr, Shapiro JL, Thurman GH, et al. Disseminated histoplasmosis: clinical and pathologic correlations. Medicine (Baltimore). 1980;59:1.

Hage CA, Davis TE, Fuller D, et al. Diagnosis of histoplasmosis by antigen detection in BAL fluid. Chest. 2010;137:623.

Hage CA, Ribes JA, Wengenack NL, et al. A multicenter evaluation of tests for diagnosis of histoplasmosis. Clin Infect Dis. 2011;53:448.

Johnson PC, Wheat LJ, Cloud GA, et al. Safety and efficacy of liposomal amphotericin B compared with conventional amphotericin B for induction therapy of histoplasmosis in patients with AIDS. Ann Intern Med. 2002;137:105.

Litvintseva AP, Lindsley MD, Gade L, et al. Utility of (1-3)-β-D-glucan testing for diagnostics and monitoring response to treatment during the multistate outbreak of fungal meningitis and other infections. Clin Infect Dis. 2014;58:622.

Loyd JE, Tillman BF, Atkinson JB, Des Prez RM. Mediastinal fibrosis complicating histoplasmosis. Medicine (Baltimore). 1988;67:295.

McKinsey DS, Kauffman CA, Pappas PG, et al. Fluconazole therapy for histoplasmosis. The National Institute of Allergy and Infectious Diseases Mycoses Study Group. Clin Infect Dis. 1996;23:996.

Putnam LR, Sutliff WD, Larkin JC, et al. Histoplasmosis cooperative study: chronic pulmonary histoplasmosis treated with amphotericin B alone and with amphotericin B and triple sulfonamide. Am Rev Respir Dis. 1968;97:96.

Richer SM, Smedema ML, Durkin MM, et al. Improved diagnosis of acute pulmonary histoplasmosis by combining antigen and antibody detection. Clin Infect Dis. 2016;62:896.

Scheel CM, Samayoa B, Herrera A, et al. Development and evaluation of an enzyme-linked immunosorbent assay to detect histoplasma capsulatum antigenuria in immunocompromised patients. Clin Vaccine Immunol. 2009;16:852.

Swartzentruber S, Rhodes L, Kurkjian K, et al. Diagnosis of acute pulmonary histoplasmosis by antigen detection. Clin Infect Dis. 2009;49:1878.

Theel ES, Jespersen DJ, Harring J, et al. Evaluation of an enzyme immunoassay for detection of histoplasma capsulatum antigen from urine specimens. J Clin Microbiol. 2013;51:3555.

Tran T, Beal SG. Application of the 1,3-β-D-glucan (fungitell) assay in the diagnosis of invasive fungal infections. Arch Pathol Lab Med. 2016;140:181.

Wheat LJ, Batteiger BE, Sathapatayavongs B. Histoplasma capsulatum infections of the central nervous system. A clinical review. Medicine (Baltimore). 1990;69:244.

Wheat LJ, Conces D, Allen SD, et al. Pulmonary histoplasmosis syndromes: recognition, diagnosis, and management. Semin Respir Crit Care Med. 2004;25:129.

Wheat LJ, Freifeld AG, Kleiman MB, et al. Clinical practice guidelines for the management of patients with histoplasmosis: 2007 update by the Infectious Diseases Society of America. Clin Infect Dis. 2007;45:807.

Wheat J, MaWhinney S, Hafner R, et al. Treatment of histoplasmosis with fluconazole in patients with acquired immunodeficiency syndrome. National Institute of Allergy and Infectious Diseases Acquired Immunodeficiency Syndrome Clinical Trials Group and Mycoses Study Group. Am J Med. 1997;103:223.

Wheat J, Wheat H, Connolly P, et al. Cross-reactivity in histoplasma capsulatum variety capsulatum antigen assays of urine samples from patients with endemic mycoses. Clin Infect Dis. 1997;24:1169.

CASE 29

A 44-year-old man with Crohn disease receiving antitumor necrosis factor-alpha (TNFα) therapy presents to the ED with fevers, chills, sweats, dyspnea, chest pain, and a productive cough with blood-tinged sputum. His vital signs on presentation are T 101.5°F, HR 132, BP 103/66, RR 18, and O$_2$ saturation 88% on 6 L/min supplement O$_2$ via nasal cannula. The patient also has developed a skin lesion (Image 29-2). The patient developed mild symptoms about 4 to 5 weeks ago and was treated unsuccessfully with two courses of antibiotics for outpatient pneumonia. He reports no work exposure and no tuberculosis (TB) risk factors, and he was tested for TB before starting therapy for Crohn disease. He spent about 3 weeks backpacking in Wisconsin recently with two friends, during which he went hunting and camping while traveling down a local riverway. One of his friends was recently diagnosed with pneumonia as well. He takes a bowel regimen regularly but otherwise does not take any medications outside of his anti-TNFα monoclonal antibody.

The patient is admitted to the medical ICU and rapidly deteriorates. He is intubated for increased work of breathing and respiratory muscle fatigue. He subsequently undergoes chest imaging.

His chest imaging and skin lesion are shown below in Images 29-1 and 29-2, respectively.

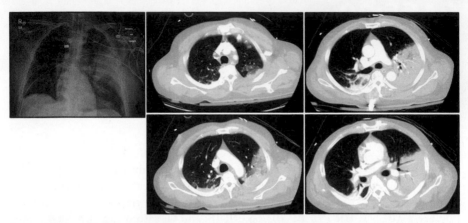

Image 29-1 • Chest radiograph and CT images for the patient in **Case 29**.

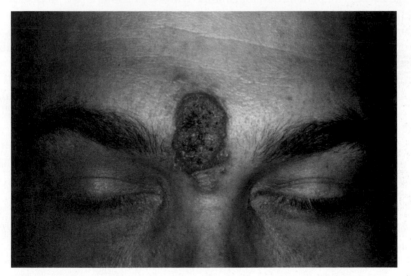

Image 29-2 • Skin lesion seen on examination of the patient in **Case 29**. (*Reproduced with permission from Grippi MA, Elias JA, Fishman JA, et al: Fishman's Pulmonary Diseases and Disorders, 5th ed. New York, NY: McGraw Hill; 2015.*)

QUESTIONS

Q29-1: How would you describe the abnormalities on the chest radiograph above?

A. Diffuse interstitial infiltrates
B. Right upper lobe cystic lung lesion
C. Right upper lobe loculated effusion
D. Left upper lobe consolidation
E. Scattered nodular opacities
F. Left upper lobe atelectasis

Q29-2: How would you describe the skin lesion in Image 29-2?

A. Ulceration
B. Xanthomatous
C. Lichenification
D. Verrucous
E. Telangiectasias

Q29-3: Given the patient's immunocompromised status, bronchoscopy with BAL and transbronchial biopsy is performed. A biopsy specimen of the lesion is shown in Image 29-3.

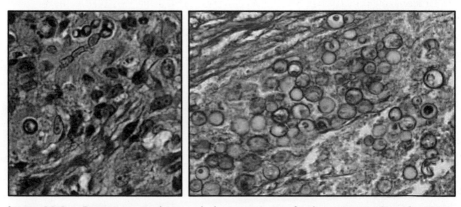

Image 29-3 • Representative histopathology specimens for the patient in **Question 29-3**.

What is the likely diagnosis?

A. Coccidioidomycosis
B. Blastomycosis
C. Histoplasmosis
D. *Mycobacterium* tuberculosis
E. Sarcoidosis

Q29-4: What is the most common extrapulmonary organ system to be involved in blastomycosis?

A. Bone marrow
B. Bone
C. Skin
D. Central nervous system
E. Genitourinary tract
F. Lymph nodes
G. Parotid gland

Q29-5: The patient undergoes a lumbar puncture, which demonstrates no evidence of infection. What is the recommended initial treatment for this patient?

A. Liposomal amphotericin B
B. Itraconazole
C. Fluconazole
D. Voriconazole
E. Ketoconazole

Q29-6: A pregnant woman presents with acute pulmonary blastomycosis. Her symptoms are mild to moderate. What is the best treatment option?

A. Liposomal amphotericin B
B. Itraconazole
C. Fluconazole
D. Voriconazole
E. Ketoconazole

ANSWERS

Q29-1: D
Left upper lobe consolidation

Rationale: This patient presented with a large left upper lobe consolidative opacity with air bronchograms clearly visible, even on the patient's chest radiograph. There is some opacification of the right posterior upper lobe as well on the CT scan, but the predominant abnormality is on the left. There is no evidence of a loculated effusion or cystic lesions, and there are no diffuse infiltrates or micronodular disease. Note that on the chest radiograph, an endotracheal tube may be seen. The presence of air bronchograms, the irregular shape of the opacification, and lack of volume loss suggest that this is not atelectasis of the left upper lobe.

Q29-2: D
Verrucous

Rationale: The lesions have an irregular, pebbled, or rough surface that may resemble a wart. The lesion is raised from the surface of the skin. There is no apparent ulceration present, and this is not a xanthomatous lesion (waxy). Lichenification is a thickening of the skin with normal skin marking. Telangiectasias are small, dilated blood vessels.

Q29-3: B
Blastomycosis

Rationale: The patient is immunosuppressed and presents with a consolidative opacity (what appears to be community-acquired pneumonia that has failed outpatient antibiotics) and a skin lesion that has a verrucous appearance. He is immunocompromised and was traveling in an area endemic for blastomycosis. The diagnosis of blastomycosis is based on direct visualization of the organism in respiratory, bodily fluid, or tissue samples and the ability to grow *Blastomyces* from culture material. The H&E stain shows a granuloma with neutrophils and epithelioid cells, consistent with a suppurative granulomatous inflammation, and here one can actually see a single nonbudding yeast cell as well as the conidia form (balloon-shaped like scedosporium, septate hyphae with single microconidia present). They can form focal micro-abscesses as well, but suppurative granulomas are very common. The periodic acid–Schiff (PAS) stains show thick-walled, spherical, single budding yeast with broad-based budding (rather than narrow-based budding seen in *Histoplasma*).

Predominant in North America, endemic in Ohio, Mississippi, and the St. Lawrence River Valley, and similar to *Coccidioides*, *Blastomyces* are inhaled via the soil. While endemic in the environment, *Blastomyces* is an opportunistic organism in patients with compromised immune systems, including patients with AIDS, organ transplantation, and those patients on immunosuppressive medications, especially the patient's prescribed anti-TNFα inhibitors.

Acute infection mimics that of other common pulmonary ailments (community-acquired bacterial or viral pneumonia) and is likely underreported as a result. The chest imaging in acute blastomycosis typically demonstrates focal or lobar consolidative opacities or tree-in-bud opacities with ground glass. This is more commonly seen in the upper lobes because this is where the mycelia are distributed. These opacities may have cavitations. However, patients may also present with multifocal disease or a more micronodular or reticulonodular appearance. Unlike coccidioidomycosis or histoplasmosis, hilar lymphadenopathy is not commonly encountered. Acute respiratory distress syndrome (ARDS) has also been reported in blastomycosis. Similar to other fungal infections, blastomycosis may also lead to the development of more chronic lung disease, with findings similar to acute pneumonia, and it is more likely to involve the upper lobes.

The definitive diagnosis of blastomycosis is direct visualization of the organism in a respiratory or tissue specimen (CSF, urine, skin biopsy, lung biopsy, biopsy of the respiratory epithelium from upper airway), or a positive culture from such a specimen (or from the bloodstream in the case of disseminated disease). Unfortunately, standard wet preparations have a low diagnostic yield (less than 50%). At body temperature, the yeast form dominates and can be identified by the single, broad-based budding yeast in which the daughter cell is nearly equal in size to the parent. Gomori methenamine silver (GMS) or Papanicolaou stains are often used for cytologic analysis, while H&E or PAS stains are used on histologic samples. The common pathology seen is granulomatous inflammation. The yeast forms have refractile walls. Unlike cryptococcus species, they do not contain a capsule.

Serologic testing is generally not used for a diagnosis of blastomycosis. None of the available immunodiffusion, complement fixation, or ELISA tests provide both the necessary sensitivity and specificity. Nucleic acid identification via PCR has been used in the literature but is not commonly available. An antigen test is available and may be performed using blood or other bodily fluids. It provides greater than 90% sensitivity but is also plagued by some cross-reactivity with antigens from *Histoplasma*, reducing the specificity to 70% to 80%.

Q29-4: C
Skin

Rationale: Blastomycosis may be asymptomatic in immunocompromised hosts, or it may cause acute or chronic pulmonary disease. Additionally, immunocompromised hosts may develop disseminated disease. The lungs are the primary site of infection (90%), followed by the skin (20%), bone (less than 5%), CNS (less than 1%), genitourinary tract (1%-2%), and lymph nodes (1%). The most common presenting symptoms include productive cough, dyspnea, fever, and pleuritic chest pain. Patients may also experience other constitutional symptoms (weight loss, chills, night sweats), arthralgia/myalgia, and fatigue. The most common skin manifestation of blastomycosis is the presence of irregular verrucous lesions, which are purple in color. Patients may also have ulcerative lesions or subcutaneous nodules (most common in disseminated disease).

Like in other fungal infections, CNS disease is seen almost exclusively in immuno-compromised hosts and presents as meningitis or intracranial abscesses. Osteomyelitis is the most common form of bone-related blastomycosis.

Q29-5: A
Liposomal amphotericin B

Rationale: This patient, who is immunocompromised, would receive induction with amphotericin B followed by maintenance therapy with either itraconazole or voriconazole most likely. Unlike coccidioidomycosis or histoplasmosis, the majority of patients with blastomycosis receive antifungal therapy. The treatment of blastomycosis again depends on the severity of the presentation, host immunocompetency, and the organ systems involved. For mild or moderate pulmonary disease, itraconazole is the treatment of choice, and it is used for 6 to 12 months. In all cases below, the liposomal formulation of amphotericin B is preferred based on reduced toxicity. For patients with severe pulmonary disease, amphotericin B induction (typically 2 weeks) and itraconazole maintenance therapy is recommended. For patients with mild or moderate disseminated/extrapulmonary disease, itraconazole is recommended, while amphotericin B induction and itraconazole or voriconazole maintenance are prescribed. Any patient with CNS involvement typically receives 6 weeks of amphotericin induction followed by an undetermined length of either voriconazole or itraconazole maintenance (typically at least 12 months). For immunocompromised patients, induction with amphotericin B and indefinite maintenance/suppressive therapy with either itraconazole or another azole is recommended.

Q29-6: A
Liposomal amphotericin B

Rationale: For pregnant women, amphotericin B (lipophilic preparation) is used because azoles are contraindicated during pregnancy.

References

Bariola JR, Hage CA, Durkin M, et al. Detection of *Blastomyces dermatitidis* antigen in patients with newly diagnosed blastomycosis. Diagn Microbiol Infect Dis. 2011;69:187.

Bariola JR, Perry P, Pappas PG, et al. Blastomycosis of the central nervous system: a multicenter review of diagnosis and treatment in the modern era. Clin Infect Dis. 2010;50:797.

Chapman SW, Dismukes WE, Proia LA, et al. Clinical practice guidelines for the management of blastomycosis: 2008 update by the Infectious Diseases Society of America. Clin Infect Dis. 2008;46:1801.

Johnson MD, Perfect JR. Fungal infections of the bones and joints. Curr Infect Dis Rep. 2001;3:450.

Li RK, Ciblak MA, Nordoff N, et al. In vitro activities of voriconazole, itraconazole, and amphotericin B against *Blastomyces dermatitidis*, *Coccidioides immitis*, and *Histoplasma capsulatum*. Antimicrob Agents Chemother. 2000;44:1734.

Limper AH, Knox KS, Sarosi GA, et al. An official American Thoracic Society statement: treatment of fungal infections in adult pulmonary and critical care patients. Am J Respir Crit Care Med. 2011;183:96.

Martynowicz MA, Prakash UB. Pulmonary blastomycosis: an appraisal of diagnostic techniques. Chest. 2002;121:768.

Parker JD, Doto IL, Tosh FE. A decade of experience with blastomycosis and its treatment with amphotericin B. A National Communicable Disease Center Cooperative Mycoses Study. Am Rev Respir Dis. 1969;99:895.

Perfect JR. Treatment of non-*Aspergillus* moulds in immunocompromised patients, with amphotericin B lipid complex. Clin Infect Dis. 2005;40:S401.

Saccente M, Woods GL. Clinical and laboratory update on blastomycosis. Clin Microbiol Rev. 2010;23:367.

Sidamonidze K, Peck MK, Perez M, et al. Real-time PCR assay for identification of *Blastomyces dermatitidis* in culture and in tissue. J Clin Microbiol. 2012;50:1783.

Wheat LJ. Antigen detection, serology, and molecular diagnosis of invasive mycoses in the immunocompromised host. Transpl Infect Dis. 2006;8:128.

CASE 30

A 32-year-old man presents to the ED with acute hypoxemic respiratory failure. He is an occasional smoker, smoking two to three cigarettes daily. He does not use drugs, but he does drink alcohol three to five times per week. He has a history of GERD, for which he takes a proton pump inhibitor (PPI), and hypothyroidism, for which he takes levothyroxine. He is a minister at a church in Colorado, and last month he traveled to New Mexico to build a new school as part of a church missionary trip. He spent about 6 weeks there and returned about 2 weeks ago. He started feeling more fatigued before returning, but since he returned home he developed a cough and some mild pleuritic pain, for which he was treated with azithromycin and a short course of steroids for pneumonia and reactive airway disease. He felt much worse thereafter and developed significant dyspnea with exertion over the last 24 hours, prompting his presentation. He has been having low-grade fevers as well as some chills. His vital signs are: T 101.3°F, HR 103, BP 121/78, RR 23, and O_2 saturation 96% on room air.

A tuberculin purified protein derivative (PPD) is placed, and a *M. tuberculosis* interferon-γ release assay (ie, QuantiFERON GOLD) is negative. An HIV study is negative. His chest radiogram is shown in Image 30-1.

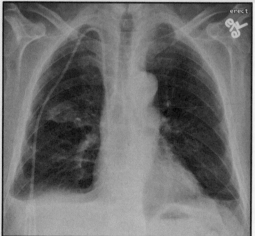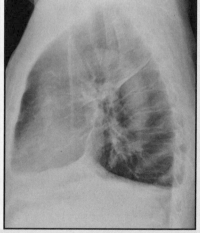

Image 30-1 • Chest radiographs (PA and lateral) for the patient in **Question 30-1**.

QUESTIONS

Q30-1: What is the primary abnormality on the imaging in Image 30-1?

A. Cystic lung lesion
B. Cavitary lung lesion
C. Focal consolidation
D. Atelectasis
E. Lung mass

Q30-2: The patient's laboratory values are notable for a WBC count of $12.4 \times 10^3/\mu L$, with a mild left shift (85% neutrophils). The patient is admitted to the hospital and undergoes a CT scan of chest, abdomen, and pelvis to evaluate for a source of infection. The CT images are shown in Image 30-2.

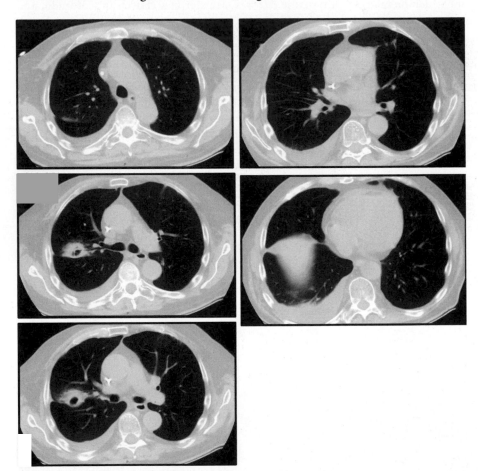

Image 30-2 • Chest CT images for the patient in **Question 30-2**.

Which abnormalities are present on the patient's CT scan?

A. Cystic lung lesion
B. Cavitary lung lesion
C. Right pleural effusion
D. Pericardial effusion
E. Centrilobular emphysema
F. A and C
G. B and C
H. C and D
 I. B, C, and E

Q30-3: The patient undergoes bronchoscopy with transbronchial biopsies. The result of the HIV antibody test is negative. The results are shown in Image 30-3.

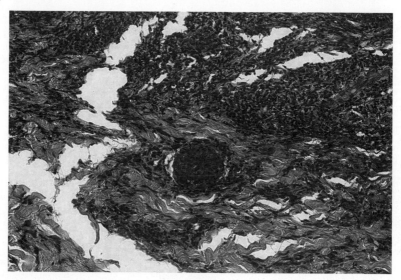

Image 30-3 • Representative histopathology specimen for the patient in **Question 30-3**.

What is the likely diagnosis?

A. Histoplasmosis
B. Coccidioidomycosis
C. Paracoccidioidomycosis
D. Blastomycosis
E. Aspergilloma
F. Mucormycosis

Q30-5: Which factor in this patient's history is most important to narrowing the differential diagnosis?

A. Smoking history
B. Family history
C. Travel history
D. Medical history
E. Recent sick contacts

Q30-6: Which test is most commonly used to diagnose acute focal pulmonary coccidioidomycosis?

A. Serum antigen
B. Serum serology (IgM antibody)
C. Radiographic findings
D. Skin test
E. Serum procalcitonin

Q30-7: Which treatment is indicated for patients with coccidioidomycosis complicated by meningitis?

A. Intravenous amphotericin B
B. Fluconazole
C. Metronidazole
D. Flucytosine
E. Itraconazole

Q30-8: If the patient's bronchoscopy had demonstrated the findings shown in Image 30-4, what would be the likely diagnosis?

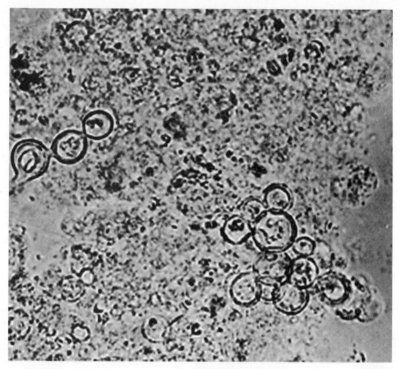

Image 30-4 • Representative findings on cytologic examination of bronchoalveolar lavage (BAL) fluid from the patient in **Question 30-8**. *(Reproduced with permission from Riedel S, Hobden JA, Miller S, et al: Jawetz, Melnick, & Adelberg's Medical Microbiology, 28th ed. New York, NY: McGraw Hill; 2019.)*

A. Histoplasmosis
B. Coccidioidomycosis
C. Paracoccidioidomycosis
D. Blastomycosis
E. Aspergilloma
F. Mucormycosis

ANSWERS

Q30-1: B
Cavitary lung lesion

Rationale: On the CXR there is a large cavitary lung lesion near the right hilum and perhaps some interstitial opacities on the right. The CXR shows a lesion with a thick wall, so this is not a cystic lesion. There are no focal consolidations or plate-like atelectasis. Although this could be construed as a lung mass with central cavitation, the better term to describe the lesion is a *cavitary lung lesion*.

Q30-2: G – B and C
Cavitary lung lesion and Right pleural effusion

Rationale: The patient's CT scan shows a thick-walled cavitary lesion on the right, with perhaps some surrounding ground glass. The lesion is thick walled and consistent with a cystic lesion. This is an important distinction because the differential diagnoses for cystic and cavitary lesions are quite different. It is also important to differentiate cystic and cavitary lesions from emphysematous changes in the lung, as demonstrated in **Image 30-5**.

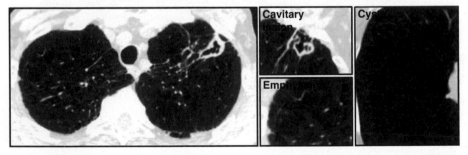

Image 30-5 • Examples of cavitary lesions, cysts, and emphysematous lesions as seen on CT chest imaging (lung windows).

There is also a right-sided pleural effusion present on this patient's CT scan. Given that the cavitary lesion and the effusion are on the same side, it is likely that this effusion is related to the process ongoing in the cavitary lesion. There is no evidence of a pericardial effusion (although without mediastinal windows, this is difficult to rule out entirely). Additionally, there is no significant evidence of centrilobular emphysema on the patient's CT scan.

Q30-3: B
Coccidioidomycosis

Rationale: The H&E sections, at body temperature, the fungi is present in tissue in large thick-walled spherules containing numerous endospores, which are released when the spherule ruptures. One such spherule can be seen at the center of the biopsy specimen above, with numerous fungal elements present surrounding the spherule. The histopathology of the other organisms mentioned here will discussed in other cases in this book.

Q30-5: C
Travel history

Rationale: This is a common presentation of coccidioidomycosis occurring after exposure in an endemic location (southwestern United States). Primary pulmonary coccidiomycosis, often called "valley fever," is a fungal infection caused by either *Coccidioides immitis* or *Coccidioides posadasii* species. *Coccidioides* species exist as a mold at room temperature and in spherule form at body temperature. *Coccidioides* species are endemic in desert climates, and in the United States it is most often found in the southwestern states, along with Central and South America. It is estimated that 100,000 to 200,000 coccidioidal infections occur annually in the United States, though it is difficult to estimate because more than 50% of such infections are never reported and resolve with mild symptoms. Innoculation occurs via inhalation of arthroconidia from the desert soil (3-5 μm in diameter), which may then develop into these large spherules that can be up to 60 to 80 μm in diameter. Patients who develop primary pulmonary infection have symptoms similar to those seen in community-acquired pneumonia, with fever, cough, congestion, fatigue, and malaise often reported. Some patients may develop extrapulmonary symptoms, including rheumatologic and dermatologic manifestations. These are believed to be the result of immune response to the infection and do not necessarily represent disseminated disease. In immunocompetent hosts, most patients will recover on their own without treatment, though patients can also develop chronic disease, particularly with cavitary lesions or other structural lung disease. This patient was treated with steroids, which may have led to worsening of his condition via immunosuppression. The usual findings are cavitary lung lesions, nodular opacities, and consolidation. Disseminated disease is rare and is seen most commonly in immunocompromised patients. Patients will often present with a miliary pattern of disease similar to that seen in miliary TB. These patients may also have adenopathy, effusions, cavitations, and other complications including empyema, pneumothorax, and bronchopleural fistulas. Involvement of the CNS can lead to formation of brain abscesses or meningoencephalitis. Disseminated disease may involve the CNS, skin, liver, adrenal glands, pericardium, heart, and eyes, among other organs. Radiographic findings are nonspecific, and diagnosis relies on histopathology, culture, and serologic testing.

Blastomycosis is common in the Ohio River Valley region and upper Midwest, while histoplasmosis is common in the southeastern United States, the Mississippi River Valley, regions of Pennsylvania, and in regions of the northeastern United States near the Great Lakes. *Aspergillus* species are generally found throughout the United States.

Q30-6: B
Serum serology (IgM antibody)

Rationale: Serum serology is the most commonly used and likely the most sensitive test for the diagnosis of acute focal coccidiomycosis, particularly in outpatients with mild or moderate disease. Similar to aspergillosis, coccidiomycosis may cause focal or diffuse acute pneumonia, chronic fibrocavitary pulmonary disease, or disseminated disease; the choice of which test to use depends on the particular presentation. The antigen test is slightly less sensitive at this point, but it can be obtained from urine and serum samples and is used more frequently in patients with disseminated disease. Serology testing is initially performed using enzyme immunoassay (EIA) and then confirmed using either immunodiffusion or complement fixation. The IgM antibody appears in after 1 to 3 weeks of illness (typically about the time patients develop symptoms), with an IgG antibody developing after 3 to 6 weeks and titer quickly dropping thereafter. However, in disseminated disease, the IgG titer does not drop until the disease is cleared. While direct visualization of the organisms in a tissue or respiratory specimen is the most specific test available, identification of spherules requires special preparations (ie, Papanicolaou staining, potassium hydroxide preparations, GMS or PAS stains), so some prior suspicion is usually necessary. Cultures from respiratory specimens, or blood cultures in disseminated disease, may also be useful. PCR is currently only available at reference laboratories, but one would expect this technology to be readily available in the future. Immunocompromised patients are at increased risk for severe disease, and depending on the etiology of their immunocompromised state, they may not have IgM antibodies present. In these patients, direct visualization of the organism from respiratory or biopsy specimens or via culture are more commonly used. A skin test has been developed to screen asymptomatic patients for immunity, but it is not currently used to diagnose acute disease. Procalcitonin may be elevated in coccidioidomycosis, but it is not specific. Similarly, the radiographic findings are nonspecific and may been seen in most endemic fungal infections as well as in community or nosocomial pneumonia.

Q30-7: B
Fluconazole

Rationale: Fluconazole remains the primary treatment for coccidioidal meningitis because evidence for amphotericin B is lacking (though it has been used as salvage therapy). Itraconazole is an alternative option. *Intrathecal* amphotericin B has been used for patients during the first trimester of pregnancy to reduce potential teratogenicity from treatment. Importantly, patients presenting with coccidiomycosis with a new diagnosis of HIV, or those patients with HIV not on highly active antiretroviral therapy (HAART) currently, are often started on antifungal therapy for several weeks before the initiation of HAART to prevent immune reconstitution inflammatory syndrome (IRIS), as this has been reported in the past.

Immunocompetent patients with focal mild-to-moderate pulmonary disease and no evidence of respiratory compromise often do not require treatment. Patients with focal acute disease and more severe presentations and those with diffuse pulmonary disease are often treated with fluconazole or itraconazole. Patients with chronic pulmonary disease may require a prolonged course of antifungal therapy. There is some evidence of the use of amphotericin B for induction therapy (or in combination with an azole) in patients with severe presentations including acute respiratory distress syndrome (ARDS), and in immunocompromised patients, with fluconazole as consolidation therapy. Check the Infectious Diseases Society of America (IDSA) guidelines for current recommendations regarding specific treatment regimens for specific patient groups.

Q30-8: C
Paracoccidioidomycosis

Rationale: These are large, multiply-budding yeasts, consistent with paracoccidioidomycosis. This fungi may also cause pulmonary manifestations, though it is not commonly associated with an acute pneumonia. Spores are inhaled and may form granulomas that remain dormant for long periods, but they have the potential to reactivate, leading to chronic pulmonary disease or even disseminated disease. A very small population of patients will develop an acute or subacute pneumonia-like process.

References

Arsura EL, Kilgore WB. Miliary coccidioidomycosis in the immunocompetent. Chest. 2000;117:404.

Benedict K, Thompson GR 3rd, Deresinski S, Chiller T. Mycotic Infections Acquired outside Areas of Known Endemicity, United States. Emerg Infect Dis. 2015;21:1935.

Campion JM, Gardner M, Galgiani JN. Coccidioidomycosis (valley fever) in older adults: an increasing problem. Arizona Geriatr Soc J. 2003;8:3.

Catanzaro A, Cloud GA, Stevens DA, et al. Safety, tolerance, and efficacy of posaconazole therapy in patients with nonmeningeal disseminated or chronic pulmonary coccidioidomycosis. Clin Infect Dis. 2007;45:562.

Galgiani JN, Ampel NM, Blair JE, et al. 2016 Infectious Diseases Society of America (IDSA) Clinical Practice Guideline for the Treatment of Coccidioidomycosis. Clin Infect Dis. 2016;63:e112.

Galgiani JN, Catanzaro A, Cloud GA, et al. Comparison of oral fluconazole and itraconazole for progressive, nonmeningeal coccidioidomycosis. A randomized, double-blind trial. Mycoses Study Group. Ann Intern Med. 2000;133:676.

Kassis C, Zaidi S, Kuberski T, et al. Role of coccidioides antigen testing in the cerebrospinal fluid for the diagnosis of coccidioidal meningitis. Clin Infect Dis. 2015;61:1521.

Kim MM, Vikram HR, Kusne S, et al. Treatment of refractory coccidioidomycosis with voriconazole or posaconazole. Clin Infect Dis. 2011;53:1060.

Kuberski T, Myers R, Wheat LJ, et al. Diagnosis of coccidioidomycosis by antigen detection using cross-reaction with a Histoplasma antigen. Clin Infect Dis. 2007;44:e50.

Martins TB, Jaskowski TD, Mouritsen CL, Hill HR. Comparison of commercially available enzyme immunoassay with traditional serological tests for detection of antibodies to Coccidioides immitis. J Clin Microbiol. 1995;33:940.

Mertz LE, Blair JE. Coccidioidomycosis in rheumatology patients: incidence and potential risk factors. Ann N Y Acad Sci. 2007;1111:343.

Nesbit LA, Knox KS, Nguyen CT, et al. Immunological characterization of bronchoalveolar lavage fluid in patients with acute pulmonary coccidioidomycosis. J Infect Dis. 2013;208:857.

Saubolle MA, McKellar PP, Sussland D. Epidemiologic, clinical, and diagnostic aspects of coccidioidomycosis. J Clin Microbiol. 2007;45:26.

Stevens DA, Rendon A, Gaona-Flores V, et al. Posaconazole therapy for chronic refractory coccidioidomycosis. Chest. 2007;132:952.

Thompson GR 3rd, Bays DJ, Johnson SM, et al. Serum (1->3)-β-D-glucan measurement in coccidioidomycosis. J Clin Microbiol. 2012;50:3060.

Valdivia L, Nix D, Wright M, et al. Coccidioidomycosis as a common cause of community-acquired pneumonia. Emerg Infect Dis. 2006;12:958.

CASE 31

A 44-year-old man presents with dyspnea, hypoxemia, fever, fatigue/malaise, and a skin rash. He reports that the symptoms started about 1 week ago and have slowly worsened. He is currently taking carvedilol for HTN and pantoprazole for gastroesophageal reflux disease (GERD), and he started allopurinol a few months ago for gout. He does not smoke or use illicit drugs, and he drinks one to two alcoholic beverages a week. On examination, the patient has some enlarged lymph nodes in the inguinal region. His chest radiograph and an image of the skin rash are shown (Images 31-1 and 31-2, respectively). There is no mucosal involvement of the rash. He has taken no other antibiotics, over-the-counter medications, or herbal supplements, and no other medications have been prescribed other than those listed previously. He denies any environmental exposures and has not changed any home-cleaning or clothes-washing products. The patient's vitals signs are T 38.3°C, HR 104, BP 110/83, RR 19-23, and requiring 3 L of O_2 on NC at rest to maintain his oxygen saturation above 90%. He is started on antibiotics for community-acquired pneumonia and is pan-cultured.

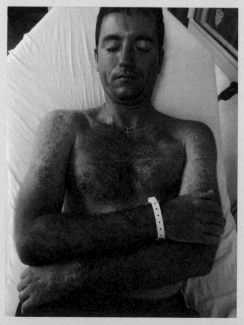

Image 31-1 • Dermatologic abnormalities discovered on examination of the patient in **Questions 31-1** and **31-2**. (*Reproduced with permission from Jameson J, Fauci AS, Kasper DL, et al: Harrison's Principles of Internal Medicine, 20th ed. New York, NY: McGraw Hill; 2018.*)

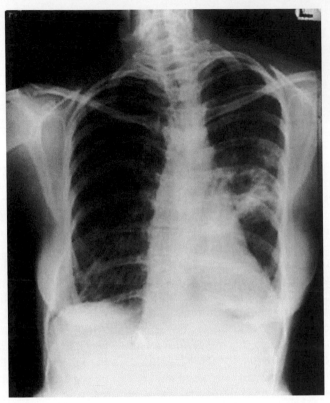

Image 31-2 • Chest radiograph (AP) for the patient in **Questions 31-1** and **31-2**. (*Reproduced with permission from Papadakis MA, McPhee SJ, Rabow MW: Current Medical Diagnosis & Treatment 2021. New York, NY: McGraw Hill; 2021.*)

QUESTIONS

Q31-1: How would you describe the abnormalities on the chest radiograph in Image 31-2?

A. Loculated pleural effusion
B. Linear interstitial opacities
C. Reticulonodular interstitial opacities
D. Focal infiltrate/consolidation
E. Diffuse alveolar infiltrates

Q31-2: The patient's laboratory data results demonstrate the following abnormalities: creatinine is slightly elevated at 1.6 mg/dL from 1.0 baseline; alanine aminotransferase (ALT) is elevated at 120 U/L; alkaline phosphatase (AP) is elevated at 220 U/L; and the WBC count is normal (7800/μL) with 21% eosinophils.

What is the likely diagnosis?

A. Community-acquired pneumonia
B. Stevens-Johnson syndrome
C. Drug eruption with eosinophilia and systemic symptoms (DRESS)
D. Acute cutaneous lupus erythematosus
E. Hypersensitivity pneumonitis

Q31-3: A 30-year-old man presents with severe hypoxemic respiratory failure. He has no medical history. He noted the onset of symptoms 2 days ago, with no apparent prodrome. He is experiencing fevers, dyspnea, a dry cough, pleuritic chest pain, fatigue, and malaise. He takes no medications and denies any occupational exposures, environmental exposures, or new medications. He takes no illicit drugs. He had previously smoked 1 pack of cigarettes per day for about 10 years and quit a year ago, but he began smoking again about 3 weeks ago. He has taken acetaminophen but no other medications. His examination demonstrates polyphonic wheezing and diffuse inspiratory crackles. He has no skin rash. His chest film and CT scan are shown in Images 31-3 and 31-4. He was intubated in the ED for respiratory distress and admitted to the medical ICU.

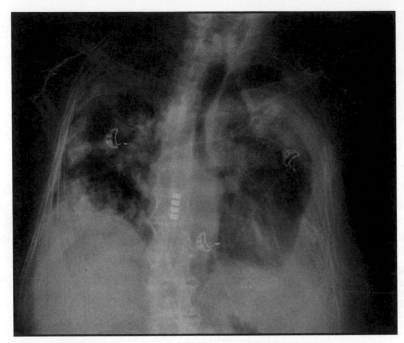

Image 31-3 • Chest radiograph (AP) for the patient in **Question 31-3**.

How would you describe the patient's chest X-ray abnormalities in Image 31-3?

A. Reticulonodular interstitial opacities
B. Linear interstitial opacities
C. Diffuse alveolar and interstitial opacities
D. Atelectasis
E. Bilateral pleural effusions
F. C and E

Q31-4: How would you describe the primary abnormality on the patient's CT scan as shown in Image 31-4?

A. Diffuse micronodular opacities
B. Perihilar cavitary lung lesions
C. Interlobular and intralobular septal thickening
D. Honeycombing
E. Scattered ground-glass opacities, pleural effusions and consolidation
F. Focal atelectasis

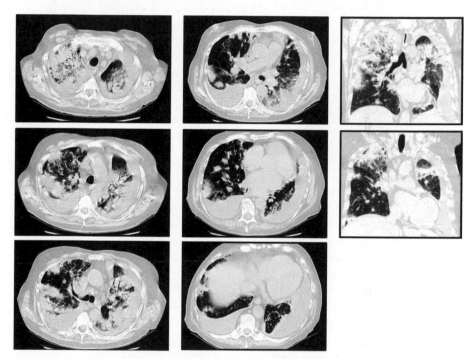

Image 31-4 • Chest CT images for the patient in **Question 31-4**.

Q31-5: The patient's QuantiFERON gold study for tuberculosis (TB) is negative. He has an HIV study that is negative. His respiratory viral panel is negative. He undergoes a bronchoscopy with transbronchial biopsies. The results of the additional testing are shown in the table below and in Image 31-5.

Gram:	Negative	**Cell Count**		**Blood Smear**	
KOH:	Negative	Neutrophil	15%	Neutrophil	80%
AFB:	Negative	Macrophage	30%	Lymphocyte	8%
Silver:	Negative	Eosinophil	40%	Monocyte	8%
		Lymphocyte	15%	Eosinophil	4% (500/uL)

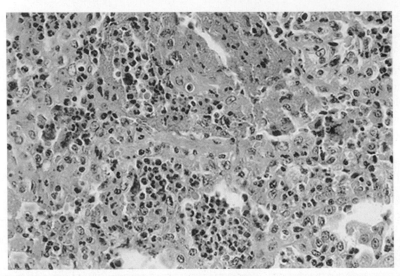

Image 31-5 • Biopsy result (H&E stain). (*Reproduced with permission from Stone JH: Current Diagnosis & Treatment: Rheumatology, 4th ed. New York, NY: McGraw Hill; 2021.*)

Special stains for all organisms are negative. An extended respiratory viral panel from the BAL is negative. What is the most likely diagnosis?

A. Nonspecific interstitial pneumonia (NSIP)
B. Acute respiratory distress syndrome (ARDS)
C. Adenovirus pneumonia
D. Acute eosinophilic pneumonia (AEP)
E. Cryptogenic organizing pneumonia (COP)
F. Respiratory bronchiolitis–related interstitial lung disease (RB-ILD)
G. Desquamative interstitial pneumonia (DIP)

Q31-6: What is the primary treatment for AEP?

A. Antibiotic therapy
B. Plasmapheresis
C. Antihistamines
D. Monoclonal anti-IgE therapy
E. Corticosteroid therapy

Q31-7: A 44-year-old man presents to the clinic with progressively worsening symptoms of dyspnea and nocturnal cough. He reports that the symptoms started about 4 to 5 months ago and he has been experiencing some low-grade fevers, intermittent wheezing, and a nonproductive cough. He has lost approximately 10 lb unintentionally over that time. He has seen his primary care physician twice and received antibiotics without improvement. He had a PPD that was negative, as well as an HIV test that was also negative. He does not smoke, use illicit drugs, or drink alcohol. He is currently an airplane mechanic in the military. He spent nearly 8 years living in Southeast Asia before returning to the United States about 12 months ago. On examination, he has scattered rales and polyphonic wheezing. He was started on albuterol which has helped to some degree. His chest radiograph is shown in Image 31-6.

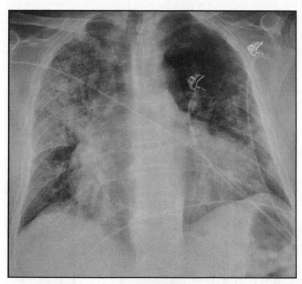

Pulmonary Function Testing:

FEV1	58%
FVC	72%
Ratio	70%
TLC	75%
VC	71%
RV	66%
DLCO	69%

Image 31-6 • Chest radiograph for the patient in Question 31-7.

The patient's PFTs indices are shown as well. The patient's initial laboratory work from his clinic visit is as follows: peripheral blood count 13,000/μL; cell differential reported as 55%, eosinophils, 25% neutrophils, 20% lymphocytes; serum IgG level 2400 IU/mL, serum IgE level 2100 IU/mL. The patient undergoes bronchoscopy with 60% eosinophils in the lavage fluid. The typical studies from the BAL are negative, including Gram stain, KOH, and AFB stain, as well as an extended respiratory viral panel. What test would you request next?

A. ESR
B. Antifilarial antibodies (*Wuchereria bancrofti, Brugia malayi*)
C. Nocardia culture
D. PET-CT
E. Serum galactomannan
F. BAL beta-D-glucan

Q31-8: The testing for antibodies against *W. bancrofti* returns positive at 1:64. What is the next step in management for the patient?

A. Itraconazole
B. Corticosteroids
C. Trimethoprim
D. Diethylcarbamazine
E. Anti-TNF-alpha therapy

Q31-9: A 40-year-old woman presents to the clinic with several months of dyspnea, drenching night sweats, a 20-lb weight loss, and an intractable cough with intermittent wheezing. She has been undergoing an extensive evaluation with her primary care physician for a possible malignancy. She had a negative PPD, a negative HIV study, a negative acute hepatitis panel, and negative serologies for rheumatologic disease. The patient works as a homemaker and has three children without medical issues. She does not smoke, drink alcohol, or use illicit drugs. She recalls no environmental exposures. She has no relevant travel history and lives in the northwest United States. Images from the CT are shown in Image 31-7.

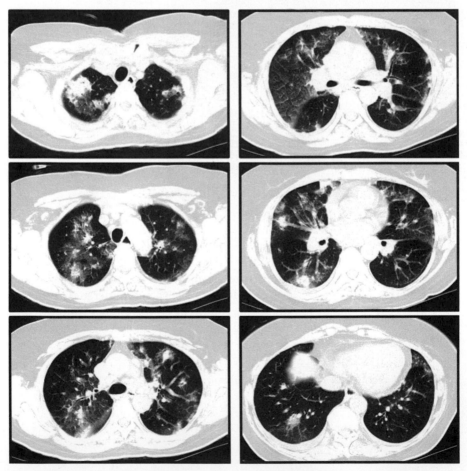

Image 31-7 • Chest CT images for the patient in **Question 31-9**.

Her additional laboratory testing revealed peripheral eosinophilia (20%), thrombocytosis, and an elevated ESR. The serum IgE is elevated. The patient is sent for bronchoscopy with BAL. The differential from the BAL fluid had a 70% eosinophil predominance. The Gram stain, KOH, and AFB smear are negative. Special stains for fungal and viral etiologies in the biopsy specimen are negative, and a respiratory viral panel is negative.

What is the likely diagnosis?

A. Acute eosinophilic pneumonia (AEP)
B. Chronic eosinophilic pneumonia (CEP)
C. Tropical pulmonary eosinophilia (TPE)
D. Invasive pulmonary aspergillosis (IPA)
E. Pulmonary histoplasmosis

ANSWERS

Q31-1: D
Focal infiltrate/opacity/consolidation

Rationale: There is a focal left-sided infiltrate likely in the lingula. This is highly nonspecific and could be consistent with lobar pneumonia.

Q31-2: C
Drug eruption with eosinophilia and systemic symptoms (DRESS)

Rationale: DRESS is a delayed hypersensitivity reaction (usually occurring 2-6 weeks after initiation of therapy), yielding a skin rash, fevers, lymphadenopathy, peripheral eosinophilia, elevated transaminases, and, in some cases, pulmonary infiltrates. It was originally described in patients taking antiepileptic medications, but it has been associated with a number of other medications, including sulfasalazine and allopurinol. This patient started allopurinol a few months ago, placing him in the appropriate window for the development of this condition. His rash is a macular rash that is almost morbilliform in nature, which is the typical early finding. This may progress to a more erythematous, papular rash that becomes confluent. The rash will typically cover more than 50% of the body surface area and may include facial edema and scaling. Systemic symptoms include diffuse adenopathy, elevated transaminases with hepatomegaly, and kidney injury, among others. Pulmonary infiltrates may occur in up to half of patients. DRESS is a subtype of Loeffler syndrome.

Loeffler syndrome, or simple pulmonary eosinophilia, is an acute presentation of eosinophilic pneumonia resulting from parasitic infection, drugs, or other exposures characterized by fleeting pulmonary infiltrates, peripheral eosinophilia, and respiratory symptoms. Common drugs known to cause Loeffler syndrome include amiodarone, cocaine (inhalation), bleomycin, daptomycin, ethambutol, methotrexate, montelukast, and nitrofurantoin, among others.

Drug-induced eosinophilic pneumonia may be acute or subacute in nature and do not necessarily correlate to the duration of therapy or the cumulative dose.

Q31-3: F
Diffuse alveolar and interstitial opacities and bilateral pleural effusions

Rationale: There are diffuse abnormalities with both interstitial opacities and fluffy alveolar opacities. There is also a moderate-sized left-sided pleural effusion and likely a small right-sided pleural effusion (given how obscured the costophrenic angle is in **Image 31-3**).

Q31-4: E
Scattered ground-glass opacities, pleural effusions and consolidation

Rationale: There are also air bronchograms noted. There are no nodular opacities, and there is no evidence of cysts of cavitation. Bilateral pleural effusions are also seen. There is no apparent honeycombing at the bases (although this may be obscured by the effusions to some degree). There are no cavitary lesions present. There may be some areas of atelectasis present as a result of the effusions, however this is not the primary abnormality present.

Q31-5: D
Acute eosinophilic pneumonia (AEP)

Rationale: The BAL shows a predominance of eosinophils (often greater than 25% in AEP). While the peripheral blood film does not have peripheral eosinophilia, this is often absent early in the course of AEP. The pathology specimen shown in **Image 31-5** shows a significant eosinophilic infiltrate into the interstitium and filling of the alveolar spaces with an exudative process (hyaline membrane deposition in pink). There are no giant cells or granulomas, and the pathology and radiographic findings are not consistent with RB-ILD, DIP, COP, or NSIP. The primary differential diagnosis for AEP includes ARDS and disseminated infection. The presentation is usually abrupt, occurring in younger patients (ages 20-40) with a male predominance, and rapid progression to hypoxemia and respiratory failure is common. Often patients will report they recently started smoking before the onset of symptoms. Approximately 70% of patients who develop AEP have a history of tobacco use.

The prodrome is very similar to that of an infection, with fevers, nonproductive cough, dyspnea, and myalgias. Radiographic findings vary from patchy opacities to a reticulonodular interstitial pattern diffuse alveolar infiltrates mimicking ARDS. Pleural effusions are common. CT imaging may show ground-glass opacities, interlobular septal thickening, scattered areas of consolidation, or micronodular opacities. Given the lack of a clear inciting event, this would be classified as idiopathic AEP. AEP is a diagnosis of exclusion. Having excluded a granulomatous process and an infectious etiology, the pathology shows a predominance of eosinophils, suggesting AEP rather than ARDS or one of the idiopathic interstitial pneumonias (IIPs).

Q31-6: E
Corticosteroid therapy

Rationale: Steroid therapy is highly effective for the treatment of idiopathic AEP, with the vast majority of patients responding to steroids in 12 to 48 hours with resolution of their fevers and respiratory symptoms and complete improvement in pulmonary function and resolution of imaging abnormalities within a month. Intravenous steroids are initially dosed every 6 hours. With resolution of the respiratory failure, steroids are transitioned to oral and tapered over several weeks. If there is a suspected inciting etiology, the primary treatment is first removal of the offending agent following by steroid therapy. There is no role for antibiotics, though they are often continued in patients until reversal of the respiratory failure. Monoclonal antibody therapy against IgE (eg, Xolair or omalizumab) is a potential steroid-sparing agent in patients with chronic, but not acute, eosinophilic pneumonia. AEP generally does not relapse, unlike chronic eosinophilic pneumonia, which is prone to relapse.

Q31-7: B
Antifilarial antibodies

Rationale: This patient has a significant eosinophilia, both in the peripheral blood and in BAL specimens, an infiltrate on chest radiograph, a significantly elevated serum IgE, and his symptoms that include a paroxysmal nocturnal cough. The patient has spent considerable time recently in an endemic area for filarial disease. This presentation is highly consistent with tropical pulmonary eosinophilia (TPE), caused most commonly by *W. bancrofti* and *B. malayi*. While the differential is quite broad, and it would be ideal to include a number of additional tests, the presence of elevated titers of antibodies against filarial species would be of particular interest.

TPE is a hypersensitivity reaction to microfilarial antigens that occurs months to years after the infection. It presents with fevers, weight loss, a nocturnal dry cough, dyspnea, wheezing, and peripheral eosinophilia.

Q31-8: D
Diethylcarbamazine

Rationale: This is the preferred treatment for patients with filarial infection, including TPE. It has limited side effects, and a trial of treatment will often lead to rapid clinical improvement. The duration of therapy is generally 14 to 21 days, and this is generally curative.

Q31-9: B
Chronic eosinophilic pneumonia (CEP)

Rationale: As opposed to AEP or Loeffler syndrome, CEP typically presents in a subacute fashion, with progressive dyspnea, cough, and constitutional symptoms. Peripheral eosinophilia is commonly seen but not required. The BAL differential is typically dominated by eosinophils (greater than 25% eosinophils). An elevated IgE level is seen in half of all patients with CEP. Radiographic findings include the progressive development of peripheral-based ground-glass opacities and areas of consolidation, often described as the "photographic negative" of what would be expected in patients with pulmonary edema. The mid- and upper lung zones are more commonly involved.

The diagnosis is dependent on clinical, radiographic, and bronchoscopy findings and is typically a diagnosis of exclusion. The differential includes eosinophilic granulomatosis with polyangiitis (EGPA), Loeffler syndrome, sarcoidosis, COP, DIP,

ABPA, infections (fungal, parasitic), hypereosinophilic syndrome (HES), AEP, and lymphangitic spread of malignancy. HES is a syndrome marked by persistent peripheral hypereosinophilia with diffuse organ infiltration by eosinophils.

Many patients with CEP have a history of asthma. PFTs in CEP may show obstruction or restriction or may even be normal; therefore, PFTs are not helpful in diagnosing CEP, but they are helpful in monitoring a patient's response to treatment.

Similar to treatment for AEP, the primary treatment for CEP is systemic corticosteroids. A response to glucocorticoids is measured by resolution of symptoms, improvement in the peripheral eosinophilia, improvement in radiographic abnormalities, and improvement in PFTs. There are no guidelines on steroid dosing or the duration of therapy; some patients require treatment for only a few months, while others require dosing for a year. Although CEP has a good long-term prognosis, relapse is common and occurs in over 50% of cases. Relapse may occur after steroids are discontinued or while the steroid dose is being lowered.

Alternatives to steroids in patients with relapses of CEP include omalizumab, which is a monoclonal antibody to IgE, and mepolizumab, which is a monoclonal antibody to IL-5. There is no substantial evidence suggesting these drugs work in CEP; rather there have been case reports of these drugs being used.

References

Allen J. Acute eosinophilic pneumonia. Semin Respir Crit Care Med. 2006;27:142.

Allen JN, Davis WB. Eosinophilic lung diseases. Am J Respir Crit Care Med. 1994;150:1423.

Arter ZL, Wiggins A, Hudspath C, et al. Acute eosinophilic pneumonia following electronic cigarette use. Respir Med Case Rep. 2019;27:100825.

Badesch DB, King TE Jr, Schwarz MI. Acute eosinophilic pneumonia: a hypersensitivity phenomenon? Am Rev Respir Dis. 1989;139:249.

Balbi B, Fabiano F. A young man with fever, dyspnoea and nonproductive cough. Eur Respir J. 1996;9:619.

Chesnutt AN, Chesnutt MS, Prendergast NT, Prendergast TJ. Eosinophilic pulmonary syndromes. In: Papadakis MA, McPhee SJ, Rabow MW, eds. Current Medical Diagnosis & Treatment 2021. McGraw-Hill; 2021. https://accessmedicine.mhmedical.com/content.aspx?bookid=2957&sectionid=249370107

Crowe M, Robinson D, Sagar M, Chen L, Ghamande S. Chronic eosinophilic pneumonia: clinical perspectives. Ther Clin Risk Manag. 2019;15:397.

De Giacomi F, Vassallo R, Yi E, Ryu J. Acute eosinophilic pneumonia: causes, diagnosis, and management. Am J Respir Crit Care Med. 2018;197:728.

Ebara H, Ikezoe J, Johkoh T, et al. Chronic eosinophilic pneumonia: evolution of chest radiograms and CT features. J Comput Assist Tomogr. 1994;18:737.

Glazer CS, Cohen LB, Schwarz MI. Acute eosinophilic pneumonia in AIDS. Chest. 2001;120:1732.

Jeong YJ, Kim KI, Seo IJ, et al. Eosinophilic lung diseases: a clinical, radiologic, and pathologic overview. Radiographics. 2007;27:617.

Jhun BW, Kim SJ, Kim K, Lee JE. Clinical implications of initial peripheral eosinophilia in acute eosinophilic pneumonia. Respirology. 2014;19:1059.

Jhun BW, Kim SJ, Kim K, Lee JE. Outcomes of rapid corticosteroid tapering in acute eosinophilic pneumonia patients with initial eosinophilia. Respirology. 2015;20:1241.

Johkoh T, Müller NL, Akira M, et al. Eosinophilic lung diseases: diagnostic accuracy of thin-section CT in 111 patients. Radiology. 2000;216:773.

Kaya H, Gümüş S, Uçar E, et al. Omalizumab as a steroid-sparing agent in chronic eosinophilic pneumonia. Chest. 2012;142:513.

Micheletti R, Rosenbach M, Wintroub BU, Shinkai K. Cutaneous drug reactions. In: Jameson J, Fauci AS, Kasper DL, Hauser SL, Longo DL, Loscalzo J, eds. *Harrison's Principles of Internal Medicine*. 20th ed. McGraw-Hill; 2018. https://accessmedicine.mhmedical.com/content.aspx?bookid=2129&sectionid=159214349

Minakuchi M, Niimi A, Matsumoto H, et al. Chronic eosinophilic pneumonia: treatment with inhaled corticosteroids. Respiration. 2003;70:362.

Nesbit LA, Knox KS, Nguyen CT, et al. Immunological characterization of bronchoalveolar lavage fluid in patients with acute pulmonary coccidioidomycosis. J Infect Dis. 2013;208:857.

Oyama Y, Fujisawa T, Hashimoto D, et al. Efficacy of short-term prednisolone treatment in patients with chronic eosinophilic pneumonia. Eur Respir J. 2015;45:1624.

Philit F, Etienne-Mastroïanni B, Parrot A, et al. Idiopathic acute eosinophilic pneumonia: a study of 22 patients. Am J Respir Crit Care Med. 2002;166:1235.

Rochester CL. The eosinophilic pneumonias. In: Grippi MA, Elias AJ, Fishman JA, et al, eds. *Fishman's Pulmonary Diseases and Disorders*. 5th ed. McGraw-Hill; 2015. https://accessmedicine.mhmedical.com/content.aspx?bookid=1344&sectionid=8119230

Uppal P, LaPlante KL, Gaitanis MM, et al. Daptomycin-induced eosinophilic pneumonia – a systematic review. Antimicrob Resist Infect Control. 2016;5:55.

Watanabe K, Fujimura M, Kasahara K, et al. Acute eosinophilic pneumonia following cigarette smoking: a case report including cigarette-smoking challenge test. Intern Med. 2002;41:1016.

Zimhony O. Photographic negative shadow of pulmonary oedema. Lancet. 2002;360:33.

CASE 32

A 55-year-old woman presents to the clinic for evaluation of worsening dyspnea over the last 6 months. She has a history of hypothyroidism, is currently taking levothyroxine, and has HTN, for which she takes amlodipine. She states she was well until approximately 6 months ago when she first noticed some shortness of breath when taking her daily 3-mile walk. She denies any wheezing but says she developed a nonproductive cough. A trial of an albuterol inhaler did not help. She now has some dyspnea with minimal activity. She also notes increasing fatigue, almost to the point where she has trouble simply getting up from a chair. She has never smoked tobacco, and she does not use alcohol or illicit drugs. The patient's vital signs are T 37.0°C, HR 71, BP 144/62, RR 14 at rest, and oxygen saturation 91% on room air at rest. The patient's chest radiograph is shown in Image 32-1.

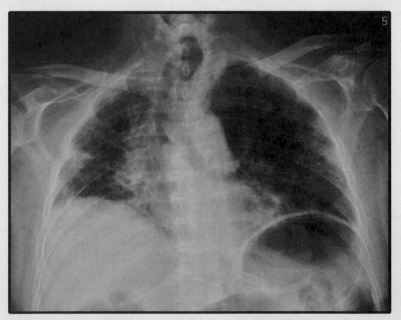

Image 32-1 • Chest radiograph (AP) for the patient in **Question 32-1**.

QUESTIONS

Q32-1: How would you describe the above abnormalities on the chest radiograph?

A. Linear interstitial opacities
B. Reticulonodular interstitial opacities
C. Diffuse alveolar infiltrates
D. Hyperinflation
E. Cystic lung lesions

Q32-2: Corresponding CT findings are provided in Image 32-2.

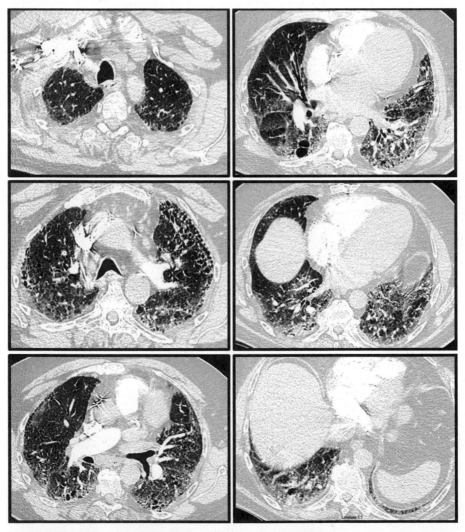

Image 32-2 • Chest CT images for the patient in **Question 32-2**.

How would you describe the primary abnormalities on the above CT scan (chose only ONE)?

A. Diffuse nodular opacities
B. Cystic lung lesions
C. Scattered areas of ground-glass opacities and consolidations
D. Centrilobular emphysema
E. Diffuse reticular opacities with interlobular and intralobular septal thickening

Q32-3: The patient undergoes PFT. Based on the patient's radiographic findings, which set of PFTs would you expect?

	A	B	C	D	E
FEV1	66%	90%	66%	80%	66%
FVC	91%	100%	68%	100%	70%
Ratio	69%	90%	97%	80%	99%
TLC	110%	89%	59%	79%	69%
VC	68%	99%	66%	80%	66%
RV	140%	70%	40%	30%	66%
DLCO	70%	35%	35%	88%	93%

Q32-4: The patient's examination demonstrates bibasilar crackles. Additionally, you discover the following on examination (see Images 32-3 and 32-4):

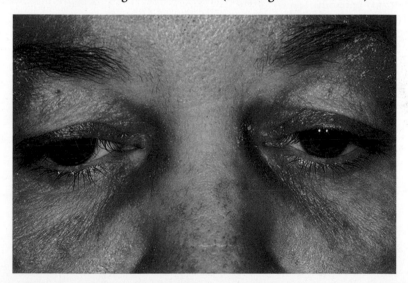

Image 32-3 • Dermatologic abnormalities identified on examination of the patient in **Question 32-4.** (*Reproduced with permission from Usatine RP, Smith MA, Mayeaux EJ, et al: The Color Atlas and Synopsis of Family Medicine, 3rd ed. New York, NY: McGraw Hill; 2019. Photo contributor: Richard P. Usatine, MD.*)

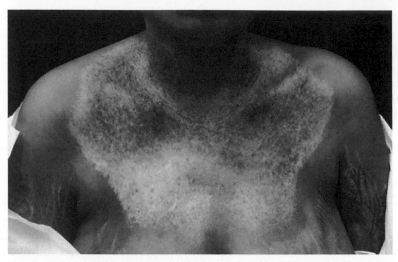

Image 32-4 • Dermatologic abnormalities identified on examination of the patient in **Question 32-4**. (*Reproduced with permission from Kelly AP, Taylor SC, Lom HW, et al: Taylor and Kelly's Dermatology for Skin of Color, 2nd ed. New York, NY: McGraw Hill; 2016.*)

Based on these skin findings, which laboratory test do you anticipate being positive?

A. Anti-Scl70 antibody
B. Anti-Jo1 antibody
C. Anti-double stranded DNA antibody
D. Serum precipitins to bird feather antigens
E. Anti-CCP antibody

Q32-5: What is the name of the abnormality also associated with dermatomyositis (see Image 32-5)?

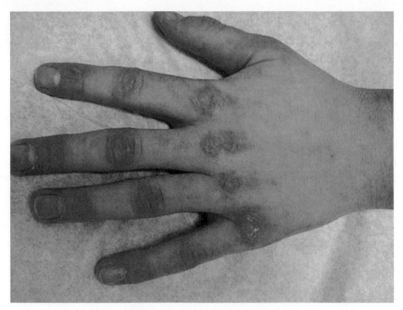

Image 32-5 • Dermatologic abnormalities identified on examination of the patient in **Question 32-5**. (*Reproduced with permission from Zaoutis LB, Chiang VW: Comprehensive Pediatric Hospital Medicine, 2nd ed. New York, NY: McGraw Hill; 2018.*)

A. Mechanic's hand
B. Gottron papules
C. Heberden nodes
D. Boutonniere deformities
E. Gardener's hand

Q32-6: The patient has abnormalities on the neurologic examination, including proximal weakness, most notable in her arms. What test would be the most useful next step to confirm the diagnosis?

A. Open lung biopsy
B. Transbronchial lung biopsy
C. Serum creatinine kinase (CK)
D. Serum aldolase
E. MRI
F. Electromyogram (EMG)

Q32-7: What is the utility of a lung biopsy in this patient?

A. Rule out an infectious cause of the abnormalities on chest imaging.
B. There is no utility.
C. Determine the most appropriate treatment option.
D. Evaluate for malignancy given the increased risk in dermatomyositis.

ANSWERS

Q32-1: B
Reticulonodular interstitial opacities

Rationale: Reticulonodular interstitial opacities are present throughout the lung fields, though they are more predominant in the right lung and at the bases.

Q32-2: E
Diffuse reticular opacities with interlobular/intralobular septal thickening

Rationale: The abnormalities seen on CT are diffuse reticular opacities with interlobular/intralobular septal thickening as well as honeycomb changes. Note the subpleural distribution. There is also some traction bronchiectasis, suggesting architectural distortion. This represents more chronic and likely irreversible changes in the lung parenchyma. The traction bronchiectasis should not be confused with cavitary or cystic lesions. There may be some ground glass opacities micronodular opacities present, however this is not the most striking abnormality present. There are no changes consistent with centribolular emphysema.

Q32-3: C

Rationale: The radiographic findings would be most concerning for restrictive physiology resulting from interstitial lung disease (ILD), which would also present with a reduced DLCO. Option A is consistent with an obstructive physiology based on an FEV1/FVC ratio less than 70% and evidence of air trapping and hyperinflation. Given the elevated TLC and RV, option B would be consistent with an isolated issue with the diffusing capacity of oxygen, such as may be seen in a patient with pulmonary arterial hypertension. Option D represents a patient with likely extrapulmonary restriction from excess weight (note that the reduction in RV is far in excess of that observed for the VC or TLC). Option E would be a PFT from a patient with extrathoracic restriction from neuromuscular disease such as amyotrophic lateral sclerosis (ALS).

Q32-4: B
Anti-Jo1 antibody

Rationale: The images represent the classic heliotrope rash and poikiloderma seen in dermatomyositis. Note that the poikiloderma is distributed in sun-exposed areas. The anti-Jo1 antibody is a member of a larger set of anti-tRNA synthetase antibodies that are commonly positive in DM/PM. Other tests that are typically positive include CK, aldolase, ESR, and ANA. In patients with overlapping syndromes, anti-Scl70 and anti-RNP may be positive, but these are not seen as frequently as anti-Jo1. The dsDNA antibody is specific to systemic lupus erythematosus (SLE), while the anti-CCP is specific to rheumatoid arthritis (RA).

Q32-5: B
Gottron papules

Rationale: These are violaceous, sometimes erythematous lesions common in dermatomyositis that are most prominent over the joint spaces of the hand and fingers (periungual telangiectasias). These abnormalities can extend to the nailbed as well. Mechanic's hand is another abnormality sometimes seen in dermatomyositis and is characterized by hyperkeratotic eruptions on the ulnar aspect of the thumb and the radial aspect of the index finger, with associated desquamation. Heberden nodes and boutonniere deformities are seen in arthritic conditions. Gardener's hand is not a clinical condition.

Q32-6: E
MRI

Rationale: Because the primary concern in this patient with proximal muscle weakness, ILD, the above skin findings, and a positive Jo-1 antibody is dermatomyositis or polymyositis, the next step in the evaluation would be an MRI of the proximal muscle groups where there was noted weakness on examination. Although an EMG would also be useful, MRI with T2-weighted images and short tau inversion recovery (STIR) is proving superior to identify a location for biopsy. The CK and aldolase are not specific for dermatomyositis or polymyositis and will not aid in confirming a diagnosis. A lung biopsy would help to identify the type of ILD present but will not identify the underlying autoimmune disease.

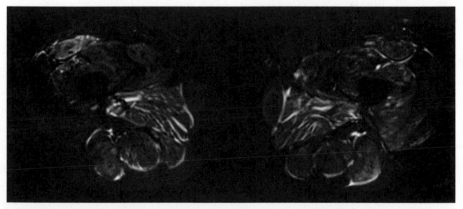

Image 32-6 • Short-TI inversion recovery MRI of the proximal thigh in a patient with dermatomyositis, demonstrating marked enhancement in the thighs, which is symmetric. *(Reproduced with permission from Stone JH: Current Diagnosis & Treatment: Rheumatology, 4th ed. New York, NY: McGraw Hill; 2021.)*

Inflammatory myopathies are rare, with a prevalence of 1 in 100,000. Patients present with symmetrical proximal muscle weakness that progresses over a course of weeks to months. They may report difficulty climbing stairs, rising from a seated position, or washing or brushing their hair. A rash is typical in dermatomyositis (ie, the heliotrope rash, Gottron papules, or the Shawl sign). Other signs or symptoms in dermatomyositis or polymyositis include constitutional symptoms, dysphagia, tachyarrhythmias, cardiomyopathy, ILD, subcutaneous calcifications, and synovitis.

Diagnosing an inflammatory myopathy requires a muscle biopsy showing lymphocytic inflammatory infiltration of the muscle tissue. CK is the muscle enzyme that often correlates with disease activity. Other muscle enzymes that can be elevated in these diseases include LDH and aldolase. Although EMGs and MRIs are helpful in the evaluation of a potential inflammatory myopathy, they are not diagnostic.

Initial treatment is usually corticosteroids; however, most patients require additional immunosuppression to manage their disease. Azathioprine, methotrexate, calcineurin inhibitors (tacrolimus, cyclosporine) and mycophenolate mofetil are commonly used drugs. In patients with refractory disease to the above two-drug approach, cyclophosphamide, intravenous immune globulin (IVIG) therapy (with or without plasmapheresis), and rituximab are also considerations. Newer therapies such as tofacitinib (Janus Kinase inhibitor) and Basilixumab (anti-CD25 or anti-IL2 receptor alpha antibody) has also been used in patients with DM/PM who have refractory disease with some benefit.

Prognosis is generally excellent for patients with dermatomyositis or polymyositis, with a 5-year survival rate of about 95% and a 10-year survival rate of approximately 84%. The prognosis is worse for patients with ILD.

Q32-7: D
Determine the most appropriate treatment option

Rationale: This patient's imaging is most consistent with nonspecific interstitial pneumonia (NSIP) or usual interstitial pneumonia (UIP). NSIP is the most common type of ILD seen in dermatomyositis or polymyositis. Recall that it can occur in a cellular, fibrotic, or mixed picture, with the cellular subtype thought to be the more treatment-responsive of these subtypes. Alternatively, patients may have a pathology that is consistent with pulmonary capillaritis (diffuse alveolar opacities on imaging) or organizing pneumonia (focal consolidations/opacities or scattered alveolar infiltrates on imaging), and the biopsy can be useful to help determine the best treatment option and likely prognosis.

ILD occurs in 5% to 30% of patients with dermatomyositis or polymyositis. The ILD associated with dermatomyositis or polymyositis occurs more commonly in women. It is also associated with the anti-Jo-1 antibody, which is positive in approximately 50% of patients with dermatomyositis- or polymyositis-associated ILD.

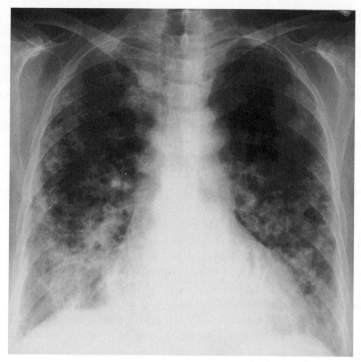

Image 32-7 • CXR of a patient with polymyositis and acute respiratory symptoms, demonstrating diffuse alveolar and interstitial opacities that are most prominent in the lower lobes. The patient's pathology is consistent with organizing pneumonia, which usually responds well to corticosteroid therapy. (*Reproduced with permission from Grippi MA, Elias JA, Fishman JA, et al: Fishman's Pulmonary Diseases and Disorders, 5th ed. New York, NY: McGraw Hill; 2015.*)

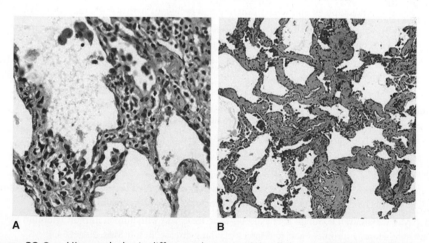

Image 32-8 • Histopathologic difference between (A) cellular and (B) fibrotic subtypes of nonspecific interstitial pneumonia. In A, the patient has lymphocytic infiltrate in the interstitial space expanding the interstitium, whereas in B, there is less cellular infiltrate and more hyaline deposition, leading to thickening of the interstitium. (*Reproduced with permission from Travis WD, Colby TV, Koss MN, et al: Atlas of Nontumor Pathology: Volume 2: Non-Neoplastic Disorders of the Lower Respiratory Tract, American Registry of Pathology; 2002.*)

References

Arakawa H, Yamada H, Kurihara Y, et al. Nonspecific interstitial pneumonia associated with polymyositis and dermatomyositis: serial high-resolution CT findings and functional correlation. Chest. 2003;123:1096.

Bradley B, Branley HM, Egan JJ, et al. Interstitial lung disease guideline: the British Thoracic Society in collaboration with the Thoracic Society of Australia and New Zealand and the Irish Thoracic Society. Thorax. 2008;63 Suppl 5:v1.

Brink DS. Pathology of restrictive lung diseases. In: Lechner AJ, Matuschak GM, Brink DS, eds. *Respiratory: An Integrated Approach to Disease.* McGraw-Hill; 2012. https://accessmedicine. mhmedical.com/content.aspx?bookid=1623&sectionid=105764671

Brulhart L, Waldburger JM, Gabay C. Rituximab in the treatment of antisynthetase syndrome. Ann Rheum Dis. 2006;65:974.

Chen Z, Wang X, Ye S. Tofacitinib in amyopathic dermatomyositis-associated interstitial lung disease. N Engl J Med. 2019;381:291.

Dalakas MC. Polymyositis, dermatomyositis, and inclusion body myositis. In: Kasper D, Fauci A, Hauser S, Longo D, Jameson J, Loscalzo J, eds. *Harrison's Principles of Internal Medicine.* 19th ed. McGraw-Hill; 2014. https://accessmedicine.mhmedical.com/content. aspx?bookid=1130&sectionid=79750722

Dalakas MC. Inflammatory muscle diseases. N Engl J Med. 2015;372:1734.

Dasa O, Ruzieh M, Oraibi O. Successful treatment of life-threatening interstitial lung disease secondary to antisynthetase syndrome using Rituximab: a case report and review of the literature. Am J Ther. 2016;23:e639.

Douglas WW, Tazelaar HD, Hartman TE, et al. Polymyositis-dermatomyositis-associated interstitial lung disease. Am J Respir Crit Care Med. 2001;164:1182.

Endo Y, Koga T, Suzuki T, et al. Successful treatment of plasma exchange for rapidly progressive interstitial lung disease with anti-MDA5 antibody-positive dermatomyositis: a case report. Medicine (Baltimore). 2018;97:e0436.

Fathi M, Vikgren J, Boijsen M, et al. Interstitial lung disease in polymyositis and dermatomyositis: longitudinal evaluation by pulmonary function and radiology. Arthritis Rheum. 2008;59:677.

Fischer A, Brown KK, Du Bois RM, et al. Mycophenolate mofetil improves lung function in connective tissue disease-associated interstitial lung disease. J Rheumatol. 2013;40:640.

Grippi MA, Senior RM, Callen JP. Approach to the patient with respiratory symptoms. In: Grippi MA, Elias JA, Fishman JA, et al, eds. *Fishman's Pulmonary Diseases and Disorders.* 5th ed. McGraw-Hill; 2015. https://accessmedicine.mhmedical.com/content.aspx?bookid=1344&sectionid=81186194

Gupta N, Matta EJ, Oldham SA. Cardiothoracic imaging. In: Elsayes KM, Oldham SA, eds. *Introduction to Diagnostic Radiology.* McGraw-Hill; 2014. https://accessmedicine.mhmedical.com/ content.aspx?bookid=1562&sectionid=95876454

Gutsche M, Rosen GD, Swigris JJ. Connective tissue disease-associated interstitial lung disease: a review. Curr Respir Care Rep. 2012;1:224.

Hayashi S, Tanaka M, Kobayashi H, et al. High-resolution computed tomography characterization of interstitial lung diseases in polymyositis/dermatomyositis. J Rheumatol. 2008;35:260.

Huapaya JA, Hallowell R, Silhan L, et al. Long-term treatment with human immunoglobulin for antisynthetase syndrome-associated interstitial lung disease. Respir Med. 2019;154:6.

Johnson C, Pinal-Fernandez I, Parikh R, et al. Assessment of mortality in autoimmune myositis with and without associated interstitial lung disease. Lung. 2016;194:733.

Kalluri M, Sahn SA, Oddis CV, et al. Clinical profile of anti-PL-12 autoantibody. Cohort study and review of the literature. Chest. 2009;135:1550.

Koreeda Y, Higashimoto I, Yamamoto M, et al. Clinical and pathological findings of interstitial lung disease patients with anti-aminoacyl-tRNA synthetase autoantibodies. Intern Med. 2010;49:361.

Mammen AL, Truong A, Christopher-Stine L. Dermatomyositis, polymyositis, and immune-mediated necrotizing myopathy. In: Imboden JB, Hellmann DB, Stone JH, eds. *Current Diagnosis and Treatment: Rheumatology*. 3rd ed. McGraw-Hill; 2013. https://accessmedicine.mhmedical. com/content.aspx?bookid=506&sectionid=42584912

Marie I, Hachulla E, Chérin P, et al. Interstitial lung disease in polymyositis and dermatomyositis. Arthritis Rheum. 2002;47:614.

Marie I, Josse S, Decaux O, et al. Comparison of long-term outcome between anti-Jo1- and anti-PL7/PL12 positive patients with antisynthetase syndrome. Autoimmun Rev. 2012;11:739.

Mukae H, Ishimoto H, Sakamoto N, et al. Clinical differences between interstitial lung disease associated with clinically amyopathic dermatomyositis and classic dermatomyositis. Chest. 2009;136:1341.

Nambu Y, Mouri M, Toga H, et al. Gender and underlying diseases affect the frequency of the concurrence of adult polymyositis/dermatomyositis and interstitial pneumonia. Chest. 1994;106:1931.

Sharma N, Putman MS, Vij R, et al. Myositis-associated interstitial lung disease: predictors of failure of conventional treatment and response to tacrolimus in a US Cohort. J Rheumatol. 2017;44:1612.

Sharp C, McCabe M, Dodds N, et al. Rituximab in autoimmune connective tissue disease-associated interstitial lung disease. Rheumatology (Oxford). 2016;55:1318.

Swigris JJ, Olson AL, Fischer A, et al. Mycophenolate mofetil is safe, well tolerated, and preserves lung function in patients with connective tissue disease-related interstitial lung disease. Chest. 2006;130:30.

Tillie-Leblond I, Wislez M, Valeyre D, et al. Interstitial lung disease and anti-Jo-1 antibodies: difference between acute and gradual onset. Thorax. 2008;63:53.

Tiniakou E, Mammen AL. Idiopathic inflammatory myopathies and malignancy: a comprehensive review. Clin Rev Allergy Immunol. 2017;52:20.

Tsuji H, Nakashima R, Hosono Y, et al. Multicenter prospective study of the efficacy and safety of combined immunosuppressive therapy with high-dose glucocorticoid, tacrolimus, and cyclophosphamide in interstitial lung diseases accompanied by anti-melanoma differentiation-associated gene 5-positive dermatomyositis. Arthritis Rheumatol. 2020;72:488.

Vandenbroucke E, Grutters JC, Altenburg J, et al. Rituximab in life threatening antisynthetase syndrome. Rheumatol Int. 2009;29:1499.

Vij R, Strek ME. Diagnosis and treatment of connective tissue disease-associated interstitial lung disease. Chest. 2013;143:814.

Wells AU, Flaherty KR, Brown KK, et al. Nintedanib in patients with progressive fibrosing interstitial lung diseases-subgroup analyses by interstitial lung disease diagnosis in the INBUILD trial: a randomised, double-blind, placebo-controlled, parallel-group trial. Lancet Respir Med. 2020;8:453.

Yamasaki Y, Yamada H, Yamasaki M, et al. Intravenous cyclophosphamide therapy for progressive interstitial pneumonia in patients with polymyositis/dermatomyositis. Rheumatology (Oxford). 2007;46:124.

Zou J, Li T, Huang X, et al. Basiliximab may improve the survival rate of rapidly progressive interstitial pneumonia in patients with clinically amyopathic dermatomyositis with anti-MDA5 antibody. Ann Rheum Dis. 2014;73:1591.

CASE 33

A 58-year-old White woman presents to the clinic for evaluation of dyspnea with exertion that has worsened over the last 12 months. She was previously running 3 miles three times a week but now feels like she can only run about ½ a mile at a time before becoming quite dyspneic. She did note some increased cough recently that is nonproductive. She denies any fevers, chills, sweats, hemoptysis, or pleuritic chest pain. She has not gained weight recently, and in fact, she believes she may have lost a few pounds. She worked until the age of 55 as a medical transcriptionist, at which point she retired. She denies any other environmental or occupational exposures. She lives in the midwest United States. Her vital signs are T 36.5°C, HR 63, BP 108/67, RR 13, oxygen saturation 95% on room air at rest. Her primary care physician ordered a set of PFTs as well as chest imaging. These are shown in Image 33-1.

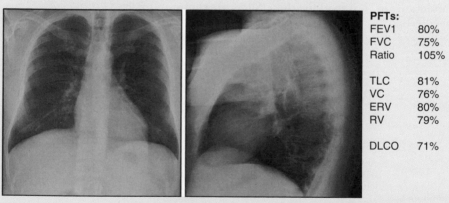

PFTs:

FEV1	80%
FVC	75%
Ratio	105%
TLC	81%
VC	76%
ERV	80%
RV	79%
DLCO	71%

Image 33-1 • Chest radiographs (PA and lateral) for the patient in **Question 33-1**.

QUESTIONS

Q33-1: What abnormalities are present in the patient's chest radiograph?

A. Hilar adenopathy
B. Diffuse parenchymal calcifications
C. Normal
D. Kerley B lines
E. Pulmonary artery enlargement

Q33-2: Which disease process would best fit the abnormalities on the PFT seen in Image 33-1?

A. Pulmonary arterial hypertension (PAH, World Health Organization [WHO] group I pulmonary hypertension)
B. Asthma
C. Chronic obstructive pulmonary disease (COPD)
D. Nonspecific interstitial pneumonia (NSIP)
E. Diffuse alveolar hemorrhage (DAH)
F. Morbid obesity
G. None; this represents normal PFT

Q33-3: Given the concern for possible interstitial lung disease (ILD), the patient undergoes a CT scan of the chest. Slices are shown in Image 33-2.

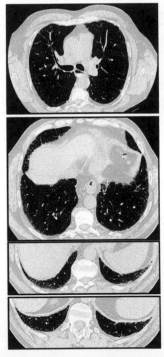

Image 33-2 • Chest CT images for the patient in **Question 33-3**.

What abnormalities are present in the CT scan?

A. Cystic lesions
B. Mosaic attenuation
C. Reticular interstitial opacities
D. Miliary nodular opacities
E. Pleural effusion

Q33-4: On examination, the patient has bibasilar crackles and a dry cough. The patient's husband has also noticed she has some skin changes, as shown in Image 33-3 below.

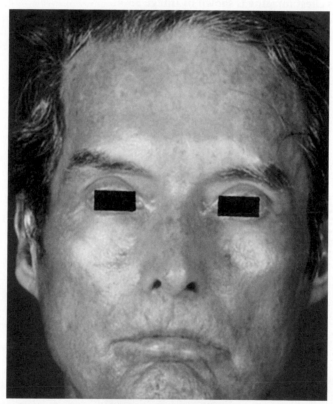

Image 33-3 • Dermatologic abnormalities representative of those found during examination of the patient in **Question 33-4**. (*Reproduced with permission from Jameson J, Fauci AS, Kasper DL, et al: Harrison's Principles of Internal Medicine, 20th ed. New York, NY: McGraw Hill; 2018.*)

Which test would you expect to be positive in this patient?

A. Anti-double-stranded DNA antibody (dsDNA)
B. Rheumatoid factor (Rf)
C. Anti-ribonucleoprotein (RNP) antibody
D. Anti-Jo1-antibody
E. Anti-Scl70 antibody

Q33-5: Aside from ILD, what is the other common pulmonary complication of scleroderma/systemic sclerosis (SSc)?

A. Airway hyperreactivity and obstructive lung disease
B. Cavitary lung lesions
C. PAH (WHO group I pulmonary hypertension)
D. Pleural effusions
E. Bronchiectasis

Q33-6: Another patient with scleroderma is referred for evaluation after frequent admissions over the last 2 years with reported "flares" of ILD. A portion of the patient's chest imaging is shown in Image 33-4.

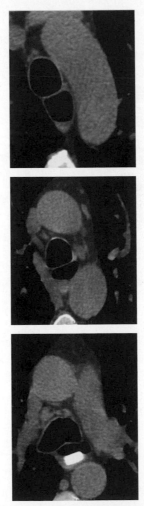

Image 33-4 • CT chest images (mediastinal windows) for the patient in **Question 33-4**.

What is the likely cause of the patient's recurrent admission to the hospital?

A. Pulmonary hypertension
B. Pericardial effusion
C. Pleural effusions
D. Aspiration pneumonia
E. Mucous impaction in the trachea
F. ILD

Q33-7: Match the following additional abnormalities associated with the limited form of scleroderma with Images 33-5 through 33-13.

A. Digital gangrene/necrosis
B. Calcinosis cutis
C. Sclerodactyly
D. Telangiectasia
E. Dyspigmentation
F. Acro-osteolysis
G. Esophageal dilatation
H. Raynaud phenomenon

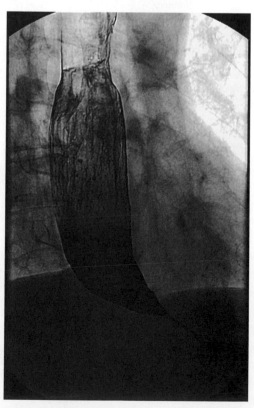

Image 33-5 • *(Reproduced with permission from Doherty GM: CURRENT Diagnosis & Treatment Surgery, 15th ed. New York, NY: McGraw Hill; 2020.)*

Q33-8.

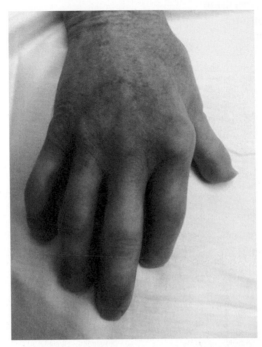

Image 33-6 • *(Reproduced with permission from Stone JH: Current Diagnosis & Treatment: Rheumatology, 4th ed. New York, NY: McGraw Hill; 2021.)*

Q33-9.

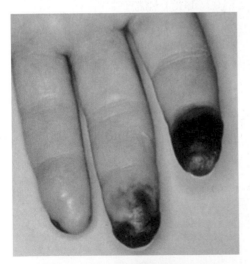

Image 33-7 • *(Reproduced with permission from Jameson J, Fauci AS, Kasper DL, et al: Harrison's Principles of Internal Medicine, 20th ed. New York, NY: McGraw Hill; 2018.)*

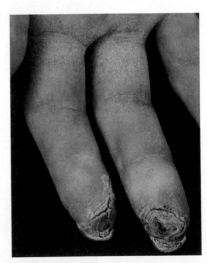

Image 33-8 • *(Reproduced with permission from Wolff K, Johnson RA, Saavedra AP, et al: Fitzpatrick's Color Atlas and Synopsis of Clinical Dermatology, 8th ed. New York, NY: McGraw Hill; 2017.)*

Q33-10.

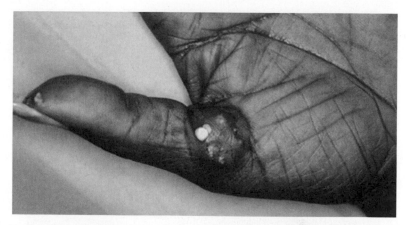

Image 33-9 • (*Reproduced with permission from Jameson J, Fauci AS, Kasper DL, et al: Harrison's Principles of Internal Medicine, 20th ed. New York, NY: McGraw Hill; 2018.*)

Q33-11.

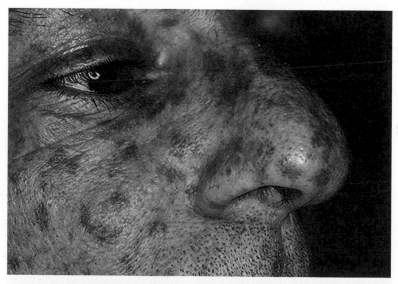

Image 33-10 • (*Reproduced with permission from Jameson J, Fauci AS, Kasper DL, et al: Harrison's Principles of Internal Medicine, 20th ed. New York, NY: McGraw Hill; 2018.*)

Q33-12.

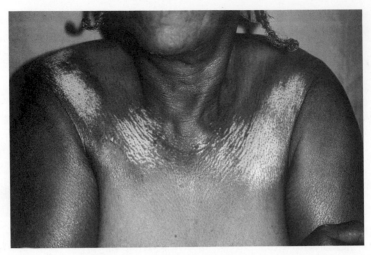

Image 33-11 • *(Reproduced with permission from Grippi MA, Elias JA, Fishman JA, et al: Fishman's Pulmonary Diseases and Disorders, 5th ed. New York, NY: McGraw Hill; 2015).*

Q33-13.

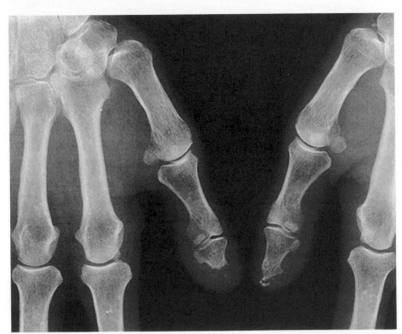

Image 33-12 • *(Reproduced with permission from Jameson J, Fauci AS, Kasper DL, et al: Harrison's Principles of Internal Medicine, 20th ed. New York, NY: McGraw Hill; 2018).*

Q33-14.

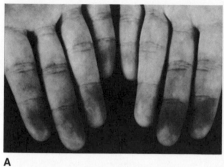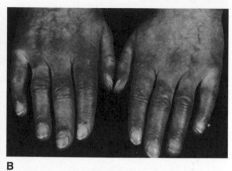

A   B

Image 33-13 • *(Reproduced with permission from Kang S, Amagai M, Bruckner AL, et al: Fitzpatrick's Dermatology, 9th ed. New York, NY: McGraw Hill; 2019.)*

Q33-15: What is the preferred primary treatment for patients with scleroderma-associated ILD?

A. Cyclophosphamide
B. Mycophenolate
C. Cyclosporine
D. Anti-TNF therapy
E. Plasmapheresis
F. Lung transplantation

ANSWERS

Q33-1: C
Normal

Rationale: This is a relatively normal chest radiograph. The mediastinal boards are crisp, the right and left heart borders are easily recognizable, and there is no enlargement of the cardiac silhouette. The pulmonary arteries are not enlarged. The pulmonary vessels are more visible in zones 2 and 3 of the lung than in zone 1 (upper), though they are still visible in the upper lung fields. There are no obvious Kerley B lines or calcifications.

Q33-2: D
Nonspecific interstitial pneumonia (NSIP)

Rationale: The PFT shows an abnormal FVC, with a normal ratio (FEV1/FVC) and a mildly reduced TLC, VC, RV, and DLCO, consistent with a restrictive lung process that is also associated with reduced oxygen-diffusing capacity. Although a concomitant obstructive lung disease cannot be completely ruled out without analyzing the flow-volume loop, one would primarily suspect that restrictive lung disease is present. PAH (WHO group I pulmonary hypertension) is associated with an isolated reduced DLCO without restriction (though pulmonary hypertension may also complicate restrictive lung disease, and this is termed *WHO group III disease*). Diffuse alveolar hemorrhage may occur in restrictive lung diseases as well, but it may be associated with an increase in the diffuse capacity of oxygen. As there is blood in the alveolar space, oxygen is more readily taken up by hemoglobin because there is no added barrier to diffusion through the basement membrane. Morbid obesity is also associated with restriction, though the ERV and RV are usually reduced out of proportion to the TLC and VC, and the DLCO should not (in theory) be reduced as severely as the lung volumes unless there is considerable atelectasis.

Q33-3: C
Reticular interstitial opacities

Rationale: There are no cystic lesions or nodular opacities present, and there is no pleural effusion visible. These subpleural reticulations are often an early sign of evolving ILD and typically cannot be visualized clearly on plain radiographs. This demonstrates the importance of high-resolution CT scanning in patients with potential ILD.

Q33-4: E
Anti-Scl70 antibody

Rationale: Image 33-3 shows skin thickening and tightening yielding an expressionless, mask-like facies (the latter is similar to that seen in Parkinson disease). The skin changes are more pronounced around the nose and mouth. This is consistent with systemic sclerosis, a form of scleroderma. The anti-Scl70 (topoisomerase) antibody is quite specific for ILD in patients with scleroderma. Although other antibodies (including those against ribonucleoprotein [RNP]) can be seen in patients with scleroderma and ILD, the diagnostic utility is unclear. Anti-dsDNA is specific for systemic lupus erythematosus (SLE), Rf for rheumatoid arthritis, anti-RNP for mixed connective tissue disease (a mixture of features between SLE, scleroderma, and polymyositis). Anti-centromere B antibodies are also positive in patients with scleroderma.

Q33-5: C
PAH (WHO group I pulmonary hypertension)

Rationale: PAH is a common complication of scleroderma. Although pulmonary hypertension may also develop as a complication of ILD in patients with scleroderma (classified as WHO group III pulmonary hypertension), patients may also develop "primary" pulmonary hypertension, termed *pulmonary arterial hypertension*, as a direct consequence of vascular remodeling of the pulmonary arterioles. Although ILD is more commonly seen in patients with systemic sclerosis, PAH is more commonly seen in patients with limited disease. The development of PAH is often associated with anti-ribonucleoprotein (RNP) antibodies, and it is also associated with a very poor prognosis when compared with patients with idiopathic PAH (see **Image 33-14**).

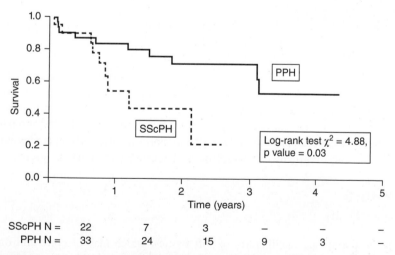

Image 33-14 • Kaplan-Meier survival estimates of patients with SScPH and PPH. (*Reproduced with permission from Kawut SM, Taichman DB, Archer-Chicko CL, Palevsky HI, Kimmel SE. Hemodynamics and survival in patients with pulmonary arterial hypertension related to systemic sclerosis, Chest 2003 Feb;123(2):344-350.*)

Q33-6: D
Aspiration pneumonia

Rationale: Recall that scleroderma is also associated with esophageal dysmotility and a patulous/dilated esophagus, a significant factor that prevents many patients with scleroderma from being eligible for lung transplantation because of the considerable risk for aspiration. This patient's CT demonstrates a large dilated/patulous esophagus.

Q33-7: G
Esophageal dilatation

Not to be confused with esophageal dilation (a procedure to dilate the esophagus), esophageal dilatation – or a patulous esophagus – is a frequent observation in patients with SSc. Patients with a patulous esophagus are at higher risk for microaspiration and gastroesophageal reflux disease.

Q33-8: C
Sclerodactyly

Sclerodactyly is the hardening of the skin in the hand and digits that cause retraction of the fingers toward the palm. This occurs in three phases: (1) the edematous phase; (2) the indurative phase; and (3) the atrophic phase. The edematous phase involves typical findings of edematous digits and mild arthralgias, and may last for a few months. This is followed by the indurative phase, in which the skin becomes thickened and may appear shiny. Patient's may note a loss of the skin folds in the digits and the palms. In limited cutaneous disease, this may persist for years. During the atrophic phase, the skin becomes more fragile (end-stages of disease).

Q33-9: A
Digital gangrene/necrosis

Digital gangrene and necrosis (as a complication of Raynaud phenomenon). Raynaud's phenomenon consists of periodic episodes of vascular constriction in the hands, most commonly limited to the distal tips of the digits, but may extend to the hand and wrist in some cases. The hand may appear cyanotic, be cool to the touch, and patients may experience pain or paresthesia during these episodes. Repeated episodes over the course of life may eventually lead to episodes of necrosis and digital gangrene.

Q33-10: B
Calcinosis cutis

This is the pathologic calcification of soft tissues, which may ulcerate and drain a chalky white substance. Superinfection of ulcerated lesions is common.

Q33-11: D
Telangiectasia

These are dilated blood vessels that are often present in an acral distribution (ie, face, hands, feet, forearms), but may also involve the truncal areas.

Q33-12: E
Dyspigmentation

Dyspigmentation of the skin may also be seen in both the limited and diffuse cutaneous forms of SSc.

Q33-13: F
Acro-osteolysis

Acro-osteolysis (due to digital ischemia in Raynaud phenomenon). This is the result of a resportive process in the distal tips of the digits, in which the terminal tuft of the digit is most commonly affected.

Q33-14: H
Raynaud phenomenon

Skin and digital vascular abnormalities are very common in SSc, and it is imperative to understand the scope of abnormalities that may raise clinical suspicion for SSc. The CREST syndrome (calcinosis, Raynaud's syndrome, esophageal dysmotility, sclerodactyly, and telangiectasia syndrome) is also referred to as limited cutaneous scleroderma (of limited cutaneous SSc). The skin involvement in the disease is primarily in acral areas (ie, face, hands, feet). These patient's may also have typical nailfold capillary changes. While these patient rarely develop renal disease, these patients may develop pulmonary hypertension or interstitial lung disease late in the disease course. Patients with diffuse cutaneous scleroderma (or diffuse cutaneous SSc) may have more widespread skin involvement including the truncal areas, and often have much early evidence of systemic disease including the pulmonary gastrointestinal, and renal systems.

Q33-15: B
Mycophenolate

Rationale: Although corticosteroids and cyclophosphamide had been the primary means of treatment for patients with SSc-associated ILD, recent evidence suggests that mycophenolate is equally as effective and associated with fewer complications or adverse events, and it is now the mainstay of treatment. Additional research is underway regarding the use of monoclonal therapies targeting IL-6 (ie, tocilizumab). Lung transplantation may be considered in patients with progressive ILD or PAH associated with scleroderma, though issues related to esophageal dysmotility and aspiration often prevent this. Cyclophosphamide and azathioprine remain alternative options to mycophenolate.

For patients with progressive disease despite these therapies, there are additional options. Nintedanib, a promiscuous tyrosine kinase inhibitor initially approved for the treatment of idiopathic pulmonary fibrosis (IPF), has been approved for use in patients with SSc-ILD. Date demonstrated that nintedanib helps to slow the progression of disease in patients failing monotherapy with mycophenolate or cyclophosphamide. Rituximab is another agent that may be added to standard maintenance therapy for patients with progressive disease, although this has not received FDA approval at the time this case was created.

References

Cosgrove GP, Schwarz MI. Pulmonary manifestations of the collagen vascular diseases. In: Grippi MA, Elias JA, Fishman JA, et al, eds. *Fishman's Pulmonary Diseases and Disorders.* 5th ed. McGraw-Hill; 2015. https://accessmedicine.mhmedical.com/content.aspx?bookid=1344&sectionid=81191284

Grippi MA, Senior RM, Callen JP. Approach to the patient with respiratory symptoms. In: Grippi MA, Elias JA, Fishman JA, et al, eds. *Fishman's Pulmonary Diseases and Disorders.* 5th ed. McGraw-Hill; 2015. https://accessmedicine.mhmedical.com/content.aspx?bookid=1344&sectionid=81186194

Jameson J, Fauci AS, Kasper DL, Hauser SL, Longo DL, Loscalzo J. *Harrison's Principles of Internal Medicine.* 20th ed. McGraw-Hill; 2018. https://accessmedicine.mhmedical.com/content.aspx?bookid=2129&sectionid=159213747

Kawut SM, Taichman DB, Archer-Chicko CL, et al. Hemodynamics and survival in patients with pulmonary arterial hypertension related to systemic sclerosis. Chest. 2003;123:344.

Moinzadeh P, Denton CP, Black CM, Krieg T Systemic sclerosis. In: Kang S, Amagai M, Bruckner AL, eds. *Fitzpatrick's Dermatology.* 9th ed. McGraw-Hill; 2019. https://accessmedicine.mhmedical.com/content.aspx?bookid=2570&sectionid=210426516

Schlottmann F, Patti MG. Esophagus and diaphragm. In: Doherty GM, ed. *Current Diagnosis and Treatment: Surgery.* 15th ed. McGraw-Hill. https://accessmedicine.mhmedical.com/content.aspx?bookid=2859&sectionid=242157241

The skin in immune, autoimmune, autoinflammatory, and rheumatic disorders. In: Wolff K, Johnson R, Saavedra AP, Roh EK, eds. *Fitzpatrick's Color Atlas and Synopsis of Clinical Dermatology.* 8th ed. McGraw-Hill; 2017. https://accessmedicine.mhmedical.com/content.aspx?bookid=2043&sectionid=154898980

Yazdany J, Manno R, Hellmann DB, Imboden JB Jr. Scleroderma (systemic sclerosis). In: Papadakis MA, McPhee SJ, Rabow MW, eds. *Current Medical Diagnosis & Treatment 2021.* McGraw-Hill; 2021. https://accessmedicine.mhmedical.com/content.aspx?bookid=2957&sectionid=249383286

CASE 34

A 55-year-old man presents for evaluation of persistent dyspnea and cough. He has been experiencing a progressive worsening of shortness of breath over the last 12 months, if not longer. The cough is nonproductive, and he denies hemoptysis. He initially had symptoms only with heavy exertion but is now short of breath with minimal exertion. He has a history of hypertension and hypercholesterolemia, and he takes amlodipine and simvastatin. He has never smoked or used illicit drugs. He drinks two to three alcoholic beverages a week. He worked as a lawyer until recently, when he retired because of his health concerns. His primary care physician ordered a chest radiograph, which he was told was "normal." He has lost about 2 to 3 lb over the last 2 months. He denies any fevers, chills, sweats, or abdominal pain. His vital signs are T 36.5°C, HR 81, BP 151/67, RR 12, oxygen saturation 95% on room air. He has some joints that bother him, but he claims this has been a chronic issue. The chest imaging is shown in Images 34-1 and 34-2.

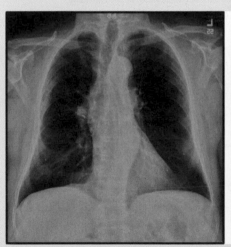 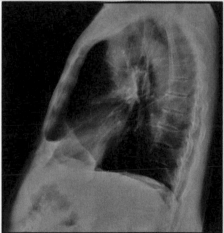

Image 34-1 • Chest radiograph for the patient in **Question 34-1**.

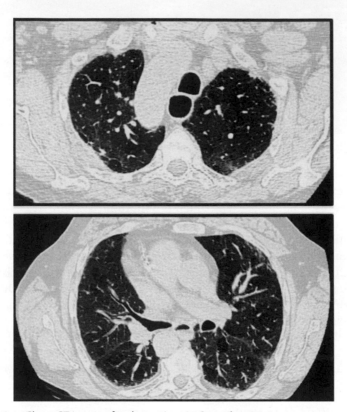

Image 34-2 • Chest CT images for the patient in **Question 34-1**.

QUESTIONS

Q34-1: Which is the best description of the abnormalities demonstrated in the patient's chest imaging?

A. Reticulonodular interstitial opacities with honeycombing and traction bronchiectasis
B. Cylindrical bronchiectasis and tree-in-bud opacities
C. Hyperinflation with a mosaic pattern of attenuation and ground-glass opacities
D. Miliary pattern of micronodular interstitial opacities
E. Cystic lung lesions with air-fluid levels

Q34-2: On examination, the patient has diminished breath sounds throughout, with an intermittent inspiratory wheeze. His PFT and flow-volume loop is shown in Image 34-3 below.

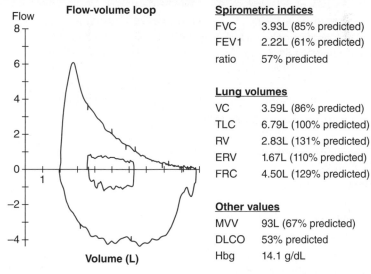

Flow-volume loop

Spirometric indices	
FVC	3.93L (85% predicted)
FEV1	2.22L (61% predicted)
ratio	57% predicted

Lung volumes	
VC	3.59L (86% predicted)
TLC	6.79L (100% predicted)
RV	2.83L (131% predicted)
ERV	1.67L (110% predicted)
FRC	4.50L (129% predicted)

Other values	
MVV	93L (67% predicted)
DLCO	53% predicted
Hbg	14.1 g/dL

Image 34-3 • Pulmonary function testing results for the patient in **Question 34-2**.

What is the primary abnormality of the patient's PFT?

A. Pulmonary vascular disease
B. Extrapulmonary restrictive disease
C. Restrictive lung disease
D. Obstructive lung disease

Q34-3: The patient has the following abnormalities on his musculoskeletal examination (Images 34-4 and 34-5).

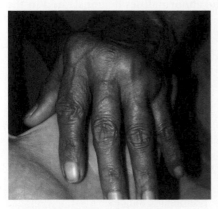

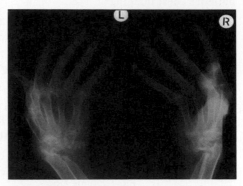

Image 34-4 • Musculoskeletal abnormalities identified on exam for the patient in **Question 34-3.** (*Used with permission from Richard P. Usatine, MD.*)

Image 34-5 • Hand radiographs for the patient in **Question 34-3.** (*Reproduced with permission from Mitra R: Principles of Rehabilitation Medicine. New York, NY: McGraw Hill; 2019.*)

What laboratory test would you send to aid in confirming the patient's diagnosis?

A. Erythrocyte sedimentation rate (ESR)
B. C-reactive protein (CRP)
C. Anti-double-stranded DNA (dsDNA) antibody
D. Ant-Jo1 antibody
E. Rheumatoid factor (Rf)

Q34-4: What is the likely diagnosis of the patient's lung disease?

A. Usual interstitial pneumonia (UIP)
B. Nonspecific interstitial pneumonia (NSIP)
C. Cryptogenic organizing pneumonia (COP)
D. Obliterative bronchiolitis
E. Follicular bronchiolitis
F. Lymphocytic interstitial pneumonia (LIP)
G. Necrotic lung nodules

Q34-5: A 62-year old-woman with RA presents with progressively worsening dyspnea over the course of 3 weeks as well as a cough and some low-grade fevers. She was started on methotrexate approximately 8 months ago. She takes a daily folic acid supplement as well. She has had no recent sick contacts. She recently started smoking cigarettes again after having quit for approximately 10 years. She has mild COPD, which has been well controlled on tiotropium bromide and budesonide/formoterol with just PRN albuterol. She is admitted to the hospital and ends up in the ICU on high-flow supplemental oxygen. A BAL shows lymphocytosis, and the cultures are negative. CT of her chest is shown in Image 34-6.

What is the predominant finding on her chest imaging (Image 34-6)?

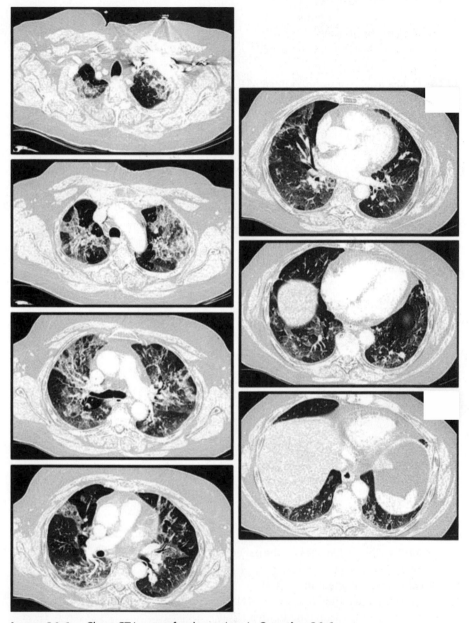

Image 34-6 • Chest CT images for the patient in **Question 34-6**.

A. Scattered areas of ground-glass opacities
B. Focal consolidation with air bronchograms
C. Honeycombing and traction bronchiectasis
D. Pleural effusions
E. Bronchiectasis with tree-in-bud opacities

Q34-6: What is the most likely diagnosis?

A. RA-interstitial lung disease (ILD)
B. Methotrexate pneumonitis
C. Pulmonary embolism
D. Community-acquired pneumonia

Q34-7: The most common pattern of RA-ILD seen on high-resolution CT of the chest is shown in Image 34-7. What pattern is this?

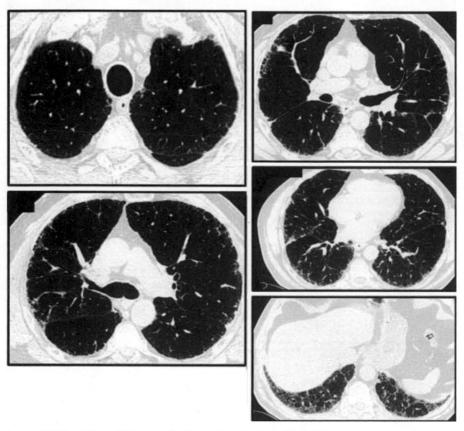

Image 34-7 • Chest CT images for the patient in **Question 34-7**.

A. Usual interstitial pneumonia (UIP)
B. Nonspecific interstitial pneumonia (NSIP)
C. Cryptogenic organizing pneumonia (COP)
D. Obliterative bronchiolitis
E. Follicular bronchiolitis
F. Lymphocytic interstitial pneumonia (LIP)

Q34-8: A 57-year-old man with RA is referred to a pulmonologist for the abnormal imaging shown in Image 34-8.

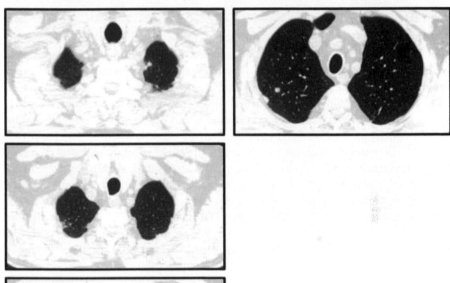

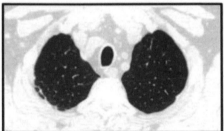

Image 34-8 • Chest CT images for the patient in **Question 34-8**.

He was diagnosed with RA over 20 years ago. He has been managed with methotrexate for the last 3 years (he previously refused treatment). He has typical findings of RA, including ulnar deviation in his hands and subcutaneous nodules. He has no history of tuberculosis or any risk factors for the disease. He is a never smoker. From a respiratory standpoint, he is completely asymptomatic. What is the most likely diagnosis?

A. Malignancy
B. Rheumatoid nodule
C. Tuberculosis
D. Septic emboli
E. Pulmonary abscess

ANSWERS

Q34-1: C
Hyperinflation with a mosaic pattern of attenuation and ground glass-opacities

Rationale: The chest radiograph demonstrates no obvious parenchymal abnormalities, but there is some evidence of hyperinflation with flattening of the diaphragms (at least the portions that can be seen). The CT scan shows a mixed pattern of attenuation, with some areas of higher attenuation (ground-glass opacities) mixed with those of low attenuation areas. This mixed pattern of attenuation is termed *mosaic*. It is a nonspecific finding that can be associated with a number of diseases, including hypersensitivity pneumonitis (HP) and other airway-centric diseases. The important issue is to determine which area is abnormal (the low- or high-attenuation areas). During expiration, the lung parenchyma volume is reduced, and the appearance of normal lung tissue has a higher attenuation than during full inspiration, and this higher attenuation may look like ground glass. In these cases, the areas of lung with lower attenuation may in fact be the abnormal portion, such as in airway diseases like COPD. Although most radiology studies are performed in full inspiration with a breath hold, specific studies may be performed in expiration as well. The above CT scan is an expiratory film. This can be determined by examining the shape of the trachea, although it is difficult from this two-image view to determine this here. During expiration, the posterior wall of the trachea will be displaced anteriorly, in contrast to inhalation when the trachea is filled with air the posterior wall may be flat or displaced posteriorly.

Q34-2: D
Obstructive lung disease

Rationale: First, the flow-volume loop demonstrated a concave pattern, with worsening expiratory airflow at lower lung volumes. Additionally, the spirometric indices show obstruction, with a FEV1/FVC ratio of 57% predicted. The lung volumes demonstrate a pattern consistent with hyperinflation, in which the precent-predicted value of the RV (residual volume, 131% predicted here) is greater than the TLC (total lung capacity, 100% predicted here), with the vital capacity (VC < 86% predicted), less than both the above. Also note that the patient's FRC is 129% predicted, indicating that the patients tidal breathing occurs at higher lung volumes, also indicating air trapping is present. This is consistent with obstructive lung disease. The TLC is normal, so there is no restrictive lung disease present. The MVV is reduced at 67%. However, this reduction in the MVV is appropriate for the degree of the patient's obstructive lung disease. One would expect an MVV in the range of 66-73L given the patient's FEV1 of 2.22L (assuming 30-33 breaths per minute during the MVV maneuver). Therefore, the MVV is appropriate for this patient and does not suggest neuromuscular disease. The DLCO is substantially reduced despite a normal hemoglobin, so this is not due to anemia. This pattern of abnormalities is most consistent with obstructive lung disease as the underlying cause. Pulmonary vascular disease, in isolation, should present with an isolated reduction in the DLCO.

Q34-3: E
Rheumatoid factor (Rf)

Rationale: This patient's musculoskeletal examination demonstrates class changes seen in rheumatoid arthritis (RA), with ulnar deviation at the metacarpophalangeal joint. Therefore, a rheumatoid factor (Rf) or an anticyclic citrullinated peptide (CCP) antibody study would be most appropriate. The ESR and CRP will often be positive in patients with active musculoskeletal disease, but these are nonspecific. The ds-DNA is specific for systemic lupus erythematosus (SLE), while the anti-Jo1 is more specific for polymyositis.

Q34-4: D
Obliterative bronchiolitis (bronchiolitis obliterans)

Rationale: Importantly, all the entities listed may be seen as pulmonary complications in patients with RA. UIP, NSIP, COP, and LIP are parenchymal lung diseases. Obliterative and follicular bronchiolitis are airway-centric diseases associated with obstruction on PFT. Obliterative bronchiolitis is a disease associated with the small airways (bronchioles) and is marked by significant expiratory airflow obstruction, wheezing, dyspnea, fatigue, and dry cough. It is a complication of bone marrow transplantation as well as a form of chronic rejection in lung transplantation; however, it may also occur as a result of toxic inhalational exposures and connective tissue disorders. Chest radiograph findings generally show a mosaic pattern of attenuation that is termed a *perfusion pattern*, in which the vessels in the hypoattenuated areas of lung are smaller in size than in the surrounding regions. Patients may also have evidence of central bronchiectasis. Follicular bronchiolitis, another complication of RA, is marked by bronchial wall thickening and bronchiectasis as well as a centrilobular distribution of lung nodules (see **Image 34-9** below) or interstitial opacities. The pathology of follicular (or respiratory) bronchiolitis demonstrates dense lymphocyte and plasma cell infiltrates around the small airways.

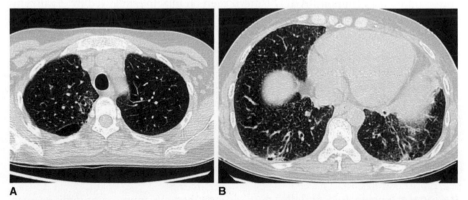

Image 34-9 • Follicular bronchiolitis. (*Reproduced with permission from Lu J, Ma M, Zhao Q, et al: The Clinical Characteristics and Outcomes of Follicular Bronchiolitis in Chinese Adult Patients, Sci Rep 2018 May 8;8(1):7300.*)

Q34-5: A
Scattered areas of ground-glass opacities

Rationale: The CT scan of the patient's chest shows patchy areas of ground-glass opacities. There are no focal consolidations, nor is there any evidence of honeycombing. There are no pleural effusions or overt bronchiectasis present

Q34-6: B
Methotrexate pneumonitis

Rationale: Although methotrexate pneumonitis generally occurs within the first year of therapy and higher doses may be associated with increased risk (though data on this are variable), it may occur at any point in time while on therapy. This patient started methotrexate 8 months before presentation, which is within the typical timeframe. Methotrexate pneumonitis occurs in up to 11% of patients treated with the drug. Risk factors for the development of pneumonitis include age older than 60, chronic kidney disease, preexisting lung disease, male sex, and diabetes. The pneumonitis generally presents in an acute to subacute fashion with fevers, shortness of breath, cough, and infiltrates on imaging. Bronchoalveolar lavage is often done to evaluate for infection. It may reveal lymphocytosis. Treatment for methotrexate pneumonitis includes stopping the methotrexate. In more severe cases, patients may need to be treated with corticosteroids. Restarting methotrexate after recovery is not recommended because pneumonitis recurs in approximately 25% of cases.

Q34-7: A
Usual interstitial pneumonia (UIP)

Rationale: UIP is the most common pattern of RA-ILD seen on high-resolution CT, occurring in 40% to 60% of cases. UIP on imaging is characterized by subpleural reticular abnormalities with honeycombing and traction bronchiectasis. NSIP is the second most common RA-ILD pattern seen on imaging, followed by organizing pneumonia. Pulmonary nodules ("rheumatoid" nodules) is another potential presentation, and these may be cavitary or solid.

ILD is quite prevalent in patients with RA. It presents with shortness of breath and cough. It is more common in men, patients with high rheumatoid factor levels, older patients, smokers, and in patients with later-onset disease. Subclinical ILD is suspected in about 30% of patients with RA.

Q34-8: B
Rheumatoid nodule

Rationale: Rheumatoid nodules are rare, but they are more commonly seen in patients with longstanding disease, smokers, men, patients with high rheumatoid factors, patients with subcutaneous nodules, and in patients with active joint disease. A patient may have a single nodule or several nodules noted on imaging. These nodules have a predilection for the upper or mid lung zones. Rheumatoid nodules range from a few millimeters in size to several centimeters. They may cavitate or rupture, resulting in pulmonary abscess formation, pleural effusion, or a pneumothorax. Generally, however, rheumatoid nodules are asymptomatic. Although they may spontaneously regress or at least improve with RA therapies, rheumatoid nodules may also enlarge with treatment of the disease, especially if the treatment is with methotrexate.

It is important, particularly in patients with a smoking history, to thoroughly evaluate for malignancy before attributing a pulmonary nodule to a manifestation of RA. Rheumatoid nodules generally have little to no uptake on PET scans.

References

Al Nokhatha SA, Harrington R, Conway R. Methotrexate and the lung in rheumatoid arthritis. EMJ Rheumatol. 2020;7:80.

Cosgrove GP, Schwarz MI. Pulmonary manifestations of the collagen vascular diseases. In: Grippi MA, Elias JA, Fishman JA, et al, eds. *Fishman's Pulmonary Diseases and Disorders.* 5th ed. McGraw-Hill; 2015. https://accessmedicine.mhmedical.com/content.aspx?bookid=1344&sectionid=81191284

Hansell DM, Bankier AA, MacMahon H, McLoud TC, Muller NL, Remy J. Fleischner Society: glossary of terms for thoracic imaging. Radiology. 2008;246:697.

Kim EJ, Collard HR, King TE Jr. Rheumatoid arthritis-associated interstitial lung disease: the relevance of histopathologic and radiographic patterns. Chest. 2009;136:1397.

Lu J, Ma M, Zhao Q, et al. The clinical characteristics and outcomes of follicular bronchiolitis in Chinese adult patients. Scientific Reports. 2018;8:1.

Pellegrino R, Viegi G, Brusasco V, et al. Interpretative strategies for lung function tests. Eur Respir J. 2005;26:948.

Shaw M, Collins BF, Ho LA, Raghu G. Rheumatoid arthritis-associated lung disease. Eur Respir Rev. 2015;24:1.

Webb WR. Thin-section CT of the secondary pulmonary lobule; anatomy and the image — the 2004 Fleischner lecture. Radiology. 2006;239:322.

Yazdany J, Manno R, Hellmann DB, Imboden JB Jr. Rheumatoid arthritis. In: Papadakis MA, McPhee SJ, Rabow MW, eds. *Current Medical Diagnosis & Treatment 2021.* McGraw-Hill; 2021. https://accessmedicine.mhmedical.com/content.aspx?bookid=2957&sectionid=249383117

CASE 35

A 23-year-old White man presents for evaluation for recurrent episodes of bronchitis. He reports that the issues began approximately 4 years ago and he has subsequently experienced three to four episodes a year of bronchitis, requiring antibiotics. He states that has no other known medical issues but he experienced respiratory infections more frequently than his brother throughout childhood. He also has experienced moderate worsening dyspnea on exertion over the last 2 years. He has no occupational exposures and is currently in graduate school. He has a 4- to 5-year history of smoking. On examination, the patient has some mild expiratory wheezes and crackles at the bases. He has a resting O_2 saturation of 99% and an O_2 saturation of 94% with moderate activity. He has some mild clubbing. There is no cyanosis. He has a BMI of 21 kg/m². He was recently seen by a physician at his school's health clinic and was referred to you. His current CXR is shown in Image 35-1 below.

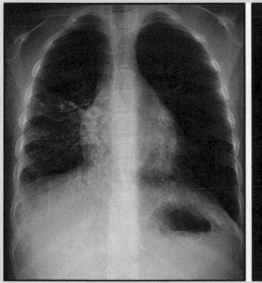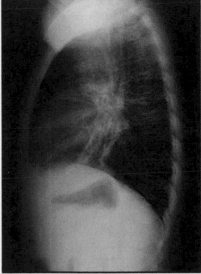

Image 35-1 • Chest radiographs (PA and lateral) for the patient in **Question 35-1**.

QUESTIONS

Q35-1: Which abnormality is seen on the chest film?

A. Bronchial wall thickening
B. Bilateral pleural effusions
C. Hyperinflation
D. Cavitary lung lesions

Q35-2: The patient undergoes a CT scan (Image 35-2), which demonstrates the following:

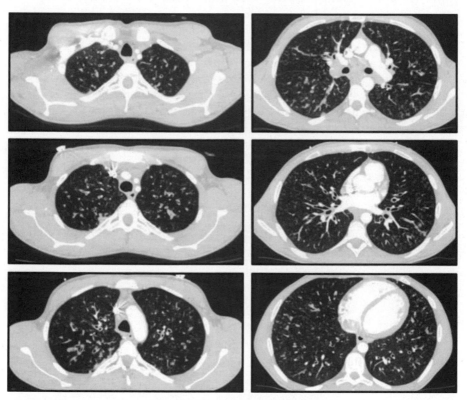

Image 35-2 • Chest CT images for the patient in **Question 35-2**.

Which abnormalities are seen in the CT scan images?

A. Tree-in-bud opacities
B. Cystic bronchiectasis
C. Bronchial wall thickening
D. All of the above
E. None of the above

Q35-3: The patient's spirometry is shown in Image 35-3 below.

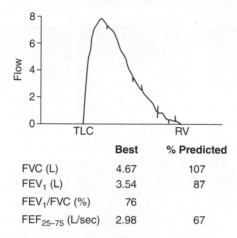

	Best	% Predicted
FVC (L)	4.67	107
FEV$_1$ (L)	3.54	87
FEV$_1$/FVC (%)	76	
FEF$_{25-75}$ (L/sec)	2.98	67

Image 35-3 • Expiratory flow loop and spirometric indices for the patient in Question 35-3. (*Reproduced with permission from Lechner AJ, Matuschak GM, Brink DS: Respiratory: An Integrated Approach to Disease. New York, NY: McGraw Hill; 2012.*)

Which abnormality is demonstrated above?

A. Reduced diffusing capacity of oxygen
B. Hyperinflation
C. Restrictive lung disease
D. Variable intrathoracic obstruction
E. Small airways disease

Q35-4: Given the patient's history and clinical findings, which test would be the most appropriate study to diagnose the patient's condition?

A. Transbronchial lung biopsy
B. Open (surgical) lung biopsy
C. Echocardiogram
D. Alpha-1-antitrypsin enzyme level (A1AT)
E. Antinuclear antibody (ANA) titer
F. Sweat chloride test (pilocarpine iontophoresis)
G. Cystic fibrosis transmembrane receptor (CFTR) mutation test
H. Sputum cultures

Q35-5: What is the most common CFTR mutation seen in patients in the United States?

A. G551D
B. G542X
C. F508del
D. W1282X
E. I507del

Q35-6: Match the following radiographs from patients with CF shown in Images 35-4 to 35-6 to the corresponding abnormality.

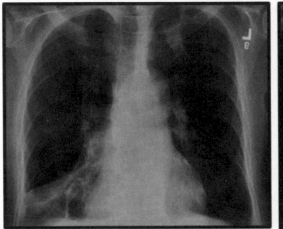
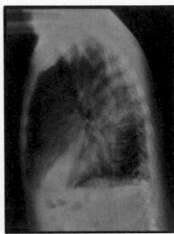

Image 35-4 •

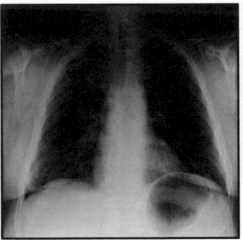
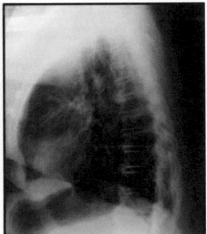

Image 35-5 •

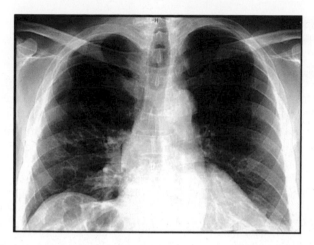

Image 35-6 •

A. Infiltrate
B. Pneumothorax
C. Blebs
D. Atelectasis

Q35-7: Which CFTR modulator is approved for use in patients with CF in the United States?

A. Ivacaftor
B. Dornase alfa
C. Pancrelipase
D. Azithromycin
E. Tobramycin
F. A and B
G. A, C, and E
H. A, D, and E
I. B and C

ANSWERS

Q35-1: A
Bronchial wall thickening

Rationale: The chest radiograph shows bronchial wall thickening bilaterally, with a slight prominence of the pulmonary vasculature and likely some cystic changes in the middle lung fields, more notable on the right than the left. The bronchial wall thickening with a patent central airway produces the "tram-track" appearance classically seen in bronchiectasis.

Q35-2: D
All of the above

Rationale: There are clear areas of bronchial wall thickening as well as bronchiectasis and tree-in-bud opacities. As a general rule, the bronchioles should have a diameter similar to their accompanying pulmonary arteriole. Bronchiectasis can produce a "signet-ring" sign, in which the smaller pulmonary artery/arteriole sitting adjacent to a much larger airway has an appearance of a gemstone on a ring (example shown in **Image 35-7** in white circle).

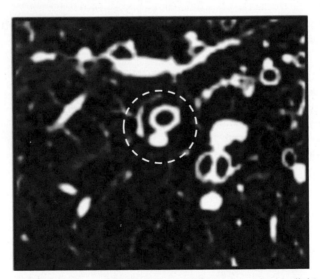

Image 35-7 • Example of signet ring sign associated with bronchial wall thickening and bronchiectasis.

Q35-3: E
Small airways disease

Rationale: Importantly, this shows only spirometry, so there is no formal testing of lung volumes or diffusing capacity here. Therefore, it would be difficult to diagnosis hyperinflation, restrictive lung disease, or reduced diffusing capacity of oxygen (carbon monoxide as a surrogate); however, the FVC is normal, suggesting no significant restriction is present. There is no evidence of variable intrathoracic obstruction (which could be seen in the expiratory portion of a flow loop). And while the patient's FVC and FEV1 are normal and the FEV1/FVC ratio is greater than 70%, the FEF25-75 is abnormal at 67%, and the flow loop shows that there is worsening obstruction at lower lung volumes (ie, the curve is more concave as you approach residual volume). This is commonly the first abnormality seen in patients with evolving obstructive lung diseases.

Note: To determine if obstructive lung disease is present, one should preferably use the lower limits of normal (LLN) if available, which represents the 95% confidence interval for healthy nonsmokers of a similar age.

Q35-4: F
Sweat chloride test

Rationale: The patient presents with progressively worsening dyspnea and recurrent infections, with a prominent CT finding of bronchiectasis. The patient has no known pancreatic insufficiency or liver disease, but cystic fibrosis (CF) must be ruled out as the cause of the patient's bronchiectasis before exploring non–CF-related causes of bronchiectasis. Although more than 90% of patients with CF are diagnosed before the age of 18, one must be aware of atypical presentations in adulthood. The appropriate test is the sweat chloride test because it is independent of the mutation present. Current CFTR mutation tests are limited to common or known mutations at the time the test was developed and often do not include rare mutations. Although next-generation sequencing techniques may eventually impact this, current testing for CFTR mutations alone risks a false negative. Lung biopsy is not necessary at this point. An echocardiogram may demonstrate early evidence of pulmonary hypertension. A1AT is a good thought that this point, but it is more commonly associated with panlobular emphysema in addition to bronchiectasis. Similarly, while connective tissue disorders and other autoimmune disorders are associated with bronchiectasis, an ANA would not be necessary until CF was ruled out. Sputum cultures will be helpful but would not confirm a diagnosis.

CF is an autosomal recessive disease with the highest incidence in White people at 1 in 3000. CF results from a mutation in the CF transmembrane conductance regulator (*CFTR*) gene. Currently, there are more than 2000 different mutations known to cause CF, with F508del (a three-base deletion that results in the deletion of a phenylalanine) being the most common mutation.

Typically, the diagnosis of CF is made in a patient with a history and symptoms consistent with CF by performing a sweat chloride test. If the sweat chloride test is positive, a CF mutation analysis may be pursued, though a negative analysis does not rule out cystic fibrosis.

Q35-5: C
Delta F508

Rationale: The most common mutation in CF is the delta F508 mutation. Currently, there are more than 2000 different mutations known to cause cystic fibrosis.

There are six classes of CFTR mutations:

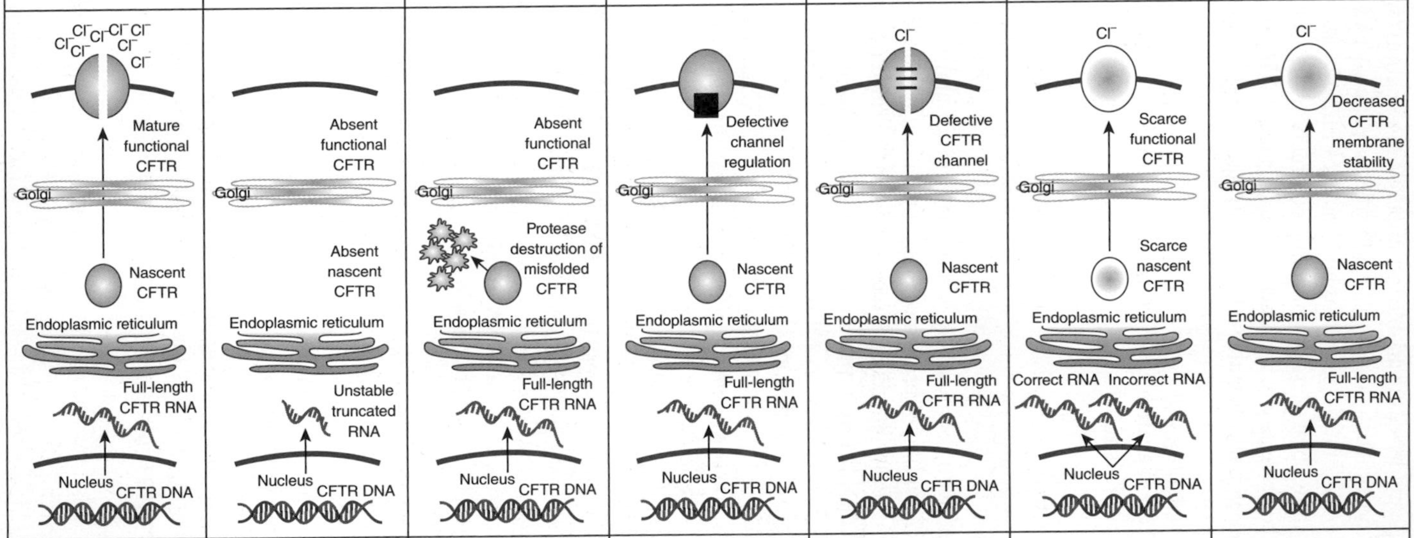

	Normal	I	II	III	IV	V	VI
CFTR defect		No functional CFTR protein	CFTR trafficking defect	Defective channel regulation	Decreased channel conductance	Reduced synthesis of CFTR	Decreased CFTR stability
Type of mutations		Nonsense; frameshift; canonical splice	Missense; aminoacid deletion	Missense; aminoacid change	Missense; aminoacid change	Splicing defect; missense	Missense; aminoacid change
Specific mutation examples		Gly542X Trp1282X Arg553X 621+1G→T	Phe508del Asn1303Lys Ile507del Arg560Thr	Gly551Asp Gly178Arg Gly551Ser Ser549Asn	Arg117His Arg347Pro Arg117Cys Arg334Trp	3849+10kbC→T 2789+5G→A 3120+1G→A 5T	4326delTC Gln1412X 4279insA

Image 35-8 • Classifications of CFTR mutations. (Reproduced with permission from Boyle MP, De Boeck K. A new era in the treatment of cystic fibrosis: correction of the underlying CFTR defect, Lancet Respir Med 2013 Apr;1(2):158-163.)

Q35-6: Image 35-6 – D
Atelectasis

Rationale: These images show right middle lobe atelectasis. On the PA image, there is an opacification in the right lung. The lateral image shows a wedge-shaped or triangular opacification overlying the cardiac shadow, consistent with right middle lobe atelectasis.

Q35-6: Image 35-7 – A
Infiltrate

Rationale: There is a hazy opacification in the right lower lobe.

Q35-6: Image 35-8 – B
Pneumothorax

Rationale: There is a clear loss of lung markings on the right along the lateral chest wall, consistent with a pneumothorax.

Outside of classic bacterial infection, there is a multitude of potential pulmonary complications that may arise in patients with CF, including atelectasis, hemoptysis, pneumothoraces, ABPA/fungal infection, mycobacterial infection, and both hypoxemic and hypercarbic respiratory failure.

Nonpulmonary complications include, but are not limited to, intestinal obstruction (meconium ileus in infants, distal intestinal obstruction syndrome [DIOS] in children and adults), liver disease, immotile sperm/infertility, and depression and anxiety.

Q35-7: A
Ivacaftor

Rationale: Ivacaftor (VX-770; Kalydeco) was the first CFTR modulator approved for use in the United States. Although the other medications listed are commonly used in the treatment of CF, none are CFTR modulators. Currently, four drugs targeting the mutated *CFTR* gene are FDA approved in the United States. Ivacaftor was the first drug approved in the United States. Ivacaftor is a CFTR potentiator, initially tested for efficacy against the G551D mutation. It is approved for use in patients with at least one copy of any of the following CFTR mutations: E56K, G178R, S549R, K1060T, G1244E, P67L, E193K, G551D, A1067T, S1251N, R74W, L206W, G551S, G1069R, S1255P, D110E, R347H, D579G, R1070Q, D1270N, D110H, R352Q, S945L, R1070W, G1349D, R117C, A455E, S977F, F1074L, R117H, S549N, F1052V, and D1152H. Ivacaftor is approved for use in patients 2 years of age or older. Dose adjustments are necessary for patients with Child-Pugh class B or C hepatic disease or those with stage IV and V chronic kidney disease. Ivacaftor is metabolized by the CYP3A4 enzyme, and therefore strong inducers such as rifampin may significantly reduce ivacaftor levels. The most common side effects are headache, nausea, rash, rhinitis, dizziness, transaminitis, and arthralgia. Aspartate transaminase (AST) and alanine transaminase (ALT) should be monitored during treatment initiation.

Lumacaftor/ivacaftor (Orkambi) is a combination drug. Lumacaftor is a CFTR corrector. This combination drug is indicated for patients 6 years of age and older who have at least one copy of the F508del CFTR mutation. Dosage adjustments are necessary because of the presence of ivacaftor. Common side effects included dyspnea, nausea, diarrhea, fatigue, and rash. Transaminitis and elevations of serum creatine kinase have been observed. Liver enzymes should be monitored every 3 months during the first year of therapy.

Tezacaftor/ivacaftor (Symdeko) is a combination drug. Tezacaftor is a CFTR corrector. The combination drug is indicated for patients 12 years of age or older with two copies of the F508del mutation or at least one of the following mutations: E56K, R117C, A455E, S945L, R1070W, 3272-26A→G, P67L, E193K, S977F, F1074L, 3849+10kbC→T, R74W, L206W, D579G, F1052V, D1152H, D110E, R347H, 711+3G→G, K1060T, D1270N, D110H, R352Q, E831X, A1067T, 2789+5G→A. Similar to the above, Tezacaftor/Ivacaftor requires dosage adjustment in patients with liver impairment and those taking strong inducers of the CYP3A4 system. Headache, nausea, and dizziness are the most common side effects. Monitoring of liver enzymes is necessary every 3 months for the first year of therapy.

Elexacaftor/tezacaftor/ivacaftor (Trikafta) is a triple-combination drug made up of two CFTR correctors (elexacaftor, which is a next generation corrector, and the corrector tezacaftor) and a potentiator (ivacaftor). This medication is approved for patients 12 years of age or older with at least one copy of the F508del mutation. Monitoring of liver enzymes is necessary every 3 months for the first year of therapy and annually thereafter. As above, it requires dosage adjustment in patients with liver impairment and in those taking strong inducers of the CYP3A4 system.

In addition to the CFTR modulators discussed above, other mainstays of therapy for the pulmonary disease in patients with CF include airway clearance (ie, chest vest, flutter valve, acapella), mucolytics (ie, Pulmozyme), inhaled hypertonic saline, inhaled antibiotics, inhaled bronchodilators, and oral azithromycin.

Exacerbations of CF may be treated with intravenous or oral antibiotics as dictated by sputum cultures and the severity of symptoms. Exacerbations are generally treated with a 14-day course of antibiotics.

Some typical radiographic findings in CF are also shown in **Image 35-9**, with an example of advanced disease shown in **Image 35-10**.

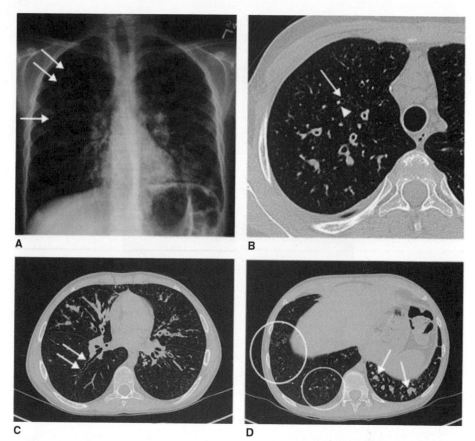

Image 35-9 • Classic chest radiograph and CT findings in CF: (A) bronchial wall thickening and bronchiectasis with tram-track appearance. To determine the difference between cystic parenchymal lesions and cystic bronchiectasis, one needs to demonstrate that the cystic structures follow the expected pattern of bronchioles. (B) Bronchiectasis and signet-ring appearance (*arrow*). (C) Bronchial wall thickening. (D) Tree-in-bud opacities, ground-glass opacities. As the disease progresses, patients may develop apical blebs, severe fibrotic changes with reticulonodular opacities, honeycomb changes, and interlobular and intralobular septal thickening (**Image 35-10**). (*Reproduced with permission from Elsayes KM, Oldham SA: Introduction to Diagnostic Radiology. New York, NY: McGraw Hill; 2014.*)

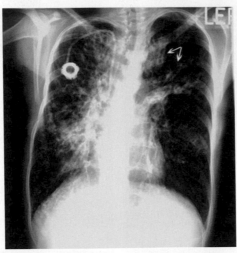

Image 35-10 • Fibrotic changes in advanced disease in CF. (*Reproduced with permission from Papadakis MA, McPhee SJ, Rabow MW: Current Medical Diagnosis & Treatment 2021. New York, NY: McGraw Hill; 2021.*)

References

Chesnutt AN, Chesnutt MS, Prendergast NT, Prendergast TJ. Bronchiectasis. In: Papadakis MA, McPhee SJ, Rabow MW, eds. *Current Medical Diagnosis & Treatment 2021*. McGraw-Hill; 2021. https://accessmedicine.mhmedical.com/content.aspx?bookid=2957&sectionid=249369726

Cystic Fibrosis Foundation, Borowitz D, Robinson KA, et al. Cystic Fibrosis Foundation evidence-based guidelines for management of infants with cystic fibrosis. J Pediatr. 2009;155:S73.

Elborn JS. Cystic fibrosis. Lancet. 2016;388:2519.

Flume PA, O'Sullivan BP, Robinson KA, et al. Cystic fibrosis pulmonary guidelines: chronic medications for maintenance of lung health. Am J Respir Crit Care Med. 2007;176:957.

Flume PA, Robinson KA, O'Sullivan BP. Cystic fibrosis pulmonary guidelines: airway clearance therapies. Respir Care. 2009;54:522.

Gupta N, Matta EJ, Oldham SA. Cardiothoracic imaging. In: Elsayes KM, Oldham SA, eds. *Introduction to Diagnostic Radiology*. McGraw-Hill; 2014. https://accessmedicine.mhmedical.com/content.aspx?bookid=1562&sectionid=95876454

Lahiri T, Hempstead SE, Brady C, et al. Clinical practice guidelines from the cystic fibrosis foundation for preschoolers with cystic fibrosis. Pediatrics. 2016;137.

Middleton PG, Mall MA, Drevinek P, et al. Elexacaftor-tezacaftor-ivacaftor for cystic fibrosis with a single Phe508del allele. NEJM. 2019;381:1809.

Mogayzel PJ Jr, Naureckas ET, Robinson KA, et al. Cystic fibrosis pulmonary guidelines. Chronic medications for maintenance of lung health. Am J Respir Crit Care Med. 2013;187:680.

Noyes BE, Lechner AJ. Presentation and management of cystic fibrosis. In: Lechner AJ, Matuschak GM, Brink DS, eds. *Respiratory: An Integrated Approach to Disease*. McGraw-Hill; 2012. https://accessmedicine.mhmedical.com/content.aspx?bookid=1623&sectionid=105765527

Ren CL, Morgan RL, Oermann C, et al. Cystic Fibrosis Foundation Pulmonary Guidelines: use of cystic fibrosis transmembrane conductance regulator modulator therapy in patients with cystic fibrosis. Ann Am Thorac Soc. 2018;15:271.

Stoltz DA, Meyerholz DK, Welsh MJ. Origins of cystic fibrosis lung disease. N Engl J Med. 2015;372:351.

Voynow JA, Mascarenhas M, Kelly A, Scanlin TF. Cystic fibrosis. In: Grippi MA, Elias JA, Fishman JA, et al, eds. *Fishman's Pulmonary Diseases and Disorders*. 5th ed. McGraw-Hill; 2015. https://accessmedicine.mhmedical.com/content.aspx?bookid=1344&sectionid=81189522

CASE 36

A 65-year-old man with a history of coronary artery disease status post three-vessel coronary artery bypass grafting (CABG) 10 years ago, chronic obstructive pulmonary disease (COPD), hyperlipidemia, hypertension, and type 2 diabetes mellitus presents to the ED reporting dyspnea and orthopnea. He presented initially to his primary care physician 3 days ago with an increased cough and shortness of breath. He has some scant sputum production, which is at baseline, and the color of the sputum is clear to white, also unchanged, though the patient describes it as "frothy." He denies any chest pain, abdominal pain, nausea, emesis, fevers, chills, sweats, or new rashes. He endorses paroxysmal nocturnal dyspnea (PND), orthopnea, and mildly increased symmetric lower extremity edema. He takes metformin, losartan, metoprolol, amlodipine, spironolactone and uses an albuterol inhaler in addition to a fluticasone/salmeterol inhaler. His vitals are T 99.1°F, HR 108, BP 110/70, RR 23, and saturation 93% on 2 L NC. He has some mild expiratory wheezing and lower-lobe predominant inspiratory crackles on examination. He denies any environmental or occupational exposures. His father had COPD and coronary artery disease (CAD) and died of lung cancer at the age of 81. He was a long-time smoker. His mother died of breast cancer at the age of 79. The patient has a prior history of smoking tobacco use, approximately 20 pack-years, but he quit 12 years ago at the time of his initial CAD diagnosis.

The patient's chest radiograph is shown in Image 36-1 below.

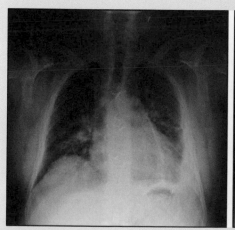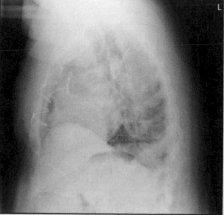

Image 36-1 • Chest radiograph for the patient in Question 36-1.

QUESTIONS

Q36-1: Which abnormality is present on the chest radiographs shown in Image 36-1? Select all that apply.

A. Kerley A lines
B. Kerley B lines
C. Kerley C lines
D. Kerley D lines
E. Pneumothorax
F. Pleural effusion
G. Hyperinflation
H. Peribronchial cuffing
I. Cardiomegaly
J. Pulmonary vascular prominence

Q36-2: The patient has a procalcitonin level that returns less than 0.015 pg/mL (ULN 0.25). His creatinine is 1.1 mg/dL, and his WBC count is 4.5×10^9/mL with 67% neutrophils and no band forms. The patient's electrolytes are within normal limits. The patient's D-dimer is mildly elevated, so he undergoes a pulmonary embolism (PE)-protocol CT scan, and images are obtained with and without contrast. The CT angiogram portion is negative for PE. The noncontrasted CT portion is shown below.

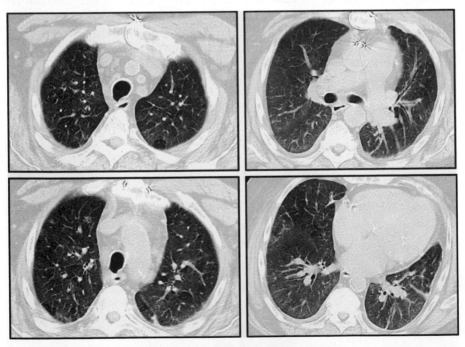

Image 36-2 • CT scan for the patient in **Question 36-2**.

Which abnormality is present on the CT scan shown in Image 36-2? Select all that apply.

A. Ground-glass opacities
B. Consolidation
C. Atelectasis
D. Interlobular and septal thickening
E. Bronchial wall thickening
F. Cystic lesions
G. Traction bronchiectasis
H. Honeycomb changes
I. Hyperinflation/air trapping

Q36-3: The blood work shows that the patient's troponin level is undetectable and the creatine kinase (CK)–MB is within normal limits. What is the most appropriate diagnostic test for this patient to aid in determining the cause of his dyspnea and hypoxia?

A. D-dimer
B. C-reactive protein (CRP)
C. Procalcitonin
D. Brain (B-type) natriuretic peptide (BNP)
E. Blood urea nitrogen (BUN)
F. Respiratory viral panel

Q36-4: The patient's BNP returns 454 pg/mL (ULN 100 pg/mL). The patient's right ventricle has a normal diameter and function with no tricuspid regurgitation. Which finding on point-of-care ultrasound would support a diagnosis of cardiogenic pulmonary edema?

A. A lines on pulmonary examination
B. B lines on pulmonary examination
C. Pleural effusion on pulmonary examination
D. IVC 1.5 cm in diameter with greater than 50% collapse with respiration
E. IVC 2.5 cm with no collapse with respiration
F. Lung point

Q36-5: You successfully diagnose the patient with cardiogenic pulmonary edema. Which etiology is not commonly associated with cardiogenic pulmonary edema?

A. Myocardial infarction/ischemia
B. Acute mitral regurgitation
C. Hypertensive urgency/emergency
D. Mitral stenosis
E. Cor pulmonale
F. LV systolic failure
G. LV diastolic failure
H. Volume overload

Q36-6: Match the following chest radiographs shown in Image 36-3 to the appropriate stage of cardiogenic pulmonary edema.

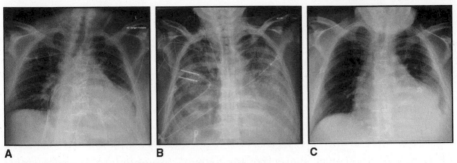

A   B   C

Image 36-3 • Chest radiographs for **Question 36-6**.

1. Redistribution. Answer _____
2. Interstitial Edema. Answer _____
3. Alveolar Edema. Answer _____

Q36-7: A 26-year-old man presents to the ED with acute onset of shortness of breath. He has no medical history. He denies any recent trauma. He denies any risk factors for PE as well. He has inspiratory crackles on examination. The patient's vitals are BP 140/80, RR 20, and saturation 85% on room air. He is afebrile and has a dry cough that began two days ago while hiking and slowly progressed over the next 2 days. The chest radiograph is shown in Image 36-4 below.

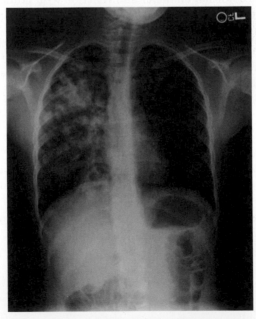

Image 36-4 • Chest radiograph for the patient in **Question 36-7**. (*Reproduced with permission from Tintinalli J, Ma O, Yealy DM, et al: Tintinalli's Emergency Medicine: A Comprehensive Study Guide. 9th ed. New York, NY: McGraw Hill; 2020.*)

What is the likely diagnosis?

A. Lobar pneumonia
B. Cardiogenic pulmonary edema
C. Noncardiogenic pulmonary edema
D. PE

Q36-8: A 26-year-old woman presents to the ED with the acute onset of shortness of breath. She has no medical history. She denies any recent trauma. She denies any risk factors for PE as well. She has inspiratory crackles on examination and is tachypneic with increased accessory muscle usage. The patient's vital signs are BP 220/100, RR 35, and saturation 85% on room air. She is afebrile with a dry cough. The symptoms started suddenly this morning. The patient has no lower extremity edema. The chest radiograph is shown below in Image 36-5.

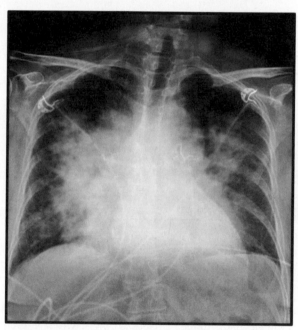

Image 36-5 • Chest radiograph for the patient in **Question 36-8**.

What is the likely diagnosis?

A. Lobar pneumonia
B. Cardiogenic pulmonary edema
C. Noncardiogenic pulmonary edema
D. PE

ANSWERS

Q36-1: A; B; C; F; H; I; J
Kerley B lines; Kerley C lines; Pleural effusion; Peribronchial cuffing; Cardiomegaly; Pulmonary vascular prominence

Rationale: The abnormalities listed above are demonstrated in **Image 36-6**.

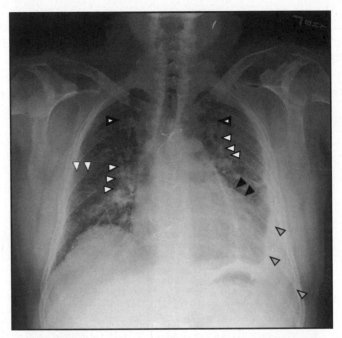

Image 36-6 • Annotated chest radiograph for the patient in **Question 36-1**. *Black arrows*, cardiomegaly; *gray arrows*, left-sided pleural effusion; *white arrows*, fullness/prominence of the pulmonary vasculature with evidence of peribronchial cuffing; *thick arrows*, Kerley A lines; *thin arrow*, Kerley B lines.

First, one should note that this is a PA and lateral film. On the PA film, there is enlargement of the cardiac silhouette (*black arrows*) with the presence of sternal wires, consistent with cardiomegaly and prior CABG. There is also a moderate left-sided pleural effusion present (*gray arrows*) with blunting of the costophrenic angle and a meniscus sign. There is no evidence of hyperinflation based on the appearance of the right hemidiaphragm. Additionally, there is no pneumothorax present. The pulmonary vasculature also appears hazy and more prominent (*white arrows*), and there are bronchi visible in this region with what appear to be thickened wall ("peribronchial cuffing").

In terms of the air spaces, there are diffuse linear interstitial opacities. Linear interstitial opacities can be seen in numerous conditions, including cardiogenic and noncardiogenic pulmonary edema, lymphangitic carcinomatosis, early-stage interstitial lung disease, and viral/atypical pneumonitis, among others. Moreover, linear interstitial opacities can be difficult to distinguish from reticular (curvilinear) opacities in some instances. Linear interstitial opacities arise from thickening of the interstitium (from edema, inflammation, fibrosis), yielding an indistinctness or haziness. The pattern may be either axial (running from the hilum to the periphery, along the bronchovascular bundle), predominantly peripheral, or mixed. This interstitial thickening gives rise to the Kerley A, B, and C lines (there are no Kerley D lines). Kerley A lines are linear interstitial opacities oriented from the periphery toward to the hila along bronchovascular bundles and arise from congestion of lymphatics. These are best seen in the upper lobes (*thick arrows*). Kerley B lines (*thin arrows*) appear to arise from and run perpendicular to the pleural surface. Kerley B lines represent thickening of the interlobular septa usually caused by edema. Kerley C lines are Kerley B lines out-of-plane of the film; these are seen as reticular interstitial opacities on CXR due to a reduction from three to two dimensions, giving the appearance that they overlap. One can see something similar here in the periphery of the lung on the right, particularly in the right middle and lower lobes.

Q36-2: A; D; E

Ground-glass opacities; Interlobular and septal thickening; Bronchial wall thickening. The abnormalities are annotated in Image 36-7.

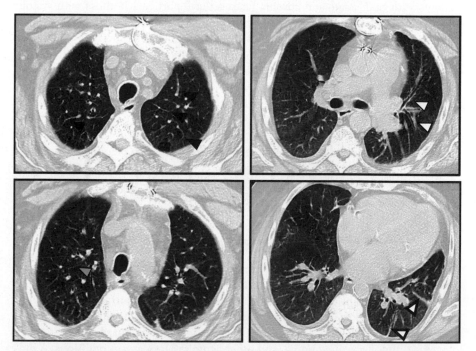

Image 36-7 • Noncontrasted CT (inspiratory) of the chest for the patient in **Question 36-2**. *Black arrows*, interlobular septal thickening; *gray arrow*, interlobular septal thickening surrounded by ground glass (the ground-glass opacities are diffuse here, with only small patches of normal-appearing lung tissue); *white arrows*, bronchial wall thickening (peribronchial cuffing); *thick arrows*, septal thickening.

The patient's CT scan of the chest is shown with coronal cuts. The study is non-contrasted, and by the appearance of the trachea, the study is a standard inspiratory film (which is not particularly useful to determine hyperinflation). There is diffuse ground glass present with no evidence of overt consolidation or masses, though there are some scattered nodular opacities. There is interlobular (*gray and black arrows*) and septal (*thick arrows*) thickening present, which gives rise to the Kerley A, B, and C lines present on chest radiographs. Additionally, there is bronchial wall thickening (*white arrows*), which leads to the appearance of peribronchial cuffing. There are no significant atelectasis or cystic lesions present. There is no architectural distortion or traction bronchiectasis, and there are no honeycomb changes.

Q36-3: D
B-type natriuretic peptide (BNP)

BNP is a hormone secreted by cardiomyocytes in response to increased wall strain in the ventricles of the heart, which is typically caused by volume overload. BNP is a biologically active peptide with activity similar to ANP and is formed from the precursor proBNP. After synthesis, proBNP is cleaved to yield the N-terminal fragment (NT-proBNP) and BNP. Clinical tests exist for both NT-proBNP and BNP, and both have been shown to have significant diagnostic as well as prognostic value in patients with both acute and chronic heart failure, particularly those with systolic heart failure. Additionally, they may be used to guide diuretic therapy in selected patients, though studies are ongoing. Both values may be falsely low in obese patients with heart failure and elevated in patients with renal failure or RV strain due to PE or pulmonary hypertension, among others. A D-dimer would be useful to rule out a PE as the cause if it is negative, but it is not diagnostic, and given the patient's chest radiograph, cardiogenic pulmonary edema should be higher on the differential diagnosis. A CRP is nonspecific and, again, would not yield a diagnosis. A procalcitonin or respiratory viral panel would be helpful if the primary concern was for infection. A BUN would be of interest if the patient had large bilateral pleural effusions or a pericardial effusion as the cause of the respiratory distress. However, with a normal CK–MB, this would be less useful here.

Q36-4: E
IVC 2.5 cm with no collapse with respiration

Rationale: Point-of-care ultrasound is quickly gaining traction to aid in the diagnosis of acute cardiopulmonary conditions. On thoracic examination, A lines are normal and represent an artifact, indicating a normal lung surface. B lines, while helpful, simply indicate the presence of interstitial edema. Interstitial edema can be seen in a number of conditions, including cardiogenic pulmonary edema, noncardiogenic pulmonary, pneumonia, and other acute inflammatory conditions. A lung point is used to diagnose a pneumothorax. A pleural effusion, while supportive, again is not specific for cardiogenic pulmonary edema. Measurement of the IVC 1 to 2 cm proximal to the hepatic vein with inspiration and expiration can provide an estimate of the patient's central venous pressure (CVP). For a patient with an IVC diameter less than 1.5 cm and total collapse of the IVC with respiration, the CVP is likely 0 to 4 cm H_2O. A patient with an IVC 1.5 to 2.5 cm and 50% collapse may have a CVP between 5 and 15 cm H_2O, while a patient with a dilated IVC (2.5 cm or greater) and less than 50% collapse with respiration is likely to have a CVP above ~18 cm H_2O. Because of the finding of normal RV size and RV function and no tricuspid regurgitation, there is no evidence for decompensated right-sided heart failure or pulmonary hypertension. Therefore, the CVP may be a decent estimate for the left-sided filling pressures.

Q36-5: E
Cor pulmonale

Rationale: RV failure (cor pulmonale) and pulmonary hypertension (with the exception of World Health Organization [WHO] group II disease, due to left-sided heart failure) do not typically lead to issues with pulmonary edema. However, if the RV becomes sufficiently dilated and dysfunctional, it can impede LV function in instances. Cardiogenic pulmonary edema may result from any condition that acutely increases preload (volume overload, acute aortic or mitral regurgitation), decreased contractility or chronotropy (ischemic, infarction, high-degree AV block, beta-blocker overdose), or increases the afterload (systemic hypertension/hypertensive urgency, mitral stenosis, aortic stenosis).

Q36-6: C - Redistribution; A - Interstitial Edema; B - Alveolar Edema

Rationale: Cardiogenic pulmonary edema is primarily due to increased left-sided filling pressures, which causes pulmonary venous and capillary congestion, while non-cardiogenic pulmonary edema is more commonly associated with increased capillary leak/permeability (it is likely not this black and white, however). In the first stages of pulmonary edema, when the left-ventricular end-diastolic pressure (LVEDP) is 13 to 18 cm H_2O, there is an increase in the pulmonary venous vasculature, and fluid backs up into the lymphatics. On chest radiograph, this most commonly appears as hazy, prominent pulmonary vascular bundles. The increased venous pressure also means increased blood flow to zone 1, as the pulmonary venous pressures approach the alveolar pressures. The increased drainage through the lymphatics makes the pulmonary bronchovascular bundles more apparent, and this is most noticeable in the upper lobes (zone 1), where blood is traditionally slower than in zones 2 and 3. This is sometimes referred to as *cephalization* (**Image 36-3C**). As the LVEDP rises above 18 cm H_2O and the lymphatics become overwhelmed, the fluid leaks first into the interstitial spaces. This interstitial edema causes bronchial wall thickening, giving rise to peribronchial cuffing and interlobular and septal thickening that yield Kerley A, B, and C lines. The contours of the pulmonary veins and arteries become hazier (**Image 36-3A**). Eventually, fluids leak into the alveoli, yielding alveolar opacities, consolidation with air bronchograms, and pleural effusions (**Image 36-3B**). One important factor that determines how symptomatic a patient will be is the chronicity of illness. Patients with chronic congestive heart failure are more likely to have a more adapted lymphatic system that prevents the rapid onset of edema, while patients with no prior history of heart failure or cardiogenic edema are more likely to present in extremis with minimal volume overload.

An example of a patient progressing through the stages of cardiogenic pulmonary edema is shown in **Image 36-8** below.

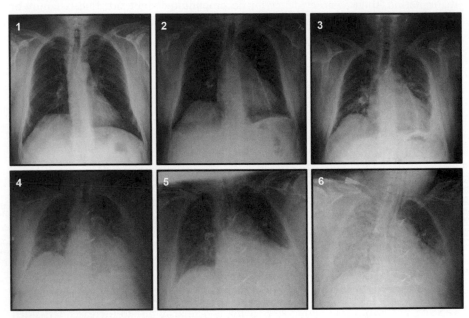

Image 36-8 • Progression of cardiogenic pulmonary edema from baseline (1), through redistribution (2), mild interstitial edema (3), moderate interstitial edema (4), transition to alveolar edema (5), and alveolar edema (6).

Q36-7: C
Non-cardiogenic pulmonary edema

Rationale: This will be discussed further in the next question.

Q36-8: B
Cardiogenic pulmonary edema

Rationale: As discussed previously, pulmonary edema may be classified in multiple ways, though the most common method is to determine the etiology of the edema first. Cardiogenic edema is edema that develops as a result of pulmonary venous hypertension, whereas noncardiogenic edema is caused by conditions leading to increased pulmonary capillary permeability. In noncardiogenic pulmonary edema, the pattern is marked by diffuse or focal areas of patchy airspace disease with more involvement of the periphery and a lack of linear interstitial opacities or cardiomegaly. Noncardiogenic edema may be seen in patients with acute respiratory distress syndrome (ARDS), high-altitude pulmonary edema, near-drowning, trauma, transfusion-related acute lung injury (TRALI), fat/amniotic embolism, and sepsis. CT scan will show an alveolar filling pattern similar to diffuse alveolar hemorrhage (DAH).

The patient in **Question 36-7** likely has high-altitude pulmonary edema (HAPE), as he was recently hiking. HAPE is noncardiogenic edema that occurs when non-acclimatized people experience a significant and rapid change in altitude (greater than 3000 meters). The development of this pulmonary edema is multifactorial and thought to involve "stress failure" of the vascular endothelium under conditions of reduced alveolar pressure and hypoxemic pulmonary vasoconstriction. Treatment involves returning to normal living altitude, supplemental oxygen, and hyperbaric treatment when needed. Nifedipine has been used for prevention, while phosphodiesterase inhibitors and dexamethasone have also been used for treatment.

The patient in **Question 36-8** has flash pulmonary edema, a common complication of hypertensive emergency/urgency, leading to acute respiratory distress and hypoxemia. This is commonly seen in patients with acute increases in afterload or preload. Unlike patients with chronic volume overload, the lymphatics are not capable of handling the acute increase in venous pressure, and they more quickly progress to alveolar edema. The CXR has the classic "batwing" appearance of perihilar predominant hazy airspace opacities with sparing of the periphery of the lung. Treatment is with nitroglycerin, diuresis, supplemental oxygen, and positive airway pressure (ie, bi-level positive airway pressure [BiPAP] or continuous positive airway pressure [CPAP]).

References

Adams KF Jr, Fonarow GC, Emerman CL, et al. Characteristics and outcomes of patients hospitalized for heart failure in the United States: rationale, design, and preliminary observations from the first 100,000 cases in the Acute Decompensated Heart Failure National Registry (ADHERE). Am Heart J. 2005;149:209.

Al Deeb M, Barbic S, Featherstone R, et al. Point-of-care ultrasonography for the diagnosis of acute cardiogenic pulmonary edema in patients presenting with acute dyspnea: a systematic review and meta-analysis. Acad Emerg Med. 2014;21:843.

Baggish AL, Siebert U, Lainchbury JG, et al. A validated clinical and biochemical score for the diagnosis of acute heart failure: the ProBNP Investigation of Dyspnea in the Emergency Department (PRIDE) Acute Heart Failure Score. Am Heart J. 2006;151:48.

Dickstein K, Cohen-Solal A, Filippatos G, et al. ESC Guidelines for the diagnosis and treatment of acute and chronic heart failure 2008: the Task Force for the Diagnosis and Treatment of Acute and Chronic Heart Failure 2008 of the European Society of Cardiology. Developed in collaboration with the Heart Failure Association of the ESC (HFA) and endorsed by the European Society of Intensive Care Medicine (ESICM). Eur Heart J. 2008;29:2388.

Gandhi SK, Powers JC, Nomeir AM, et al. The pathogenesis of acute pulmonary edema associated with hypertension. N Engl J Med. 2001;344:17.

Heart Failure Society of America, Lindenfeld J, Albert NM, et al. HFSA 2010 Comprehensive Heart Failure Practice Guideline. J Card Fail. 2010;16:e1.

Hunt SA, Abraham WT, Chin MH, et al. 2009 focused update incorporated into the ACC/AHA 2005 Guidelines for the Diagnosis and Management of Heart Failure in Adults: a report of the American College of Cardiology Foundation/American Heart Association Task Force on Practice Guidelines: developed in collaboration with the International Society for Heart and Lung Transplantation. Circulation. 2009;119:e391.

Lagu T, Pekow PS, Shieh MS, et al. Validation and comparison of seven mortality prediction models for hospitalized patients with acute decompensated heart failure. Circ Heart Fail. 2016;9.

Maisel AS, Krishnaswamy P, Nowak RM, et al. Rapid measurement of B-type natriuretic peptide in the emergency diagnosis of heart failure. N Engl J Med. 2002;347:161.

Mebazaa A, Yilmaz MB, Levy P, et al. Recommendations on pre-hospital & early hospital management of acute heart failure: a consensus paper from the Heart Failure Association of the European Society of Cardiology, the European Society of Emergency Medicine and the Society of Academic Emergency Medicine. Eur J Heart Fail. 2015;17:544.

Nieminen MS, Böhm M, Cowie MR, et al. Executive summary of the guidelines on the diagnosis and treatment of acute heart failure: the Task Force on Acute Heart Failure of the European Society of Cardiology. Eur Heart J. 2005;26:384.

Ponikowski P, Voors AA, Anker SD, et al. 2016 ESC Guidelines for the diagnosis and treatment of acute and chronic heart failure: The Task Force for the diagnosis and treatment of acute and chronic heart failure of the European Society of Cardiology (ESC). Developed with the special contribution of the Heart Failure Association (HFA) of the ESC. Eur J Heart Fail. 2016;18:891.

Rimoldi SF, Yuzefpolskaya M, Allemann Y, Messerli F. Flash pulmonary edema. Prog Cardiovasc Dis. 2009;52:249.

Ware LB, Matthay MA. Clinical practice. Acute pulmonary edema. N Engl J Med. 2005;353:2788.

WRITING COMMITTEE MEMBERS, Yancy CW, Jessup M, et al. 2013 ACCF/AHA guideline for the management of heart failure: a report of the American College of Cardiology Foundation/ American Heart Association Task Force on practice guidelines. Circulation. 2013;128:e240.

CASE 37

A 56-year-old woman is referred for evaluation of dyspnea on exertion and chronic productive cough. She has a history of gout and hypertension and a 50- to 60-pack-year history of smoking, which is ongoing. She notes that she began experiencing shortness of breath approximately 2 years ago, which has progressively worsened since that time. She has a cough, which started about 1 year ago and is productive of clear sputum, worse in the morning. She denies any occupational or environmental exposures. She has no family history of lung disease or malignancy. On examination, she is thin with a BMI of 20 kg/m². Her vital signs are HR 85, BP 120/60, RR 12, and O₂ saturation is 94% on room air. She has diminished breath sounds bilaterally at the apices. There are no crackles on examination. She has a mild expiratory wheeze. There is no cyanosis or edema; mild clubbing is present. The results of the patient's PFT are shown in Image 37-1 below.

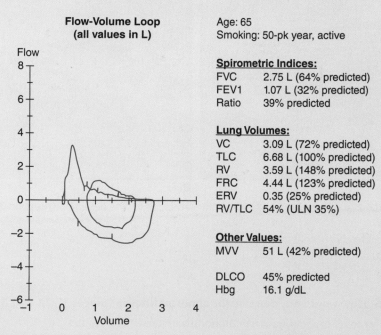

Flow-Volume Loop
(all values in L)

Age: 65
Smoking: 50-pk year, active

Spirometric Indices:
FVC   2.75 L (64% predicted)
FEV1   1.07 L (32% predicted)
Ratio   39% predicted

Lung Volumes:
VC   3.09 L (72% predicted)
TLC   6.68 L (100% predicted)
RV   3.59 L (148% predicted)
FRC   4.44 L (123% predicted)
ERV   0.35 (25% predicted)
RV/TLC   54% (ULN 35%)

Other Values:
MVV   51 L (42% predicted)

DLCO   45% predicted
Hbg   16.1 g/dL

Image 37-1 • Flow volume loop and pulmonary function testing indices for the patient in **Question 37-1**.

QUESTIONS

Q37-1: Which abnormalities are present on the pulmonary function testing?

A. Obstructive lung disease
B. Restrictive lung disease
C. Hyperinflation
D. None of the above
E. A and B
F. A and C
G. B and C

Q37-2: If this patient's postbronchodilator response showed an increase in her FEV1 of 300 mL (to 1.27 L or 42% predicted) and an increase in her FVC of 600 mL (to 3.35 L or 78% predicted) with a postbronchodilator ratio of 38% predicted, how would you describe her obstructive lung disease?

The patient chest imaging is shown below.

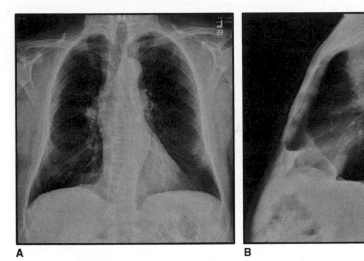

A   B

Image 37-2 • Chest radiographs (PA, A; and lateral; B) for the patient in **Question 37-2**.

A. Completely reversible
B. Partially reversible
C. Irreversible

Q37-3: How would one describe the abnormalities in Images 37-2A and B?

A. Lower lobe–predominant reticulonodular interstitial opacities
B. Upper lobe cavitary lesions
C. Hyperinflation
D. Pleural plaques
E. Diffuse alveolar infiltrates

Q37-4: How would one describe the primary abnormality seen on the chest CT shown in Image 37-3?

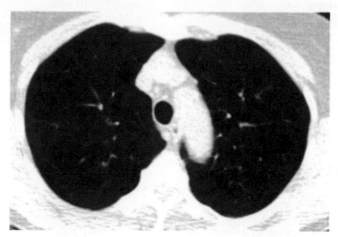

Image 37-3 • Chest CT image for the patient in **Question 37-4**. (*Reproduced with permission from Durawa A, Dziadziuszko K, Jelitto-Górska M, et al: Emphysema - The review of radiological presentation and its clinical impact in the LDCT screening era, Clin Imaging 2020 Aug;64:85-91.*)

A. Paraseptal emphysema
B. Panlobular emphysema
C. Centrilobular emphysema
D. Honeycombing with traction bronchiectasis
E. Bronchomalacia

Q37-5: Given the patient's smoking history and imaging findings, she is diagnosed with smoking-related COPD. The patient's COPD Assessment Test score is 13, and the patient has one to two exacerbations per year. What is the patient's GOLD classification?

A. Gold Class A
B. Gold Class B
C. Gold Class C
D. Gold Class D

Q37-6: A 34-year-old man with a 5–pack-year history of smoking presents with dyspnea and a productive cough. He has had progressively worsening symptoms since he started smoking 5 years ago. He denies any other medical problems and has no significant family history of pulmonary disease, rheumatologic disease, or malignancy. He denies any environmental exposures or occupational exposures. He has a negative HIV study and a normal immunoglobulin level. PFTs demonstrate obstruction with a mild decrease in his DLCO. His chest imaging is shown in Image 37-4.

What is the most appropriate study to send to aid in diagnosis?

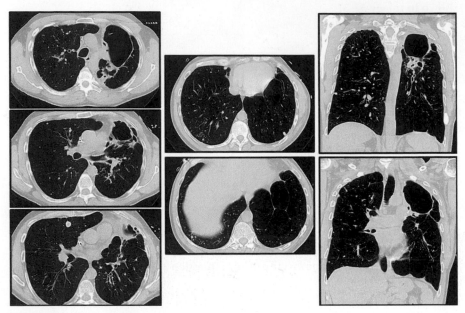

Image 37-4 • Chest CT images for the patient in **Question 37-6**.

A. Rheumatoid factor
B. Antinuclear antibody titer
C. Alpha-1-antitrypsin (A1AT) enzyme level
D. Glucose-6-phosphate dehydrogenase (G6PDH) enzyme level
E. Procalcitonin
F. Arterial blood gas
G. Alpha-fetoprotein (AFP) level

Q37-7: Which COPD patient group has an improved survival with lung-volume reduction surgery (LVRS)?

A. Upper lobe–predominant disease; high exercise capacity
B. Diffuse disease; low exercise tolerance
C. Upper lobe–predominant disease; low exercise capacity
D. Lower lobe–predominant disease; high exercise capacity

Q37-8: Aside from smoking cessation, what other medical treatment for patients with COPD is associated with a survival benefit?

A. Maintenance use of long-acting beta-agonist
B. Nebulized albuterol
C. Prophylactic antibiotics
D. Phosphodiesterase inhibitors (eg, roflumilast)
E. Supplemental oxygen for all patients
F. Supplemental oxygen for patients with resting hypoxemia

ANSWERS

Q37-1: F
A and C

Rationale: First, observe the flow-volume loop. The shape of the flow-volume is quite concave, indicating that as the lung volume decreases, there is worsening obstruction to expiratory airflow. This is reflected in the patients spirometric indices as well. This is consistent with obstructive lung disease. The patient has a reduced FEV1/FVC ratio (39%), with a normal TLC and an extremely elevated RV (residual volume; 150%) and RV/TLC ratio (54% predicted), indicative of significant air trapping or hyperinflation, also consistent with obstructive lung disease There is no evidence of restrictive lung disease as the TLC (total lung capacity) is normal. Although the patient's MVV (maximal minute ventilation) is reduced (51 L, 42% predicted), the value is appropriate for the severity of this patient's expiratory airflow obstruction. Also note that this patients FRC is elevated at 123% predicted, also reflective of air trapping. An appropriate MVV for this patient can be determined by multiplying the patient's FEV1 by an expected rate of 30 breaths per minute during the MVV maneuver. So here, we would expect the patient's MVV to be around 32 L. This is indicates that while the patient has a reduced MVV, it is unlikely to be due to neuromuscular disorder. The DLCO is also substantially reduced (45% predicted), and the patient's hemoglobin is normal (if not elevated, likely reflective of secondary polycythemia) so the reduction in the DLCO is not due to anemia.

Q37-2: B
Partially reversible

Rationale: The patient's postbronchodilator response is positive, defined as at least 200 mL and 12% predicted improved in either the FEV1 or FVC when comparing the data. This patient has a 14% increase in FVC with a 600 mL total improvement in total. Thus, the patient has significant reversibility of the airflow obstruction; however, as the FEV1/FVC ratio, the FEV1, and the FVC do not return to normal after bronchodilator therapy, there is some degree of irreversibility. Therefore, the patient has partially reversible airflow obstruction.

Q37-3: C
Hyperinflation

Rationale: The chest film shown in **Images 37-2A** and **B** demonstrates marked hyperinflation with bilateral flattening of the diaphragms. There is no evidence of upper lobe cavitary lesions, lower lobe reticulonodular opacities, pleural plaques, or diffuse alveolar infiltrates.

Q37-4: C
Centrilobular emphysema

Rationale: Patients with chronic obstructive pulmonary disease (COPD) may present with a number of abnormal findings on a CT scan, with the most common finding being centrilobular emphysema.

Severe centrilobular emphysema can be difficult to discern from panlobular emphysema when seen in the upper lobes. Smoking-related COPD is commonly associated with upper lobe–predominant disease.

Recall the structure of the secondary pulmonary lobule (**Image 37-5**):

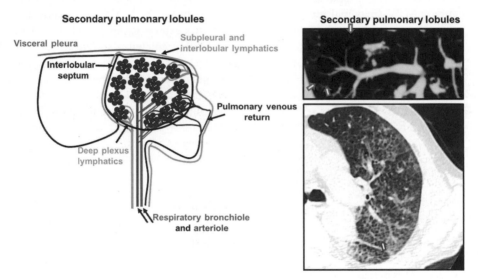

Image 37-5 • Structure of the secondary lobule.

Traveling through the center of the lobule are the terminal bronchiole and the pulmonary arteriole, leading to the alveoli and capillaries. The pulmonary veins travel on the periphery through the interlobular septum of the secondary lobules, while the lymphatics are present both centrally and peripherally. Smoking-related COPD is an airway-centric disease, and therefore the predominant areas of destruction are at the center of the secondary lobules, hence the term *centrilobular* or *centriacinar*. The other two subtypes of emphysema are paraseptal (distal acinar) emphysema and panlobular emphysema. Paraseptal emphysema predominantly involves the alveoli bordered on at least one side by the pleural surface. Pure paraseptal emphysema is associated with the formation of bullae, is usually asymptomatic, and is associated with an increased risk of iatrogenic pneumothorax. However, paraseptal emphysema is often seen in patients with severe centrilobular emphysema as well. Panlobular emphysema is classically associated with alpha-1-antitrypsin disease, and the entire secondary lobule is typically involved. Examples of the different imaging findings in emphysema are shown in **Image 37-6**. Patients with COPD may have evidence of a saber-sheath trachea (**Image 37-7**). This is nearly pathognomonic for COPD. This is defined as the narrowing of coronal diameter of the trachea with a widening of the sagittal diameter, typically yielding a ratio greater than 1:2. There may also be calcifications of the tracheal cartilage present. Patients with COPD may also have bronchomalacia seen on CT of the chest expiratory images where the mainstem bronchi collapse during expiration as compared with inspiration. The image above shows bronchomalacia as seen during a bronchoscopy where the posterior membrane of the trachea moves anteriorly, almost abutting the anterior tracheal wall (**Image 37-8**). Additionally, patients with emphysema may have evidence of air trapping on expiratory films with a mosaic attenuation pattern (**Image 37-9**). Again, this is not specific to COPD or emphysema.

In patients with a chronic bronchitis subtype of COPD, a chest radiograph may show predominantly linear or reticular interstitial opacities consistent with likely bronchial wall thickening, though significant overlap exists between the two.

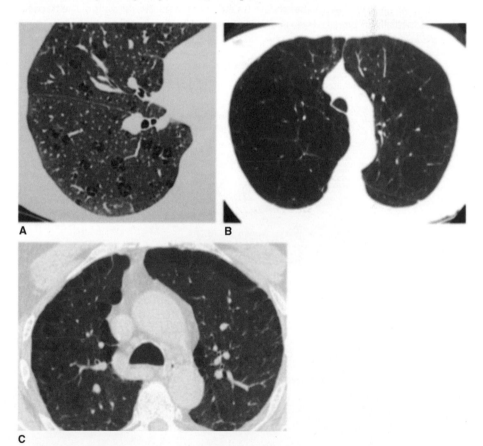

Image 37-6 • Examples of the distribution of emphysematous changes seen on CT imaging. (A) centrilobular emphysema; (B) panlobular emphysema; (C) paraseptal emphysema. (*Reproduced with permission from Washko GR. Diagnostic imaging in COPD, Semin Respir Crit Care Med 2010 Jun;31(3):276-285.*)

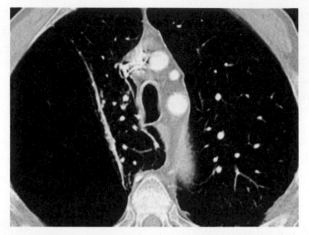

Image 37-7 • Example of a saber-sheath trachea in COPD. Patients with COPD may have what has been described as a "saber sheath trachea," where the lateral walls of the trachea compress medially. (*Reproduced with permission from Kugler C, Stanzel F. Tracheomalacia, Thorac Surg Clin 2014 Feb;24(1):51-58.*)

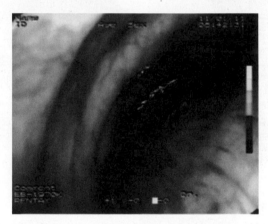

Image 37-8 • Example of bronchomalacia diagnosed during bronchoscopy. (*Reproduced with permission from Kugler C, Stanzel F. Tracheomalacia, Thorac Surg Clin 2014 Feb;24(1):51-58.*)

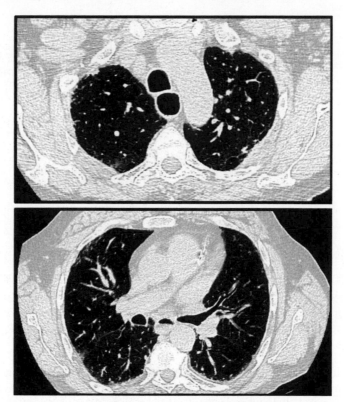

Image 37-9 • Example of air-trapping seen on expiratory chest CT images. Air trapping is indicated by the retention of air (black areas) during expiration. Air trapping occurs due to premature closing of the airways during expiration, resulting from destruction and inflammation in the airways. During expiration, as the lung volumes are reduced, the airways are no longer stented open and due to loss of structural integrity the airways may close before air has had to opportunity to be exhaled. This results in trapped air within the lung, surrounded by areas of more dense (gray), normal parenchyma.

Q37-5: D
Gold Class D

The GOLD classification system is based on patient characteristics, including the severity of airflow obstruction, the number of exacerbations per year, and the score on one of two subjective assessment tools (COPD assessment tool [CAT] and the modified Medical Research Council [mMRC] dyspnea scale).

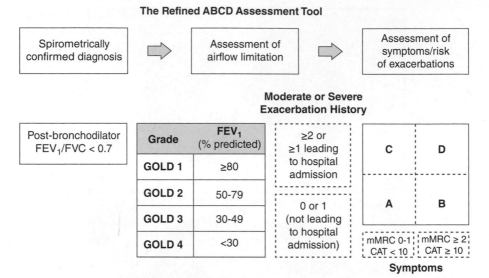

Image 37-10 • GOLD COPD classification. (*Reproduced with permission from Global Initiative for Chronic Obstructive Lung Disease. Global Strategy for the Diagnosis, Management and Prevention of Chronic Obstructive Pulmonary Disease (2021 Report). ©2020 Global Initiative for Chronic Obstructive Lung Disease, Inc.*)

This patient has Gold stage IV (very severe) airflow obstruction based on her FEV1 less than 30% predicted, a CAT score great than or equal to 10, and one to two exacerbations per year, placing her in the GOLD Class D category overall. The GOLD classification is important to identify patients at risk for frequent hospitalization as well as to determine appropriate step-wise maintenance medications for treatment.

COPD is a progressive inflammatory lung disease marked by the destruction of the pulmonary parenchyma and further characterized by irreversible airflow obstruction. Airflow obstruction is defined as a postbronchodilator FEV1/FVC ratio below 0.7. Airflow obstruction is graded based on the postbronchodilator FEV1 and is summarized in **Image 37-10**. The obstructive ventilatory defect is not completely reversible with bronchodilators in COPD. Spirometry is necessary to confirm a diagnosis of COPD in the right clinical setting.

Risk factors for the development of COPD include smoking, exposure to biomass fuels, low socioeconomic status, and occupations that involve exposure to organic and inorganic dusts. Genetic factors also influence the risk of COPD, such as in alpha-1-antitrypsin deficiency.

Symptoms of COPD include shortness of breath, chronic cough, and recurrent lower respiratory tract infections. A chronic bronchitis phenotype is characterized by mucus hypersecretion and a chronic productive cough.

Chest radiographs may show hyperinflation, and a CT scan may show centrilobular, panlobular. or paraseptal emphysema and evidence of bronchial wall thickening. Imaging is not required to establish a diagnosis of COPD.

The goals of therapy are to reduce a patient's symptoms and mortality and to prevent disease progression and exacerbations. Management of COPD involves both pharmaceuticals and lifestyle adjustments (ie, smoking cessation, avoiding air pollution, removing or minimizing occupational exposures).

Medications may help reduce symptoms and the frequency of exacerbations and may improve a patient's exercise tolerance. A combination of short- and long-acting bronchodilators is the mainstay of pharmacologic therapy in COPD, with only the most symptomatic patients (group D) needing inhaled corticosteroids.

In patients who are on maximal inhaler therapy but who continue to have exacerbations, other therapy options include roflumilast, a macrolide, or stopping the inhaled corticosteroid. Roflumilast is to be used in patients with a chronic bronchitis phenotype and an FEV1 greater than 50% predicted. Azithromycin may also be useful, particularly in patients who are not currently smoking. Stopping the inhaled corticosteroid can be helpful if the patient is developing recurrent pneumonia because inhaled corticosteroids have been associated with an increased risk of pneumonia.

Q37-6: C
Alpha-1-antitrypsin (A1AT) enzyme level

Rationale: Current guidelines recommend testing all patients with COPD for possible alpha-1-antitrypsin disorder by testing for A1AT enzyme activity, which, if abnormal, should be followed by testing for mutations in the *A1AT* gene. A1AT can account for up to 5% of patients with COPD and should be high on the differential diagnosis in patients with atypical presentations, including patients with lower lobe–predominant emphysema, patients presenting at a young age (younger than 50 years of age) or with a trivial smoking history, patients with bronchiectasis, and a family history of lung or liver disease. In A1AT, more than 50% of patients will have mid or lower lobe–predominant disease with panlobular emphysema and blebs. Note here that that CT scan shown in **Image 37-5** demonstrated diffuse emphysematous changes with complete obliteration of the entire acinus, consistent with panlobar emphysema. An additional example is shown in **Image 37-11**.

Alpha-1-antitrypsin is a proteinase inhibitor that inactivates proteolytic enzymes. Without adequate amounts of alpha-1-antitrypsin, proteolytic enzymes destroy the pulmonary parenchyma, resulting in disease.

Approximately 100,000 people in the United States are believed to have a severe alpha-1-antitrypsin deficiency. It is an autosomal recessive disorder associated with pulmonary, liver, and skin disease. Patients with severe alpha-1-antitrypsin deficiency are likely to be homozygous for the Z allele (ZZ) and to have markedly low levels of alpha-1-antitrypsin (less than 15% of normal). Family members of patients with the disease should be screened for the deficiency as well.

In the lung, alpha-1-antitrypsin deficiency may result in chronic obstructive pulmonary disease, asthma, or bronchiectasis. Respiratory symptoms including dyspnea, cough, and wheezing are the most common presenting symptoms in patients with alpha-1-antitrypsin deficiency.

The treatments used for smoking-related COPD are also used in alpha-1-antitrypsin deficiency; however, in alpha-1-antitrypsin deficiency, patients may also receive weekly infusions of alpha-1-antitrypsin (augmentation therapy).

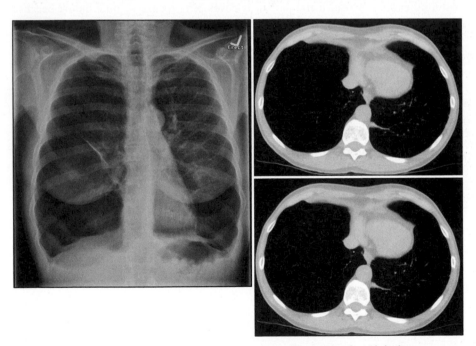

Image 37-11 • Another example of a patient with A1AT-associated panlobular emphysema.

Q37-7: C
Upper lobe–predominant disease; low exercise capacity

Rationale: Patients with upper lobe–predominant disease and low exercise tolerance at baseline, despite attempts at rehabilitation, receive both a survival benefit and an improvement in functional status with LVRS, while patients with upper lobe disease and high exercise capacity at baseline have no change in survival.

Q37-8: F
Supplemental oxygen for patients with resting hypoxemia

Rationale: Supplemental oxygen for patients with resting daytime hypoxemia is associated with a survival benefit, whereas the remaining options are not associated with a survival benefit.

References

Durawa A, Dziadziuszko K, Jelitto-Gorska M, Szurowska E. Emphysema—the review of radiological presentation and its clinical impact in the LDCT screening era. Clin Imaging. 2020;64:85.

Global Initiative for Chronic Obstructive Lung disease: global strategy for the diagnosis, management, and prevention of chronic obstructive pulmonary disease (2021 report).

Gupta N, Matta EJ, Oldham SA. Cardiothoracic imaging. In: Elsayes KM, Oldham SA, eds. *Introduction to Diagnostic Radiology.* McGraw-Hill; 2014. https://accessmedicine.mhmedical.com/content.aspx?bookid=1562&sectionid=95876454

Kohnlein T, Welte T. Alpha-1 antitrypsin deficiency: pathogenesis, clinical presentation, diagnosis, and treatment. Am J Med. 2008;121:3.

Kugler C, Stanzel F. Traceomalacia. Thorac Surg Clin. 2014;24:51.

Senior RM, Pierce RA, Atkinson JJ. Chronic obstructive pulmonary disease: epidemiology, pathophysiology, pathogenesis, and α1-antitrypsin deficiency. Grippi MA, Elias JA, Fishman JA, et al, eds. *Fishman's Pulmonary Diseases and Disorders.* 5th ed. McGraw-Hill; 2015. https://accessmedicine.mhmedical.com/content.aspx?bookid=1344&sectionid=81188304

Washko GR. Diagnostic imaging in COPD. Semin Respir Crit Care Med. 2010;31:276.

CASE 38

A 66-year-old man presents to the ED with fevers, chills, a productive cough, and new leukocytosis. The patient has no significant medical history but does not follow with a health care provider routinely. He denies any sick contacts or environmental or occupational exposures, and he does not smoke or use illicit drugs. He reports the onset of symptoms 3 days ago, starting with general malaise and some mild back pain on the right. He developed some fevers, chills, and rigors during the day, and this morning he developed a productive cough with yellow sputum. He denies any hemoptysis, diarrhea, nausea, or emesis. A few days before the onset of symptoms, he was camping with his grandchildren and was caught in a rainstorm for a few hours. His vital signs in triage are T 101.4°F, HR 125, BP 88/54, RR 22, and O_2 saturation 84% on room air, improved to 94% on 4 L NC. He has dullness at the right base on percussion, and there are bronchial breath sounds present. His WBC count is 17 × 10^9/L with 30% bands. He has an acute kidney injury with a creatinine level of 2.2 mg/dL and a BUN of 48 mg/dL. He is hyponatremic to 127 mEq/L. His ABG shows a slight metabolic acidosis with a pH 7.30, $PaCO_2$ 28, and PaO_2 of 58 mm Hg. His chest radiograph and point-of-care ultrasound findings are shown in Images 38-1 and 38-2 below.

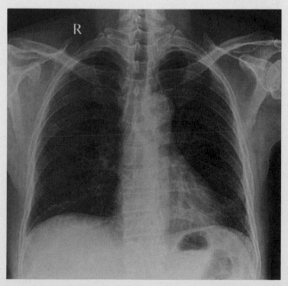

Image 38-1 • Chest radiograph (AP) for the patient in **Question 38-1**. (*Reproduced with permission from Hoan L, Hang LM, Thanh Hong DT,et al: A 69-Year-Old Man With Chronic Cough and Recurrent Pneumonia, Chest 2020 Dec;158(6):e283-e287.*)

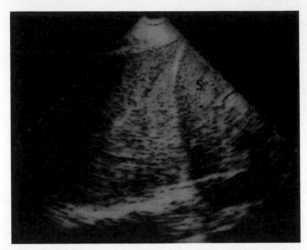

Image 38-2 • Thoracic ultrasound image for the patient in **Question 38-1**. (*Reproduced with permission from Lichtenstein D. Novel approaches to ultrasonography of the lung and pleural space: where are we now? Breathe 2017 Jun;13(2):100-111.*)

QUESTIONS

Q38-1: What is the primary abnormality seen on the chest radiography and ultrasound?

A. Left lower lobe atelectasis
B. Left lower lobe consolidation
C. Left-sided pleural effusion
D. Left lower lobe pulmonary abscess
E. Septic emboli
F. Both A and C
G. Both B and C

Q38-2: Which of the following abnormalities is present in both the chest images shown in Images 38-3A and B?

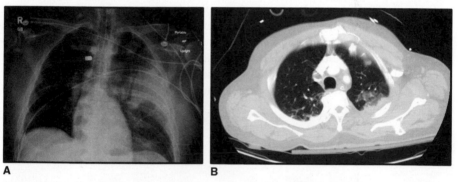

A   **B**

Image 38-3 • A. Chest radiograph for the patient in **Question 38-2**. B. Chest CT image for the patient in **Question 38-2**.

A. Cavitary lung lesions
B. Bronchial wall thickening
C. Endobronchial lesion
D. Air bronchograms
E. Pleural effusions

Q38-3: The patient is presumptively diagnosed with community-acquired pneumonia (CAP). What is the patient's 30-day mortality risk based on the above data using the CURB-65 criteria?

A. 0.7% (CURB-65 score: 0 points)
B. 2.1% (1 point)
C. 9.2% (2 points)
D. 14.5% (3 points)
E. 40% (4 points)

Q38-4: What is the most appropriate antibiotic regimen for the patient?

A. Azithromycin
B. Ceftriaxone
C. Amoxicillin/clavulonate
D. Pipercillin/tazobactam plus tobramycin IV
E. Ceftriaxone plus azithromycin

Q38-5: A 57-year-old woman presents to the ED with 6 days of malaise, fevers, chills, and productive cough. She was recently admitted to the hospital for pain control related to her underlying rheumatoid arthritis, for which she takes chronic glucocorticoids. She was discharged 10 days ago. She smokes 0.5 packs of cigarettes daily. She has diabetes mellitus type 2, which is diet controlled. She is up to date on her vaccinations. She is confused on examination, and her sister provides the history. The patient developed some mild confusion and malaise 6 days ago, with a nonproductive cough. Four days before that, she began experiencing diarrhea, and the cough turned productive. At that point, her primary care doctor started her on augmentin, but she only continued to worsen. Her laboratory test results are notable for a WBC count of 2.1×10^9L with 95% neutrophils, a sodium level of 121 mEq/L, and AST and ALT levels of approximately 200 U/L each (1:1 ratio). Her kidney function is normal. The patient's procalcitonin is positive. She has no prior infectious disease history. The chest radiograph is shown below in Image 38-4.

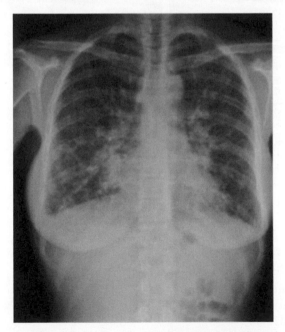

Image 38-4 • Chest radiograph for the patient in **Question 38-5**. (*Reproduced with permission from Tintinalli J, Ma O, Yealy DM, et al: Tintinalli's Emergency Medicine: A Comprehensive Study Guide. 9th ed. New York, NY: McGraw Hill; 2020.*)

What is the likely etiology for the patient's clinical presentation?

A. *Streptococcus pneumoniae*
B. *Mycoplasma pneumoniae*
C. *Legionella pneumophilia*
D. Methicillin-resistant *Staphylococcus aureus*
E. Human metapneumovirus (hMPV)
F. Respiratory syncytial virus (RSV)

Q38-6: Match each patient vignette to the most specific diagnosis.

A. CAP
B. Hospital-acquired pneumonia (HAP)
C. Ventilator-associated pneumonia (VAP)
D. Health care–associated pneumonia

Case 1: A 56-year-old man with a history of COPD presents to the ED with respiratory failure. He is hypoxemic and hypercarbic. His chest radiographon presentation shows some linear interstitial opacities that appear chronic. His pro-calcitonin test is positive. He is treated for COPD exacerbation with steroids, albuterol, and antibiotics. He fails a trial of bi-level positive airway pressure (BiPAP) and requires intubation. He has a history of multiple COPD exacerbations. His microbiology data in the electronic chart show a culture positive for *P. aeruginosa* 3 years ago. Two months ago, he was hospitalized for 4 days for a COPD exacerbation. He lives at home. He does not have any other diagnoses. He does not take chronic steroids or other immunosuppressives. On hospital day 3, his chest radiograph shown in Image 38-5 demonstrates the following:

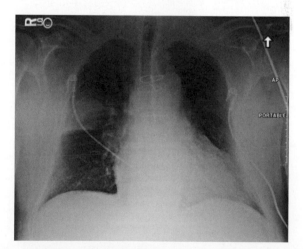

Image 38-5 • Chest radiograph for the patient in **Question 38-6**. (*Reproduced with permission from Mittal S, Singh AP, Gold M, et al: Thoracic Imaging Features of Legionnaire's Disease, Infect Dis Clin North Am 2017 Mar;31(1):43-54.*)

Diagnosis? _____

Case 2: A 44-year-old man with a history of alcoholism was admitted to the ICU 8 days ago for severe alcohol withdrawal with delirium tremens. He required intubation 6 days ago for airway protection in the setting of recurrent seizures. His chest radiograph at the time was clear. He had been maintained on minimal ventilator settings until today. On hospital day 8 the patient developed a right lower lobe infiltrate, with an increased oxygen requirement. Endotracheal suction samples return positive for 3+ white blood cells, it is a sputum sample so they report the quantity of white blood cells using qualitative measures: none, 1+, 2+, 3+, 4+, and many gram-negative bacilli.

Diagnosis? _____

Case 3: A 44-year-old man with a history of alcoholism was admitted to the ICU 8 days ago for severe alcohol withdrawal. He was doing well until yesterday, when he suddenly developed respiratory failure and was intubated. Today, his chest radiograph shows a right lower lobe infiltrate. Endotracheal suction samples return positive for 3+ white blood cells, it is a sputum sample so they report the quantity of white blood cells using qualitative measures: none, 1+, 2+, 3+, 4+, and many gram-negative bacilli.

Diagnosis? _____

ANSWERS

Q38-1: B
Left lower lobe consolidation

Rationale: The chest film shows a focal lobular opacity in the left lower lobe. The infiltrate or opacity is heterogeneous in appearance and does not appear consistent with classic atelectasis. There are no apparent cavities to suggest an abscess, and there are no multiple diffuse opacities as would be seen with septic emboli. In this case, the ultrasound provides very valuable evidence of lung consolidation without evidence of a pleural effusion. In the ultrasound image, the diaphragm is the echogenic curvilinear line on the right side, with the spleen to the right and consolidated lung to the left. Note that the consolidated lung has an appearance very similar to that of the liver or other body tissue. An alternative finding of consolidation on lung ultrasound is shown below, called the "shred sign," in which the lung tissue has the appearance of being shredded into chunks, with areas of hyper- and hypoechogenic tissue (*black arrows* in **Image 38-6A**). Comet tails may also be seen (**Image 38-6B**).

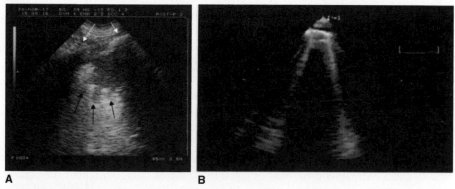

A   **B**

Image 38-6 • A. Shred sign on thoracic ultrasound. (*Reproduced with permission from Lichtenstein D. Novel approaches to ultrasonography of the lung and pleural space: where are we now? Breathe 2017 Jun;13(2):100-111.*) B. **Comet tail sign on thoracic ultrasound indicating the presence of interstitial edema.** (*Reproduced with permission from Agricola E, Bove T, Oppizzi M, et al: "Ultrasound comet-tail images": a marker of pulmonary edema: a comparative study with wedge pressure and extravascular lung water, Chest 2005 May;127(5):1690-1695.*)

Q38-2: D
Air bronchograms

Rationale: The chest radiograph and the corresponding CT scan of the chest demonstrate air bronchograms in a dense left lower lobe infiltrate. Air bronchograms are air-filled bronchi that are made more apparent by surrounding opacification and are commonly seen in lobar pneumonia. These are proximal airways supported by cartilage. This is commonly seen in pulmonary consolidation but may also be seen in atelectasis, pulmonary infarction, pulmonary hemorrhage, cryptogenic or other organizing pneumonia, and severe (alveolar) pulmonary edema.

Q38-3: D
14.5% 30-day mortality

Rationale: The CURB-65 is a clinical prediction tool for patients with CAP to aid in determining the most appropriate patient disposition (outpatient management, inpatient management, ICU admission). The CURB-65 score is based on the following criteria, with one point counted for each question answered "yes": confusion (yes/no); urea (is the BUN greater than 20 mg/dL); respiratory rate (is the RR greater than 30 breaths/min); blood pressure (is the systolic blood pressure less than 90 mm Hg or is the diastolic blood pressure less than 60 mm Hg; if either is positive, the answer is "yes"); and age (is the patient 65 years of age or older?). This patient has a score of 3 (answered "yes" to the BUN, blood pressure, and age questions). This patient has a 14.5% 30-day mortality based on the available studies and should be admitted to the inpatient unit.

Other clinical prediction tools utilized for determining the severity of CAP include the Pneumonia Severity Index (PSI, or PORT score), which is a far more complicated tool that requires additional objective data, including an ABG. This patient's PSI evaluation places him in class V (the higher the class, the higher the risk of mortality), which is associated with a 27% to 29% risk of 30-day mortality. A number of additional tools exist to determine the severity of CAP, with a particular focus on determining which patients should be admitted to the ICU. These include the SMART-COP and SCAP scoring systems. Additionally, the Infectious Disease Society of America (IDSA)/ American Thoracic Society (ATS) have provided guidelines based on major and minor criteria to determine which patients should be admitted to the ICU. Using the IDSA/ATS criteria, this patient has neither of the major criteria (septic shock requiring vasopressor support or need for mechanical ventilation), but he does meet three of the minor criteria: hypotension requiring fluid support, PaO_2/FIO_2 ratio less than or equal to 250, and a BUN level great than or equal to 20 mg/dL, suggesting that the patient has severe CAP and should be admitted to the ICU. Other minor criteria include a respiratory rate of greater than or equal to 30 breaths/min, multilobular infiltrates, altered mental status, WBC count less than 4000 cells/mm³, platelet count less than 100,000 cells/mm³, core temperature less than 36°C. This has become of increasing interest as multiple studies have focused on the use of adjunctive corticosteroids for the treatment of severe CAP, with some studies suggesting a mortality benefit. However, no randomized controlled trial data exist to truly guide their use at this point.

Q38-4: E
Ceftriaxone plus azithromycin

Rationale: The current IDSA guidelines recommend antibiotics based on two primary criteria: (1) treatment setting (outpatient, inpatient, ICU); and (2) risk factors for *Pseudomonas aeruginosa*, *Staphylococcus aureus*, or other commonly resistant organisms. Patients being treated as outpatients should receive treatment with either a macrolide, a doxycycline, or a respiratory fluoroquinolone, depending on prior antibiotic exposure and other comorbidities.

For inpatients, therapy is determined by the presence of risk factors for resistant organisms, namely *P. aeruginosa* and methicillin-resistant *S. aureus* MRSA, though any history of a resistant organism (or significant prior antibiotic exposure) remains a risk factor as well. For inpatients without risk factors for resistant organisms, a combination of third-generation or later beta-lactam plus a macrolide (or a respiratory fluoroquinolone) versus a respiratory fluoroquinolone as monotherapy is recommended. For inpatients with risk factors for *Pseudomonas*, MRSA, or other resistant organisms, regimens should be based on prior antibiotic exposure, prior patient-specific microbiologic data, local resistance patterns, and drug availability.

This patient presents with severe CAP, requiring inpatient admission with consideration for ICU admission. He has no known risk factors for MRSA or *P. aeruginosa*, nor does he have a history of prior resistant organisms. Some risk factors for multidrug-resistant gram-negative bacteria and MRSA include a recent hospitalization that lasted longer than 48 hours (in the prior 90 days), recent antibiotic use (within 90 days), immunosuppression, and severe COPD or bronchiectasis.

Answer (A) would be appropriate for outpatient therapy. Answers (B) and (C) fail to cover atypical organisms and are not recommended as monotherapy for CAP. Likewise, while answer (D) does provide coverage for *Pseudomonas* infection, this patient has no risk factors for a *Pseudomonas* infection, and this regimen again fails to cover atypical organisms. Answer (E) is the most appropriate.

Although there are some data that support the use of combination therapy in severe CAP over the use of monotherapy with a respiratory fluoroquinolone, these data are based on meta-analyses of observational studies performed during the early 1990s, and no randomized control trials have been performed to confirm them. In fact, the CAP-START trial published in 2015 (randomized, cross-over, noninferiority trial) demonstrated similar 90-day mortality outcomes between beta-lactam/macrolide combination therapy and fluoroquinolone monotherapy (though this not an outcome directly examined in the trial). There are observational data to suggest that beta-lactam monotherapy is ineffective for the treatment of CAP requiring inpatient admission (Rodrigo et al).

Q38-5: C
Legionella pneumophilia

Rationale: This patient presents with symptoms of an infection and on chest radiograph has diffusely distributed patchy infiltrates, most consistent with an atypical infection. The patient is an older adult, a chronic smoker, and immunosuppressed (chronic glucocorticoid use, diabetes mellitus), all of which are risk factors associated with Legionnaire disease (*Legionella* pneumonia). The patient is demonstrating classic symptoms of *Legionella* pneumonia with encephalopathy, hyponatremia, gastrointestinal symptoms (namely diarrhea), and elevated transaminases. The positive procalcitonin with normal kidney function suggests a bacterial rather than viral etiology, though the appearance on chest radiography would be consistent with viral pneumonia as well (particularly with her immunosuppression). *Streptococcus* pneumonia can cause all of the same symptoms and may present with a similar radiographic pattern in some instances. However, the patient's symptoms progressed despite what would be appropriate therapy for *S. pneumoniae*. Augmentin does not cover atypical organisms such as *Legionella*.

Although MRSA remains on the differential diagnosis as well, there is nothing in the history, examination, or other objective findings to suggest this as the cause (eg, cavitary lesions). *M. pneumoniae* and *Hemophilus influenza* are the other atypical organisms to consider based on the positive procalcitonin and the chest radiograph; however, given the clinical presentation, *Legionella* must be suspected. *Mycoplasma* pneumonia has been associated with hemolytic anemia, thrombocytopenia, encephalopathy, myocarditis, and Stevens-Johnson syndrome as well as multiple neurologic complications, including cerebellar ataxia. Although *Legionella* pneumonia accounts for less than 1% of all CAP cases, the critical factor here is identifying both the risk factors and common clinical presentation for *Legionella* pneumonia because appropriate therapy with azithromycin would be critical.

L. pneumoniae may be transmitted via aerosolized water droplets, so etiologic clues for possible *Legionella* infection would be exposure to mist machines, evaporative cooling systems, large-scale air-conditioning systems, fountains, pools or hot tubs, and large-scale water systems such as in hotels, conference centers, hospitals, and nursing homes. However, *Legionella* pneumonia may also develop from simple aspiration of oral secretions or from soil exposures. The urine antigen test for *Legionella* is specific to *L. pneumoniae* serogroup 1, and there are several other causes of false-negative results. Additionally, a positive result may indicate a prior infection because patients may shed the antigen for up to 12 months.

Both *Legionella* pneumonia and *Streptococcus* pneumonia may present as a focal lobar, multifocal, or diffuse infection.

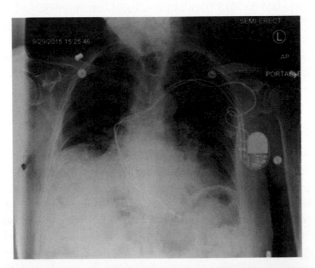

Image 38-7 • A Example of a chest radiograph in *Legionella* pneumonia presenting with multifocal involvement. An example of *Legionella pneumonia* resulting in a multifocal (bibasilar) infection. (*Reproduced with permission from Mittal S, Singh AP, Gold M, et al: Thoracic Imaging Features of Legionnaire's Disease, Infect Dis Clin North Am 2017 Mar;31(1):43-54.*)

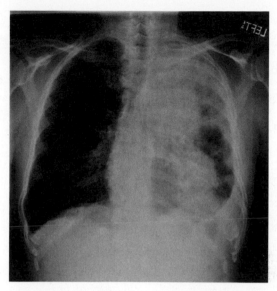

Image 38-8 • Example of a chest radiograph in Legionella pneumonia presenting with focal non-segmental involvement. An example of *Legionella* pneumonia presenting as lobar pneumonia (left upper lobe) with air bronchograms and an associated left-sided pleural effusion. (*Reproduced with permission from Mittal S, Singh AP, Gold M, et al: Thoracic Imaging Features of Legionnaire's Disease, Infect Dis Clin North Am 2017 Mar;31(1):43-54.*)

Although the chest radiographs may provide some insight as to possible organisms or etiologies, keep in mind that a definitive diagnosis requires a positive diagnostic test either based on antigens, PCR, or culture, depending on the organism.

Q38-6: A
CAP

Rationale: Although this patient does meet the 2005 American Thoracic Society/ Infectious Disease Society of America (ATS/IDSA) guideline definition for health care–associated pneumonia (HCAP), the current American Thoracic Society/ Infectious Disease Society of America guidelines, published in 2016, has abandoned this term. The diagnosis of HCAP was initially developed to identify patients at risk for *P. aeruginosa, S. aureus*, of other hospital-acquired or multidrug-resistant organisms to ensure appropriate empiric antibiotics were initiated early. Several studies since 2005 have suggested that this broad definition of HCAP led to overtreatment of many patients, resulting in increased morbidity associated with adverse events, *C. difficile* infection, and increasing antibiotic resistance in the community, among others. The current ATS/IDSA, as well as the combined European/Latin American guidelines, have refined the diagnoses of pneumonia to include CAP, HAP, and VAP. Therefore, despite the patient's hospitalization 2 months ago and his *P. aeruginosa* infection 3 years ago, he would be diagnosed with CAP with risk factors for pathogens resistant to usual treatment. His treatment would likely include antibiotics to cover *P. aeruginosa* as well as MRSA because of his risk factors, including his underlying COPD, recent hospitalization (less than 90 days before this admission and a stay of more than 2 days), and likely recent use of antibiotics (during his recent admission).

Q38-6: C
Ventilator-associated pneumonia (VAP)

Rationale: See discussion below.

Q38-6: B
Hospital-acquired pneumonia (HAP)

Rationale: Regarding **Case 2** and **Case 3**, the ATS/IDSA guidelines provide the following definitions for VAP and HAP:

HAP – A pneumonia that develops at least 48 hours following admission and was not present or suspected at the time of admission

VAP – A pneumonia that develops at least 48 hours following endotracheal intubation and was not present or suspected at the time of the intubation

Technically, VAP is a hospital-acquired pneumonia, though the term *VAP* is more specific. The patient in **Case 2** developed symptoms of pneumonia after 6 days of intubation; therefore, this would be classified as VAP for the sake of treatment. The patient in **Case 3** developed symptoms of pneumonia less than 2 days after intubation. However, the patient had been hospitalized for at least 2 days before the onset of symptoms and thus meets the criteria for HAP.

Although the Centers for Disease Control and Prevention (CDC) has provided additional definitions for ventilator-associated conditions, infection-related ventilator-associated complications, possible VAP, and probable VAP, these terms are not used by the ATS/IDSA, and they should not be used to determine treatment. These definitions were developed for the purposes of surveillance and epidemiologic studies only.

VAP has been more extensively studied than HAP, in large part because of the ability to obtain adequate sputum cultures in the former via either endotracheal suctioning, bronchoalveolar lavage, or a protected brush specimen. The common causes of HAP/VAP, epidemiologic data, risk factors for VAP, risk factors for multidrug-resistant organisms, and treatment recommendations for HAP/VAP are provided below. Treatment for CAP, HAP, and VAP should be based on guideline recommendations, the severity of illness, patient-specific risk factors for gram-negative bacilli, MRSA, and multidrug-resistant organisms, as well as local resistance patterns.

Common risk factors for *Pseudomonas* infection (or other gram-negative bacilli):
- Recent antibiotic use
- Recent hospitalization
- Structural lung disease (COPD, bronchiectasis, cystic fibrosis)
- Immunosuppression
- Chronic alcoholism or chronic aspiration
- Prior microbiological data demonstrating previous infection

Common risk factors for MRSA infection (including community-acquired):

- Recent antibiotic use
- Recent influenza infection
- MRSA colonization or prior infection
- End-stage kidney disease
- Intravenous drug use
- Presence of cavitary lung lesions on chest imaging
- Treatment in an ICU or hospital ward where more than 20% of *S. aureus* organisms are methicillin-resistant or the resistant rates are unknown

Risk factors for multidrug-resistant organisms in HAP:

- IV antibiotics in the past 3 months

Risk factors for multidrug-resistant organisms in VAP:

- IV antibiotic use in previous 3 months
- Concomitant presence of ARDS or septic shock
- More than 5 days of hospitalization before the onset of VAP or initiation of acute kidney replacement therapy before the onset of VAP
- Treatment in an ICU in which more than 10% of gram-negative isolates are multidrug resistant or the resistant rates are unknown

Common pathogens in HAP/VAP include *S. pneumoniae, H. influenzae,* methicillin-sensitive *S. aureus, Enterobacteriaceae, Escherichia coli, Klebsiella pneumoniae, Proteus* spp., *Enterobacter* spp., and *Serratia marcescens* with *P. aeruginosa, S. aureus,* and *Enterobacteriaceae* being the most common causes of VAP.

Multidrug-resistant pathogens causing HAP/VAP include *P. aeruginosa,* MRSA, *Acinetobacter,* extended-spectrum beta-lactamase (ESBL)-positive bacteria, carbapenem-resistant bacteria, *Burkholderia cepacia,* among others.

Risk factors for VAP include aspiration, acid reflux, intubation, prolonged antibiotic use, and prolonged mechanical ventilation. Prevention strategies include elevating the head of the bed, avoiding prolonged courses of antibiotics and intubation, if possible, and avoiding early percutaneous tracheostomy in those patients who do end up intubated.

Treatment for HAP/VAP depends on whether or not the patient has risk factors for resistant gram-negative organisms. In patients without risk factors, piperacillin-tazobactam, cefepime, or levofloxacin are reasonable choices. In patients with risk factors for gram-negative organisms, combination therapy is recommended.

References

Agricola E, Bove T, Oppizzi M, et al. Ultrasound comet-tail images: a marker of pulmonary edema. Chest. 2005;127:1690.

American Thoracic Society, Infectious Diseases Society of America. Guidelines for the management of adults with hospital-acquired, ventilator-associated, and healthcare-associated pneumonia. Am J Respir Crit Care Med. 2005;171:388.

Anderson E, French S, Maloney GE. Community-acquired pneumonia, aspiration pneumonia, and noninfectious pulmonary infiltrates. In: Tintinalli JE, Ma O, Yealy DM, et al, eds. *Tintinalli's Emergency Medicine: A Comprehensive Study Guide*. 9th ed. McGraw-Hill; 2020. https://accessmedicine .mhmedical.com/content.aspx?bookid=2353&sectionid=219642145

Chalmers JD, Rother C, Salih W, Ewig S. Healthcare-associated pneumonia does not accurately identify potentially resistant pathogens: a systematic review and meta-analysis. Clin Infect Dis. 2014;58:330.

Hoan L, Hang LM, Hong DTT, et al. A 69-year-old man with chronic cough and recurrent pneumonia. Chest. 2020;158:e283.

Kalil AC, Metersky ML, Klompas M, et al. Management of adults with hospital-acquired and ventilator-associated pneumonia: 2016 clinical practice guidelines by the Infectious Diseases Society of America and the American Thoracic Society. Clin Infect Dis. 2016;63:e61.

Klompas M. Complications of mechanical ventilation—the CDC's new surveillance paradigm. N Engl J Med. 2013;368:1472.

Lichtenstein D. Novel approaches to ultrasonography of the lung and pleural space: where are we now? Breathe. 2017;13:100.

Magiorakos AP, Srinivasan A, Carey RB, et al. Multidrug-resistant, extensively drug-resistant and pandrug-resistant bacteria: an international expert proposal for interim standard definitions for acquired resistance. Clin Microbiol Infect. 2012;18:268.

Mandell, LA, Wunderink, RG, Anzueto, A, et al. Infectious Diseases Society of America/American Thoracic Society consensus guidelines on the management of community-acquired pneumonia in adults. Clin Infect Dis. 2007;44 (Supp 2):S27-S72, https://doi.org/10.1086/511159.

Mittal S, Singh AP, Gold M, Leung AN, Haramati LB, Katz DS. Thoracic imaging features of legionnaire's disease. Infect Dis Clin N Am. 2017;31:43.

Postma DF, van Werkhoven CH, van Elden LJ, et al; CAP-START Study Group. Antibiotic treatment strategies for community-acquired pneumonia in adults. N Engl J Med. 2015;372:1312.

Rodrigo C, Mckeever TM, Woodhead M, Lim WS; British Thoracic Society. Single versus combination antibiotic therapy in adults hospitalised with community acquired pneumonia. Thorax. 2013;68:493.

Stout JE, Yu VL. Legionellosis. N Engl J Med. 1997;337:682.

Torres A, Niederman MS, Chastre J, et al. International ERS/ESICM/ESCMID/ALAT guidelines for the management of hospital-acquired pneumonia and ventilator-associated pneumonia: guidelines for the management of hospital-acquired pneumonia (HAP)/ventilator-associated pneumonia (VAP) of the European Respiratory Society (ERS), European Society of Intensive Care Medicine (ESICM), European Society of Clinical Microbiology and Infectious Diseases (ESCMID) and Asociación Latinoamericana del Tórax (ALAT). Eur Respir J. 2017;50.

CASE 39

A 51-year-old investment banker presents to the clinic because of issues with fatigue and dyspnea on exertion. He has a history of hypertension and is currently taking amlodipine 10 mg daily. He had asthma as a child, but this resolved during adolescence. He is a very active individual, exercising three to five times a week. He is married with two children, is a never-smoker, and does not drink alcohol or use illicit drugs. He has worked in the banking industry since graduating from business school approximately 25 years ago. He first noticed some mild dyspnea on exertion several months ago, which was only noticeable when he was at peak exercise. This was associated with a mild, nonproductive cough. He denies any fevers, chills, wheezing, pleuritic chest pain, substernal chest pain, diaphoresis, nausea, emesis, or changes in bowel habits. The symptoms have progressively worsened over the last 6 months, and he now becomes short of breath with only mild exertion. His exercise tolerance is significantly diminished as well. The patient's vital signs are T 36.5°C, HR 101, BP 120/80, RR 15, oxygen saturation 90% on room air at rest.

QUESTIONS

Q39-1: The patient has mild, symmetric lower extremity edema that is pitting on examination. His brain (B-type) natriuretic peptide (BNP) is 88 pg/mL (normal: 0-100). His chest radiograph is shown in Image 39-1.

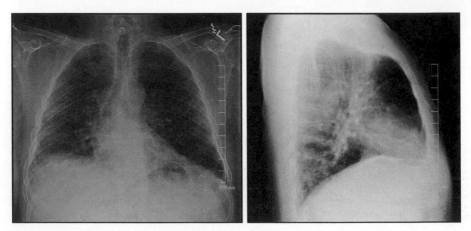

Image 39-1 • Chest radiographs (PA and lateral) for the patient in **Question 39-1**.

Additional laboratory testing is as follows:

Hemoglobin (Hgb):	14.0 g/dL
WBC:	6.0/µL
Creatinine (cr):	1.0 mg/dL
Rheumatoid factor (Rf):	<20 U/mL
ANA:	Negative
ANCA:	Negative

What is the most likely cause for this patient's worsening dyspnea on exertion?

A. Pulmonary arterial hypertension
B. Cardiogenic pulmonary edema
C. Asthma
D. Centrilobular chronic obstructive pulmonary disease (COPD)
E. Pulmonary fibrosis
F. Lobar pneumonia

Q39-2: What would you expect to hear on lung examination in a patient with pulmonary fibrosis?

A. Vesicular
B. Rhonchus
C. Bronchial
D. Fine crackles
E. Coarse crackles

Q39-3: What study would you perform next in this patient to further confirm your suspicion?

A. Echocardiogram
B. Flexible bronchoscopy
C. CT scan of the chest with IV contrast
D. CT scan of the chest without IV contrast
E. Barium swallow

Q39-4: Which CT image (Images 39-2 to 39-5) would you expect to find in this patient?

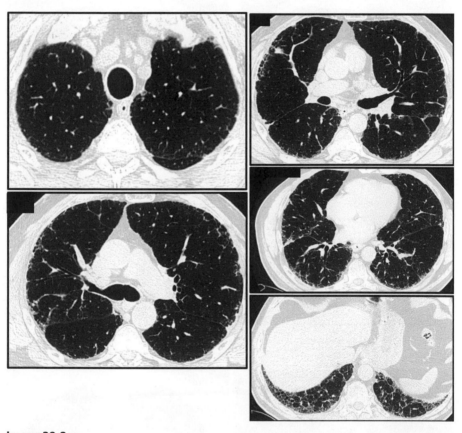

Image 39-2 •

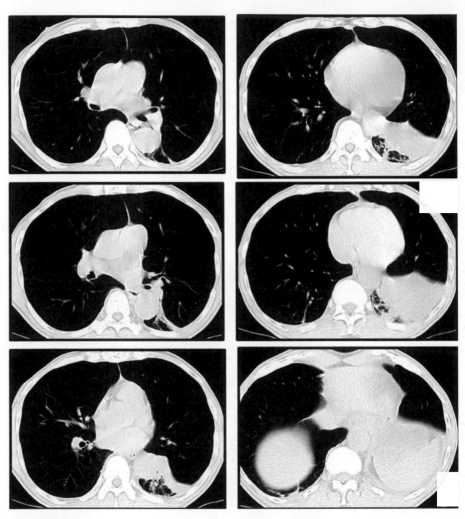

Image 39-3 •

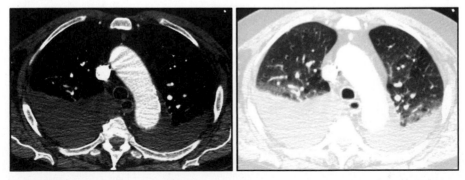

Image 39-4 •

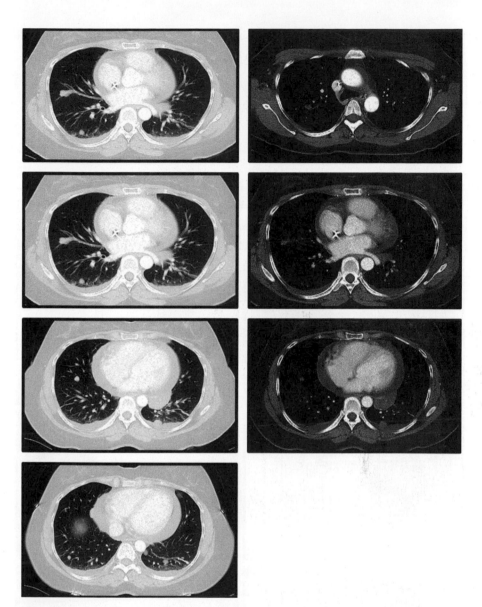

Image 39-5 •

Q39-5: What pulmonary function testing (PFT) would you expect from this patient?

	A	B	C	D	E
FEV1 (% predicted)	80	50	65	40	90
FVC (% predicted)	90	80	70	55	100
Ratio	80	60	95	85	90
TLC (% predicted)	105	80	70	60	95
RV (% predicted)	85	130	30	40	100
DLCO (% predicted)	95	75	80	30	20

Q39-6: Which medication has been shown to impact mortality in patients with IPF in initial clinical trials?

A. Prednisone
B. Azathioprine
C. *N*-acetylcysteine (NAC)
D. Nintedanib
E. Pirfenidone
F. Cyclophosphamide

Q39-7: Identify each image as A: consistent with UIP; B: probable UIP; C: indeterminate for UIP; D: alternate diagnosis.

1.

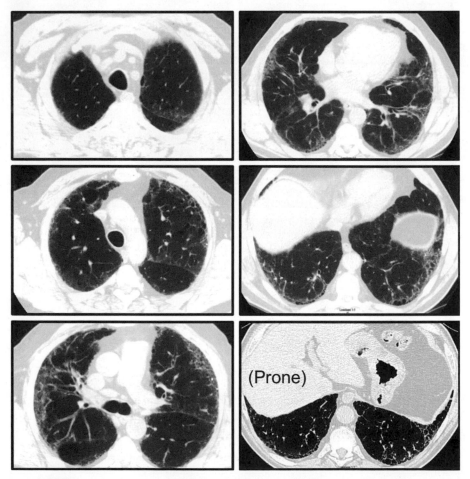

Image 39-6 •

2.

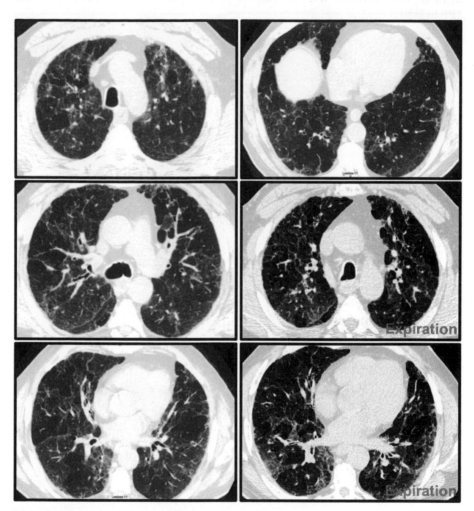

Image 39-7 •

3.

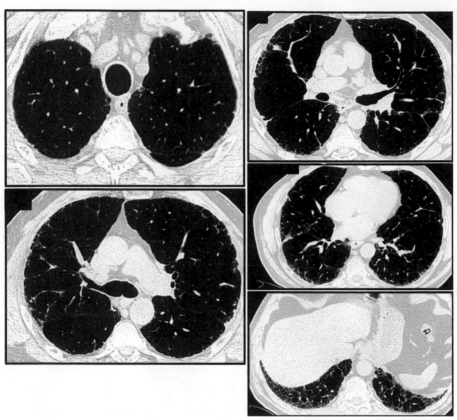

Image 39-8 •

ANSWERS

Q39-1: E
Pulmonary fibrosis

Rationale: The chest radiograph demonstrates diffuse bilateral interstitial opacities casting a net-like appearance (often termed "reticular") as well as slight flattening of the diaphragms. This is most consistent with pulmonary fibrosis. The lung parenchyma is typically normal in pulmonary arterial hypertension (World Health Organization [WHO] group 1), with prominence of the pulmonary arteries. In asthma, the chest radiograph may show mild hyperinflation but not reticular opacities. Centrilobular COPD is usually marked by hyperinflation and flattening of the diaphragms, in addition to possible loss of lung markings, most commonly in the upper lobes. Lobar pneumonia presents with lobar consolidation and associated air bronchograms. Cardiogenic pulmonary edema can have a similar appearance, but the patient's normal BNP, cardiac silhouette, and the lack of Kerley B lines on the chest radiograph argue against this.

Q39-2: D
Fine crackles

Rationale: Fine crackles would be typical of pulmonary fibrosis.

Q39-3: D
CT scan of the chest without IV contrast

Rationale: High-resolution CT (HRCT) radiography has revolutionized the diagnosis of interstitial lung diseases (ILDs), including pulmonary fibrosis. HRCT is very useful in discriminating between potential causes of pulmonary fibrosis, in particular for idiopathic pulmonary fibrosis (IPF). Contrast is not needed for these studies and can obscure the air trapping or hyperinflation seen in some airway-centric ILDs, such as hypersensitivity pneumonitis. An echocardiogram, while useful, would not provide additional information about the patient's lung disease outside of the development of secondary pulmonary hypertension. A barium swallow could also be useful in this patient because chronic aspiration may lead to the development of pulmonary fibrosis; however, a CT scan to better characterize the pulmonary fibrosis would be more useful. Similarly, a flexible bronchoscopy may be useful to identify the cause of the patient's fibrosis if the patient's CT scan is not consistent with IPF because it may identify other potential causes (eg, sarcoidosis).

Q39-4: Image 39-2

Rationale: Image 39-2 is consistent with a diagnosis of IPF, demonstrating peripheral subpleural reticular opacities (interlobular septal thickening), traction bronchiectasis, and subpleural honeycombing. Given the patient's history, laboratory testing, and chest imaging, this makes the most sense. **Image 39-3** demonstrates left lower lobe collapse or atelectasis and emphysema. **Image 39-4** demonstrates bilateral pleural effusions, while **Image 39-5** demonstrates multiple bilateral pulmonary nodules.

Q39-5: Column D

Rationale: This patient has IPF, a restrictive lung disease associated with a reduction in both FEV1 and FVC (as well as in measured lung volumes such as TLC [total lung capacity] and RV [residual volume]), a normal FEV1/FVC ratio, and a reduction in the diffusing capacity of carbon monoxide (DLCO), a surrogate for how well oxygen diffuses from the alveoli to blood. The PFT values from column A are consistent with a healthy patient or perhaps a patient with asthma without active symptoms. Column B represents the PFTs of a patient with COPD, with a reduction in FEV1 greater than FVC consistent with airflow obstruction, an increased residual volume consistent with air trapping, and a slightly reduced DLCO. Column C is consistent with restriction as well; however, the reduction in the residual volume is out of proportion to the reduction in the lung volumes, and the DLCO is normal. This is consistent with extrathoracic restriction from obesity. Column E shows normal airflow and lung volumes with a drastically reduced DLCO, which is classic for pulmonary arterial hypertension. Column D shows the expected pattern for IPF, with significant reductions in FEV1, FVC, TLC, and RV (all in relative proportion), a normal FEV1/FVC ratio, and a significant reduction in DLCO.

Q39-6: E
Pirfenidone

Rationale: In addition to showing promise in slowing disease progression in IPF, pirfenidone has shown a potential reduction in all-cause and IPF-related mortality in patients with mild-to-moderate IPF. However, note that these results are limited to a select population of patients with IPF with mild-to-moderate reductions in lung volumes and DLCO and are not generalizable to all patients with IPF, particularly those with advanced disease. All the other listed therapies have shown no mortality benefit in IPF, though nintedanib has demonstrated potential in slowing disease progression.

Q39-7: Image 39-6: B
Probable UIP

Rationale: There are subpleural reticular changes with the suggestion of early honeycombing at the bases and some traction bronchiectasis, but there are also some areas of ground-glass opacities.

Image 39-7: D
Alternate diagnosis

Rationale: Given the lack of honeycombing, the marked mosaic attenuation seen on the expiratory images, and the predominant ground-glass opacities seen throughout both lungs, this set of images suggests a diagnosis other than UIP.

Image 39-8: A
UIP

Rationale: This set of images shows traction bronchiectasis, subpleural reticular changes, and honeycombing at the bases. To definitely diagnosis UIP on an HRCT of the chest, honeycombing must be present. UIP is generally basilar predominant, though upper lobe involvement may occur. Ground-glass opacities are not a common finding.

During the evaluation of a patient with possible pulmonary fibrosis, HRCT of the chest is of significant value. Based on the ATS guidelines, HRCT of the chest can be separated into four different patterns or categories when evaluating for pulmonary fibrosis: UIP, probable UIP, indeterminate for UIP, and alternative diagnosis suggested. See the table in **Image 39-9**.

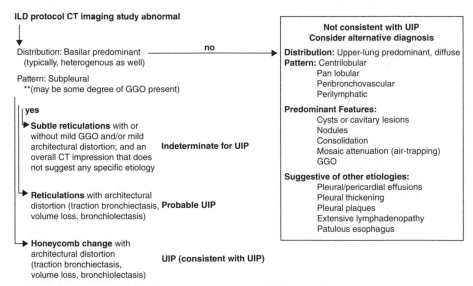

Image 39-9 • Algorithm for clinical and radiographic diagnosis of IPF. (*Developed based on the figures and data from Raghu G, Remy-Jardin M, Myers JL, et al: Diagnosis of Idiopathic Pulmonary Fibrosis. An Official ATS/ERS/JRS/ALAT Clinical Practice Guideline, Am J Respir Crit Care Med 2018 Sep 1;198(5):e44-e68.*)

IPF is diagnosed if the following criteria are fulfilled:

1. Other causes of ILDs are excluded
   And the patient has either a
2. UIP pattern on HRCT of the chest or
3. Lung biopsy findings and HRCT of the chest findings in specific combinations suggestive of IPF

IPF is marked by progressive scarring of the lungs. The disease results in respiratory failure and death, with a median survival of 2 to 5 years from diagnosis.

Patients with IPF are typically over 60 years old and present with shortness of breath and a dry cough. A physical examination may reveal fine bibasilar inspiratory crackles, and a chest radiograph may show signs of fibrosis, or early on, it may be normal.

Epidemiologic data suggest IPF is more common in men than in women, though the exact incidence and prevalence of the disease has been difficult to determine given the limited available data and recent changes to diagnostic criteria.

Possible risk factors for IPF include age, male sex assigned at birth, a history of smoking, acid reflux, and environmental exposures (metal particulate, wood dust). Familial cases have also been observed.

When evaluating a patient for idiopathic pulmonary fibrosis, it is important to rule out other causes of ILD, such as connective tissue diseases, hypersensitivity pneumonitis, organizing pneumonia, eosinophilic pneumonia, respiratory bronchiolitis-associated ILD, and nonspecific interstitial pneumonia, among others. Laboratory data that may be useful in evaluating for these alternative diagnoses include a C-reactive protein, erythrocyte sedimentation rate, antinuclear antibodies, rheumatoid factor, anticyclic citrullinated peptide, and a myositis panel. Other specific rheumatologic tests may be obtained as indicated by the patient's history and physical. There is no specific laboratory test for idiopathic pulmonary fibrosis.

Bronchoalveolar lavage is not required in the evaluation of IPF unless alternative diagnoses are being considered (ie, infection, sarcoidosis).

Early on, imaging may only show subtle changes, with chest radiographs showing peripheral, predominantly lower lobe, reticular opacities. Although chest radiographs may be normal early on in the disease, HRCT of the chest generally reveals evidence of fibrosis. HRCT chest findings are as previously discussed.

Surgical lung biopsies do play a role in evaluating for IPF, particularly when imaging shows probable, indeterminate, or alternate diagnosis patterns, but they are no longer required to formalize a diagnosis of IPF.

Nintedanib, a tyrosine kinase inhibitor, and pirfenidone, an antifibrotic, are recommended for the treatment of IPF. Gastrointestinal side effects are common with both of these medications. Pirfenidone has also been associated with photosensitivity. Given the high prevalence of acid reflux in patients with IPF, treatment with an antacid is recommended. Patients should also be on supplemental oxygen if needed. They should also stop smoking and be vaccinated against respiratory diseases.

References

Canestaro WJ, Forrester SH, Raghu G, et al. Drug Treatment of idiopathic pulmonary fibrosis: systematic review and network meta-analysis. Chest. 2016;149:756.

Costabel U, Albera C, Glassberg MK, et al. Effect of pirfenidone in patients with more advanced idiopathic pulmonary fibrosis. Respir Res. 2019;20:55.

Faghu G, Rochwerg B, Zhang Y, et al. An official ATS/ERS/JRS/ALAT clinical practice guideline: treatment of idiopathic pulmonary fibrosis. Am J Respir Crit Care Med. 2015;192:e3.

Harari S, Caminati A, Poletti V, et al. A real-life multicenter national study on nintedanib in severe idiopathic pulmonary fibrosis. Respiration. 2018;95:433.

King TE Jr, Bradford WZ, Castro-Bernardini S, et al. A phase 3 trial of pirfenidone in patients with idiopathic pulmonary fibrosis. N Engl J Med. 2014;370:2083.

King TE Jr, Pardo A, Selman M. Idiopathic pulmonary fibrosis. Lancet. 2011;378:1949.

Laurenson S, Sidhu R, Goodall M, Adler AI. NICE guidance on nintedanib for treating idiopathic pulmonary fibrosis. Lancet Respir Med. 2016;4:176.

Lynch DA, Godwin JD, Safrin S, et al. High-resolution computed tomography in idiopathic pulmonary fibrosis: diagnosis and prognosis. Am J Respir Crit Care Med. 2005;172:488.

Nathan SD, Albera C, Bradford WZ, et al. Effect of pirfenidone on mortality: pooled analyses and meta-analyses of clinical trials in idiopathic pulmonary fibrosis. Lancet Respir Med. 2017;5:33.

Noble PW, Albera C, Bradford WZ, et al. Pirfenidone in patients with idiopathic pulmonary fibrosis (CAPACITY): two randomised trials. Lancet 2011;377:1760.

Noble PW, Albera C, Bradford WZ, et al. Pirfenidone for idiopathic pulmonary fibrosis: analysis of pooled data from three multinational phase 3 trials. Eur Respir J. 2016;47:243.

Raghu G, Remy-Jardin M, Myers JL, et al. Diagnosis of idiopathic pulmonary fibrosis: an official ATS/ERS/JRS/ALAT clinical practice guidelines: executive summary. Am J Respir Crit Care Med. 2018;198:563.

Raghu G, Rochwerg B, Zhang Y, et al. An Official ATS/ERS/JRS/ALAT Clinical Practice Guideline: Treatment of Idiopathic Pulmonary Fibrosis. An Update of the 2011 Clinical Practice Guideline. Am J Respir Crit Care Med. 2015;192:e3.

Richeldi L, Collard HR, Jones MG. Idiopathic pulmonary fibrosis. Lancet. 2017.

Tighe RM, Meltzer EB, Noble PW. Idiopathic pulmonary fibrosis. In: Grippi MA, Elias JA, Fishman JA, et al, eds. *Fishman's Pulmonary Diseases and Disorders.* 5th ed. McGraw-Hill; 2015. https://accessmedicine.mhmedical.com/content.aspx?bookid=1344&sectionid=81190295

Tzouvelekis A, Ntolios P, Karampitsakos T, et al. Safety and efficacy of pirfenidone in severe Idiopathic Pulmonary Fibrosis: a real-world observational study. Pulm Pharmacol Ther. 2017;46:48.

Weill D, Benden C, Corris PA, et al. A consensus document for the selection of lung transplant candidates: 2014—an update from the Pulmonary Transplantation Council of the International Society for Heart and Lung Transplantation. J Heart Lung Transplant. 2015;34:1.

Wuyts WA, Kolb M, Stowasser S, et al. First data on efficacy and safety of nintedanib in patients with idiopathic pulmonary fibrosis and forced vital capacity of ≤50 % of predicted value. Lung. 2016; 194:739.

CASE 40

A 44-year-old man with a history of alcoholism presents to the ED. He is confused and unable to provide history. He is hypoxemic and coughing frequently. His sputum is thick, putrid, and blood-tinged. On examination, he has coarse, bronchial breath sounds over the left upper lung fields, as well as dullness to percussion in this area. His vital signs are T 38.1°C, HR 133, BP 90/61, RR 25, oxygen saturation 88% on 4 L/min supplement O$_2$ via nasal cannula. His chest radiograph is shown in Image 40-1.

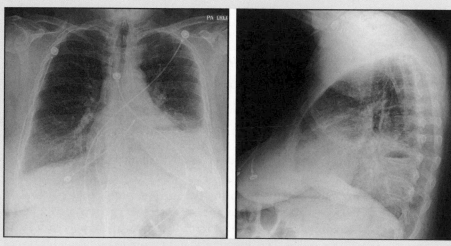

Image 40-1 • Chest radiograph (PA and lateral) for the patient in **Question 40-1**.

QUESTIONS

Q40-1: How would you describe the abnormalities in the chest imaging shown in Image 40-1? (Select ALL that may apply.)

A. Cystic lung lesion
B. Cavitary lung lesion
C. Pleural plaques and pericardial effusion.
D. Hilar adenopathy
E. Hydropneumothorax

Q40-2: The patient is intubated, and a sputum culture demonstrates 3+ gram-negative rods and numerous polymorphonuclear cells. Which antibiotic course would be most appropriate?

A. Ceftriaxone and azithromycin
B. Ceftriaxone
C. Ampicillin-sulbactam
D. Levofloxacin
E. Gentamicin

Q40-3: What is NOT a risk factor for bacterial aspiration pneumonia?

A. Recent cerebrovascular accident (stroke)
B. Scleroderma
C. Drug use
D. Older age
E. Smoking tobacco use
F. Gastroesophageal reflux disease on proton pump inhibitor (PPI) therapy

Q40-4: A 66-year-old man presents to the ED in respiratory failure following a witnessed aspiration event during an upper endoscopy approximately 2 hours ago. He progressively worsened in the postprocedure area, and Emergency Medical Services (EMS) was called. The patient was undergoing evaluation for severe reflux disease. He had stopped his PPI therapy several days ago to complete a 24-hour manometry and pH study. He had been NPO for 12 hours before the procedure. There were no apparent complications during the procedure. The patient is severely hypoxemic on arrival and intubated immediately. His PaO_2/FIO_2 ratio is 75. His chest radiograph is shown in Image 40-2.

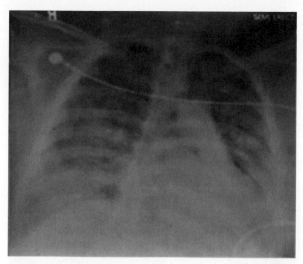

Image 40-2 • Chest radiograph (AP) for the patient in **Question 40-4**. (*Reproduced with permission from Kashif M, Patel R, Bajantri B, et al: Legionella pneumonia associated with severe acute respiratory distress syndrome and diffuse alveolar hemorrhage - A rare association, Respir Med Case Rep 2017 Mar 14;21:7-11.*)

How would you describe the abnormalities seen in the radiograph?

A. Linear interstitial opacities

B. Reticulonodular interstitial opacities

C. Multifocal opacities

D. Diffuse alveolar infiltrates

E. Atelectasis

Q40-5: A 34-year-old woman presents with respiratory distress in the setting of fevers, chills, and rigors. She is disheveled and somewhat cachectic. She is encephalopathic and unable to provide a history. EMS found the patient down on the sidewalk. She received IV fluids and naloxone en route to the hospital with considerable improvement in her level of consciousness, though she remains confused. She requires 4 L of oxygen via NC to maintain oxygen saturation above 90%. She is febrile to 101.4°F and has a significant leukocytosis. Her chest radiograph and an abnormal finding on skin examination are shown in Images 40-3 and 40-4 below. Palpation of the great toe is not painful, and the erythematous lesions are blanching.

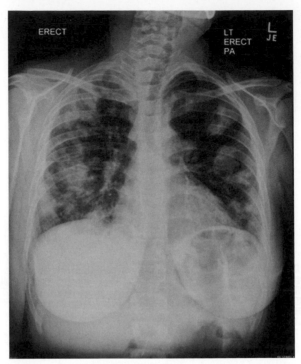

Image 40-3 • Chest radiograph (AP) for the patient in **Question 40-5**. (*Reproduced with permission from Tintinalli J, Ma O, Yealy DM, et al: Tintinalli's Emergency Medicine: A Comprehensive Study Guide. 9th ed. New York, NY: McGraw Hill; 2020.*)

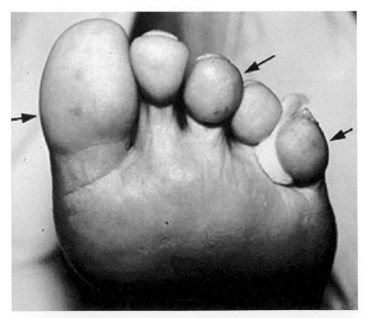

Image 40-4 • Examples of the ophthalmologic and dermatologic abnormalities seen on physical examination of the patient in **Question 40-5**. (*Reproduced with permission from Southwick FS: Infectious Diseases: A Clinical Short Course, 4th ed. New York, NY: McGraw Hill; 2020.*)

How would you describe the abnormalities on the patient's chest radiograph?

A. Reticulonodular interstitial opacities
B. Cystic lung lesions
C. Multiple cavitary nodules
D. Miliary nodular opacities
E. Focal consolidation

Q40-6: Given the patient's objective findings, which diagnosis is most likely?

A. Metastatic malignancy with numerous pulmonary metastases
B. Septic emboli secondary to infective endocarditis
C. Legionnaire disease
D. *Pneumocystis carinii* pneumonia (PCP)
E. Pulmonary embolism

Q40-7: What other condition is commonly associated with septic pulmonary emboli?

A. Aortic valve endocarditis
B. Infective aortitis
C. Infected pacemaker lead
D. Infected arterial line

ANSWERS

Q40-1: B and/or E
Cavitary lung lesion and/or Hydropneumothorax

Rationale: The chest radiographs are bit complicated in this case. The cardiac and mediastinal contours are within normal limits overall, although the heart size is borderline enlarged. There is opacification in the left lower lobe with what appears to be a clear air-fluid level without a meniscus sign present. This may represent a cavitary lung lesions or pulmonary abscess, or alternative may represent a hydropneumothorax with surround atelectasis. The air-fluid level is more clearly seen on the lateral film as a likely cavitary lung lesion. The lateral film also does not clearly demonstrate a meniscus sign to suggest that fluid collection is definitively present, although a fluid collection (hydropneumothorax) or empyema cannot be ruled out based on the chest radiographs alone. A chest CT scan is recommended (although thoracic ultrasound should also be performed)

The patient's chest CT images are shown in **Image 40-5** below. Here, we can see a small amount of layering pleural fluid on the more cranial images. However, in the left lower lobe there is a air-fluid level present which may represent with a loculated hydropneumothorax or a pulmonary absccess.

This patient underwent a contrasted CT scan as well as thoracic ultrasound and was diagnosed with a pulmonary abscess, as there was no significant fluid collection identified and there was predominantly consolidated lung seen. Differentiating between a pulmonary abscess (cavitary pneumonia) and an empyema is critical, as the management is quite different. On plain radiographs, pulmonary abscesses are typically round in shape, and form an acute angle with the chest wall or costal surfaces, whereas empyemas have a more lentiform shape (ie, convex on both sides) that is often referred to as the "split pleura" sign. Pulmonary abscess and empyema as more easily diffferentiated on CT imaging. Pulmonary abscess may be identified by the "claw sign" (**Image 40-5**). The claw sign helps to determine the origin of a mass of lesion. Here, as one moves from cranial to caudal slices of the CT, there is a "claw" of parenchyema that appears to grasp the opacity which seems to arise from the parenchyma. Additionally, in pulmonary abscess, the bronchovascular structures are absent within the abscess, whereas in an empyema, the bronchovascular structures are still seen in the atelectatic lung. In this patient, note that complete loss of bronchovascular structures in the mass. Empyema will be covered in future cases.

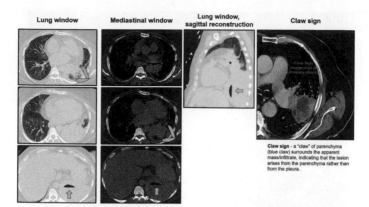

| Lung window | Mediastinal window | Lung window, sagittal reconstruction | Claw sign |

Claw sign - a "claw" of parenchyma (blue claw) surrounds the apparent mass/infiltrate, indicating that the lesion arises from the parenchyma rather than from the pleura.

Image 40-5 • Chest CT images for the patient in **Question 40-1**, demonstrating a loss of bronchovascular markings indicating a lack of significant atelectasis and, more caudally, there is the presence of the "claw" sign, indicating that the lesion appears to arise from the parenchyma rather than as result of empyema. However, a pulmonary abscess and empyema may both be present, resulting from a communication between the airways and pleural space (bronchopleural fistula). A contrasted chest CT (for pleural enhancement) and thoracic ultrasound are often helpful in these cases..

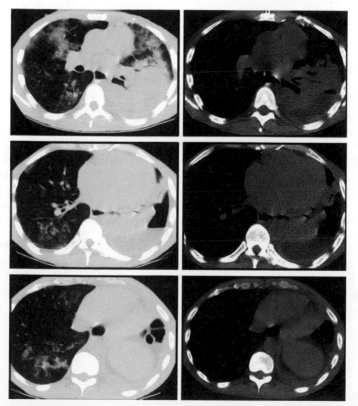

Image 40-6 • Empyema (seen in **Images 40-3** and **40-4**). Note here that the empyema (with air present laterally in **Image 40-3**) compressed the surrounding lung (yielding compressive atelectasis).

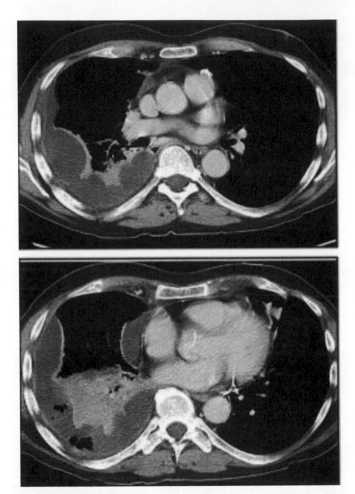

Image 40-7 • Although the visceral and parietal pleura cannot be separated on CT of a normal subject, patients with empyema will often have the "split pleura" sign (well seen in **Image 40-4**), where the fluid separating the visceral and parietal pleura allows for clear visualization of the two surfaces (better visualized on mediastinal windows). Empyemas often form obtuse angles as they connect with the parietal pleural surface rather than the acute angles often seen in isolated cavitary lesions.

As for the other answer choices, a cystic lung lesion should be thin walled rather than thick walled. Pleural plaques are typically calcified and solid throughout, and this is clearly not atelectasis. These cavitary lesions, when associated with a possible infection, are termed *pulmonary abscesses*.

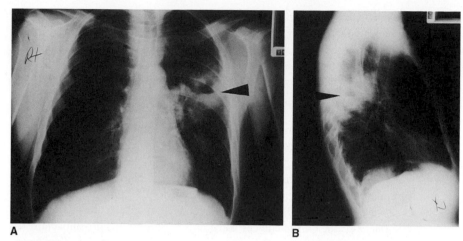

Image 40-8A and B • An example of a pulmonary abscess with an air-fluid level in the left upper lung field. Note the clear air-fluid level with the lack of a meniscus sign. (*Reproduced with permission from Karcic AA, Karcic E. Lung abscess, J Emerg Med 2001 Feb;20(2):165-166.*)

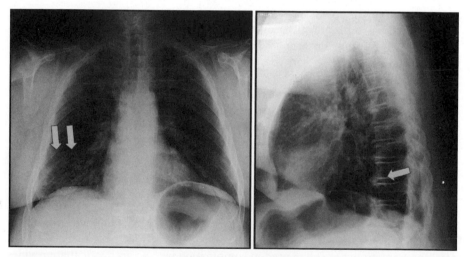

Image 40-9 • Simple aspiration pneumonia without evidence of abscess formation. Note that alveolar infiltrate in the right middle and lower lobes (gray arrows). The right middle lobe and the bilateral lower lobes are most commonly involved in aspiration events.

Q40-2: C
Ampicillin-sulbactam

Rationale: The patient presents with a pulmonary abscess likely secondary to aspiration. His history of alcoholism places him at risk for possible aspiration. The putrid sputum is concerning for possible anaerobic organisms, while the thick, blood-tinged sputum could be concerning for possible *Klebsiella pneumoniae* infection, as this case has the classic "currant jelly" appearance of sputum in alcoholics. The most common organisms involved in aspiration pneumonia that lead to the formation of pulmonary abscess are anaerobic organisms, though other culprits include *Staphylococcus aureus*, *K. pneumoniae*, *Pseudomonas aeruginosa*, *Nocardia asteroids*, *Actinomyces* species, *Mycobacterium* (eg, *M. tuberculosis*, *M. avium* complex), and fungi (eg, *Aspergillus* species), among others.

The most commonly involved anaerobes include *Bacteroides fragilis*, *Prevotella*, *Fusobacterium nucleatum*, *Peptostreptococcus*, *Clostridium* species, and *Eubacterium* species.

Given the high likelihood that the patient may have an anaerobic infection, appropriate empiric antibiotic coverage should include coverage for the appropriate organisms, which in this case would include community-acquired organisms, anaerobic organisms, and *K. pneumoniae*. Of the choices listed above, only ampicillin-sulbactam has proven in vivo anaerobic activity (with the exception of *C. difficile*) as well as coverage of gram-negative bacilli. Azithromycin has some in vitro activity against most anaerobes, but it is not sufficient anaerobic coverage. Ceftriaxone, a third-generation cephalosporin, has limited in vitro activity as well, so it is insufficient as a monotherapy or in combination with azithromycin. Some of the second-generation cephalosporins have better anaerobic activity, including cefoxitin. The aminoglycosides also have extremely limited activity against anaerobic organisms, as does aztreonam (gram-negative aerobic organisms only), trimethoprim/sulfamethoxazole, and tetracycline. And while moxifloxacin has good anaerobic coverage, levofloxacin does not have the same anaerobic activity and would also be insufficient.

Antibiotics with good anaerobic coverage include clindamycin, moxifloxacin, metronidazole, the beta-lactam/beta-lactamase inhibitor combinations (ticarcillin–clavulanate, ampicillin–sulbactam, amoxicillin–clavulanate, piperacillin–tazobactam), the carbapenems (meropenem and imipenem), and the second-generation cephalosporins. Although clindamycin and metronidazole have good anaerobic coverage, they have no activity against gram-negative aerobic organisms (or gram-positive aerobic organisms in the case of metronidazole). More importantly, studies examining the utility of metronidazole for anaerobic lung abscesses have shown very poor efficacy, thought to be due to the poor activity against anaerobic streptococci; however, it may still be used in simple bacterial aspiration pneumonia without abscess. Therefore, these antibiotics are often used in combination with an antibiotic that provides appropriate gram-positive/negative aerobic coverages (eg, ceftriaxone/clindamycin).

Although simple bacterial aspiration pneumonia may be treated for 5 to 10 days with appropriate antibiotics, a lung abscess requires prolonged treatment. Empiric therapy should be continued until culture data are available to allow for narrowing. The duration of therapy is typically in the range of 4 to 6 weeks, but it may also be dependent on response to therapy. Once patients show clinical improvement (eg, improved sputum odor, defervescence), they may be switched from parental therapy to oral therapy, with amoxicillin–clavulanate or moxifloxacin used most often. Surgery is rarely indicated unless there is failure to respond to therapy or there is uncertainty regarding the diagnosis. Percutaneous drainage is an alternative to operative intervention in some patients, but it is associated with considerable complications, including the potential for seeding the pleural space and causing empyema.

Aspiration pneumonia or lung abscesses occurring in patients during prolonged hospitalization are more likely to involve gram-negative aerobic and nosocomial organisms, and they should be treated as such. Luckily, many of the options for the treatment of anaerobic infections are also appropriate for hospital-acquired pneumonia (ie, piperacillin–tazobactam, meropenem).

Q40-3: E
Smoking

Rationale: All the remaining conditions have been associated with an increased risk of aspiration. Any neurologic condition that reduces consciousness or impacts the function of swallowing (eg, stroke, Parkinson disease) is associated with an increased risk of aspiration. Similarly, conditions that directly affect the esophagus (such as scleroderma causing achalasia) can increase the risk of aspiration. Conditions that reduce consciousness (drug use, alcohol use, general anesthesia, antipsychotic medications) increase the risk of aspiration as well. Tube feeding, the use of nasogastric tubes, and endotracheal intubation are also risk factors. The use of PPIs has been associated with an increased risk of bacterial aspiration as opposed to chemical aspiration in patients with GERD, which is independently associated with an increased risk of aspiration. Other factors include older age, near drowning, protracted vomiting, and recent procedures that disrupt glottis closure, such as endoscopy and bronchoscopy.

Q40-4: D
Diffuse alveolar infiltrate

Rationale: This is a classic presentation of acute chemical pneumonitis resulting from the aspiration of gastric acid with a pH of less than 2.5. He had stopped his GERD therapy several days ago in preparation for a procedure, and during the esophagogastroduodenoscopy, with the scope in place and the patient sedated, the patient likely experienced a massive chemical aspiration resulting in severe pneumonitis. This is also termed *Mendelson syndrome*. The changes in chemical pneumonitis occur much more rapidly than in bacterial aspiration. Treatment is supportive, with mechanical ventilation often required. Antibiotics are typically initiated empirically but are only required for superinfection.

Q40-5: C
Multiple cavitary nodules

Rationale: This patient's chest film shows multiple diffuse areas of opacities, many of which have a nodular appearance or are cavitary. The opacities vary considerably in size and are bilateral. They have a peripheral distribution as well.

Q40-6: B
Septic emboli secondary to infective endocarditis

Rationale: The patient presents with evidence of narcotic use in association with fever, hypoxemia, and encephalopathy. She has an elevated WBC count as well, consistent with likely infection. The patient's examination demonstrates Janeway lesions (nonblanching, nonpainful erythematous lesions on the soles of the foot), consistent with infective endocarditis. Intravenous drug use is associated with right-sided endocarditis, which can lead to septic pulmonary emboli as a result of seeding from the valve. PCP is associated with cystic lung lesions rather than cavitary lesions, while *Legionella* is not commonly associated with cavitary or nodular lesions. Metastatic malignancy rarely presents with cavitation, though it may occur in some adenocarcinomas or following chemotherapy as tumor necrosis occurs.

Here is the patient's accompanying CT scan of the chest (**Image 40-10**), which demonstrates multiple nodular opacities of varying size and with varying degrees of cavitation. Additionally, there is a small pleural effusion on the right, which is also very common. The nodules are diffuse and more peripheral in distribution. Patients may also have wedge-shaped lesions. Some of the lesions have feeding vessels, a sign termed the "feeding vessel sign." The primary differential diagnosis is metastatic pulmonary opacities, granulomatosis with polyangiitis (Wegener granulomatosis), necrobiotic lung nodules, and pulmonary tuberculosis.

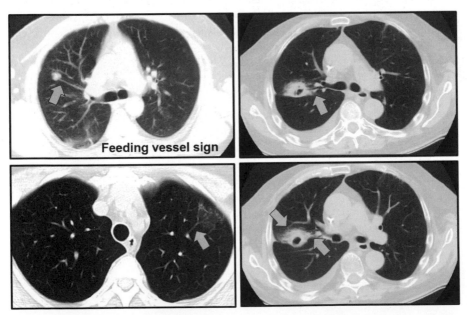

Image 40-10 • Chest CT examples of peripheral GGO, solid, and cavitary lesions with the feeding vessel sign (indicated by the gray arrows).

Q40-7: C
Infected pacemaker lead

Rationale: Septic emboli arise from venous (right-sided) sources of infection, including tricuspid valve endocarditis from intravenous drug use, infected venous catheters including pacemaker leads, infected deep vein thrombosis, or pulmonary emboli. All the alternative conditions listed are arterial side (left-sided) issues that would be anticipated to result in emboli to the skin, kidneys, brain, or other end organs. Although septic emboli can result from bronchial artery emboli, which are left-sided, this is much rarer. An example is shown in **Image 40-11** below.

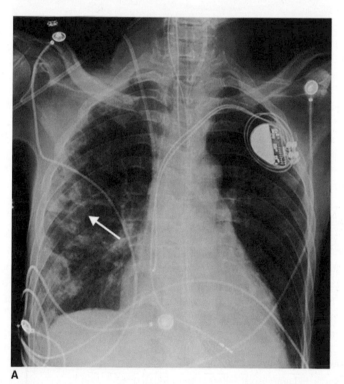

A

Image 40-11 • *(Reproduced with permission from Elsayes KM, Oldham SA: Introduction to Diagnostic Radiology. New York, NY: McGraw Hill; 2014.)*

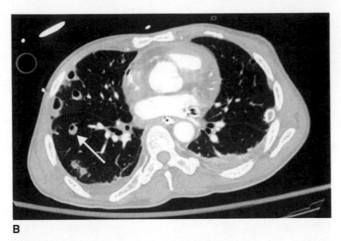

B

Image 40-11 • (Continued)

References

Akira M, Suganuma N. Acute and subacute chemical-induced lung injuries: HRCT findings. Eur J Radiol. 2014;83:1461.

Desai H, Agrawal A. Pulmonary emergencies: pneumonia, acute respiratory distress syndrome, lung abscess, and empyema. Med Clin North Am. 2012;96:1127.

DiBardino DM, Wunderink RG. Aspiration pneumonia: a review of modern trends. J Crit Care. 2015;30:40.

Fernandes AM, Pedreira DG, Janeiro S, Fera M. Lung abscess in a young patient. BMJ Case Rep. 2014;2014:bcr2013202761.

Fernández-Sabé N, Carratalà J, Dorca J, et al. Efficacy and safety of sequential amoxicillin-clavulanate in the treatment of anaerobic lung infections. Eur J Clin Microbiol Infect Dis. 2003;22:185.

Gafoor K, Patel S, Girvin F, et al. Cavitary lung diseases: a clinical-radiologic algorithmic approach. Chest. 2018;153:1443.

Goswami U, Brenes JA, Punjabi GV, LeClaire MM, Williams DN. Associations and outcomes of septic pulmonary embolism. Open Respir Med J. 2014;8:28.

Gupta N, Matta EJ, Oldham SA. Cardiothoracic imaging. In: Elsayes KM, Oldham SA, eds. *Introduction to Diagnostic Radiology*. McGraw-Hill; 2014. https://accessmedicine.mhmedical.com/content.aspx?bookid=1562&sectionid=95876454

Karcic AA, Karcic E. Lung abscess. J Emerg Med. 2001;20:165.

Kashif M, Patel R, Bajantri B, Diaz-Fuentes G. Legionella pneumonia associated with severe acute respiratory distress syndrome and diffuse alveolar hemorrhage—a rare association. Respir Med Case Rep. 2017;21:7.

Kuhajda I, Zarogoulidis K, Tsirgogianni K, et al. Lung abscess-etiology, diagnostic and treatment options. Ann Transl Med. 2015;3:183.

Mandell LA, Niederman MS. Aspiration pneumonia. NEJM. 2019;380:651.

Mansharamani NG, Koziel H. Chronic lung sepsis: lung abscess, bronchiectasis, and empyema. Curr Opin Pulm Med. 2003;9:181.

Marik PE. Aspiration pneumonitis and aspiration pneumonia. NEJM. 2001;344:665.

Nii T, Yoshikawa H, Okabe T, Tachibana I. Septic pulmonary and systemic embolism in tricuspid endocarditis. BMJ Case Rep. 2014;2014:bcr2014206569.

Ott SR, Allewelt M, Lorenz J, et al. Moxifloxacin vs ampicillin/sulbactam in aspiration pneumonia and primary lung abscess. Infection. 2008;36:23.

Perlino CA. Metronidazole vs clindamycin treatment of anerobic pulmonary infection. Failure of metronidazole therapy. Arch Intern Med. 1981;141:1424.

Said SA, Nijhuis R, Derks A, Droste H. Septic pulmonary embolism caused by infected pacemaker leads after replacement of a cardiac resynchronization therapy device. Am J Case Rep. 2016;17:507.

Scott DB. History of Mendelson's syndrome. J Int Med Res. 1978;6:47.

Snydman DR, Jacobus NV, McDermott LA, et al. Lessons learned from the anaerobe survey: historical perspective and review of the most recent data (2005-2007). Clin Infect Dis. 2010;50:S26.

Taylor JK, Fleming GB, Singanayagam A, Hill AT, Chalmers JD. Risk factors for aspiration in community-acquired pneumonia: analysis of a hospitalized UK cohort. Am J Med. 2013;126:995.

van der Maarel-Wierink CD, Vanobbergen JN, Bronkhorst EM, Schols JM, de Baat C. Risk factors for aspiration pneumonia in frail older people: a systematic literature review. J Am Med Dir Assoc. 2011;12:344.

Ye R, Zhao L, Wang C, Wu X, Yan H. Clinical characteristics of septic pulmonary embolism in adults: a systematic review. Respir Med. 2014;108:1.

CASE 41

A 45-year-old woman presents with complaints of dyspnea. She is otherwise healthy. She takes no medications. She has no significant family history. She reports that the dyspnea has progressively worsened over the last few months. She previously only experienced the dyspnea when active but now is experiencing some symptoms when she is supine. She denies any cough, fevers, chills, sweats, weight loss, changes in appetite, diarrhea, nausea, or emesis. She denies any hemoptysis. She endorses some mild lower-extremity edema that she thought may be related to her menstrual cycle, but it has been worse over the last few weeks. Her vital signs are T 36.0°C, HR 75, BP 118/65, RR 14, oxygen saturation 97% on room air. Her chest radiograph is shown in Image 41-1.

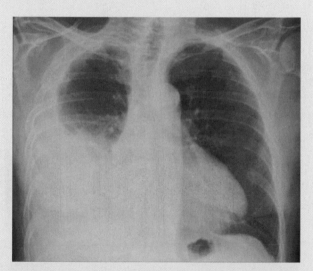

Image 41-1 • Chest radiograph for the patient in **Question 41-1**. (*Reproduced with permission from Hallifax RJ, Talwar A, Wrightson JM, et al: State-of-the-art: Radiological investigation of pleural disease, Respir Med 2017 Mar;124:88-99.*)

QUESTIONS

Q41-1: What is the primary abnormality on the patient's chest radiograph shown in Image 41-1?

A. Hydropneumothorax
B. Blunted right costophrenic angle
C. Diffuse alveolar opacities
D. Reticular interstitial opacities
E. Bilateral hilar adenopathy
F. Cardiomegaly

Q41-2: What is the most sensitive imaging method to detect the presence of a pleural effusion?

A. Upright frontal chest film
B. Upright lateral chest film
C. Ultrasound
D. CT scan
E. Supine chest film
F. C and D
G. C and E
H. D and E

Q41-3: The patient undergoes a bedside ultrasound, which is shown in Image 41-2. Her laboratory tests return with a BNP of 77 pg/mL (ULN 100) but evidence of kidney dysfunction with a creatinine level of 3.1 mg/dL. There are no prior laboratory tests in the system to determine the duration of the patient's kidney dysfunction.

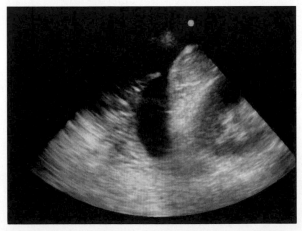

Image 41-2 • Thoracic ultrasound image obtained for the patient in **Question 41-3**.

What is the next step to determine the etiology of the patient's pleural effusion?

A. CT scan of the chest
B. Pulmonary embolism (PE)-protocol CT scan of the chest
C. CT scan of the abdomen and pelvis
D. Thoracentesis
E. Paracentesis
F. Pericardiocentesis

Q41-4: The patient undergoes a thoracentesis, and the following studies are conducted, with the primary studies shown below. The appearance of the fluid was straw-colored and clear.

Parameter	Value	Notes
pH	7.55	
Nucleated cell count	500/µL	
Differential	Macrophages, mesothelial cells, scant neutrophils	
Spun hematocrit	2	Serum value: 30
Glucose	90 mg/dL	Serum value: 110 mg/dL
Protein	1.4 g/dL	Serum value: 3.1 g/dL
LDH	45 U/L	ULN: 200 IU/L; serum value: 144 U/L

Which term best describes this pleural effusion?

A. Empyema
B. Exudative effusion
C. Parapneumonic effusion
D. Transudative effusion
E. Chylothorax
F. Hemothorax

Q41-5: Some additional laboratory test results show an albumin level of 1.4 g/dL and a 24-hour urinary excretion of creatinine of 2.8 g/dL. The patient's pleural fluid albumin is 0.7 g/dL, and the pleural fluid creatinine is 2.4 g/dL (serum 2.9 g/dL). Her thyroid-stimulating hormone (TSH) and free T4 levels are normal.

What is the likely cause of the patient's pleural effusion?

A. Urinothorax
B. Glycinothorax
C. Nephrotic syndrome
D. Cirrhosis
E. Myxedema

Q41-6: A 57-year-old man presents to the ED with dyspnea and orthopnea. He does not know his medical history, but he has the following medications with him: spironolactone, losartan, metoprolol, and aspirin. He is visiting a friend in town and has never seen anyone in the area for medical care. He is mildly hypoxemic, requiring 2 L O_2 on NC with activity. On examination, he has inspiratory crackles in the mid-lung fields, as well as egophony and dullness to percussion in the lower lung fields bilaterally. The patient is afebrile, with vital signs within normal limits. He reports no smoking history, no drug use, no alcohol use, and no occupational exposures. He retired 3 years ago from his work as the manager of a grocery store because of medical problems. His wife, who takes care of his medications and medical issues, is not present to provide additional history. The patient's chest radiograph is shown below in Image 41-3.

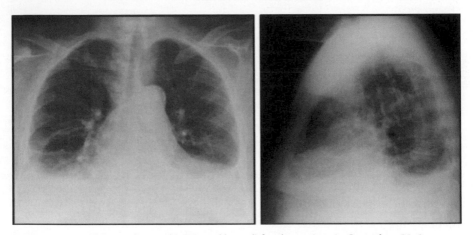

Image 41-3 • Chest radiographs (PA and lateral) for the patient in **Question 41-6**.

The patient has a complete blood count, international normalized ratio, and basic metabolic panel pending. What is the next step to determine the etiology of the patient's dyspnea?

A. D-dimer
B. Echocardiogram
C. VQ scan
D. PE-protocol CTA
E. Thoracentesis
F. Serum brain natriuretic peptide (BNP)

Q41-7: The patient undergoes diuresis for 4 consecutive days with good efficacy but continues to have dyspnea, and the effusion on the right, though it is slightly improved, remains moderate in size. Therapeutic thoracentesis is performed, and 1.2 L of fluid is removed. The team sends a basic laboratory test that reveals pH 7.55, glucose 90 mg/dL (serum glucose 110 mg/dL), and protein 1.3 mg/dL (serum protein 5.6 mg/dL), but the LDH level is 200 IU/L, with the ULN for the test of 222 IU/L, indicating a potential exudative effusion. The primary team asks if you would like to send any other laboratory tests to determine the etiology of the patient's pleural effusion. Which test is most appropriate to demonstrate that the effusions are due to congestive heart failure?

A. Pleural fluid/serum albumin ratio
B. Pleural fluid/serum protein gradient
C. Pleural fluid N-terminal proBNP
D. Pleural fluid BNP
E. Serum N-terminal proBNP

Q41-8: Match pleural fluid test results with the most appropriate diagnosis.

Diagnoses:
A. Tuberculous effusion
B. Esophageal rupture
C. Malignant pleural effusion
D. Cerebrospinal fluid leak
E. Rheumatoid pleurisy
F. Acute pancreatitis
G. Hemothorax
H. Chylothorax
I. Cholesterol effusion

Q41-8-1: pH 7.10, glucose 20 mg/dL (serum 110 mg/dL), protein 3.0 g/dL, pleural fluid amylase 110 U/L (serum value 40 U/L, ULN 220 U/L), LDH 360 IU/L (ULN 200 IU/L), 99% salivary amylase, 55,000 nucleated cells/μL, neutrophilic predominance, Gram stain positive.

Q41-8-2: pH 7.10, glucose 20 mg/dL (serum 110 mg/dL), protein 2.9 g/dL, pleural fluid amylase 1100 U/L (serum value 40 U/L, ULN 220 IU/L), 87% pancreatic amylase, 20,000 nucleated cells/μL, neutrophil predominance, Gram stain negative.

Q41-8-3: pH 7.10, glucose 5 mg/dL (serum 110 mg/dL), protein 5.0 g/dL, nucleated cell count 20,000/μL, 88% lymphocytes. Adenosine deaminase 70 IU/L. Cytology negative. Acid-fast bacilli (AFB) smear positive.

Q41-8-4: pH 7.10, glucose 5 mg/dL (serum 110), protein 3.1 g/dL, nucleated cell count 20,000/μL, 79% neutrophils, LDH 1120 IU/L (ULN 200 IU/L), cytology positive for "tadpole cells," Gram stain negative, complement levels at the lower end of normal.

Q41-8-5: pH 7.30, glucose 30 mg/dL (serum 110 mg/dL), protein 8.0 g/dL, nucleated cell count 1000/μL, 100% lymphocytes, LDH 660 IU/L (ULN 200 IU/L), cytology positive for atypical lymphocytes, flow cytometry with a monoclonal population of plasma cells, adenosine deaminase 22 IU/L.

Q41-8-6: pH 7.40, glucose 66 mg/dL (serum 90 mg/dL), protein 1.2 g/dL, positive beta-2-transferrin test. Beta-1-transferrin is found in nearly all body fluids; however, beta-2-transferrin (detected by electrophoresis) is a variant found only in the cerebral spinal fluid (CSF). Do not confuse this with beta-2-microglobulin, which is expressed by most cells in the body.

Q41-8-7: pH 7.40, glucose 90 mg/dL (serum 100 mg/dL), protein 5.9 g/dL (serum 7.0 g/dL), spun hematocrit 35 (serum 41).

Q41-8-8: pH 7.40, glucose 77 mg/dL (serum 110 mg/dL), protein 2.9 g/dL (serum 6.4 g/dL), LDH 145 IU/L (ULN 200 IU/L), cholesterol 50 mg/dL, triglycerides 220 mg/dL, chylomicrons present on electrophoresis.

Q41-9: A 56-year-old man presents with fevers, chills, fatigue, nausea, and a productive cough for the last 2 days. He is febrile to 102.7°F. He is hypoxemic and requires 4 L of O_2 on NC to maintain an oxygen saturation of 88%. He is tachycardic with an HR of 121 and a BP of 105/60. His cough is productive of yellow-green sputum with some tinges of blood but no frank hemoptysis. He reports a 10–pack-year smoking history. He has no prior occupational exposures or travel history. He has type 2 diabetes and osteoarthritis. He takes acetaminophen PRN and metformin. A bedside ultrasound is shown below in Image 41-4.

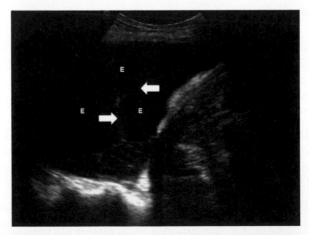

Image 41-4 • Thoracic ultrasound image obtained for the patient in **Question 41-9**. (*Reproduced with permission from Hallifax RJ, Talwar A, Wrightson JM, et al: State-of-the-art: Radiological investigation of pleural disease, Respir Med 2017 Mar;124:88-99.*)

The patient undergoes a diagnostic thoracentesis with a pH of 7.10. In addition to antibiotics, what is the next step in management?

A. Therapeutic thoracentesis
B. Chest tube placement
C. Corticosteroids
D. QuantiFERON Gold testing and airborne isolation
E. Pericardiocentesis

Q41-10: The patient's pleural fluid appears cloudy and purulent, with a nucleated cell count of 75,000/μL with a neutrophil predominance and an undetectable glucose level. The LDH is 1400 IU/L, and the protein is 3.2 g/dL. The Gram stain is positive for gram-negative rods and gram-positive rods. A chest tube is placed, but the effusion fails to drain completely based on a repeated CT scan and ultrasound, with loculations still present. What is the next step in management?

A. Surgical decortication
B. Change antibiotics
C. Instillation of alteplase (tPA) into the pleural space
D. Pleurodesis with doxycycline
E. Instillation of tPA and DNase into the pleural space

Q41-11: A 42-year-old woman with known metastatic breast cancer presents with rapidly progressive dyspnea over the last several days. The patient had noted some worsening dyspnea over the last few weeks, but over the last few days, the dyspnea has progressed rapidly. She is hypotensive on presentation with an HR of 120 and a BP of 85/60. She is saturating 89% on room air and is tachypneic (RR 22). A chest CXR and a CT scan are performed immediately upon arrival. The images are shown below in Images 41-5 and 41-6.

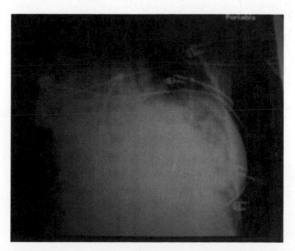

Image 41-5 • Chest radiograph (AP) for the patient in **Question 41-11**. (*Reproduced with permission from Dagrosa RL, Martin JF, Bebarta VS. Tension hydrothorax, J Emerg Med 2009 Jan;36(1):78-79.*)

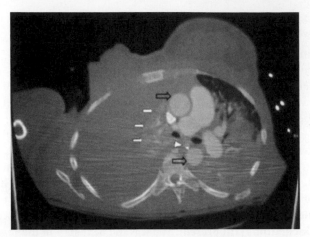

Image 41-6 • Chest CT scan image for the patient in **Question 41-11.** (*Reproduced with permission from Dagrosa RL, Martin JF, Bebarta VS. Tension hydrothorax, J Emerg Med 2009 Jan; 36(1):78-79.*)

What is the next management step for this patient?

A. Diagnostic thoracentesis
B. Chest tube placement
C. Anticoagulation
D. Thrombolytic therapy
E. Antibiotics

ANSWERS

Q41-1: B
Blunted costophrenic angle

Rationale: The patient's plain film shows a loss of the costophrenic angle on the right (**Image 41-7**). In addition, there is a loss of the hemidiaphragm. There is a meniscus on the right lateral chest wall, which would not be present if a hydropneumothorax was present, ruling out hydropneumothorax. There are no diffuse alveolar opacities or reticular interstitial opacities. There is no apparent hilar adenopathy or cardiomegaly. Although this image is most consistent with a pleural effusion (particularly given the meniscus), one must also consider that a concomitant process is ongoing in the right lower lobe, leading to the development of a pleural effusion, such as right lower lobe pneumonia, a mass, atelectasis, or a trapped lung.

A lateral decubitus film would provide more information about the presence of an effusion and whether that effusion is free flowing, and it would provide an estimate of the size of the effusion. If the effusion is free flowing, a lateral decubitus film will show the fluid accumulating along the lateral edge of the chest wall and displacing the lateral margin of the lung from the chest wall (assuming the side of the effusion is down). A supine film may also be useful when evaluating for pleural effusions. In a supine film of a free-flowing effusion, the lung may appear hazy because of the posterior fluid layers in the chest.

With left-sided pleural effusions, the separation between the gastric bubble (usually at the level of the left hemidiaphragm) and the top of the effusion can provide information regarding the size of the effusion.

In free-flowing effusions, the effusions are gravity dependent and will generally collect in the subpulmonic space.

The pleural meniscus sign seen here is suggestive of a pleural effusion. Loculated effusions arising from adhesions formed between the visceral and parietal pleura can lead to pockets of fluids that are trapped at odd locations in the pleural cavity.

Pleural effusions develop from conditions that alter the hydrostatic forces or permeability of pulmonary capillaries, processes that alter lymphatic drainage of the pleural space and affect the production of pleural fluid by the pleura, and conditions that allow communication between the pleural space and other areas of the body (eg, cerebral spinal fluid, peritoneal cavity).

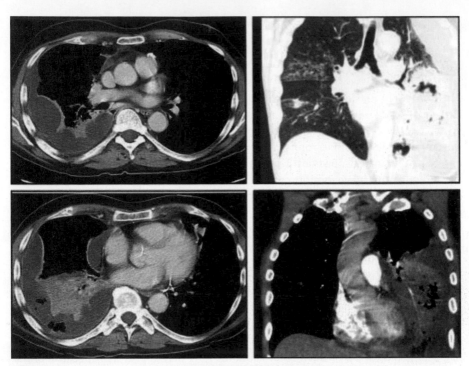

Image 41-7 • These images show examples of loculated effusions. On the axial images (left), one can appreciate that the effusion is not free flowing. The effusion is located posteriorly and laterally and almost wraps around to the anterior chest, with pockets of fluid trapped in the usual locations. In a free-flowing effusion, the fluid is gravity dependent and would layer in the posterior part of the chest. On the coronal images (right), there is atelectatic lung seen just to the right of the left heart border, and effusion is visualized both above and below the lung. Again, in a free-flowing effusion, the fluid is gravity dependent, and the pleural cavity would be expected to fill from the subpulmonic space and superiorly.

Loculated fluid collections can also collect in the interlobar fissures and produce a "pseudotumor" pattern on plain film.

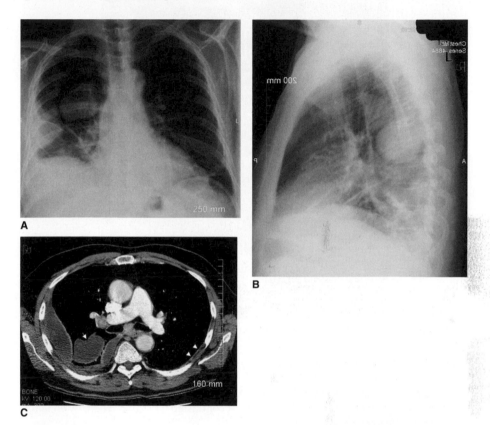

Image 41-8 • (A) shows a right-sided loculated pleural effusion and a "pseudotumor" in the right mid-lung field. The lateral chest radiograph (B) is helpful in demonstrating that the pseudotumor is located in the major fissure. The CT scan (C) confirms the presence of the loculated right-sided effusion and the pseudotumor. (*Reproduced with permission from Heffner JE, Klein JS, Hampson C. Diagnostic utility and clinical application of imaging for pleural space infections, Chest 2010 Feb;137(2):467-479.*)

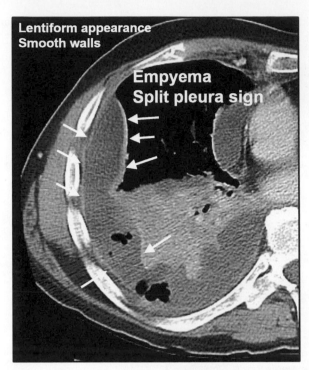

Image 41-9 • Split pleura sign indicating potential empyema. Note the separation of the visceral and parietal pleura (both indicated by arrows above) by a complex fluid collection that also contains pockets of air. This is another example of a loculated pleural effusion. On this CT scan, the pleura is enhanced, suggestive of an inflammatory process. The CT scan also demonstrates the split pleural sign, where the visceral pleural and the parietal pleura are split by the presence of the effusion. A contrasted CT scan can help by enhancing and more clearly defining the pleura.

These loculated effusions can have a varied pattern on chest imaging, depending on their orientation relative to the plane of the film and whether air is present in the loculation.

When a hydropneumothorax is present, there is air and fluid present in the pleural space. In a hydropneumothorax, there is typically no meniscus sign (see **Image 41-10**).

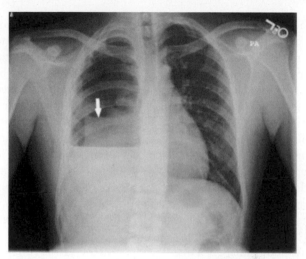

Image 41-10 • Note the loss of the meniscus sign consistent with the presence of a hydropneumothorax. (*Reproduced with permission from Heffner JE, Klein JS, Hampson C. Diagnostic utility and clinical application of imaging for pleural space infections, Chest 2010 Feb;137(2):467-479.*)

Q41-2: F
C and D

Rationale: The most sensitive methods for the detection of pleural effusions are CT scanning and ultrasound, both of which can detect pleural effusions down to an approximate volume of 5 to 10 mL. Lateral decubitus films can detect fluid volumes of approximately 25 to 50 mL, while lateral films can detect levels as low as approximately 50 to 75 mL. Supine and upright films are less sensitive, able to detect effusions down to approximately 200 mL in some patients. At approximately 500 to 600 mL, the hemidiaphragm will be obscured, while at approximately 1000 mL, the effusion will reach the level of the sternal angle. Massive effusions can lead to complete opacification of the hemidiaphragm and mediastinal shift. This can ultimately lead to tension physiology.

On supine films, free-flowing pleural effusions can be more difficult to detect because of the posterior effusion layers. They may present as haziness throughout the entire or partial lung field, and distinct blunting of the costophrenic angle may not be as obvious as it would be on an upright film.

Q41-3: D
Thoracentesis

Rationale: The indication for thoracentesis is any new or undiagnosed pleural effusion with two potential exceptions. Patients with obvious decompensated congestive heart failure with an elevated BNP can be observed during treatment to determine if the effusions resolve with therapy; if they do not, thoracentesis should be considered. The second case is in patients with clear viral pleurisy; however, given the relative uncertainty associated with this diagnosis, it is reasonable to consider thoracentesis in this patient population as well to rule out other causes of pleurisy. This patient has a normal BNP and therefore does not appear to have decompensated congestive heart failure, nor does she have symptoms of a recent viral illness. The ultrasound shows what appears to be a simple, free-flowing pleural effusion without evidence of septations or debris that would be concerning for a more complicated effusion. Ultrasound is an excellent tool for bedside examination of patients with suspected pleural effusions. The ultrasound image shows an effusion in the pleural space.

Shown below is another image of a free-flowing, simple effusion (**Image 41-11**). Note the anechoic fluid, with no artifact or evidence of septations.

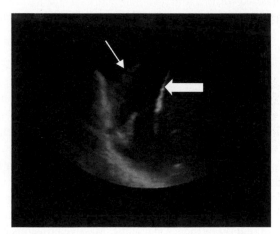

Image 41-11 • The thick arrow points to the diaphragm, and the thin arrow points to the lung. (*Reproduced with permission from Aboudara M, Maldonado F. Update in the Management of Pleural Effusions, Med Clin North Am 2019 May;103(3):475-485.*)

Q41-4: D
Transudative effusion

Rationale: To determine the etiology of a pleural effusion, one must first determine if the effusion is a transudate or an exudate because the differential diagnoses are quite different between these two groups (though not mutually exclusive). Answers A, C, E, and F are examples of exudative effusions. The primary tool used to differentiate transudative and exudative effusions are the Light criteria, though two additional sets of rules have also been proposed.

The pleural fluid pH is a critical piece of information and should be examined first. The pleural fluid pH in a healthy person is between pH 7.5 and 7.6, owing to the difference in bicarbonate concentrations. Transudative effusions usually have a pH greater than 7.40, while highly inflammatory processes (empyema, rheumatoid effusion, tuberculosis [TB] effusion) can have a pH less than 7.20. A pH less than 7.20 is an indication for evacuation of the chest cavity (either with a chest tube or surgical procedure). Most other exudative effusions will have a pH greater than 7.30. The management of effusions with a pH between 7.20 and 7.30 is less clear, and decisions about evacuation should be made on a case-by-case basis. Importantly, pH does not definitively determine the type of effusion. It is important to note that the pleural fluid pH may be artificially elevated if there is residual air in the collection syringe and may be artificially lowered if there is residual lidocaine mixed in the sample.

Light criteria: If any one of these criteria is met (ie, positive), the effusion is defined as an exudate; therefore, these criteria have a high sensitivity but lower specificity. The reason for this is that it is imperative not to miss an exudative effusion because the underlying causes are classically more morbid and may require additional procedures or surgery.

- Pleural fluid/serum protein ratio greater than 0.5 *or*
- Pleural fluid/serum LDH ratio greater than 0.6 *or*
- Pleural fluid LDH greater than (0.66) * (upper limit of normal of serum LDH laboratory study).

Two additional sets of criteria have been developed as well (termed the *two-test* and *three-test* criteria). They are similar to the Light criteria, with the exception that they include criteria for the pleural fluid cholesterol. If any **one** of the below criteria in either the two-test or the three-test criteria is positive, the effusion is considered an exudate.

Two-test rule:

- Pleural fluid cholesterol greater than 45 mg/dL *or*
- Pleural fluid LDH greater than (0.45) * upper limit of normal of serum LDH test

Three-test rule:

- Pleural fluid protein greater than 2.9 g/dL *or*
- Pleural fluid cholesterol greater than 45 mg/dL *or*
- Pleural fluid LDH greater than (0.45) * upper limit of normal of serum LDH test

As we do not have a pleural fluid cholesterol level, we will use the Light criteria first:

A. Pleural fluid/serum protein → 1.4/3.1 less than 0.50 – transudate
B. Pleural fluid/serum LDH → 45/144 less than 0.60 – transudate
C. Pleural fluid LDH/ULN of serum LDH → 0.3125 less than 0.66 (as well as less than 0.45 in the other criteria), so transudate

Since none of the above criteria is positive for an exudative effusion, the effusion is classified as a transudative effusion. An empyema is characterized by a low pH, low glucose, high protein, extremely high LDH (greater than 1000 U/L), and extremely high nucleated cell count (greater than 50,000 cells/μL), with a neutrophilic predominance. A parapneumonic effusion is similar to an empyema, with the exception that an empyema has frank pus in the pleural cavity, and a complicated parapneumonic effusion does not have pus (both can be culture positive). A chylothorax has an elevated pleural fluid triglyceride level, while a hemothorax has a spun pleural fluid hematocrit that is at least 50% of the serum hematocrit. That is not the case here.

Additionally, the appearance of the effusion can often be helpful.

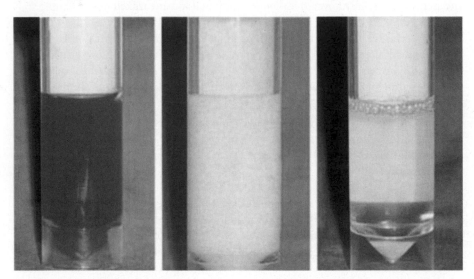

Image 41-12 • *Far left:* serosanguinous (sanguinous) effusion, consistent with an exudate. *Center:* white, milky effusion consistent with likely chylothorax or cholesterol effusion. *Right:* clear effusion consistent with a transudate. (*Reproduced with permission from Forbes CD, Jackson WF, Color Atlas and Text of Clinical Medicine, 2nd ed. London, UK: Mosby; 1997.*)

Causes of transudative effusions include volume overload states like congestive heart failure, cirrhosis, and nephrotic syndrome, among others. Some common causes of exudative effusions include malignancies, infections, pulmonary emboli, collagen vascular diseases, and medications.

Q41-5: C
Nephrotic syndrome

Rationale: The patient has an elevated creatinine, lower extremity edema, nephrotic-range proteinuria, and a severely depressed serum protein and serum albumin level with a pleural effusion. A urinothorax occurs when a pleural effusion forms secondary to obstructive uropathy and urine leaks into the pleural cavity either via lymphatics or directly through the diaphragm via a defect. In this case, the pleural fluid/serum creatinine ratio should always be greater than 1, and it is not diagnostic unless it is greater than 1.7 (here, it is less than 1). The TSH and free T4 are normal, so myxedema is unlikely. Patients with cirrhosis can develop hepatic hydrothoraces. This is most common in patients with ascites (not mentioned here), though it can occur in the absence of even mild ascites. These patients should have a large pleural fluid–serum albumin gradient (greater than 1.1 g/dL), but this patient has no evidence of cirrhosis per the case vignette, and the gradient is only 0.7 g/dL. A glycinothorax is a rare complication of procedures in which the bladder is irrigated with glycine-containing solutions. A glycinothorax can be diagnosed by a measurable glycine level in the pleural fluid in the appropriate clinical setting.

Q41-6: F
Serum brain natriuretic peptide (BNP)

Rationale: The patient's presentation is most consistent with decompensated congestive heart failure complicated by moderate bilateral pleural effusions. The patient has cephalization present on the chest film, in addition to cardiomegaly and loss or haziness of the costophrenic angles bilaterally, with some loss in the distinctness of both hemidiaphragms. The patient's medications are suggestive of a history of systolic heart failure as well. Although the general principle is to perform a thoracentesis on any new finding of a pleural effusion, a patient presenting with uncomplicated decompensated heart failure can typically be observed, and the response of the effusions can be monitored during diuretic therapy to ensure resolution. If the diagnosis of decompensated congestive heart failure is unclear, or if the patient has complicating factors, such as concomitant pneumonia, a thoracentesis would be warranted. PE should always be considered in a patient presenting to the ED with dyspnea and hypoxemia, but the abnormal chest radiology provides a reasonable alternative diagnosis. An echocardiogram would be helpful to determine the patient's heart function, but a serum BNP is a much more rapid test and provides additional prognostic information.

Q41-7: E
Serum N-terminal proBNP

Rationale: In some patients with pleural effusions caused by congestive heart failure, the pleural fluid analysis will point to an exudate, as is the case here. In some cases, this may be caused by contamination of the pleural fluid by red blood cells due to procedural complications or related to complications after coronary artery bypass grafting (CABG). In other cases, diuresis may transform a transudate to an exudate or a "pseudoexudate" by concentrating the protein or LDH in the remaining fluid. A number of tests have been proposed to discriminate which exudative effusions are associated with congestive heart failure.

The pleural fluid albumin to serum albumin gradient (greater than 1.2 g/dL), the pleural fluid protein/serum protein gradient (greater than 3.1 g/dL), and a pleural fluid/serum albumin ratio (less than 0.6) can be used in this situation, where there is a high pretest probability for congestive heart failure. Several studies have also examined the utility of pleural fluid NT-proBNP and BNP; however, the results of these studies are highly correlated with abnormalities in serum NT-proBNP and offer no advantage over the serum study with regard to diagnosis. Therefore, the optimal test remains the serum N-terminal proBNP because the pleural fluid studies will provide no further information.

Q41-8: B
Esophageal rupture

Rationale: Esophageal rupture effusions are associated with a low pH, a low pleural fluid/serum glucose ratio (usually less than 0.50), and an elevated (or detectable) pleural fluid amylase, which is predominantly salivary when fractionated. The LDH is typically elevated as well, and the fluid will have a neutrophil predominance on the differential diagnosis. Note, however, that the pleural fluid glucose could be elevated, depending on what was taken orally by the patient before the thoracentesis. Additionally, these effusions can often become empyemas because of contamination with oropharyngeal flora, so the Gram stain may be positive.

Diagnostic criteria: Pleural fluid amylase greater than the upper limit of normal of serum amylase level *or* a pleural fluid to serum amylase ratio greater than 1.

Q41-8: F
Acute pancreatitis

Rationale: Effusions associated with acute or chronic pancreatitis have findings similar to esophageal rupture, with the exception that the pleural fluid amylase is predominantly pancreatic compared with salivary and is usually greater than 1000 IU/L. Similarly, acute/chronic pancreatitis effusions (or a pancreaticopleural fistula) can develop into an empyema by seeding from an inflamed biliary tree. However, an elevated pleural fluid amylase level can also be associated with malignancy, pneumonia, cirrhosis, and ectopic pregnancy, so clinical correlation is required.

Diagnostic criteria: Pleural fluid amylase greater than the upper limit of normal of the serum amylase level *or* a pleural fluid to serum amylase ratio greater than 1.

Q41-8: A
Tuberculous effusion

Rationale: Tuberculous effusions and rheumatoid effusions are both highly inflammatory and associated with significantly reduced pleural fluid glucose levels and acidotic pH values. Tuberculous effusions are associated with very elevated protein levels (usually greater than 4 g/dL) and an elevated pleural fluid ADA level (usually greater than 40 IU/L). The cell count is usually between 10,000 and 50,000 cells/µL with a strong lymphocytic predominance. The AFB smear should be positive. Additionally, it is possible to order a QuantiFERON Gold study for these patients, which can also aid in making a diagnosis. Chest imaging is often helpful as well.

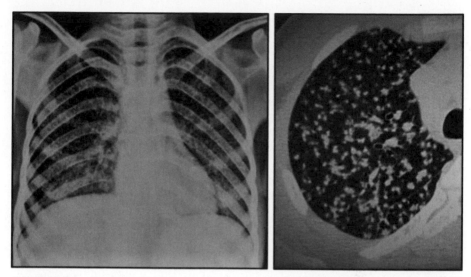

Image 41-13 • Example of a patient with miliary pattern on CT of the chest, consistent with disseminated active TB.

Q41-8: E
Rheumatoid pleurisy

Rationale: Rheumatoid effusions are difficult to differentiate from other exudates because there is no definitive diagnostic test from the pleural fluid. "Tadpole cells" are multinucleated giant cells sometimes seen on cytology that can aid in making a diagnosis, though oftentimes, a pleural biopsy is needed. In acute rheumatoid effusions, the cell differential is often neutrophilic, but it may shift toward a lymphocytic predominance over the ensuing weeks. A serum rheumatoid factor is typically positive, but this is nonspecific.

The pleural fluid glucose level and the pleural fluid rheumatoid factor are two fluid studies that can help differentiate lupus from rheumatoid pleurisy. In lupus pleuritis, the pleural glucose level is usually similar to the serum glucose level, and the pleural rheumatoid factor is low, while in rheumatoid pleuritis, the pleural fluid glucose is low (less than 30 mg/dL), and the pleural fluid rheumatoid factor is elevated. Both types of effusions are exudates with low levels of complement and high levels of immune complexes. Pleural fluid ANA levels are often positive in lupus pleuritis, while they may be positive or negative in rheumatoid pleurisy.

Q41-8: C
Malignant pleural effusion

Rationale: Malignant effusions can have a normal or acidic pH depending on the cell type. Malignant effusions are often somewhat bloody or serosanguinous in appearance, with a cell count of approximately 1000 to 5000 cells/μL and a variable differential depending on the duration and malignancy. The LDH and protein levels are typically elevated, and the glucose can be normal or low. The ADA pleural fluid test can be used to differentiate malignant effusions from TB, where malignant effusions typically have a pleural fluid ADA less than 40 IU/L. Cytology has variable sensitivity for diagnosing malignant effusions and is highly dependent on the underlying malignancy. Here, we have a very elevated protein level and an atypical, monoclonal population of lymphocytes, which would be concerning for a lymphoma, particularly multiple myeloma or Waldenstrom gammaglobulinemia.

Another differential in the case of patients with known malignancy and pleural effusion is the entity of a "paramalignant" effusion. These are effusions with negative cytology and are thought to be caused by other effects of malignancy (lymphatic obstruction) or as a consequence of the treatment of a malignancy (eg, radiation-associated pleuritis or related to treatment with chemotherapy).

Q41-8: D
Cerebrospinal fluid leak

Rationale: This can occur with a ventriculopleural fistula or shunt. A beta-2-transferrin test can aid in diagnosing a CSF-associated effusion.

Q41-8: G
Hemothorax

Rationale: A hemothorax is an exudative effusion caused by direct bleeding into the pleural space. A hemothorax is diagnosed when the spun hematocrit of the pleural fluid is greater than or equal to 50% of the value of peripheral blood hematocrit, which is present in this case. Some causes of hemothorax include coagulopathy, ruptured lung bullae, arteriovenous malformations, and trauma.

Q41-8: H
Chylothorax

Rationale: A chylothorax results from an obstruction of the lymphatic drainage back to the central venous system and is usually caused by trauma, postoperative complications, or malignancy.

The appearance of the fluid is typically milky white or lipidemic in appearance. The primary differential diagnosis is a cholesterol effusion ("pseudochylothorax," **Answer I** above). The pathogenesis of cholesterol effusions is unclear, but they can arise from rheumatoid or tuberculous pleurisy as well. Cholesterol effusions typically contain high levels of cholesterol without significant elevations in triglyceride levels because they develop as a result of the cholesterol membrane component of degenerating cells in the pleural space. A cholesterol level higher than 250 mg/dL with a cholesterol-to-triglyceride ratio greater than 1 is diagnostic of a cholesterol effusion. Additionally, cholesterol crystals are usually seen under polarized light.

Note: The above is an exercise, and in all actual cases, the history, physical examination, and radiographic imaging must be also be taken into account when formulating a differential diagnosis for patients. The pleural fluid analysis can certainly aid in making a diagnosis but should not be viewed in isolation.

Q41-9: B
Chest tube placement

Rationale: This patient has a complex pleural effusion with septations present and a pH less than 7.20. A pH less than 7.20 necessitates evacuation of the pleural cavity. A chest tube is the next step in the management of this patient. **Answers C** and **D** would be appropriate if rheumatoid or tuberculous pleurisy were suspected as the primary cause of the effusion; however, with the infectious symptoms, a parapneumonic effusion or empyema should be suspected. Effusions with significant loculations (septations, indicated by the white arrows in **Image 41-11**; pockets of effusion marked by letter "E" may be difficult to evacuate with a chest tube alone.

Ultrasound is very useful for characterizing effusions, as shown in **Image 41-14** below.

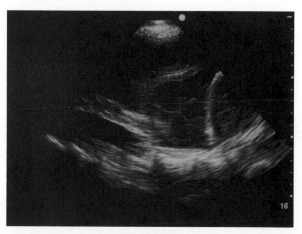

Image 41-14 • Here the diaphragm is to the right, and just adjacent (left) to the diaphragm, septations (loculations) or adhesions are seen. They form between the visceral and parietal pleura. Common causes include hemothorax, empyema/complicated parapneumonic effusion, and chylothorax.

Q41-10: E
Instillation of tPA and DNase into the pleural space

Rationale: The first step in this process is determining the cause of the effusion. The classifications of effusions associated with bacterial pneumonia are described in **Image 41-15**. This effusion is consistent with an empyema based on the gross appearance (purulent fluid), the ultrasound findings (septations), the clinical presentation with sepsis, and the pleural fluid analysis with a low pH, low glucose, high protein, high LDH, high nucleated cell count with neutrophilic predominance, and positive Gram stain.

This patient has had appropriate management to this point, but the empyema has failed to evacuate completely, meaning that the pleural space is not sterilized and the lung has not reexpanded completely. Additionally, there are persistent loculations present on the ultrasound. In prior decades, this patient would have been referred for surgical decortication to achieve the aforementioned goals. However, recent evidence suggests that instillation of tPA and DNase into the empyema cavity can reduce the need for surgery (RR 0.17) when compared with a chest tube alone, and it also decreases the hospital length of stay by nearly a week. Instillation of tPA and DNase is more effective than either therapy alone. This is performed twice a day for a total of 3 days, with a 2-hour dwell time in the empyema cavity before reopening the chest tube.

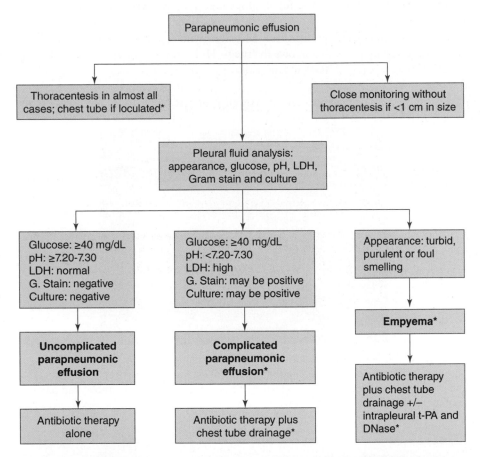

*Pulmonary consultation is recommended in these situations. Surgery consultation may be needed if persistent fever, sepsis or ongoing infection despite antibiotics and chest tube drainage.

Image 41-15 • Algorithm for the evaluation and management of parapneumonic effusions. (*Reproduced with permission from McKean SC, Ross JJ, Dressler DD, et al: Principles and Practice of Hospital Medicine, 2nd ed. New York, NY: McGraw Hill; 2017.*)

Q41-11: B
Chest tube placement

Rationale: The patient's images above demonstrate a massive space-occupying process in the right hemithorax. There is a displacement of the mediastinum to the left, with evidence of hemodynamic compromise and respiratory distress, consistent with tension physiology. The CT scan demonstrates a large effusion on the right with compressive atelectasis of the right lung (*white arrows*). Given the patient's history of metastatic breast cancer, this presentation is most consistent with a malignant pleural effusion. Malignant effusions, tuberculous effusions, and hemothorax are some of the most common causes of massive pleural effusions occupying a hemithorax and are capable of causing tension physiology. The next step in management is placement of a chest tube. Although a pulmonary embolism cannot be ruled out given complete compression of the left lung, the primary concern here is tension physiology. Anticoagulation would be a significant risk without being able to characterize the pleural effusion because it could potentially be a paramalignant hemothorax.

Lung and breast cancer are the most common malignancies associated with malignant pleural effusions.

References

Aboudara M, Maldonado F. Update in the management of pleural effusions. Med Clin N Am. 2019;103:475.

Asciak R, Rahman NM. Malignant pleural effusion: from diagnostics to therapeutics. Clin Chest Med. 2018;39:181.

Blackmore CC, Black WC, Dallas RV, et al. Pleural fluid volume estimation: a chest radiograph prediction rule. Acad Radiol. 1996;3:103.

Dagrosa RL, Martin JF, Bebarta VS. Tension hydrothorax. J Emerg Med. 2009;36:78.

Feller-Kopman D, Light R. Pleural disease. N Engl J Med. 2018;378:740.

Gopi A, Madhavan SM, Sharma SK, Sahn SA. Diagnosis and treatment of tuberculous pleural effusion in 2006. Chest. 2007;131:880.

Grabczak EM, Krenke R, Zielinska-Krawczyk M, Light RW. Pleural manometry in patients with pleural diseases—the usefulness in clinical practice. Respir Med. 2018.pii: S0954-6111(18)30023-4.

Hallifax RJ, Talwar A, Wrightson JM, Edey A, Gleeson FV. State of the art: radiological investigation of pleural disease. Respir Med. 2017;124:88.

Heffner JE, Klein JS, Hampson C. Diagnostic utility and clinical application of imaging for pleural space infections. Chest. 2010;137:467.

Hooper CE, Lee YC, Maskell NA. Interferon-gamma release assays for the diagnosis of TB pleural effusions: hype or real hope? Curr Opin Pulm Med. 2009;15:358.

Huggins JT, Sahn SA. Drug-induced pleural disease. Clin Chest Med. 2004;25:141.

Huggins JT, Sahn SA, Heidecker J, et al. Characteristics of trapped lung: pleural fluid analysis, manometry, and air-contrast chest CT. Chest. 2007;131:206.

Kraus GJ. The split pleura sign. Radiology. 2007;243:297.

Kummerfeldt CE, Pastis NJ, Huggins JT. Pleural diseases. In: McKean SC, Ross JJ, Dressler DD, Scheurer DB, eds. *Principles and Practice of Hospital Medicine*. 2nd ed. McGraw-Hill; 2017. https://accessmedicine.mhmedical.com/content.aspx?bookid=1872&sectionid=146989271

Light RW. The undiagnosed pleural effusion. Clin Chest Med. 2006;27:309.

Light RW. Pleural effusions. Med Clin North Am. 2011;95:1055.

Long AC, O'Neal HR Jr, Peng S, et al. Comparison of pleural fluid N-terminal pro-brain natriuretic peptide and brain natriuretic-32 peptide levels. Chest. 2010;137:1369.

Mayo MM, Lechner AJ. Evaluating sputum and pleural effusions. In: Lechner AJ, Matuschak GM, Brink DS, eds. *Respiratory: An Integrated Approach to Disease*. McGraw-Hill; 2012. https://accessmedicine.mhmedical.com/content.aspx?bookid=1623&sectionid=105764459

Moore CL, Copel JA. Point-of-care ultrasonography. N Engl J Med. 2011;364:749.

Moskowitz H, Platt RT, Schachar R, et al. Roentgen visualization of minute pleural effusion: an experimental study to determine the minimum amount of pleural fluid visible on a radiograph. *Radiology*. 1973;109:33-35.

Porcel JM, Azzopardi M, Koegelenberg CF, Maldonado F, Rahman NM, Lee YC. The diagnosis of pleural effusions. Expert Rev Respir Med. 2015;9(6):801-815. doi: 10.1586/17476348.2015.1098535. Epub 2015 Oct 8.

Porcel JM, Civit MC, Bielsa S, Light RW. Contarini's syndrome: bilateral pleural effusion, each side from different causes. J Hosp Med. 2012 Feb;7(2):164-165. doi: 10.1002/jhm.981. Epub 2011 Oct 31. Review.

Rahman NM, Mishra EK, Davies HE, Davies RJO, Gary LEE YC. Clinically important factors influencing the diagnostic measurement of pleural fluid pH and glucose. Am J Respir Crit Care Med. 2008;178:483-490.

Sachdeva A, Matuschak GM. Interpreting chest X-rays, CT scans, and MRIS. In: Lechner A.J., & Matuschak GM, & Brink DS, eds, *Respiratory: An Integrated Approach to Disease*. McGraw-Hill; 2012. https://accessmedicine.mhmedical.com/content.aspx?bookid=1623&sectionid=105764262

Thomas R, Lee YC. Causes and management of common benign pleural effusions. Thorac Surg Clin. 2013 Feb;23(1):25-42, v-vi. doi: 10.1016/j.thorsurg.2012.10.004. Review.

Walker SP, Morley AJ, Stadon L, De Fonseka D, Arnold DT, Medford ARL, Maskell NA. Nonmalignant pleural effusions: A prospective study of 356 consecutive unselected patients. Chest. 2017 May;151(5):1099-1105. doi: 10.1016/j.chest.2016.12.014. Epub 2016 Dec 23.

Yilmaz U, Polat G, Sahin N, et al. CT in differential diagnosis of benign and malignant pleural disease. Monaldi Arch Chest Dis. 2005;63:17.

Zielinska-Krawczyk M, Krenke R, Grabczak EM, Light RW. Pleural manometry-historical background, rationale for use and methods of measurement. Respir Med. 2018 Mar;136:21-28. doi: 10.1016/j.rmed.2018.01.013. Epub 2018 Jan 31.

CASE 42

A 55-year-old man presents with 2 days of significantly worsening dyspnea. He has a history of hypertension, for which he takes amlodipine and carvedilol. He has a 20–pack-year smoking history but quit smoking 5 years ago. He reports the onset of dyspnea immediately when he awoke 2 days ago, and it has progressively worsened since that time, to the point that he is now short of breath with minimal activity. He denies any chest pain, but he does have an intermittent dry cough. He denies any fevers, chills, sweats, weight loss, changes in appetite, or hemoptysis. He denies any abdominal or joint symptoms. He works as a mechanical engineer and is in an office setting most of the time. He recently had an injury on the job and was not working for the last 2 weeks while recovering from a severe right knee sprain. He has been more sedentary over the last several weeks. He does endorse some swelling in his right lower extremity but states his leg has been swollen since the time of the injury.

EKG shows sinus tachycardia. His chest radiograph is shown in Image 42-1 below.

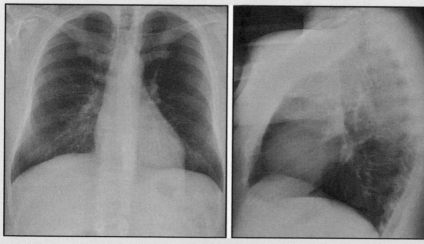

Image 42-1 • Chest radiographs (PA and lateral) for the patient in **Question 42-1**.

His vital signs are T 99.7°F, HR 110, BP 105/60, RR 24, and O$_2$ saturation 84% on room air, improved to 92% on 4 L NC. His creatine is 1.2 mg/dL. His WBC count is 11,800/µL, and his platelet count and hemoglobin are normal. His other coagulation studies and liver function panel are also normal.

QUESTIONS

Q42-1: What is the most appropriate next step in the management of this patient?

A. Arterial blood gas
B. D-dimer
C. Serum troponin determination
D. Deep vein thrombosis (DVT) ultrasound of the lower extremities
E. VQ scan
F. Pulmonary embolism (PE)-protocol CT scan of the chest

Q42-2: Match the imaging abnormalities shown in Images 42-2 through 42-6, that may be seen in acute PE to the correct terms.

A. Saddle embolus
B. Hampton hump
C. Septal flattening
D. Westermark sign
E. McConnell sign

Answer _____

What sign is indicated by the white arrowheads in Image 42-2?

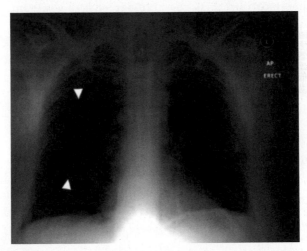

Image 42-2 • (Reproduced with permission from Sreenivasan S, Bennett S, Parfitt VJ. Images in cardiovascular medicine. Circulation 2007 Feb 27;115(8):e211.)

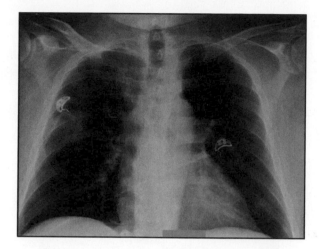

Image 42-3 •

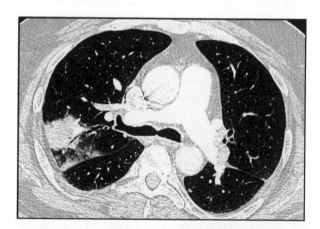

Image 42-4 •

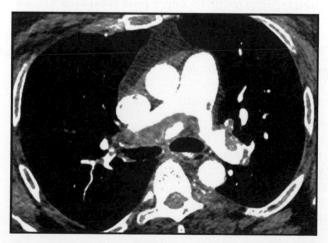

Image 42-5 •

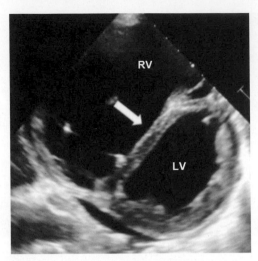

Image 42-6 • *(Reproduced with permission from Lee DW, Gopalratnam K, Ford HJ 3rd, et al: The Value of Bedside Echocardiogram in the Setting of Acute and Chronic Pulmonary Embolism, Clin Chest Med 2018 Sep;39(3):549-556.)*

Q42-3: A 29-year-old man presents with sudden-onset shortness of breath and lightheadedness. He is an athlete who typically participates in 30 to 60 minutes of highly aerobic activity a day, but when he awoke today, he was unable to catch his breath and felt lightheaded and dizzy with any activity. He recently returned from a trip overseas for work 3 days ago. He noticed his leg was somewhat painful the day after his flight, and this morning, his leg is slightly swollen. His primary care doctor had prescribed him a sleeping aid for the flight, and he states he slept the entire 11-hour trip. On presentation, he is diaphoretic, tachypneic, and hypoxemic. He is tachycardic to the 130s, and his BP is 80/50. He is given 2 L of isotonic fluids but remains hypotensive with a BP of 82/48. His O_2 requirement is a nonrebreather mask. He is started on norepinephrine. A set of stat laboratory values reveals a creatinine level of 2.6 mg/dL (baseline is 0.7 mg/dL), an elevated brain (B-type) natriuretic peptide (BNP), and a troponin-I level of 2.66 pg/mL (ULN 0.05 pg/mL). His venous lactate level is elevated at 4.2 mmol/dL (ULN 2.0 mmol/dL). A bedside ultrasound demonstrates a dilated, hypocontractile right ventricle with septal bowing into the left ventricle. He reports he had an arthroscopic knee surgery approximately 3 months ago.

What is the next step in management?

A. PE-protocol CT angiogram of the chest
B. VQ study
C. DVT ultrasound study of the lower extremities
D. Inferior vena cava (IVC) filter placement and anticoagulation
E. Systemic thrombolysis
F. Embolectomy
G. Antibiotics

Q42-4: A 44-year-old White woman presents with dyspnea. She reports that her dyspnea has progressively worsened over the last several months. She reports worsening lower extremity edema developing during this time as well. She denies any fevers, chills, or sweats. She has an appetite but is troubled by early satiety when eating. On presentation to the ED, the patient's BP is 95/60, her HR is 110, and she is requiring 4 L O_2 on NC. The patient undergoes a CXR, a VQ scan (creatinine 2.0 mg/dL), and an echocardiogram, as shown in Images 42-7 to 42-9 below.

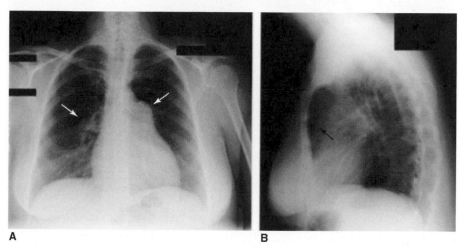

A   **B**

Image 42-7 • CXR for the patient in **Question 42-4**. (*Reproduced with permission from Forfia PR, Trow TK. Diagnosis of pulmonary arterial hypertension, Clin Chest Med 2013 Dec;34(4):665-681.*)

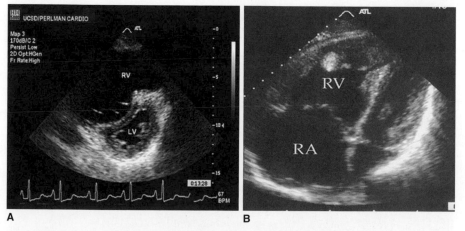

A   **B**

Image 42-8 • Echocardiogram (transthoracic). (*Reproduced with permission from Fuster V, Harrington RA, Narula J, et al: Hurst's the Heart, 14th ed. New York, NY: McGraw Hill; 2017.*)

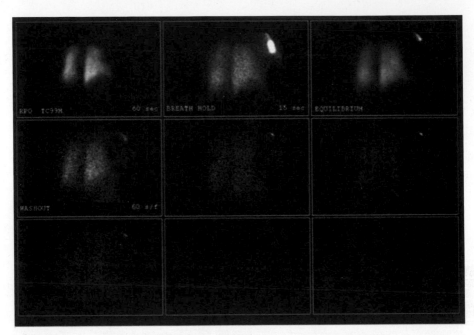

Image 42-9 • VQ scan. (*Reproduced with permission from Chen MYM, Pope TL, Ott DJ: Basic Radiology, 2nd ed. New York, NY: McGraw Hill; 2011.*)

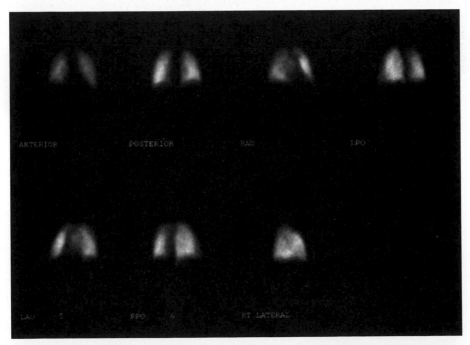

Image 42-10 • Perfusion scan. (*Reproduced with permission from Chen MYM, Pope TL, Ott DJ: Basic Radiology, 2nd ed. New York, NY: McGraw Hill; 2011.*)

Her laboratory tests return with the following: troponin I 0.01 ng/mL (upper limit of normal 0.05 ng/mL), creatine kinase-MB 2 IU/L (ULN – 10 IU/L), BNP 876 pg/mL (ULN – 100 ng/mL).

Her pulmonary function testing reveals normal spirometry, normal lung volumes, and a reduced diffusing capacity of carbon monoxide (42% predicted).

The patient has no known history of hypertension, cardiovascular disease, rheumatologic disease, or pulmonary disease. What is the most likely diagnosis?

A. Acute PE
B. Chronic thromboembolic pulmonary hypertension (CTEPH)
C. Pulmonary arterial hypertension
D. Cardiogenic pulmonary edema
E. Idiopathic pulmonary fibrosis

Q42-5: A 66-year-old woman presents with progressive dyspnea over the course of the last several years. She first noted symptoms about 4 to 5 years ago, only with strenuous exertion. Over the last 5 years, the symptoms have progressed, and she is experiencing lightheadedness and dizziness in addition to shortness of breath with even minimal exertion. She reports some mild-to-moderate symmetric lower extremity edema as well. She requires 4 L/min supplemental O_2 at rest, and 8 L/min supplemental O_2 with activity. Her BP is 104/60, her HR is 105, and she is afebrile. Her kidney function and remaining laboratory studies are normal, except for an elevated BNP. She reports that she had a PE approximately 9 years ago that was thought to be unprovoked. She completed 3 months of anticoagulation therapy, and this was stopped by her primary care doctor.

The patient's VQ scan returns abnormal, and the radiologist suggests a pulmonary angiogram be performed. The results are shown in Image 42-11. The patient's pulmonary angiogram returned the following values as well:

RA pressure: 10 mm Hg
RV pressure: 54/6 mm Hg
PA pressure: 67/22 mm Hg
mPA pressure: 40 mm Hg
Wedge pressure: 8 mm Hg

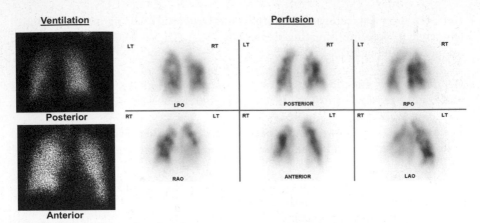

Ventilation   **Perfusion**

Posterior

Anterior

Image 42-11 • Ventilation-perfusion (VQ) scan imaging results for the patient in **Question 42-5**. The ventilation images are shown in the left-most column (top - posterior, bottom - anterior), while the perfusion projection images are shown to the right.

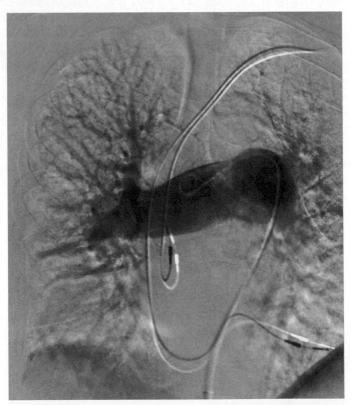

Image 42-12 • *(Reproduced with permission from Grippi MA, Elias JA, Fishman JA, et al: Fishman's Pulmonary Diseases and Disorders, 5th ed. New York, NY: McGraw Hill; 2015.)*

What is the likely etiology for the patient's persistent dyspnea and hypoxemia?

A. Acute PE
B. Chronic pulmonary emboli
C. Left-sided congestive heart failure
D. Chronic thromboembolic pulmonary hypertension (CTEPH)
E. Sleep apnea

ANSWERS

Q42-1: F
PE protocol CT scan of the chest

Rationale: The patient presents with a clinical syndrome concerning for PE. He has no significant medical history outside of hypertension, and he has recently been immobilized because of a traumatic injury of his lower extremity, which appears edematous. He has sinus tachycardia on his EKG (the most common abnormality on EKG in patients with an acute PE) and normal chest radiography, indicating no other clear cause of the patient's hypoxia. Although some patients with acute PE may have a right heart strain pattern on EKG, this is present in less than 20% of patients.

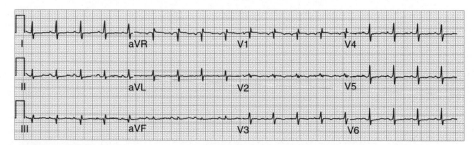

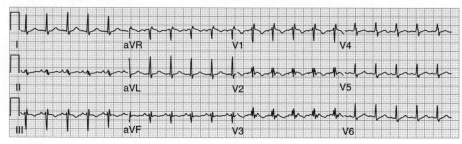

Image 42-13 • Examples of two electrocardiograms in patients with acute right heart strains secondary to pulmonary embolus. Note that both patient's ECGs demonstrate the S1-Q3-T3 pattern, with a S wave present in lead 1, a Q wave present in lead 3, and T wave flattening or inversion present in lead 3.

Importantly, while most patients with acute PE will not have significant abnormalities on chest radiography, abnormalities may be present in up to a quarter of cases, and the presence of an abnormality should not exclude PE from the differential.

In terms of the management of this patient, the next clinical consideration is hemodynamic stability. He is hemodynamically stable (no evidence of hypotension or shock). For patients with a possible PE who are hemodynamically stable on presentation, the next step is to determine the pretest probability of a PE. This is most commonly performed using the Wells criteria, the modified Wells criteria, or the Geneva score.

For this patient, the Wells criteria score would be as follows:
- Clinical signs or symptoms of a DVT – yes (+3);
- Other diagnoses are less likely than pulmonary embolism – yes (+3);

- Heart rate greater than 100 beats/min – yes (+1.5);
- Immobilization at least 3 days *or* surgery in prior month – yes (+1.5);
- Previous venous thromboembolism (DVT or PE) – no;
- Hemoptysis – no;
- Malignancy – no.

That yields a total score of 9.

The Wells criteria are used to risk-stratify hemodynamically stable patients into three groups: low risk, intermediate risk, and high risk. Low-risk patients have a Wells score less than 2, with an overall 1.3% incidence of PE on further evaluation. These patients should be further evaluated with a D-dimer study or other exclusion criteria such as the Pulmonary Embolism Rule-out Criteria (PERC) criteria before considering an imaging study. Patients with an intermediate risk have a Wells score of 2 to 6, with a 16.2% incidence of PE. These patients should have a D-dimer study and, pending the result, undergo diagnostic imaging. Patients in the high-risk group (Wells score greater than 6) have a 40.6% incidence of PE, and they should undergo diagnostic imaging without the need for a D-dimer study. The preferred imaging modality for the diagnosis of PE is a PE-protocol CT angiogram of the chest. In patients with impaired renal function, a ventilation–perfusion (VQ) study is an appropriate alternative that does not require intravenous contrast. A VQ study is often performed in conjunction with a DVT ultrasound study of the lower extremities.

In patients who present with hemodynamic instability (hypotension or evidence of shock) but are quickly able to be resuscitated and remain stable, initiation of anticoagulation is appropriate before obtaining a diagnosis via imaging. The anticoagulant of choice is heparin because it may be stopped quickly if the patient progresses to hemodynamic instability and shock, necessitating the need for systemic or local thrombolytic therapy. Oral anticoagulation with a direct thrombin inhibitor is not recommended in this patient population in the acute setting, though this would be appropriate for maintenance therapy at the time of discharge. Alternative options would include enoxaparin or an intravenous direct thrombin inhibitor.

Q42-2: D
Westermark sign

Rationale: This can be a very subtle finding in which the area of the lung distal to a PE or emboli demonstrates reduced pulmonary vascular markings (oligemia). This results from dilatation of the pulmonary arteries proximal to the occlusion and collapse of the vessels distal to the blockage, yielding a discrete or abrupt change in appearance. Here, the area between the two white arrowheads has considerably fewer pulmonary vascular markings than the left.

The black arrow indicates a prominent pulmonary artery. This is known as the *Palla sign*.

Q42-2: B
Hampton hump

Rationale: This is a wedge-shaped area of pulmonary infarction resulting from a PE. The base of the infarct typically rests on the pleural surface and is best visualized on a CT scan (even in cases when it may not be visible on CXR).

Q42-2: A
Saddle embolus

Rationale: The term *saddle embolus* is used to describe a PE that straddles the main pulmonary artery with extension into either or both the right and left pulmonary arteries.

Q42-2: C
Septal flattening

Rationale: Septal flattening refers to the flattening of the interventricular septum (indicated by the white arrow) due to RV pressure overload. This should not be confused with the McConnell sign (RV free wall hypokinesis or akinesis with sparing of the apex), which can also be seen in acute PE.

Q42-3: E
Systemic thrombolysis

Rationale: The patient is at high risk for a PE with a clear inciting event (recent air travel and immobility) and no other obvious cause to explain his symptoms. This patient is hemodynamically unstable and has failed efforts at resuscitation with IV fluids, and he is requiring a vasopressor/inotrope to support his hemodynamics. Additionally, he has evidence of shock physiology with an elevated lactate level and kidney failure. His echocardiogram and cardiac biomarkers are consistent with acute right heart failure (cor pulmonale), and immediate intervention is indicated.

The patient's Wells criteria score is very high (7.5), indicating a 40% incidence of PE. While not necessary in patients with suspected PE and hemodynamic instability, the PE severity index (PESI) is a score that can be used to estimate 30-day mortality in patients presenting with acute PE, and it is sometimes used to determine patient disposition in the ED. This patient's PESI score is 129, placing him in the highest-risk category (class V), with a 10% to 24.5% risk of death.

Points are allotted in the PESI score based on age, sex assigned at birth, a history of cancer, underlying heart failure or chronic pulmonary disease, a heart rate of 110 beats/min or higher, systolic blood pressure less than 100 mm Hg, a respiratory rate of 30 breaths/min or higher, a temperature less than 96.8°F, altered mental status, and an O_2 saturation less than 90% on room air. The PESI score estimates the risk of death in the subsequent 30 days.

Additional diagnostic testing is not indicated in a patient with a high probability of PE and hemodynamic instability. This patient has a massive PE, and systemic thrombolysis should be pursued immediately, assuming there are no contraindications to systemic thrombolysis. Absolute and relative contraindications to systemic thrombolysis are listed in **Image 42-14.**

Absolute contraindications
Hemorrhagic stroke or stroke of unknown origin at any time
Ischemic stroke in preceding 6 months
CNS damage or neoplasm
Recent major trauma, surgery, or head injury (within preceding 3 weeks)
GI bleed within the past month
Known bleeding
Relative contraindications
Transient ischemic attacks in the preceding 6 months
Oral anticoagulant therapy
Pregnancy or within 1 week postpartum
Noncompressible punctures
Traumatic resuscitation
Refractory hypertension (systolic blood pressure ≥ 180 mm Hg)
Advanced liver disease
Infective endocarditis
Active peptic ulcer

Abbreviations: CNS, central nervous system; GI, gastrointestinal.

Image 42-14 • (*Reproduced with permission from Fuster V, Harrington RA, Narula J, et al: Hurst's the Heart, 14th ed. New York, NY: McGraw Hill; 2017.*)

As the patient has no contraindications, systemic thrombolysis is the next appropriate step. Embolectomy is reserved for hemodynamically unstable PE patients in whom systemic thrombolysis is contraindicated or has been unsuccessful. Antibiotics would not be appropriate here because the patient does not present with symptoms of sepsis. Anticoagulation is appropriate if recombinant tPA is used as the thrombolytic agent. An IVC filter is only recommended in patients who have contraindications to systemic anticoagulation.

Much of the current research is directed at the most appropriate treatment course for patients with submassive acute PE. Submassive PE is defined as evidence of right ventricular strain without hemodynamic instability. RV strain may be identified in a number of ways, including the RV/LV ratio on CT scan or echocardiographic evidence of RV dilation or dysfunction. However, it has been postulated that there are subgroups within the submassive category that may benefit from a more aggressive approach to reduce RV strain. A number of studies are underway that are examining the utility of more targeted approaches, including percutaneous embolectomy catheters and local low-dose tPA infusion via a pulmonary artery catheter, among many others. Further testing is needed to identify the appropriate patient populations (submassive versus massive) and indications for these modalities.

Q42-4: C
Pulmonary arterial hypertension

Rationale: The patient's clinical presentation is most consistent with a diagnosis of pulmonary arterial hypertension. The patient's chest radiography (**Images 42-7A** and **B**) shows an enlargement of pulmonary arteries bilaterally (note again that the pulmonary arteries sit inferior to the pulmonary veins). Additionally, there is a paucity of distal pulmonary vasculature on the film overall, termed "pruning." However, there is no evidence of pulmonary edema or reticulonodular changes on the chest imaging to suggest answers (D) or (E). On the echocardiogram in **Image 42-8**, the RV is much larger than the left ventricle LV, and the septum is flattened and appears to be bowing into the left ventricle. On the VQ scan in **Image 42-9**, there is no evidence of a perfusion defect seen (note the ventilation defect associated with the positioning of the heart is matched in the ventilation and perfusion [**Image 42-10**] images), so a diagnosis of CTEPH or acute pulmonary embolism is unlikely. The clinical presentation is consistent with pulmonary arterial hypertension (World Health Organization [WHO] group I pulmonary hypertension).

The WHO has described five groups of pulmonary hypertension: group 1 is pulmonary arterial hypertension, which may be idiopathic, heritable, associated with collagen vascular disease or congenital heart defects, or portopulmonary hypertension; group 2 disease is pulmonary hypertension secondary to left heart disease; group 3 pulmonary hypertension is attributable to underlying pulmonary disease; group 4 pulmonary hypertension is a result of chronic thromboembolic disease; and group 5 pulmonary hypertension is a miscellaneous group (disease secondary to sarcoidosis, sickle cell anemia, and other poorly understood etiologies).

The evaluation of pulmonary hypertension should include a history and physical, chest radiography, an echocardiogram, pulmonary function tests, a CT scan of the chest, a V/Q scan, and a laboratory evaluation for autoantibodies, HIV, and liver disease.

Q42-5: D
Chronic thromboembolic pulmonary hypertension (CTEPH)

Rationale: The patient's clinical presentation is most consistent with a diagnosis of chronic thromboembolic pulmonary hypertension (CTEPH), rather than an acute pulmonary embolism (PE). The patient's right heart catheterization numbers demonstrate a normal wedge pressure (a surrogate for the left-ventricular end-diasolic pressure, or LVEDP) with a significantly elevated mean pulmonary artery (PA) pressure, consistent with pulmonary hypertension. Additionally, the patient has a prior history of pulmonary embolus that was treated with anticoagulation and stopped, although the etiology for the PE was never identified. The patient then presented with protracted or chronic onset of dyspnea and reduced exercise tolerance that has progressively worsened over the last several years, rather than the days to-weeks time course commonly seen in acute PE. The patient's VQ scan (**Image 42-11**) is highly abnormal, with multiple un-matched perfusion filling defects seen bilaterally. This makes isolated pulmonary arterial hypertension or PH due to WHO group II or III indications unlikely. The pulmonary arteriogram (**Image 42-12**) demonstrates delayed or absent flow to large branches of the pulmonary vasculature resulted from clot organization and deposition along the endothelium, known as a pouch defect. Additionally, there is evidence of "pruning" of the distal vasculature tree due to organized clot and reduced blood flow. This is in contrast to the typically jagged, intraluminal filling defects seen in acute pulmonary emboli.

The important differential here is between left-sided heart failure, PVOD (pulmonary veno-occlusive disease), CTEPH, and chronic pulmonary emboli. The presence of perfusion abnormalities on the VQ scan and a normal wedge pressure make left-sided heart failure (WHO group II disease) or group I disease unlikely. Although abnormalities may be seen on CT, such as dilation of the central pulmonary arteries with organized thrombi adherent to the walls of the pulmonary artery, VQ scanning followed by pulmonary angiography is preferred to establish a diagnosis of CTEPH.

CTEPH is a distinct subgroup of pulmonary hypertension that evolves following repeated episodes of pulmonary emboli, although may also arise from isolated untreated PEs or even from submassive or massive Pes with appropriate treatment. Within the WHO classification system for pulmonary hypertension, CTEPH is considered group IV disease and current does have both medical and surgical options for treatment. CTEPH is characterized by the organization of fibrinous tissues along endothelial walls, particular in the medium-to-small vessels, leading to an arteriopathy. This eventually leads to the development of pulmonary hypertension and right heart failure over time. On imaging, patients with CTEPH have findings that are distinctly different from those in acute PE and pulmonary hypertension not due to WHO group IV disease. Patients with CTEPH will have unmatched perfusion abnormalities on VQ scanning, typically in a more mild pattern than that seen in acute PE but this is non-specific (**Images 42-15D** and **42-12**, respectively). Patients with CTEPH are more likely to have changes consistent with long-standing PH, including prominent pulmonary vasculature and enlarged right heart borders than those in acute PE (**Images 42-15A** and **C**, respectively). On CT imaging, patients with CTEPH may have mosaic attenuation due to differences in perfusion or peripheral infarcts (**Image 42-15B**). Contrasted CT imaging will often demonstrate more eccentric thrombi organized along the vessel wall as opposed to the central, jagged intraluminal defects seen in acute PE (**Images 42-15B and E**, respectively). Additionally, contrasted CT imaging will often demonstrate dilatation of the central pulmonary arteries with "pruning" of the distal pulmonary arterioles and intraluminal fibrous webs. CT imaging may also show evidence of "pouch" defects as discussed above. Similar to acute PE, patients with CTEPH will have elevated RV/LV ratios, and depending on hemodynamics, septal bowing may be present.

The importance in identifying a patient with CTEPH versus that with acute PE is essential, as the management is significantly different. Acute PE is managed with anticoagulation alone in most cases, although the use of targeted thrombolytics or mechanical disaggregation continues to be explored. Systemic thrombolysis is an option for patients with massive acute PE. In CTEPH, the thrombus is organized, and such approaches are not feasible. While anticoagulation is mainstay of treatment, CTEPH is best managed with surgical thrombectomy if possible. Patient's not eligible for surgery may also be managed medically with diuretics, PDE-5 inhibitors, endothelin receptor antagonists, oral/inhaled prostanoids, or macitentan depending on the experience of treating center and the patient's eligibility for surgical thrombectomy.

A – CTEPH

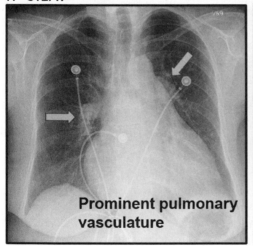
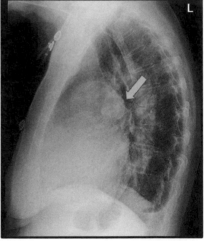

Image 42-15 • (A) Example of a chest radiograph for a patient with CTEPH, demonstrating prominent pulmonary vasculature and an enlarged right heart border.

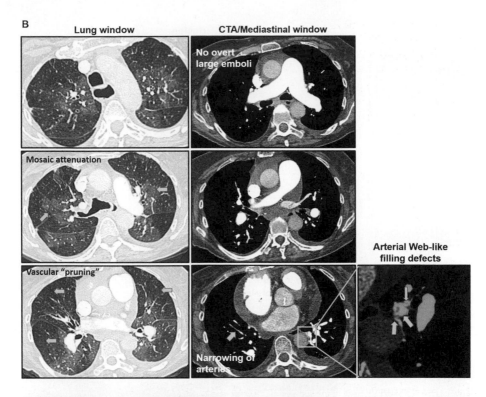

B

Lung window

CTA/Mediastinal window

No overt large emboli

Mosaic attenuation

Vascular "pruning"

Arterial Web-like filling defects

Narrowing of arteries

C – Acute Pulmonary Embolism (PE)

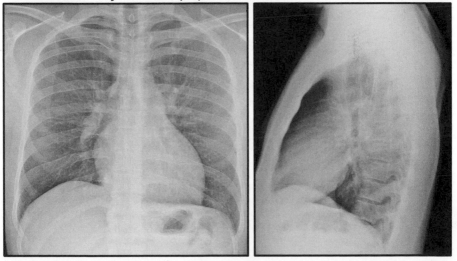

Image 42-15 • (B) Example of chest CT images in CTEPH, displaying mosaic attenuation, eccentric/organized thrombus with a lack of clear intra-luminal filling defects in the large pulmonary arteries, fibrous webs in the small arteries, and mild pruning of the distal vasculature. (C) Example of a chest radiograph in acute PE, with perhaps mild enlargement of the pulmonary vasculature.

D – VQ scan in Acute PE

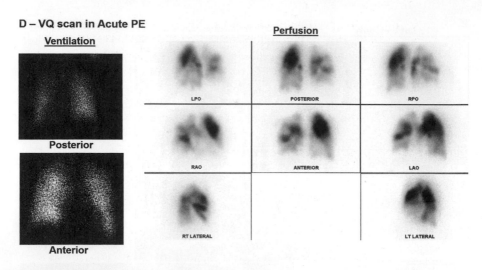

Ventilation

Posterior

Anterior

Perfusion

LPO POSTERIOR RPO

RAO ANTERIOR LAO

RT LATERAL LT LATERAL

E – CTA and Pulmonary Angiography in Acute PE

Lung window   CTA/Mediastinal window

Pulmonary angiogram

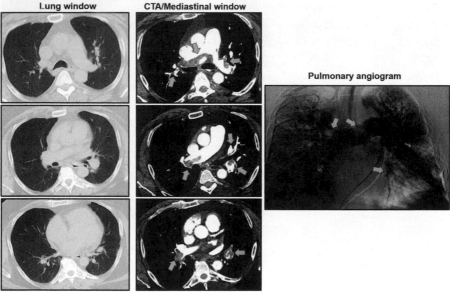

Image 42-15 • (D) Example of a VQ scan image in acute PE with large, distinct defects in perfusion as compared to the somewhat more subtle or at least less-jagged defects seen in **Image 42-12**. (E) Chest CT and pulmonary angiography imaging for a patient with acute PE, demonstrating the jagged central intraluminal defects, without evidence of significant pruning in unaffected areas or mosaic attenuation.

References

Aujesky D, Obrosky DS, Stone RA, et al. Derivation and validation of a prognostic model for pulmonary embolism. Am J Respir Crit Care Med. 2005;172:1041.

Aujesky D, Roy PM, Verschuren F, et al. Outpatient versus inpatient treatment for patients with acute pulmonary embolism: an international, open-label, randomised, non-inferiority trial. Lancet. 2011;378:41.

Benza RL, Miller DP, Barst RJ, et al. An evaluation of long-term survival from time of diagnosis in pulmonary arterial hypertension from the REVEAL Registry. Chest. 2012;142:448.

Chatterjee S, Chakraborty A, Weinberg I, et al. Thrombolysis for pulmonary embolism and risk of all-cause mortality, major bleeding, and intracranial hemorrhage: a meta-analysis. JAMA. 2014;311:2414.

Chiles C, Gulla SM. Radiology of the chest. In: Chen MM, Pope TL, Ott DJ, eds. *Basic Radiology.* 2nd ed. McGraw-Hill; 2011. https://accessmedicine.mhmedical.com/content .aspx?bookid=360&sectionid=39669011

Donzé J, Le Gal G, Fine MJ, et al. Prospective validation of the Pulmonary Embolism Severity Index. A clinical prognostic model for pulmonary embolism. Thromb Haemost. 2008;100:943.

Elmoselhi A, Seif M. Electrophysiology of the heart. In: Elmoselhi A, ed. *Cardiology: An Integrated Approach.* McGraw-Hill; 2017. https://accessmedicine.mhmedical.com/content .aspx?bookid=2224&sectionid=171660003

Fernandez-Jimenez R, Tapson V, Fuster V, Ibanez B. Pulmonary embolism. In: Fuster V, Harrington RA, Narula J, Eapen ZJ, eds. *Hurst's The Heart.* 14th ed. McGraw-Hill; 2017. https://accessmedicine. mhmedical.com/content.aspx?bookid=2046&sectionid=176562734

Fishman AJ, Moser KM, Fedullo PF. Perfusion lung scans vs pulmonary angiography in evaluation of suspected primary pulmonary hypertension. Chest. 1983;84:679.

Forfia PR, Trow TK. Diagnosis of pulmonary arterial hypertension. Clin Chest Med. 2013;34:665-681.

Gopalan D, Blanchard D, Auger WR. Diagnostic evaluation of chronic thromboembolic pulmonary hypertension. Ann Am Thorac Soc. 2016;13:S239.

Hampton AO, Castleman B. Correlation of postmortem chest teleroentgenograms with autopsy findings. Am J Roentgenol Radium Ther. 1940:34;305.

Kabrhel C, Jaff MR, Channick RN, et al. A multidisciplinary pulmonary embolism response team. Chest. 2013;144:1738.

Kearon C, Akl EA, Comerota AJ, et al. Antithrombotic therapy for VTE disease: antithrombotic therapy and prevention of thrombosis, 9th ed: American College of Chest Physicians Evidence-Based Clinical Practice Guidelines. Chest. 2012;141:e419S.

Kearon C, Akl EA, Ornelas J, et al. Antithrombotic therapy for VTE disease: CHEST guideline and expert panel report. Chest. 2016;149:315.

Lee DW, Gopalratnam K, Ford HJ, Rose-Jones LJ. The value of bedside echocardiogram in the setting of acute and chronic pulmonary embolism. Clin Chest Med. 2018;39:549.

Luke SGEH, Steven B, Robin C, et al. British Thoracic Society Guideline for the initial outpatient management of pulmonary embolism (PE). Thorax. 2018;73:ii1.

McCann C, Gopalan D, Sheares K, Screaton N. Imaging in pulmonary hypertension, part 1: clinicaly perspectives, classification, imaging techniques and imaging algorithm. Postgrad Med J. 2012;88:271.

McConnell MV, Solomon SD, Rayan ME, Come PC, Goldhaber SZ, Lee RT. Regional right ventricular dysfunction detected by echocardiography in acute pulmonary embolism. Am J Cardiol. 1996;78:469.

Nicod P, Peterson K, Levine M, et al. Pulmonary angiography in severe chronic pulmonary hypertension. Ann Intern Med. 1987;107:565.

Rali PM, Criner GJ. Concise clinical review: submassive pulmonary embolism. Am J Respir Crit Care Med. 2018;198:588.

Rich S (ed). Executive summary from the World Symposium on Primary Pulmonary Hypertension, Evian, France, September 6-10, 1998, co-sponsored by The World Health Organization.

Shahani L. S1Q3T3 pattern leading to early diagnosis of pulmonary embolism. BMJ Case Rep. 2012;2012:bcr2012006569.

Simonneau G, Gatzoulis MA, Adatia I, et al. Updated clinical classification of pulmonary hypertension. J Am Coll Cardiol. 2013;62:D34.

Sreenivasan S, Bennett S, Parfitt VJ. Westermark's and Palla's signs in acute pulmonary embolism. Circulation. 2007;115:e211.

Stein PD, Beemath A, Matta F, et al. Clinical characteristics of patients with acute pulmonary embolism: data from PIOPED II. Am J Med. 2007;120:871.

Tunariu N, Gibbs SJ, Win Z, et al. Ventilation-perfusion scintigraphy is more sensitive than multi-detector CTPA in detecting chronic thromboembolic pulmonary disease as a treatable cause of pulmonary hypertension. J Nucl Med. 2007;48:680.

van Belle A, Buller HR, Huisman MV, et al. Effectiveness of managing suspected pulmonary embolism using an algorithm combining clinical probability, D-dimer testing, and computed tomography. JAMA. 2006;295:172.

Wan S, Quinlan DJ, Agnelli G, Eikelboom JW. Thrombolysis compared with heparin for the initial treatment of pulmonary embolism: a meta-analysis of the randomized controlled trials. Circulation. 2004;110:744.

Wells PS, Anderson DR, Rodger M, et al. Excluding pulmonary embolism at the bedside without diagnostic imaging: management of patients with suspected pulmonary embolism presenting to the emergency department by using a simple clinical model and d-dimer. Ann Intern Med. 2001;135:98.

Wolf SJ, McCubbin TR, Feldhaus KM, Faragher JP, Adcock DM. Prospective validation of Wells Criteria in the evaluation of patients with suspected pulmonary embolism. Ann Emerg Med. 2004;44:503.

Worsley D, Alavi A, Aronchick J, Chen J, Greenspan R, Ravin C. Chest radiographic findings in patients with acute pulmonary embolism: observations from the PIOPED Study. Radiology. 1993;189:133.

CASE 43

A 55-year-old man with no medical problems and who takes no medications except acetaminophen (over the counter) for intermittent headaches presents to your office for evaluation. He was referred by his primary care provider for increasing dyspnea on exertion and abnormalities discovered on routine chest imaging. The patient first reported symptoms approximately 18 months ago, when he developed a dry, intermittent cough that was worse when he was at home and improved when he was at work. His primary care provider started the patient on fluticasone nasal spray for postnasal drip/upper airway cough syndrome, with minimal improvement. He then underwent spirometry with some mild restriction present, which was attributed to the patient's weight (body mass index 29 kg/m^2). He was trialed on albuterol with some improvement in the cough. However, approximately 6 months later, he developed worsening dyspnea with exercise. He had just retired from his job and assumed that his exercise tolerance was poor because of inactivity. He did not seek evaluation until the dyspnea began affecting his daily activities. Currently, the patient reports he cannot walk more than 200 feet without stopping to catch his breath. His vital signs are T 97.8°F, HR 95, BP 129/55, RR 18, O$_2$ saturation 91% on RA at rest, and 85% on room air with walking, improved to 94% on 2 L/min supplemental O$_2$. On examination, he has bilateral inspiratory crackles, with mild clubbing. There is no cardiac murmur present, and the patient has no evidence of lower extremity edema, cyanosis, or an elevated jugular vein pressure. His abdominal examination is normal, and there are no skin changes, joint effusions, or abnormalities. His neurologic examination is intact.

He denies any exposures. Before his retirement 12 months ago, he worked as a sales representative for a supermarket chain and visited stores on a daily basis, but he had no sustained exposures. He denies any new pets. He is a never-smoker and uses no drugs. He drinks three to five alcoholic beverages per week, with no history of dependence. He does not farm, perform woodworking, and do anything that generates aerosols. He does not use a humidifier. He lives in an area of the state with a significant amount of moisture and flooding. He does not garden or use organic chemicals, and he does not handle birds or animals.

The patient's CXR and CT scan are shown in Images 43-1 and 43-2, respectively.

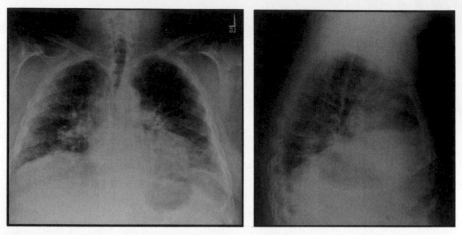

Image 43-1 • Chest radiogram for the patient in **Case 43**.

QUESTIONS

Q43-1: How would you describe the abnormalities in the chest radiogram?

A. Focal consolidative opacities in the right and left upper lobes
B. Low lung volumes
C. Diffuse reticulonodular opacities
D. Diffuse hazy and consolidative alveolar opacities
E. Upper lobe–predominant cavitary lesions
F. A and B
G. B and D
H. B and E
I. C and E
J. B and C

Q43-2: Here is the patient's corresponding interstitial lung disease (ILD)-protocol CT scan, which includes standard inspiratory imaging performed on standard chest CT scans in addition to prone inspiratory and supine expiratory images.

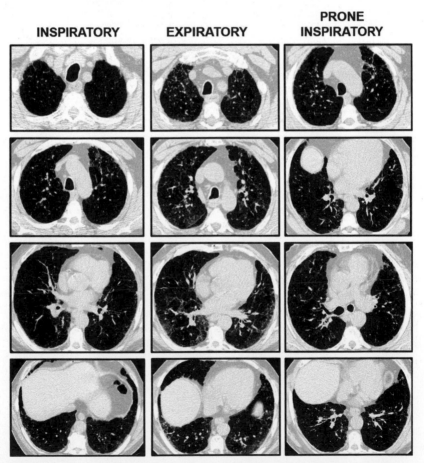

Image 43-2 • Interstitial lung disease–protocol CT scan of the patient in **Case 43**.

Which is the best description of the abnormalities seen on the patient's CT scan?

A. Upper lobe–predominant nodules, cavitary nodules, and cysts

B. Lower lobe–predominant septal thickening, traction bronchiectasis, and basilar-predominant subpleural honeycomb changes

C. Diffuse, mosaic pattern of air trapping with septal and interlobular septal thickening, ground-glass opacities, without honeycomb changes

D. Diffuse alveolar consolidative opacities

E. Centrilobular emphysema

Q43-3: Given the above imaging findings, the patient undergoes a bronchoscopy with bronchoalveolar lavage (BAL) and transbronchial biopsies, in addition to laboratory testing. The BAL returns with 35% lymphocytes, 2% neutrophils, and 60% macrophages. All the microbiology testing is negative, including acid-fast bacillus (AFB) staining. The transbronchial biopsies are pending, as are additional laboratory studies. The patient undergoes pulmonary function testing, which is shown in Image 43-3 below. What is the appropriate interpretation of the studies?

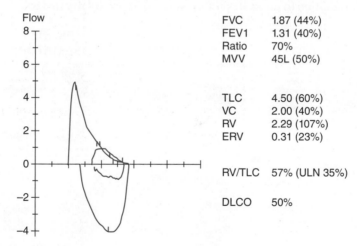

FVC	1.87 (44%)		
FEV1	1.31 (40%)		
Ratio	70%		
MVV	45L (50%)		
TLC	4.50 (60%)		
VC	2.00 (40%)		
RV	2.29 (107%)		
ERV	0.31 (23%)		
RV/TLC	57% (ULN 35%)		
DLCO	50%		

Image 43-3 • Pulmonary function testing for the patient in **Case 43.**

A. Mixed restrictive and obstruction with evidence of air trapping and a reduced DLCO

B. Restrictive defect with a reduced DLCO

C. Obstructive defect with air trapping and a normal DLCO

D. Normal spirometry, lung volumes, and a reduced DLCO

E. An elevated DLCO concerning for alveolar hemorrhage or polycythemia

Q43-4: The patient's rheumatologic workup returns negative. The pathology report returns with the following: "areas of chronic, cellular, and fibrotic nonspecific interstitial pneumonia (NSIP), with a few scattered areas of usual interstitial pneumonia (UIP). There is no evidence granulomatous inflammation." Given the pathology report and the aforementioned information, what is the likely diagnosis?

A. Sarcoidosis
B. Idiopathic pulmonary fibrosis
C. Desquamative interstitial pneumonia
D. Berylliosis
E. Miliary tuberculosis
F. Chronic hypersensitivity pneumonitis
G. Chester-Erdheim disease

Q43-5: What has been associated with a reduced risk of developing HP?

A. Cardiovascular exercise
B. Vitamin D supplementation
C. Nebulized *N*-acetylcysteine
D. Suppressive antibiotics
E. Tobacco smoking
F. Azithromycin

Q43-6: Which histopathologic pattern is associated with the worst prognosis in patients with chronic HP?

A. UIP
B. Cellular NSIP
C. Bronchiolitis obliterans-organizing pneumonia (BOOP)
D. Respiratory bronchiolitis (RB)

Q43-7: Because antigen avoidance is the most important aspect of treatment, you next aim to determine the antigen causing the patient's lung disease. Given the temporal relationship of the patient's disease progression and his environmental/occupational exposures, what would you ask the patient to do next?

A. Ask his prior employer to check ventilation systems in supermarkets.
B. Have the house inspected to look for evidence of water damage or mold.
C. Check for radon levels at his house.
D. Check for termites at his house.
E. Move to a new state.

Q43-8: The patient has his house professionally cleaned as well as his heating and air-conditioning system. He has a special contractor examine the crawl-spaces where mold is discovered and removed. The patient is started on gluco-corticoids and has some improvement in his symptoms and pulmonary function testing. However, as his prednisone dose is weaned from 20 mg/day to 15 mg/day, his symptoms appear to worsen, and his spirometry worsens as well. He has also developed some vision issues, which he reports are due to new cataracts. What is the best course of action?

A. Continue to wean the patient's prednisone dose to 10 mg/day given the development of cataracts.

B. Continue the patient on the current prednisone dose of 15 mg/day.

C. Increase the patient's prednisone dose to 20 mg/day, and start the patient on myco-phenolate with a goal of tapering the prednisone once his symptoms improve.

D. Prescribe plasmapheresis with rituximab and carfilzomib to target antibody production by B cells and plasma cells.

E. Prescribe intravenous immune globulin (IVIG).

F. Recommend transplantation.

ANSWERS

Q43-1: J
B and C

Rationale: Here, the chest radiogram shows approximately seven rib spaces. Assuming there is no issue with the patient's effort or ability to follow the instructions, this would be consistent with low lung volumes from a pathologic process. The CXR also demonstrates relatively diffuse, though likely upper lobe–predominant, reticulonodular opacities, with a more reticular appearance overall. There are no focal consolidative opacities, and there are no apparent cavitary lesions (cysts can be more difficult to identify than cavitary lesions on chest radiograms). Hazy alveolar and consolidative opacities generally have a more confluent appearance, as shown in **Image 43-4** below.

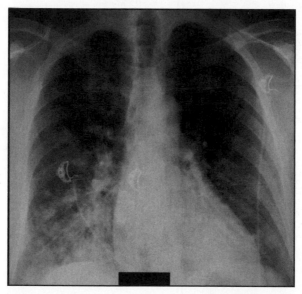

Image 43-4 • Example of a chest radiograph more consistent with "hazy" alveolar opacities.

Q43-2: C
Diffuse, mosaic pattern of air trapping with septal and interlobular septal thickening, ground-glass opacities, without honeycomb changes

Rationale: In an ILD-protocol CT scan, one can identify areas of air trapping by comparing the inspiratory and expiratory films. At inspiration, the lung is distended with air and appears less radiodense (ie, more black). On expiration, the lung is less distended, with the bronchovascular structures in closer proximity approximately, and the lung appears more radiodense (ie, more grayscale). Air trapping is identified when there are persistent areas of lung that appear similar to the inspiratory film. Here, this is indicated by darker/black areas of the lung on the expiratory film that are surrounded by areas of more dense/grayscale lung tissue. This pattern is sometimes referred to as "head-cheese." The prone imaging is used to identify areas of basilar honeycomb changes or architectural distortion that may be missed on supine imaging because of gravity and restriction. Here, we see a relatively diffuse process. The pattern is termed *mosaic* because it looks like a heterogenous process with areas of unaffected lung tissue mixed with areas of ground glass and septal thickening. There may be some micronodular opacities. There are no apparent cysts or cavitary nodules. Additionally, there is no evidence of a lower lobe–predominant process or honeycomb changes at the bases. There are no alveolar consolidative opacities (see example in **Image 43-2**). **Answer (E)** is not necessarily incorrect because the imaging has the appearance of possible centrilobular emphysema; however, this is not a complete descriptor of the abnormalities present.

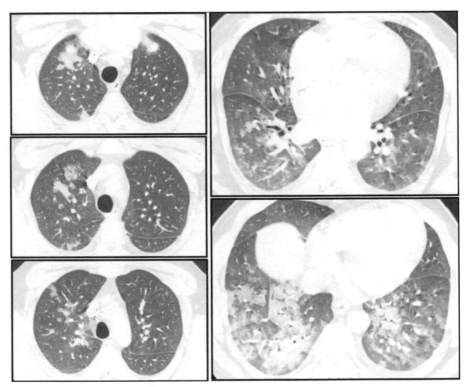

Image 43-5 • Example of hazy (ground-glass) and consolidative alveolar opacities. This is an example of a patient with diffuse alveolar hemorrhage after bone marrow transplantation.

Q43-3: A
Mixed restrictive and obstruction with evidence of air trapping and a reduced DLCO

Rationale: First, examining the spirometric indices and the flow-volume loop, there is evidence of both restrictive and obstructive defects. The FVC is low, suggesting possible restriction, and while the FEV1/FVC ratio is borderline normal (70%), the flow-volume loop clearly has a concave shape, suggesting worsening airflow obstruction at lower lung volumes, consistent with an obstructive defect. This is an example of pseudonormalization of the FEV1/FVC ratio. This is encountered mostly in restrictive lung disease, where the FVC is reduced out of proportion to the FEV1. The lung volumes show a reduced TLC (60%) consistent with at least moderate restriction of the lung volume excursion. The patient's RV is elevated (107%), and the RV/TLC ratio is considerably elevated at 57%, both suggesting that air trapping is present. The ERV is low and is reduced out of proportion to the remaining lung volumes, which may be consistent with obesity, poor effort, or difficulty with the maneuver. The MVV, while low at 45 L/min, is appropriate for the patient's reduced FEV1 (30*FEV1 = 39.3 L/min expected), so there is no evidence of neuromuscular disease. The DLCO is substantially reduced.

Q43-4: F
Chronic hypersensitivity pneumonitis

Rationale: This is a typical presentation of chronic hypersensitivity pneumonitis (HP). The chest imaging is classic for chronic hypersensitivity pneumonitis, with a mosaic pattern of air trapping, ground-glass opacities, and septal thickening. As the disease progresses, the patient may transition from a more cellular/reversible process to a more fibrotic-appearing CT scan (**Image 43-6**).

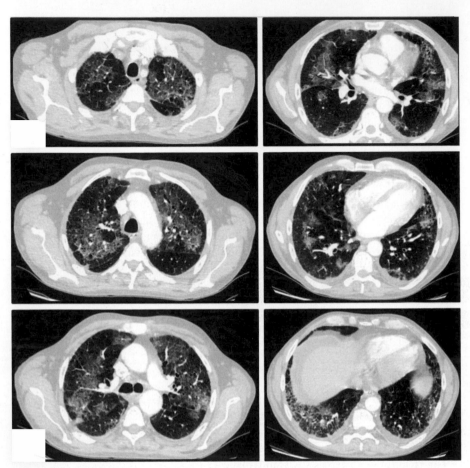

Image 43-6 • A more cellular-appearing case of subacute/chronic hypersensitivity pneumonitis with ground-glass opacities (inspiratory film only). One would expect the pathology here to show cellular interstitial pneumonitis, granulomatous inflammation, and perhaps cellular nonspecific interstitial pneumonia.

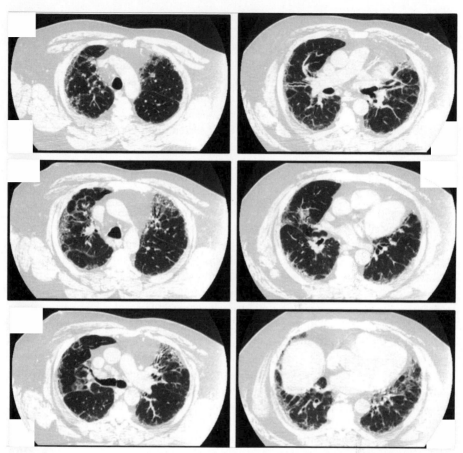

Image 43-7 • Example of a CT scan with a more fibrotic appearance, with markedly fewer ground-glass opacities and more significant septal thickening and some traction bronchiectasis (inspiratory film only).

HP (also referred to as *extrinsic allergic alveolitis*) is an immune response to an organic allergen and may be seen in acute, subacute, and chronic forms. However, it should be noted that not all presentations of HP fit nicely into this schema. Some of the more well-known variants of HP are bird fancier's disease and farmer's lung disease. Animal dander, aerosolized molds/fungi, organic chemical compounds, and many other compounds have been implicated as antigens in HP. There have been reported outbreaks of HP as well, typically associated with contaminated water supply systems or water damage leading to the development of mold. Isocyanates have most commonly been associated with asthma and HP in chemical manufacturing or other industrial processing. Infection or colonization with *Mycobacterium avium* complex has also been associated with the development in HP in patients with prolonged hot water exposure, often termed "hot-tub lung." Acute HP is covered in **Case 10**.

In subacute and chronic HP, the most common abnormality is a reduced DLCO. Most patients have some degree of restrictive lung disease, though patients with more evidence of air trapping may have a predominant obstructive pattern with an elevated RV and RV/TLC ratio. For the most part, patients have a mixed restrictive and obstructive pattern. It is important to look at the shape of the flow-volume curve on expiration and not only the spirometric indices because significant restriction can cause a pseudonormalization of the FEV1/FVC ratio (the percent reduction in FVC is typically impacted more significantly than the FEV1 in restriction), and the presence of underlying obstruction can be missed and untreated.

HP is believed to represent either a type 3 (acute/subacute) or type 4 (subacute/chronic) hypersensitivity reaction. Recall that type 3 reactions involve the development of immune complexes (IgG antigen-antibody-complement), and type 4 reactions involve CD4 T-cell–mediated delayed reactions (such as with the purified protein derivative test). Overall, testing for specific antigens in HP is somewhat limited. There are serum precipitin tests that may be performed to identify the presence of IgG antibodies against specific antigens. However, there are a number of limitations to testing: (1) these antibodies are often found in asymptomatic subjects with prior exposure to the antigens and who have no evidence of lung disease; (2) there is a significant risk of false-negative testing; and (3) there is an infinite number of potential antigens, but currently testing is limited to fewer than approximately 200 antigens through the National Jewish Hospital, and there must be some a priori knowledge of the antigen to narrow the search. This latter limitation is of particular importance in patients with chronic HP, where the exposure may be more indolent and not easily recognizable. It is possible to obtain environmental samples and test them against a patient's blood to determine if an immune complex forms; however, this is limited to specific reference laboratories and likely also depends on the purity of the environmental samples obtained. For subacute and chronic HP, there are no widely available lymphocyte proliferation tests, which, again, would require a significant number of antigens. Skin testing is not useful because this is a test of antigen-specific IgE antibodies, representing a different hypersensitivity mechanism (type 1). Other acute phase or inflammatory marker testing (ESR, CRP, LDH, procalcitonin) is generally not useful in the diagnosis of HP.

In subacute and chronic HP, clinicians usually start with exposure history, imaging, pulmonary function testing, and laboratory testing for rheumatologic conditions. If there is a clear and obvious antigen history and the imaging and laboratory testing supports the diagnosis, a trial of antigen exposure may help strengthen the case for HP, particularly early in the disease process. A transbronchial biopsy may be effective early in the disease process for a definitive diagnosis of HP, whereas bronchoalveolar lavage is nonspecific (a significant lymphocytosis, usually greater than 20%, can support the diagnosis) and generally used to rule out an infectious process. Transbronchial biopsies are also very important in ruling out sarcoidosis and other granulomatous diseases. The diagnostic yield of a transbronchial biopsy is likely around 50% and is less efficacious in patients with fibrotic changes. Patients in whom the diagnosis remains unclear after this approach may require video-assisted thoracoscopic surgery (VATS) or open surgical lung biopsy. The pathology in acute and subacute HP generally shows noncaseating granulomatous inflammation in the respiratory bronchioles with lymphocytes and monocytes present in the peribronchiolar regions (ie, cellular bronchiolitis and pneumonitis). In the end stages of the disease, the pathology may show UIP, cellular or fibrotic NSIP, or areas of organizing pneumonia.

Q43-5: E
Tobacco smoking

Rationale: Tobacco smoking is associated with a decreased risk of developing HP; however, once a diagnosis of HP is established, smoking does not appear to attenuate the disease process. Patients with HP who smoke tobacco have generally shown a more rapid decline in lung function. The mechanism by which tobacco smoking reduces the risk of HP is unclear, though it may be associated with a reduced generation of antibodies to allergens introduced through the lung.

Q43-6: A
UIP

Rationale: This is consistent across interstitial pneumonias; the presence of UIP carries the worst prognosis.

Q43-7: B
Have the house inspected to look for evidence of water damage or mold

Rationale: In this case, the temporal association is important. The patient's initial symptoms were worse when he was at home and improved when at work. Additionally, once the patient retired and was at home more often, his symptoms significantly accelerated. He adopted no new hobbies and has no other clear exposure to animal dander/excreta, chemical compounds, or organic dusts, so this would raise concern for a possible source in the house. One should check for the use of humidifiers or vaporizers, pipes, continuous positive airway pressure (CPAP) or bi-level airway pressure (BiPAP) machines that have not been cleaned, and use of hot tubs or swimming pools. Most importantly, one should inquire about potential water damage and mold contamination in the house. In addition, many clinicians recommend patients have their houses professionally cleaned. Here is a common list of items to inquire about regarding potential antigen exposure:

1. Presence of mold or water damage in the house or place of employment: This may arise from multiple sources, including heat and air-conditioning systems, swimming pools, hot tubs, and humidifiers. Often, patients may not be aware of water damage in the house, and it should be recommended to have crawl and attic spaces inspected as well as the ventilation system.
2. Exposure to farms or farm animals, as well as exposure to bird droppings or bird dander. Essentially, any prolonged exposure to animal dander or droppings may lead to the development of HP, including, potentially, household pets. Note that there is a condition known as *organic dust toxic syndrome* that is similar to acute berylliosis in that it requires a high antigen exposure load over a short period of time (ie, 1 day), whereas farmer's lung disease (HP) results from a more subacute or prolonged exposure to the antigen.
3. Exposure to any processing of organic materials that are associated with the development of aerosolized particles, including woodworking/lumber processing, granaries, flour mills, and tobacco processing plants.

4. Exposure to any organic chemical vapors with particular attention to isocyanates or plastics: It is important to differentiate HP from inhalation fever ("metal fume fever") as well.

5. Exposure to textiles manufacturing: This is controversial, and some clinicians consider textile-related lung injury to be a process separate from HP. However, this aspect of the patient's exposure history must also be addressed.

6. Of course, it is important to address exposures more commonly associated with other types of lung disease (coal dust, beryllium in aerospace or electronics manufacturing, silica) to aid in narrowing the differential diagnosis.

Q43-8: B
Increase the patient's prednisone dose to 20 mg/day, and start the patient on mycophenolate (CellCept) with a goal of tapering the prednisone once his symptoms improve

Rationale: Patients with progressive disease or those with a more cellular inflammatory appearance (ie, ground glass as opposed to fibrosis on imaging or on pathology) who have found no improvement or patients who are unable to taper below 10 mg/day of a prednisone equivalent should be considered for another steroid-sparing immunosuppressive. Mycophenolate is used most commonly, given the relatively minimal adverse effects compared with azathioprine. Rituximab has also been used in limited, nonfibrotic disease, but evidence is also lacking. Additionally, targeting B-cell responses alone may not prevent a CD4+ T-cell–driven hypersensitivity. Overall, the data for immunosuppressive are lacking. Consideration could be given to antifibrotics (nintedanib, pirfenidone). Transplantation should be reversed for patients with progressive disease despite immunosuppressives and glucocorticoids, though referral to a transplant center at this point for initial evaluation and establishing a relationship would not be out of the question because the patient now requires O_2 with activity. There is no clear role for IVIG in the treatment of HP.

In terms of his current prednisone dosing, it would not be prudent to decrease his dose (or leave his dose at the current level) in the setting of worsening lung function without starting some other steroid-sparing agent. Typically, after several weeks of tapering up the patient's mycophenolate dose, the prednisone can be further tapered down to a reasonable level (or, preferably, off).

Summary of Acute, Subacute, and Chronic HP				
	Time to Onset From Antigen Exposure	Symptoms	Radiographic Findings	Progression/Recurrence	Treatment
Acute	Several hours (4-8)	Resembles community-acquired pneumonia, with fevers, chills, malaise, dyspnea, and dry cough. Patients may have inspiratory crackles on examination.	Often normal, though patients may have reticulonodular opacities with a lower lobe predominance. Alveolar opacities can be seen in a similar pattern in severe cases. CT may demonstrate ground-glass opacities and micronodules.	Typically resolves rapidly in the absence of an antigen (1-2 days) but may recur with antigen reexposure. Not thought to be a significant risk for progression to chronic disease, assuming the antigen is avoided.	Antigen avoidance; if symptoms persist, search for an alternative antigen. A course of glucocorticoids may be necessary for patients with persistent abnormalities on imaging or pulmonary function testing or in those with continued symptoms.
Subacute	Days-weeks (typically less than 6 months)	Subacute (4-6 weeks) onset and progression of dyspnea and cough, without fever, chills, or night sweats.	As opposed to acute HP, subacute HP displays an upper lung predominance, typically with a reticulonodular pattern. CT may demonstrate ground-glass opacities and micronodules. On CT, patients may have evidence of interlobular thickening, and if expiratory imaging is performed, there may be evidence of air trapping in a mosaic pattern.	Increased risk of progression to chronic HP.	Same as above. Prednisone is typically dosed at 0.5 mg/kg/day with an unspecified period of time and tapered during follow-up based on symptoms and objective testing.

(Continued)

	Time to Onset From Antigen Exposure	Symptoms	Radiographic Findings	Progression/Recurrence	Treatment
Chronic	Typically greater than 3-6 months	Insidious onset of symptoms, often with dry cough noted and issues with exercise intolerance. Many patients do not present until the dyspnea impacts typically daily activities (ie, mowing the grass, taking out the trash, purchasing groceries). Patients may show evidence of more prolonged hypoxemia and pulmonary cachexia.	Earlier in the disease course, there is an upper-lobe predominance of patchy ground-glass opacities, again with mosaic attenuation on expiratory CT. As the disease progresses and fibrosis occurs, there may be septal thickening, architectural distortion, traction bronchiectasis, and honeycomb seen in a more diffuse distribution than in UIP.	Variable progression, monitored primarily by symptoms and pulmonary function testing longitudinally.	Antigen avoidance in patients with progressive disease or those with a more cellular inflammatory appearance (ie, ground glass as opposed to fibrosis on imaging or on pathology). If the patient finds no improvement, or if the patient is unable to be tapered below 10 mg/day of a prednisone equivalent, consideration should be made for another steroid-sparing immunosuppressive. Mycophenolate is used most commonly, given the relatively minimal adverse effects compared with azathioprine. There is a condition known as organic dust toxic syndrome that is similar to acute berylliosis in that it requires a high antigen exposure load over a short period of time (ie, one day), whereas farmer's lung disease (HP) results from a more subacute or prolonged exposure to the antigen. Rituximab has also been used in limited, nonfibrotic disease. Overall, the data for immunosuppressive are lacking. Consideration could be given to antifibrotics (nintedanib, pirfenidone).

References

Agostini C, Trentin L, Facco M, Semenzato G. New aspects of hypersensitivity pneumonitis. Curr Opin Pulm Med. 2004;10:378.

Cormier Y, Létourneau L, Racine G. Significance of precipitins and asymptomatic lymphocytic alveolitis: a 20-yr follow-up. Eur Respir J. 2004;23:523.

Fenoglio CM, Reboux G, Sudre B, et al. Diagnostic value of serum precipitins to mould antigens in active hypersensitivity pneumonitis. Eur Respir J. 2007;29:706.

Hanak V, Golbin JM, Hartman TE, Ryu JH. High-resolution CT findings of parenchymal fibrosis correlate with prognosis in hypersensitivity pneumonitis. Chest. 2008;134:133.

Johannson KA, Elicker BM, Vittinghoff E, et al. A diagnostic model for chronic hypersensitivity pneumonitis. Thorax. 2016;71:951.

Kern RM, Singer JP, Koth L, et al. Lung transplantation for hypersensitivity pneumonitis. Chest. 2015;147:1558.

Lacasse Y, Girard M, Cormier Y. Recent advances in hypersensitivity pneumonitis. Chest. 2012;142:208.

Lacasse Y, Selman M, Costabel U, et al. Clinical diagnosis of hypersensitivity pneumonitis. Am J Respir Crit Care Med. 2003;168:952.

Lentz RJ, Argento AC, Colby TV, et al. Transbronchial cryobiopsy for diffuse parenchymal lung disease: a state-of-the-art review of procedural techniques, current evidence, and future challenges. J Thorac Dis. 2017;9:2186.

Lota HK, Keir GJ, Hansell DM, et al. Novel use of rituximab in hypersensitivity pneumonitis refractory to conventional treatment. Thorax. 2013;68:780.

Mohr LC. Hypersensitivity pneumonitis. Curr Opin Pulm Med. 2004;10:401.

Morisset J, Johannson KA, Vittinghoff E, et al. Use of mycophenolate mofetil or azathioprine for the management of chronic hypersensitivity pneumonitis. Chest. 2017;151:619.

Quirce S, Vandenplas O, Campo P, et al. Occupational hypersensitivity pneumonitis: an EAACI position paper. Allergy. 2016;71:765.

Salisbury ML, Myers JL, Belloli EA, et al. Diagnosis and treatment of fibrotic hypersensitivity pneumonia. Where we stand and where we need to go. Am J Respir Crit Care Med. 2017;196:690.

Selman M. Hypersensitivity pneumonitis: a multifaceted deceiving disorder. Clin Chest Med. 2004;25:531.

Selman M, Pardo A, King TE Jr. Hypersensitivity pneumonitis: insights in diagnosis and pathobiology. Am J Respir Crit Care Med. 2012;186:314.

Sheth JS, Belperio JA, Fishbein MC, et al. Utility of transbronchial vs surgical lung biopsy in the diagnosis of suspected fibrotic interstitial lung disease. Chest. 2017;151:389.

Silva CI, Müller NL, Lynch DA, et al. Chronic hypersensitivity pneumonitis: differentiation from idiopathic pulmonary fibrosis and nonspecific interstitial pneumonia by using thin-section CT. Radiology. 2008;246:288.

Spagnolo P, Rossi G, Cavazza A, et al. Hypersensitivity pneumonitis: a comprehensive review. J Investig Allergol Clin Immunol. 25:237.

Takemura T, Akashi T, Ohtani Y, et al. Pathology of hypersensitivity pneumonitis. Curr Opin Pulm Med. 2008;14:440.

Trahan S, Hanak V, Ryu JH, Myers JL. Role of surgical lung biopsy in separating chronic hypersensitivity pneumonia from usual interstitial pneumonia/idiopathic pulmonary fibrosis: analysis of 31 biopsies from 15 patients. Chest. 2008;134:126.

Tsutsui T, Miyazaki Y, Okamoto T, et al. Antigen avoidance tests for diagnosis of chronic hypersensitivity pneumonitis. Respir Investig. 2015;53:217.

Vasakova M, Morell F, Walsh S, et al. Hypersensitivity pneumonitis: perspectives in diagnosis and management. Am J Respir Crit Care Med. 2017;196:680.

Vourlekis JS, Schwarz MI, Cool CD, et al. Nonspecific interstitial pneumonitis as the sole histologic expression of hypersensitivity pneumonitis. Am J Med. 2002;112:490.

Zacharisen MC, Schlueter DP, Kurup VP, Fink JN. The long-term outcome in acute, subacute, and chronic forms of pigeon breeder's disease hypersensitivity pneumonitis. Ann Allergy Asthma Immunol. 2002;88:175.

CASE 44

A 48-year-old White woman presents with complaints of progressive dyspnea on exertion. The symptoms have gradually worsened over the past 6 months. The patient has a history of hypertension, diabetes mellitus type 2, and hyperlipidemia. She is relatively sedentary with no regular exercise. She reports the gradual onset of dyspnea with exertion over the past 6 months, with a dry cough and some generalized fatigue. She states that she is employed as a paralegal and that the office is very clean with no concern for occupational exposure. She has no hobbies outside of the home, and she lives in a new condominium with no evidence of water damage or mold issues. She has a family history of lung cancer in her grandmother and mother, both of whom were heavy smokers. She has no history of rheumatologic disease and no signs or symptoms of such on examination. She does not use illicit drugs. She denies ever using smoking tobacco. She drinks two to three alcoholic beverages a night but has no history of aspiration or alcohol withdrawal. The patient's vital signs are T 99.1°F, HR 101, BP 121/78, RR 16, and O_2 saturation 95% on room air at rest and 92% with walking. The patient's 6-minute walk distance (6MWD) is 69% predicted. The patient has some mild expiratory wheezing and audible inspiratory crackles. There is no clubbing, cyanosis, or lower extremity edema. The patient's cardiovascular examination is otherwise unremarkable, and the joint examination demonstrates no abnormalities. The patient underwent pulmonary function testing at an outside physician's office that was reported as "mild restriction with no obstruction and a moderate reduction in the diffusing capacity of carbon monoxide." The patient underwent a chest radiograph and a CT scan. The latter is shown below in Image 44-1.

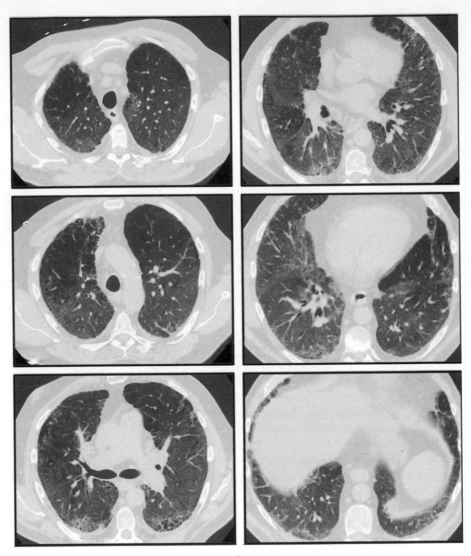

Image 44-1 • CT imaging of the patient in **Case 44**.

QUESTIONS

Q44-1: How would you describe the abnormalities on the CT scan?

A. Septal thickening, traction bronchiectasis, and subpleural bibasilar honeycombing
B. A mosaic pattern of cystic and cavitary lung lesions
C. Diffuse ground-glass and micronodular opacities
D. Tree-in-bud opacities with scattered ground glass
E. Consolidation with air bronchograms in the bilateral lower lobes

Q44-2: The patient undergoes some basic laboratory testing, as shown below. Given the patient's chest imaging and pulmonary function testing abnormalities, which treatment would you recommend next?

HIV antibodies (p24)	Negative
Purified protein derivative	0 mm
QuantiFERON Gold tuberculosis (TB) test	Nonreactive (negative)
Brain-natriuretic peptide (BNP)	34 pg/mL (ULN 100 pg/mL)
Hemoglobin	17.6 g/dL (ULN 15.0 g/dL)
Platelets	304×10^9/L
Serum bicarbonate	25 mEq/L
Procalcitonin	undetectable

A. Bronchodilator challenge with mannitol
B. Bronchodilator challenge with methacholine
C. Cardiopulmonary exercise test with pre and post arterial blood gases (ABGs)
D. Bronchoscopy with transbronchial biopsy and bronchoalveolar lavage (BAL)
E. Echocardiogram

Q44-3: The patient undergoes BAL and transbronchial biopsy, but the results are nondiagnostic. The patient is referred for a lung biopsy, and the following results are obtained. Special stains for acid-fast bacillus (AFB), fungal elements, and Cd1a are negative.

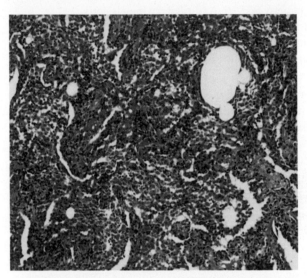

Image 44-2 • Histopathology from the patient in **Case 44**.

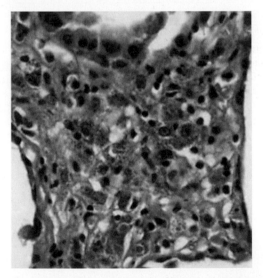

Image 44-3 • Magnified image of the interstitial infiltrate seen in **Image 44-2**.

What is the diagnosis?

A. Hypersensitivity pneumonitis (HP)
B. Respiratory bronchiolitis–associated interstitial lung disease (RB-ILD)
C. Pulmonary Langerhans cell histiocytosis (PLCH)
D. Idiopathic pulmonary fibrosis (IPF)
E. Sarcoidosis
F. Desquamative interstitial pneumonia (DIP)

Q44-4: What is the most common abnormality seen on pulmonary function testing in patients with RB-ILD or DIP?

A. Restricted ventilation defect (reduced FVC with normal FEV1/FVC ratio)
B. Obstructive airflow defect (reduced FEV1/FVC ratio)
C. Reduced diffusing capacity of carbon monoxide (DLCO)
D. Hyperinflation

Q44-5: What is the most important treatment for RB-ILD and DIP?

A. Antibiotics
B. Immunosuppression (eg, steroids)
C. Smoking cessation
D. Hyperbaric oxygen therapy
E. Noninvasive positive pressure ventilation
F. Lung transplantation

ANSWERS

Q44-1: C
Diffuse ground-glass and micronodular opacities

Rationale: In this image, there are diffuse ground-glass opacities present on a likely background of centrilobular emphysema. There is some mild septal thickening but no traction bronchiectasis or significant honeycomb changes at the bases. There are no cysts or cavitary lesions. There are some micronodular opacities, though these may be difficult to discern at this resolution. The pattern of distribution of the abnormalities is relatively diffuse.

Q44-2: D
A bronchoscopy with transbronchial biopsy and bronchoalveolar lavage (BAL)

Rationale: The patient's imaging and pulmonary function testing results are concerning for interstitial lung disease. Options (A) and (B) would be options for a patient with suspected asthma, while option (C) would be an option for a patient in whom the etiology of the dyspnea was unclear. Option (E) is appropriate in patients for whom either right or left heart failure is suspected as the source of the patient's dyspnea. Given the abnormalities in this case, bronchoscopy with biopsy and BAL would be an appropriate next step, along with additional testing for rheumatologic antibodies. One could surmise from the laboratory values that the patient does not have HIV, prior TB exposure, evidence of acute volume overload due to heart failure, or acute bacterial infection.

Q44-3: F
Desquamative interstitial pneumonia (DIP)

Rationale: The pathology specimen shows smokers macrophages (black pigment, **Image 44-3**) as a component of the peribronchiolar inflammatory response. This is common in respiratory bronchiolitis (RB) and RB-ILD. However, we also see more diffuse interstitial pneumonitis without evidence of significant fibrosis. There is some mild peribronchiolar and alveolar wall fibrosis. There are no granulomas consistent with HP or sarcoidosis and no extensive fibrosis as would be expected in UIP. The lack of CD1a staining would eliminate PLCH as a likely possibility.

The pathology of DIP is marked by smoker's macrophages in the respiratory bronchioles, with an inflammatory infiltrate of lymphocytes, plasma cells, eosinophils, and dendritic cells in the peribronchiolar interstitium, resulting in bronchiolar wall thickening. As the disease progresses, there is a more diffuse interstitial fibrosis, with the development of germinal centers/lymphoid follicles and a more inflammatory alveolar infiltrate. Generally, there is no evidence of architectural distortion. Findings of fibroblastic foci or architecture distortion should raise suspicion for NSIP or UIP. Similar to RB-ILD, DIP commonly presents in the third through fifth decades of life, almost exclusively in current/recent former smoking tobacco users, people who vape, or in people with second-hand exposure. In rare cases, DIP has been associated with rheumatologic conditions, most notably rheumatoid arthritis. DIP has also been observed in patients with genetic mutations affecting surfactant production or release. The clinical presentation of DIP is similar to RB-ILD (dyspnea, dry or productive cough, fatigue), but it is more likely to be associated with constitutional symptoms (weight loss, fever) than RB-ILD. Similar to RB-ILD, the most common examination abnormality is inspiratory crackles that are coarser than those seen in other interstitial pneumonias. Chest radiographs are typically normal, while CT will typically demonstrate reticulonodular and ground-glass abnormalities with an upper-lobe predominance.

Q44-4: C
Reduced diffusing capacity of carbon monoxide (DLCO)

Although many patients demonstrate a restrictive ventilation defect, patients may also show an obstructive airflow defect alone or a combination of obstruction and restriction (remember that many patients may have evidence of COPD as well). However, nearly all patients will show a reduction in DLCO, a surrogate for the diffusing capacity of O_2.

Q44-5: C
Smoking cessation

Rationale: Smoking cessation is the primary treatment modality in patients with RB-ILD and DIP, independent of the severity of the disease. The primary treatment for DIP is smoking cessation, which, when successful, is associated with a nearly 90% 10-year survival rate. Deaths or disease progression are more common in DIP than RB-ILD. Similar to patients with RB-ILD, patients with more severe presentations or who experience progression despite smoking cessation may be started on glucocorticoids or immunosuppressive medications (mycophenolate, azathioprine), though, again, the evidence for their efficacy is absent. Otherwise, treatment is primarily supportive, including pulmonary rehabilitation, age- and comorbidity-appropriate vaccination, treatment of underlying or existing obstructive lung disease, and, in appropriate clinical settings, supplemental O_2. The role of antifibrotic agents has not been explored in patients with more severe disease. Lung transplantation would be a reasonable option for patients with severe disease who demonstrate the ability to refrain from further smoking tobacco use. However, this is unlikely to be necessary. Lung cancer screening should be considered in patients who meet the appropriate screening criteria.

References

Bak SH, Lee HY. Overlaps and uncertainties of smoking-related idiopathic interstitial pneumonias. Int J Chron Obstruct Pulmon Dis. 2017;12:3221.

Bango-Álvarez A, Ariza-Prota M, Torres-Rivas H, et al. Transbronchial cryobiopsy in interstitial lung disease: experience in 106 cases—how to do it. ERJ Open Res. 2017;3.

Casoni GL, Tomassetti S, Cavazza A, et al. Transbronchial lung cryobiopsy in the diagnosis of fibrotic interstitial lung diseases. PLoS One. 2014;9:e86716.

Craig PJ, Wells AU, Doffman S, et al. Desquamative interstitial pneumonia, respiratory bronchiolitis and their relationship to smoking. Histopathology. 2004;45:275.

Fabre A, Treacy A, Lavelle LP, et al. Smoking-related interstitial fibrosis: evidence of radiologic regression with advancing age and smoking cessation. COPD. 2017;14:603.

Fraig M, Shreesha U, Savici D, Katzenstein AL. Respiratory bronchiolitis: a clinicopathologic study in current smokers, ex-smokers, and never-smokers. Am J Surg Pathol. 2002;26:647.

Nakanishi M, Demura Y, Mizuno S, et al. Changes in HRCT findings in patients with respiratory bronchiolitis-associated interstitial lung disease after smoking cessation. Eur Respir J. 2007;29:453.

Okada F, Ando Y, Yoshitake S, et al. Clinical/pathologic correlations in 553 patients with primary centrilobular findings on high-resolution CT scan of the thorax. Chest. 2007;132:1939.

Portnoy J, Veraldi KL, Schwarz MI, et al. Respiratory bronchiolitis-interstitial lung disease: long-term outcome. Chest. 2007;131:664.

Scheidl SJ, Kusej M, Flick H, et al. Clinical manifestations of respiratory bronchiolitis as an incidental finding in surgical lung biopsies: a retrospective analysis of a large Austrian Registry. Respiration. 2016;91:26.

Travis WD, Costabel U, Hansell DM, et al. An official American Thoracic Society/European Respiratory Society statement: update of the international multidisciplinary classification of the idiopathic interstitial pneumonias. Am J Respir Crit Care Med. 2013;188:733.

Wells AU, Nicholson AG, Hansell DM. Challenges in pulmonary fibrosis . 4: smoking-induced diffuse interstitial lung diseases. Thorax. 2007;62:904.

Woo OH, Yong HS, Oh YW, et al. Respiratory bronchiolitis-associated interstitial lung disease in a nonsmoker: radiologic and pathologic findings. AJR Am J Roentgenol. 2007;188:W412.

Yousem SA. Respiratory bronchiolitis-associated interstitial lung disease with fibrosis is a lesion distinct from fibrotic nonspecific interstitial pneumonia: a proposal. Mod Pathol. 2006;19:1474.

CASE 45

A patient presents to the clinic with complaints of worsening dyspnea, cough, and wheezing. She is a 51-year-old woman with a medical history of gastroesophageal reflux disease (treated with ranitidine), diabetes mellitus type 2 (treated with diet alone), hypertension (treated with hydrochlorothiazide and losartan), and hyper-lipidemia (treated with simvastatin). She reports that worsening reflux and some dysphagia started about 4 months ago and that the symptoms have progressed since that time. She is able to eat solids and drink liquids, but she has frequent issues with reflux. The respiratory symptoms started about 2 months ago and are improved when she is supine and worse when she is prone. She noticed some wheezing and stridor about 6 weeks ago, but she has only experienced some dyspnea with exertion at this point. She has a cough that was initially dry but is now productive of clear sputum. She denies any weight loss, fevers, chills, night sweats, or hemoptysis. She denies any chest pain. She reports no family history of malignancy or rheumato-logic disease. On examination, she has audible wheezing on expiration and perhaps very mild stridor audible on inspiration, which is position dependent. She has no other significant examination findings, including no adenopathy or masses palpa-ble in the head, neck, axilla, or upper chest. Her vital signs are T 97.6°F, HR 87, BP 144/69, RR 12, and O_2 saturation 99% on room air. There is no pertinent surgical history. The patient called and scheduled this appointment herself. She has not seen her primary care physician in approximately 6 months.

In your office, you do not have the ability to obtain a chest radiograph immediately and refer the patient to a local urgent care center for a chest radiograph after the appointment. Luckily, you have access to immediate spirometry and flow-volume loops. The patient's flow-volume loop is shown in Image 45-1.

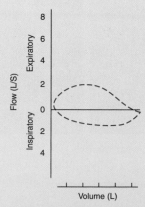

Image 45-1 • Flow-volume loop for the patient in **Case 45**.

QUESTIONS

Q45-1: Which abnormality is most consistent with the flow-volume loop shown above?

A. Variable extrathoracic airway obstruction
B. Variable intrathoracic airway obstruction
C. Lower airway obstruction (eg, asthma, chronic obstructive pulmonary disease [COPD])
D. Fixed upper airway obstruction (either intra- or extra-thoracic)
E. Normal
F. Obstructive sleep apnea

Q45-2: The patient undergoes a chest radiograph that evening, which is shown in Images 45-2A-C.

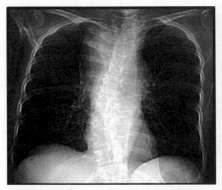
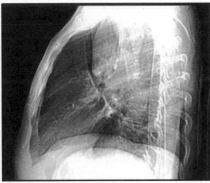

Image 45-2A • Chest radiograph for the patient in **Case 45**.

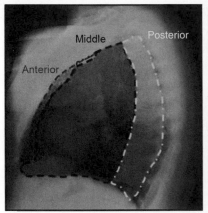
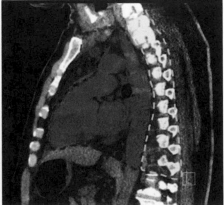

Image 45-2B • Mediastinal compartments.

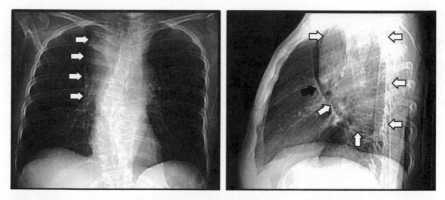

Image 45-2C • Chest radiograph for the patient in **Case 45**. Note the large middle mediastinal mass identified by the *white arrows*. Also, note the appearance of the airway at the *black arrow*.

What is the primary abnormality in the chest radiograph?

A. Anterior mediastinal mass
B. Middle mediastinal mass
C. Posterior mediastinal mass
D. Right-sided pneumothorax
E. Right-sided pleural effusion

Q45-3: Based on the patient's chest radiograph findings, you refer the patient to the ED at a local tertiary care center for further evaluation. The patient undergoes a CT scan to evaluate the mass, which is shown in Image 45-3.

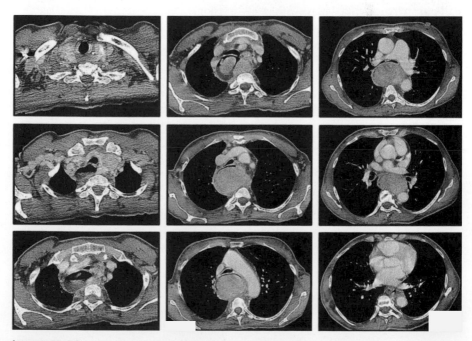

Image 45-3A • CT scan images of the patient in **Case 45**.

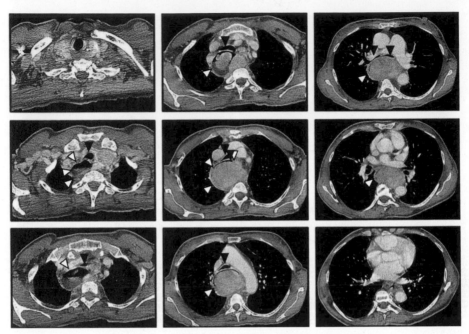

Image 45-3B • CT scan of the patient in **Case 45**, with *black arrows* indicating the well-circumscribed lesion in the middle mediastinum with air-fluid levels present. Note the critical compression of the trachea and the mainstem bronchi bilaterally (*white arrows*).

How would you describe the mass shown in Image 45-3A?

A. Heterogenous mass with calcifications and fatty tissue
B. Poorly circumscribed mass with satellite lesions
C. Homogenous mass that is well circumscribed
D. A lobulated mass with popcorn calcifications
E. A cavitary mass with air-fluid levels

Q45-4: What is the normal internal diameter of the airway at the level of the trachea?

A. 40 mm (4 cm)
B. 30 mm (3 cm)
C. 20 mm (2 cm)
D. 10 mm (1 cm)
E. 7 mm (0.7 cm)
F. 5 mm (0.5 cm)

Q45-5: At what diameter of the tracheal lumen do patients develop symptoms of dyspnea?

A. 15 mm (1.5 cm)
B. 10 mm (1 cm)
C. 7 mm (0.7 cm)
D. 5 mm (0.5 cm)
E. 2 mm (0.2 cm)

Q45-6: Based on the patient's clinical presentation and imaging results, what is the likely diagnosis?

A. Bronchogenic duplication cyst
B. Enteric duplication cyst
C. Pericardial duplication cyst
D. Esophageal adenocarcinoma
E. Small cell lung cancer
F. Diffuse large B-cell lymphoma

ANSWERS

Q45-1: D
Fixed upper airway obstruction (either intra- or extrathoracic)

Rationale: Here (**Image 45-4A**), one can see there is flow limitation and flattening of both the inspiratory and expiratory limbs of the flow-volume loop. This is consistent with upper airway obstruction (or central airway obstruction) and may be either intrathoracic (ie, below the thoracic inlet) or extrathoracic (ie, above the thoracic inlet). Generally, any flattening of the flow-volume loops on either limb or a maximum flow value that does not reach at least 2 L/S is concerning for a possible obstruction (the exception being in very severe expiratory airflow obstruction with severe air trapping; this is typically evident on physical examination).

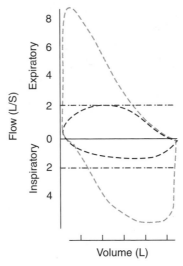

Image 45-4A • Comparison of the patient's flow-volume loop (*dark blue*) to a "normal" flow-volume loop (*blue*) for a patient of similar age and height. The *blue* dashed lines at 2 L/s of inspiratory and expiratory flow represent generalized cutoffs for identifying airflow abnormalities on pulmonary function testing.

Identification of airway obstruction via flow-volume loops is a critical skill and is often overlooked. Airway obstruction can be divided into two or three categories. *Upper airway obstruction* refers to the obstruction of airflow in the airways in the trachea and airways proximal to the trachea, while *lower airway obstruction* refers to obstruction in the lower airways, typically distal to the mainstem bronchi. A third category, *central airway obstruction*, is often used to refer to the trachea and mainstem bronchi, with some overlap with the upper airways (namely in the trachea). Upper and central airflow obstruction is most commonly seen as abnormalities in the inspiratory flow-volume loops, while lower airway obstruction is more commonly seen as abnormalities in the expiratory flow-volume loops.

This classification system can be somewhat confusing because the description of abnormalities in the flow-volume loops are typically described as intra- and extra-thoracic abnormalities rather than upper/central or lower airway abnormalities. The extrathoracic anatomy involves portions of the anatomy that are *not* exposed to the pleural pressure but rather only atmospheric pressure, while intrathoracic airways are exposed to the external pressures of the pleural space (ie, pleural pressure). The trachea is general classified as extrathoracic because part of the trachea is extrathoracic and lesions in the trachea are more commonly seen in the inspiratory flow limb or in both limbs (**Image 45-4B**).

Extrathoracic obstruction is seen during inspiration, though when fixed, it may also be seen during expiration. During inspiration, the pressure gradient created by the diaphragm and respiratory muscles (high pressure at the mouth; atmospheric; low pressure in the lower airways moving toward the alveoli), forcing air into the lungs. The alveoli and distal airways are held open by the negative intrathoracic pressure and the expansion of the lung parenchyma. The external pressure on the upper/extrathoracic airways is atmospheric (not negative intrathoracic pressure), and therefore obstruction in the upper airways is seen in the inspiratory loop. During the expiratory loop, there is a large driving pressure moving air from the lungs to a low pressure at the mouth, which is atmospheric. This high-pressure gradient helps stent the airway and lessen the effect of an obstructive extrathoracic lesion during expiration (**Image 45-4B**).

The trachea is commonly the transition point moving from the intra- to extrathoracic spaces. Obstruction in the trachea is most commonly seen in the inspiratory flow loop. The trachea has a tendency to collapse below the site of obstruction during inspiration because there is a pressure drop across the obstruction with a higher pressure in the trachea above the lesion and a lower pressure below the lesion. Once the pressure in the trachea drops below atmospheric pressure, the trachea may collapse (imagine attempting to breathe through a paper straw; the stronger the inspiratory force, the more likely the straw is to collapse; during expiration, the straw is held open by a high-pressure gradient from the mouth to the end of the straw, preventing collapse) (**Image 45-4B**).

Intrathoracic obstruction is most often seen during the expiratory limb of the flow-volume loop. The pleural space has a large negative pressure during inspiration, which has a tendency to expand the intrathoracic airways and decrease or relieve the effect of intrathoracic obstruction. However, during expiration, the airway diameters are gradually reduced, increasing the effects of the obstruction (**Image 45-4B**).

Patients with airway malacia or obstructive sleep apnea may have evidence of saw-toothing on the inspiratory or expiratory loops of the flow-volume loops (**Image 45-4B**). Additionally, patients may have a lesion that occurs at the thoracic inlet and actually moves from an intrathoracic to an extrathoracic location, depending on patient orientation or neck movement, and it may therefore have the variable appearance of the flow-volumes loops. These patients may also have a "camel-hump" appearance if the lesion moves during inspiration and expiration (**Image 45-4B**).

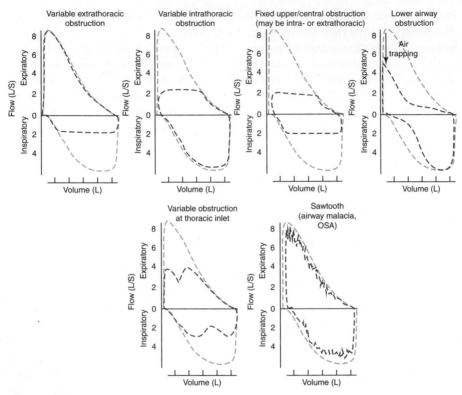

Image 45-4B • Abnormal flow-volume loops for various airway obstruction pathologies. A normal flow-volume loop is shown in blue, while the associated abnormal flow-volume loop is shown in dark blue. OSA, obstructive sleep apnea.

Q45-2: B
Middle mediastinal mass

Rationale: On this PA and lateral film, we can see mediastinal widening that is most evident on the right and superior to the heart. The lateral chest film demonstrates that the lesion originates in the middle mediastinum, though it appears to extend into the posterior mediastinum potentially (**Image 45-2B**). There is no evidence of pneumothorax or pleural effusion on the right. Note that the lesion appears well circumscribed. Also, note on the lateral film the appearance of the airway (**Image 45-2C**).

The mediastinum is the space contained within the following anatomic structures: cranially, thoracic inlet; caudally, diaphragm; left, left pleural cavity; right, right pleural cavity; anteriorly, sternum; and posteriorly, vertebral bodies (inclusive of vertebral bodies and associated structures). The mediastinum may be further subdivided into three or four categories: anterior, middle, and posterior, with superior being used in some classification systems. In 2017, the International Thymic Malignancy Interest Group (ITMIG) proposed a revised, three-compartment classification for mediastinal masses that is based on natural anatomic boundaries and is overall better suited to classification via cross-sectional imaging. We will use this classification system for the cases in this text. One primary difference between this current classification system and some prior systems is the border between the middle and posterior mediastinum. Some classification systems have used the posterior border of the pericardium or anterior border of the descending thoracic aorta; this often meant that benign cystic structures (eg, bronchogenic cysts) could be classified as either middle or posterior, despite arising from the same anatomic structures. The current system obviates these issues by using the vertebral bodies as the border between the middle and posterior compartments.

Mediastinal Compartments Definitions			
	Cranial/Caudal	Left/Right	Anterior/Posterior
Mediastinum	Cranial – thoracic inlet Caudal – diaphragm	Left and right pleural cavities	Anterior: Sternum Posterior: Transverse processes
Compartment			
Anterior (*prevascular*)	Cranial – thoracic inlet Caudal – diaphragm	Left and right pleural cavities	Anterior: Sternum Posterior: Anterior aspect of the pericardium as it wraps around the heart, not a linear plane)
Middle (*visceral*)	Cranial – thoracic inlet Caudal – diaphragm	Left and right pleural cavities	Anterior: Anterior mediastinum as defined above Posterior: Mark a point 1 cm posterior to the anterior margin of each vertebral body, and draw a line connecting the dots
Posterior (*paravertebral*)	Cranial – thoracic inlet Caudal – diaphragm	Left and right pleural cavities	Anterior: Middle mediastinum as defined above Posterior: Line drawn down the posterior aspect of the transverse processes of the spine

Q45-3: C
Homogenous mass (cystic) that is well circumscribed

Rationale: Here, we see a cystic mass arising within the lumen of the esophagus. The lesion is very well circumscribed and heterogeneous in appearance. There is an air-fluid level within the esophagus at the superior margin of the mass, but the cystic lesion itself demonstrates no air-fluid levels. There are no apparent calcifications or lobulations (**Image 45-3B**). The lesion itself is not cavitary.

Q45-4: C
20 mm (2 cm)

Rationale: The average internal diameter of the airway at the level of the trachea is approximately 20 mm (2 cm).

Q45-5: C
7 mm (0.7 cm)

Rationale: Patients with external airway compression generally have limited or no symptoms until the airway is compressed to a diameter of 0.7 cm (7 mm). That is a nearly tenfold reduction in the surface area of the airway (20 mm diameter yields an area of about 315 mm^2, whereas a 7-mm airway has a surface area of 38 mm^2). Patients generally develop dyspnea at a tracheal lumen diameter of 7 mm, with stridor developing at 4 to 5 mm diameter.

In this case, the patient had a tracheal diameter of approximately 2.7 mm on presentation, which explains her symptoms. This represents an important case of central airway obstruction (CAO). CAO may result from malignant, nonmalignant, and foreign body sources. The most common cause of central airway obstruction is primary lung malignancy, including non-small cell, small cell, and carcinoid tumors. Metastatic involvement of the airway from distant sites of malignancy is exceedingly less common. The central airways may also be compressed externally from paratracheal or peribronchial masses or lymphadenopathy. Foreign body obstruction typically results from the aspiration of food. Nonmalignant causes of central airway obstruction may result from external compression by nonmalignant lesions (duplication cysts, lymphadenopathy from granulomatous disease), tracheomalacia, inflammation, strictures, and trauma.

Although upper airway obstruction may be bypassed with a tracheostomy, central airway obstruction more often involves the distal trachea, carina, and mainstem bronchi, which makes intervention more complicated. Early identification of central airway obstruction can help clinicians avoid emergency situations. The most important aspect of treatment is to identify patients who present with acute symptoms and those who present with subacute symptoms. Patients presenting with tachypnea, tachycardia, hypotension, audible stridor, or wheezing should undergo emergency evaluation and likely necessitate specialist consultation with an anesthesiologist to secure the airway and perform emergency bronchoscopy. Depending on the location of the patient's lesion, a double-lumen endotracheal tube may be necessary, or if this is not available, the endotracheal tube may need to be advanced into one mainstem bronchi for single-lung ventilation. Noninvasive positive pressure ventilation may be used as rescue therapy while preparations are made for intubation. Importantly, the location of the lesion may identify whether cricothyroidotomy would be useful in the case of a failed intubation.

Patients with subacute presentations and stable vital signs are more capable of undergoing standard evaluation. The treatment of the various etiologies that may cause CAO is beyond the scope of this text. Treatment typically involves either an interventional pulmonologist or a thoracic surgeon. Some options include airway dilation and stenting, cryotherapy, brachytherapy, plasma coagulation, foreign body extraction, and surgical resection.

Q45-6: B
Enteric duplication cyst

Rationale: The lesion is well circumscribed, heterogenous, and fluid filled, and it appears to be arising from the esophageal lumen. There is no associated adenopathy. The patient has no constitutional symptoms. These characteristics are not consistent with malignancy. The most likely diagnosis is a duplication cyst. Given the anatomy, an enteric duplication cyst is most likely. The patient underwent an uncomplicated surgical procedure to remove the cyst, and her postoperative imaging and flow-volume studies demonstrated complete resolution of the central airway obstruction.

Differential Diagnosis for Mediastinal Masses		
Anterior	Middle	Posterior
Thymoma (approximately 50%)	Lymphoma	Neurogenic tumor (eg, neurofibroma)
Teratoma	Bronchial cyst	
Germ cell tumor (seminoma, nonseminoma)	Pericardial cyst	Meningocele
	Enteric cyst	Paravertebral abscess
Lymphoma	Granulomatous disease (eg, sarcoidosis)	Extramedullary hematopoiesis
Carcinoma (thyroid)		Discitis/osteomyelitis
Substernal goiter	Aortic pathology	
Lipoma	Diaphragmatic hernia	

References

Aboussouan LS, Stoller JK. Diagnosis and management of upper airway obstruction. Clin Chest Med. 1994;15:35.

Carter BW, Benveniste MF, Madan R, et al. ITMIG classification of mediastinal compartments and multidisciplinary approach to mediastinal masses. Radiographics. 2017;37:413.

Carter BW, Betancourt SL, Benveniste MF. MR imaging of mediastinal masses. Top Magn Reson Imaging. 2017;26:153.

Chira RI, Chira A, Mircea PA, Valean S. Mediastinal masses-transthoracic ultrasonography aspects. Medicine (Baltimore). 2017;96:e9082.

Duwe BV, Sterman DH, Musani AI. Tumors of the mediastinum. Chest. 2005;128:2893.

Ernst A, Feller-Kopman D, Becker HD, Mehta AC. Central airway obstruction. Am J Respir Crit Care Med. 2004;169:1278.

Ernst A, Silvestri GA, Johnstone D, American College of Chest Physicians. Interventional pulmonary procedures: Guidelines from the American College of Chest Physicians. Chest. 2003;123:1693.

Garcia-Pachon E. Tracheobronchomalacia: a cause of flow oscillations on the flow-volume loop. Chest 2000;118:1519.

Gascoigne AD, Corris PA, Dark JH, Gibson GJ. The biphasic spirogram: a clue to unilateral narrowing of a mainstem bronchus. Thorax 1990;45:637.

Haponik EF, Bleecker ER, Allen RP, et al. Abnormal inspiratory flow-volume curves in patients with sleep-disordered breathing. Am Rev Respir Dis. 1981;124:571.

Juanpere S, Cañete N, Ortuño P, et-al. A diagnostic approach to the mediastinal masses. Insights Imaging. 2013;4:29.

Laurent F, Latrabe V, Lecesne R, Zennaro H, Airaud JY, Rauturier JF, Drouillard J. Mediastinal masses: diagnostic approach. Eur Radiol. 1998;8:1148.

Majid A, Sosa AF, Ernst A, et al. Pulmonary function and flow-volume loop patterns in patients with tracheobronchomalacia. Respir Care. 2013;58:1521.

Modrykamien AM, Gudavalli R, McCarthy K, et al. Detection of upper airway obstruction with spirometry results and the flow-volume loop: a comparison of quantitative and visual inspection criteria. Respir Care. 2009;54:474.

Nakazono T, Yamaguchi K, Egashira R, Mizuguchi M, Irie H. Anterior mediastinal lesions: CT and MRI features and differential diagnosis. Jpn J Radiol. 2021;39:101.

Pellegrino R, Viegi G, Brusasco V, et al. Interpretative strategies for lung function tests. Eur Respir J. 2005;26:948.

Prosch H, Röhrich S, Tekin ZN, Ebner L. The role of radiological imaging for masses in the prevascular mediastinum in clinical practice. J Thorac Dis. 2020;12:7591.

Schiffman PL. A "saw-tooth" pattern in Parkinson's disease. Chest. 1985;87:124.

Stephens KE Jr, Wood DE. Bronchoscopic management of central airway obstruction. J Thorac Cardiovasc Surg. 2000;119:289.

Sterner JB, Morris MJ, Sill JM, Hayes JA. Inspiratory flow-volume curve evaluation for detecting upper airway disease. Respir Care. 2009;54:461.

Su S, Colson YL. Overview of benign and malignant mediastinal diseases. In: Adult Chest Surgery, 2nd ed, Sugarbaker DJ, Bueno R, Colson YL, et al (Eds), McGraw-Hill Education, New York, 2015. p. 1234.

Thacker PG, Mahani MG, Heider A, Lee EY. Imaging evaluation of mediastinal masses in children and adults: Practical diagnostic approach based on a new classification system. J Thorac Imaging. 2015;30:247.

Varga J, Casaburi R, Ma S, et al. Relation of concavity in the expiratory flow-volume loop to dynamic hyperinflation during exercise in COPD. Respir Physiol Neurobiol. 2016;234:79.

Watson MA, King CS, Holley AB, et al. Clinical and lung-function variables associated with vocal cord dysfunction. Respir Care. 2009;54:467.

Whitten CR, Khan S, Munneke GJ, Grubnic S. A diagnostic approach to mediastinal abnormalities. Radiographics. 2007;27:657.

CASE 46

A 61-year-old man is admitted to the hospital with complaints of dyspnea and productive cough. The patient noted the onset of symptoms approximately 4 months ago, with gradual worsening. At first, he noticed only a cough, but then he experienced the onset of some "chest pressure" as well as dyspnea with exertion. This has further progressed, and now the patient notes a productive cough intermittently, fevers, night sweats, and a 10-lb weight loss over the last several weeks. He also notes some intermittent wheezing. He denies any hemoptysis or pleuritic chest pain. He denies any dysphagia or odynophagia. He has no smoking history, does not drink alcohol, and does not use illicit drugs. He worked as an analytical chemist for 30 years before transitioning to an administrative job for the last 8 years and has no environmental or occupational exposures of note. He has a history of cholecystectomy, appendectomy, and ventral hernia repair. He also has a history of well-controlled diabetes mellitus type 2 (HbA1c 6.8%) on metformin. His body mass index is 27 kg/m². His vital signs are T 100.1°F, HR 76, BP 124/66, RR 15, and O$_2$ saturation 100% on room air.

The patient's chest radiograph is shown in Image 46-1.

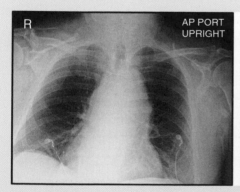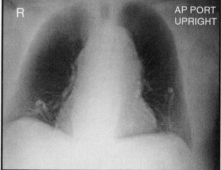

Image 46-1 • Chest radiograph (left) and enhanced (bone-reduced) image for the patient in **Case 46**.

QUESTIONS

Q46-1: How would you describe the primary abnormality in Image 46-1?

A. Cardiomegaly
B. Widened mediastinum
C. Pneumothorax on the left
D. Large pleural effusion on the right
E. Pneumomediastinum

Q46-2: The patient has normal thyroid studies, including thyroid-stimulating hormone (TSH), free T4, and T3. What would you do next to further evaluate the patient's symptoms?

A. MRI of the neck and chest with contrast
B. CT scan of the neck and chest without contrast
C. CT scan of the neck and chest with and without contrast
D. PET-CT of the skull base to mid-thigh
E. Technicium-99 (Tc-99) scan
F. Ultrasound of the neck

Q46-3: The patient undergoes a CT scan and a PET-CT scan, shown in Image 46-2.

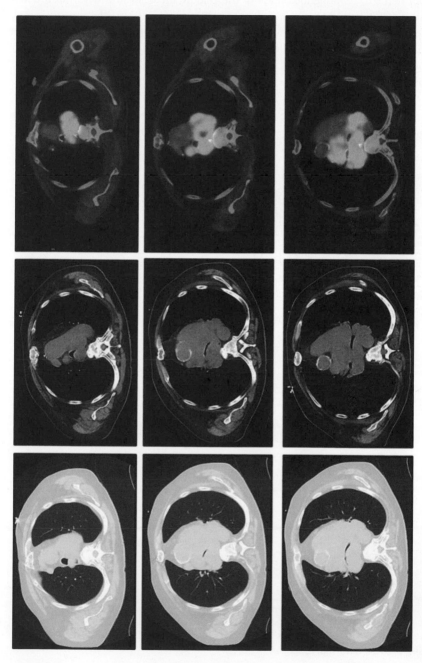

Image 46-2 • CT scan (left, lung windows; middle, mediastinal windows) and PET-CT (using fluorodeoxyglucose) of the chest for the patient in **Case 46**.

Which abnormality is present on the patient's scan shown in Image 46-2?

A. Lung mass in the right lower lobe
B. Well-defined, homogenous mass in the middle mediastinum with fluorodeoxy-glucose (FDG) avidity
C. Well-defined, homogenous mass in the middle mediastinum with no FDG avidity
D. Multiple masses in the middle mediastinum with FDG avidity
E. Pneumomediastinum
F. Posterior mediastinal mass with FDG avidity

Q46-4: Which flow-volume loop shown in Image 46-3 would you predict for the patient in Case 46?

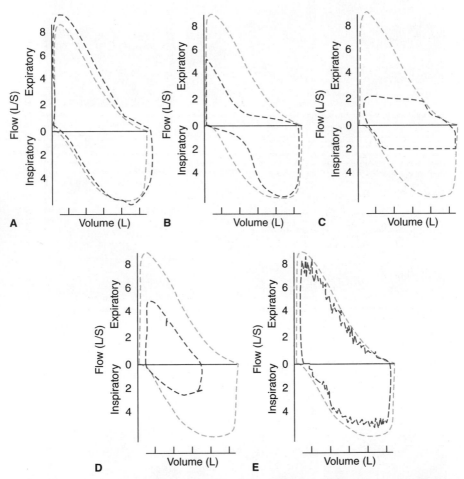

Image 46-3 • Flow-volume loops choices for **Question 46-4** in **Case 46**. The light blue loop is a predicted normal loop.

Q46-5: The patient's laboratory values return with the following results:

Laboratory Test	Value	Normal
Brain (B-type) natriuretic peptide (BNP)	34 pg/mL	1-100 pg/mL
C-reactive protein, high-sensitivity (hsCRP)	22.6 mg/L	<1.1 mg/L
Erythrocyte sedimentation rate (ESR)	115 mm/h	0-15 mm/h
Rheumatoid factor (Rf)	2 U/mL	<40 U/mL
Lactate dehydrogenase (LDH)	1152 U/mL	60-160 U/mL
Uric acid	10.2 mg/dL	2.5-8 mg/dL

Given the patient's clinical symptoms, coupled with the imaging and laboratory values provided, what is the most likely diagnosis?

A. Simple bronchogenic cyst
B. Thymoma
C. Meningocele
D. Spinal ganglioglioma
E. Non-Hodgkin lymphoma (NHL)
F. Aortic arch dissection
G. Diaphragmatic hernia
H. Germ cell tumor

Q46-6: What is the most common type of NHL?

A. Mantle cell lymphoma
B. Diffuse large B-cell lymphoma (DLBCL)
C. Hairy cell leukemia
D. Follicular lymphoma
E. Marginal cell lymphoma

ANSWERS

Q46-1: B
Widened mediastinum

Rationale: This is an AP film with no lateral film available. The mediastinum appears wide overall. There does not appear to be bulky hilar adenopathy but rather primarily a wide mediastinum. Note that the trachea, carina, and mainstem bronchi are not clearly visible below the level of the second and third thoracic ribs, which may indicate that there is a mass in the mediastinum. The heart may appear borderline enlarged; however, recall that this is an AP film, and the heart has a tendency to appear magnified compared with PA films. There is no apparent pneumomediastinum or pneumothorax. Although we cannot make out the right costophrenic angle, there is no large pleural effusion.

Q46-2: C
CT scan of the chest with contrast

Rationale: A CT is often the first imaging modality chosen because of its availability. Contrasted CT is often helpful because it will differentiate vascular structures from lymph nodes and more clearly define anatomic structures. It may also aid in identifying which vascular structures are supplying a particular mass or lesion. Therefore, a contrasted study would be preferred to a noncontrasted study. Although MRI of the chest would be considered, CT of the chest is typically the first study given its short study duration and general availability. MRI is more effective at characterizing the composition of tissue structures (eg, cystic versus solid versus fat), and it can better delineate if a mass is compressing or invading other structures, which may be necessary to determine the most appropriate treatment. MRI is particularly useful in the posterior mediastinum, where the spine and nervous system are involved. PET-CT is of somewhat limited utility in the mediastinum because of its higher propensity for false-positive results. It is often performed because it can identify distant sites of disease that may be more amenable to biopsy and may provide more staging information, but it usually has a lower overall resolution, so it is typically not used as an initial imaging study. For patients with suspected thyroid cancer or substernal goiter, a Tc-99 scan or a thyroid ultrasound (neck) may also be helpful. Although this patient's symptoms could be concerning for such pathology, his thyroid studies are normal, and CT would provide adequate information regarding a substernal thyroid goiter or thyroid cancer.

Q46-3: D
Multiple masses in the middle mediastinum with FDG avidity

Rationale: Here, we see multiple areas on the PET-CT with FDG (avidity), consistent with likely mediastinal and hilar lymph nodes. There are paratracheal, subcarinal, and hilar nodes. On the CT scan (**Image 46-4**), these nodes are a bit more difficult to differentiate from the vascular structures because of the lack of contrast on this particular series. The lesions are contained primarily in the middle mediastinum, though without visualization of the pericardium, there may be some involvement of the anterior mediastinum more superiorly. There is no involvement of the posterior mediastinum. There is no evidence of pneumomediastinum, pneumothorax, or pleural effusion.

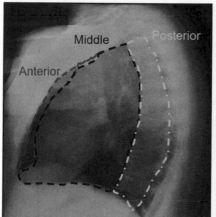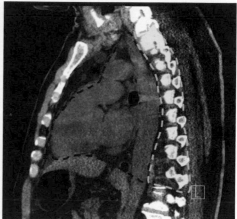

Image 46-4 • Mediastinal compartments.

Q46-4: C

Rationale: On the CT scan, note the central airway obstruction due to the mediastinal masses (**Image 46-5**).

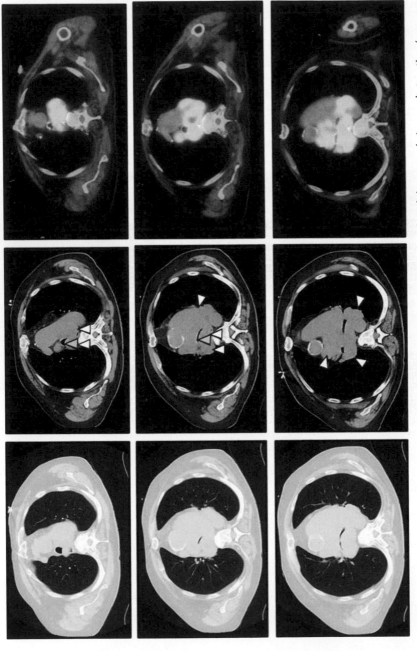

Image 46-5 • Annotated CT scan demonstrating the mediastinal masses (*white arrows*) and the central airway obstruction (*gray arrows*).

Note the compression of the airway at the distal trachea through the carina and into the mainstem bronchi. We would therefore expect this patient to have some element of central airway obstruction (CAO). This would be most consistent with the flow-volume loop in (C), which is an example of a fixed upper/central airway obstruction. Here, we see flow limitations on both the inspiratory and expiratory flow-volume loops. It would also be possible to only see flattening on the inspiratory loop with no effect on the expiratory loop; alternatively, if the mass is moving into and out of the thoracic cavity, one could also see a "double-hump" appearance of the inspiratory limb (as well as possible the expiratory limb). Flow-volume loop (A) is a normal or slightly supraphysiologic flow loop; option (B) is an example of a patient with expiratory airflow obstruction or lower airway obstruction, consistent with chronic obstructive pulmonary disease (COPD) or asthma. Option (D) is an example of a patient with restrictive lung disease, while option (E) is consistent with tracheobronchomalacia or obstructive sleep apnea.

Identification of airway obstruction via flow-volume loops is a critical skill and is often overlooked. Airway obstruction can be divided into two or three categories. *Upper airway obstruction* refers to the obstruction of airflow in the airways in the trachea and airways proximal to the trachea, while *lower airway obstruction* refers to obstruction in the lower airways, typically distal to the mainstem bronchi. A third category, *central airway obstruction*, is often used to refer to the trachea and mainstem bronchi, with some overlap with the upper airways (namely in the trachea). Upper and central airway obstruction is most commonly seen as abnormalities in the inspiratory flow-volume loops, while lower airway obstruction is more commonly seen as abnormalities in the expiratory flow-volume loops.

This classification system can be somewhat confusing because the description of abnormalities in the flow-volume loops are typically described as intra- and extra-thoracic abnormalities rather than upper/central or lower airway abnormalities. The extrathoracic anatomy involves portions of the anatomy that are *not* exposed to the pleural pressure but rather only atmospheric pressure, while intrathoracic airways are exposed to the external pressures of the pleural space (ie, pleural pressure). The trachea is general classified as extrathoracic because part of the trachea is extrathoracic and lesions in the trachea are more commonly seen in the inspiratory flow limb or in both limbs (**Image 46-6**).

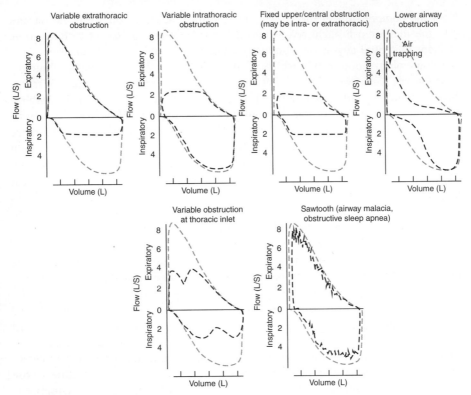

Image 46-6 • Examples of flow-volume loops in airflow obstruction.

Extrathoracic obstruction is seen during inspiration, though when fixed, it may also be seen during expiration. During inspiration, the pressure gradient created by the diaphragm and respiratory muscles (high pressure at the mouth; atmospheric; low pressure in the lower airways moving toward the alveoli) forces air into the lungs. The alveoli and distal airways are held open by the negative intrathoracic pressure and the expansion of the lung parenchyma. The external pressure on the upper/extrathoracic airways is atmospheric (not the negative intrathoracic pressure), and therefore obstruction in the upper airways is seen in the inspiratory loop. During the expiratory loop, there is a large driving pressure moving air from the lungs to a low pressure at the mouth, which is atmospheric. This high pressure gradient helps stent the airway and lessen the effect of an obstructive extrathoracic lesion during expiration (**Image 46-6**).

The trachea is commonly the transition point moving from the intrathoracic to the extrathoracic spaces. Obstruction in the trachea is most commonly seen in the inspiratory flow loop. The trachea has a tendency to collapse below the site of obstruction during inspiration because there is a pressure drop across the obstruction with higher pressure in the trachea above the lesion and lower pressure below the lesion. Once the pressure in the trachea drops below atmospheric pressure, the trachea may collapse (imagine attempting to breathe through a paper straw; the stronger the inspiratory force, the more likely the straw is to collapse; during expiration, the straw is held open by a high pressure gradient from the mouth to the end of the straw, preventing collapse) (**Image 46-6**).

Intrathoracic obstruction is most often seen during the expiratory limb of the flow-volume loop. The pleural space has a large negative pressure during inspiration, which has a tendency to expand the intrathoracic airways and decrease or relieve the effect of intrathoracic obstruction. However, during expiration, the airway diameters are gradually reduced, increasing the effects of the obstruction (**Image 46-6**).

Patients with airway malacia or obstructive sleep apnea may have evidence of saw-toothing on the inspiratory or expiratory loops of the flow-volume loops (**Image 46-6**). Additionally, patients may have a lesion that occurs at the thoracic inlet and actually moves from an intrathoracic to an extrathoracic location, depending on patient orientation or neck movement, and thus may have a variable appearance on the flow-volumes loops. These patients may also have a "camel-hump" appearance if the lesion moves during inspiration and expiration (see **Image 46-6**).

Q46-5: E
Non-Hodgkin lymphoma (NHL)

Rationale: The location of the masses in the middle mediastinum, their characteristics on CT scan, the proximity to known mediastinal and hilar lymph node stations, their FDG-avidity, and the elevated ESR, CRP, LDH, and uric acid levels would be highly concerning for a lymphoma.

Differential Diagnosis for Mediastinal Masses		
Anterior	*Middle*	*Posterior*
Thymoma (approximately 50%)	Lymphoma	Neurogenic tumor (eg, neurofibroma)
Teratoma	Bronchial cyst	
Germ cell tumor (seminoma, nonseminoma)	Pericardial cyst	Meningocele
	Enteric cyst	Paravertebral abscess
Lymphoma	Granulomatous disease (eg, sarcoidosis)	Extramedullary hematopoiesis
Carcinoma (thyroid)		Discitis/osteomyelitis
Substernal goiter	Aortic pathology	
Lipoma	Diaphragmatic hernia	

Other considerations would be a primary lung malignancy with metastatic disease to the mediastinal and hilar lymph nodes or a small cell lung cancer, particularly given the FDG avidity. A simple bronchogenic cyst (ie, not infected) should not have significant FDG avidity and should more likely appear as a single, well-circumscribed mass. A thymoma may have metastatic spread or invasion of surrounding structures, but this would be a very atypical presentation, and there is a lack of calcification as well. A meningocele and spinal ganglioglioma should arise from the posterior mediastinum. An aortic arch dissection and diaphragmatic hernia would not have this CT appearance, nor would a germ cell tumor.

Q46-6: B
Diffuse large B-cell lymphoma

Rationale: Approximately 90% of lymphomas arise in the B-cell lineage, and diffuse large B-cell lymphoma accounts for more than 30% of all NHL cases, making it the most common form. This patient has a primary mediastinal B-cell lymphoma, which is a subtype of DLBCL. This type of lymphoma, which is more common in young women, may produce fast-growing tumors that may encompass the mediastinum cavity and press on the airways and blood vessels, such as in this case. The patient was started on R-CHOP therapy (cyclophosphamide, doxorubicin, vincristine, and prednisone, plus the monoclonal antibody rituximab) with a good response initially. Unfortunately, the patient developed multiple infectious complications and elected to pursue a palliative treatment course.

Follicular lymphoma accounts for about 20% of NHL cases, mantle cell for about 5%, and marginal cell lymphoma for about 10%. Hairy cell leukemia is a rare, slowly progressive leukemia that makes up only about 2% of leukemia (not lymphoma) cases.

References

Aboussouan LS, Stoller JK. Diagnosis and management of upper airway obstruction. Clin Chest Med. 1994;15:35.

Carter BW, Benveniste MF, Madan R, et al. ITMIG classification of mediastinal compartments and multidisciplinary approach to mediastinal masses. Radiographics. 2017;37:413.

Carter BW, Betancourt SL, Benveniste MF. MR imaging of mediastinal masses. Top Magn Reson Imaging. 2017;26:153.

Chira RI, Chira A, Mircea PA, Valean S. Mediastinal masses-transthoracic ultrasonography aspects. Medicine (Baltimore). 2017;96:e9082.

Duwe BV, Sterman DH, Musani AI. Tumors of the mediastinum. Chest. 2005;128:2893.

Ernst A, Feller-Kopman D, Becker HD, Mehta AC. Central airway obstruction. Am J Respir Crit Care Med. 2004;169:1278.

Ernst A, Silvestri GA, Johnstone D, American College of Chest Physicians. Interventional pulmonary procedures: guidelines from the American College of Chest Physicians. Chest. 2003;123:1693.

Garcia-Pachon E. Tracheobronchomalacia: a cause of flow oscillations on the flow-volume loop. Chest. 2000;118:1519.

Gascoigne AD, Corris PA, Dark JH, Gibson GJ. The biphasic spirogram: a clue to unilateral narrowing of a mainstem bronchus. Thorax. 1990;45:637.

Haponik EF, Bleecker ER, Allen RP, et al. Abnormal inspiratory flow-volume curves in patients with sleep-disordered breathing. Am Rev Respir Dis. 1981;124:571.

Juanpere S, Cañete N, Ortuño P, et-al. A diagnostic approach to the mediastinal masses. Insights Imaging. 2013;4:29.

Laurent F, Latrabe V, Lecesne R, Zennaro H, Airaud JY, Rauturier JF, Drouillard J. Mediastinal masses: diagnostic approach. Eur Radiol. 1998;8:1148.

Majid A, Sosa AF, Ernst A, et al. Pulmonary function and flow-volume loop patterns in patients with tracheobronchomalacia. Respir Care. 2013;58:1521.

Modrykamien AM, Gudavalli R, McCarthy K, et al. Detection of upper airway obstruction with spirometry results and the flow-volume loop: a comparison of quantitative and visual inspection criteria. Respir Care. 2009;54:474.

Nakazono T, Yamaguchi K, Egashira R, Mizuguchi M, Irie H. Anterior mediastinal lesions: CT and MRI features and differential diagnosis. Jpn J Radiol. 2021;39:101.

Pellegrino R, Viegi G, Brusasco V, et al. Interpretative strategies for lung function tests. Eur Respir J. 2005;26:948.

Prosch H, Röhrich S, Tekin ZN, Ebner L. The role of radiological imaging for masses in the prevascular mediastinum in clinical practice. J Thorac Dis. 2020;12:7591.

Schiffman PL. A "saw-tooth" pattern in Parkinson's disease. Chest. 1985;87:124.

Stephens KE Jr, Wood DE. Bronchoscopic management of central airway obstruction. J Thorac Cardiovasc Surg. 2000;119:289.

Sterner JB, Morris MJ, Sill JM, Hayes JA. Inspiratory flow-volume curve evaluation for detecting upper airway disease. Respir Care. 2009;54:461.

Su S, Colson YL. Overview of benign and malignant mediastinal diseases. In: Adult Chest Surgery, 2nd ed, Sugarbaker DJ, Bueno R, Colson YL, et al (Eds), McGraw-Hill Education, New York 2015. p. 1234.

Thacker PG, Mahani MG, Heider A, Lee EY. Imaging evaluation of mediastinal masses in children and adults: practical diagnostic approach based on a new classification system. J Thorac Imaging. 2015;30:247.

Varga J, Casaburi R, Ma S, et al. Relation of concavity in the expiratory flow-volume loop to dynamic hyperinflation during exercise in COPD. Respir Physiol Neurobiol. 2016;234:79.

Watson MA, King CS, Holley AB, et al. Clinical and lung-function variables associated with vocal cord dysfunction. Respir Care. 2009;54:467.

Whitten CR, Khan S, Munneke GJ, Grubnic S. A diagnostic approach to mediastinal abnormalities. Radiographics. 2007;27:657.

CASE 47

A 57-year-old man with a history of diabetes mellitus type 2 (HbA1c 6.9%), hypertension, gout, and osteoarthritis presents for evaluation for an abnormal chest radiograph. The patient was involved in a car accident with airbags deployed, and during his trauma evaluation, an abnormality was identified on the patient's CXR. The patient reports no actual chest trauma during the accident. The patient was asymptomatic before this event, with no dyspnea, orthopnea, fevers, chills, sweats, weight loss, pleuritic chest pain, or cough. The patient works in a factory that produces brake pads for large vehicles and aircraft. He has worked there for the past 36 years. He lives in a condominium with no evidence of water damage. He does woodworking as a hobby but uses appropriate personal protective equipment. He does not smoke or use illicit drugs. His vital signs are T 36.7°C, HR 65, BP 104/55, RR 12, and O_2 saturation 100% on room air. His examination is notable for decreased breath sounds and dullness to percussion in the left lower lung field. He has some trace pedal edema. The patient's chest radiograph is shown in Image 47-1.

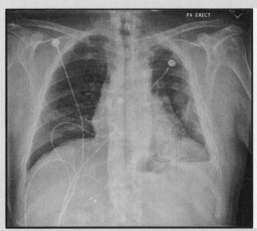 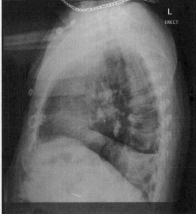

Image 47-1 • Chest radiograph for the patient in **Case 47**.

QUESTIONS

Q47-1: Which abnormalities are present in the above chest radiograph? Select all that apply.

A. Blunting of the right costophrenic angle
B. Blunting of the left costophrenic angle
C. Right-sided pneumothorax
D. Left-sided pneumothorax
E. Right-sided lung mass
F. Left-sided lung nodule

Q47-2: The patient undergoes a CT scan of the chest, shown in Image 47-2.

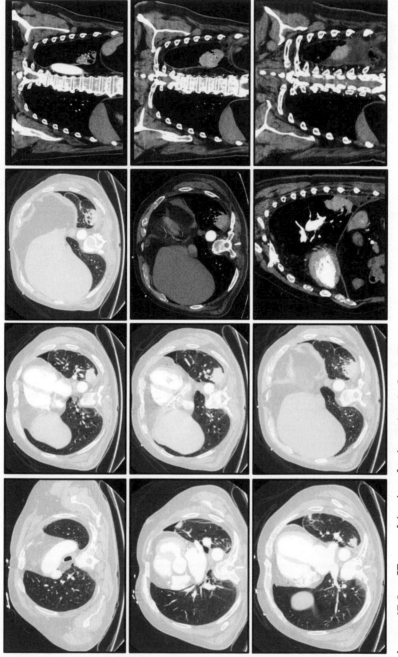

Image 47-2 • CT scan of the chest for the patient in **Case 47**.

Which abnormalities are present in the above chest CT scan? Select all that apply.

A. Right-sided pleural effusion
B. Left-sided pleural effusion
C. Left-sided atelectasis
D. Left-sided hydropneumothorax
E. Pleural plaques
F. Hiatal hernia
G. Diaphragmatic hernia
H. Left lower lobe pneumonia

Q47-3: The patient undergoes a thoracentesis, and serosanguinous fluid is found. There is an increased eosinophil count (25% total cell count). The laboratory studies show an exudative effusion with elevated lactate dehydrogenase (LDH) and protein levels and a normal glucose level. The culture data are negative, and the cytology is normal as well. The patient reports that he has never had any chest trauma or falls. The brain (B-type) natriuretic peptide (BNP) is 10 pg/mL (ULN: 100 pg/mL). Which occupational exposure may explain the abnormalities?

A. Beryllium
B. Bird dander
C. Radiation
D. Asbestos
E. Mold
F. Radon

Q47-4: What is the typical latency period between the first exposure to asbestos and the development of BAPE?

A. 1 to 3 years
B. 2 to 10 years
C. 5 to 15 years
D. 15 to 45 years
E. Random

Q47-5: Given the patient's exposure history, which disease needs to be ruled out at this point?

A. Sarcoidosis
B. Idiopathic pulmonary fibrosis (IPF)
C. Histoplasmosis
D. Alpha-1-antitrypsin (AAT) disease
E. Mesothelioma

Q47-6: Which study is the most appropriate next step in the patient's evaluation?

A. PET-CT
B. MRI of the brain with contrast
C. Echocardiogram
D. Pulmonary embolism (PE)-protocol CT scan of the chest
E. Contrasted CT scan of the sinuses and neck
F. Bronchoscopy with bronchoalveolar lavage

Q47-7: The patient's PET-CT scan is shown in Image 47-3 below.

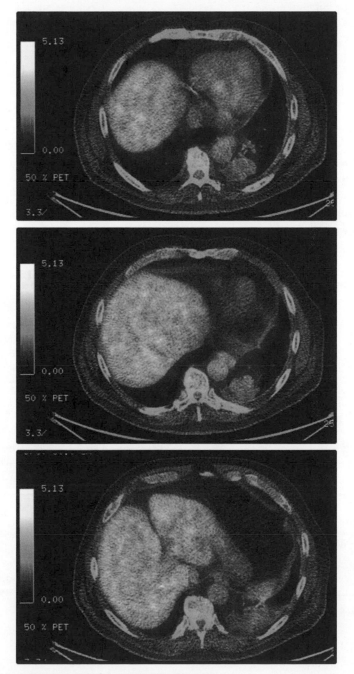

Image 47-3 • PET-CT scan of the patient in **Case 47**.

Additionally, there is physiologic uptake of fluorodeoxyglucose in the hilar and mediastinal lymph nodes. What is the next step in the patient's evaluation?

A. Referral for video-assisted thoracoscopic surgical (VATS) biopsy of the left lower lobe
B. Observation only with a repeat CT scan in 3 to 6 months
C. Indwelling pleural catheter placement with weekly fluid removal
D. A 6-week course of antibiotics
E. Extrapleural pneumonectomy
F. Pleurectomy and decortication

Q47-8: Which asbestosis-related abnormality is present in Image 47-4?

A. Asbestosis
B. Benign asbestosis-related pleural effusion
C. Hilar adenopathy
D. Focal pleural thickening
E. Pleural plaques
F. Diffuse pleural thickening

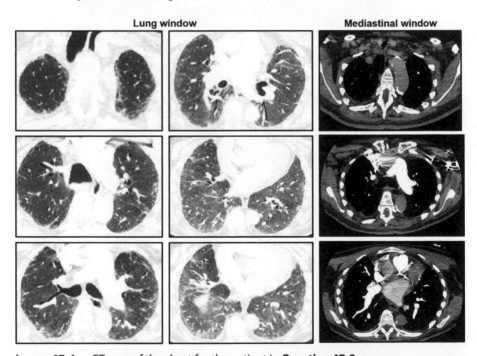

Image 47-4 • CT scan of the chest for the patient in **Question 47-8.**

Q47-9: Seven years after his initial evaluation, the same patient presents with complaints of pleuritic chest pain, fevers, and weight loss. He reports that he had a diagnosis of left-sided stage IB lung cancer 5 years ago and elected to receive radiation therapy alone rather than undergo surgical resection. He reports no symptoms until 6 or 7 months ago, when his constitutional symptoms began. The patient's chest radiograph and CT/PET-CT are shown in Images 47-5 and 47-6, respectively.

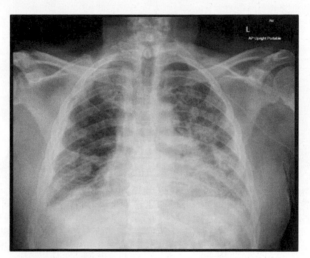

Image 47-5 • Chest radiography for the patient in **Question 47-9**.

What is the most likely diagnosis?

A. Adenocarcinoma of the lung
B. Squamous cell carcinoma of the lung
C. Small cell carcinoma of the lung
D. Carcinoid tumor of the lung
E. Erdheim-Chester syndrome
F. Mesothelioma

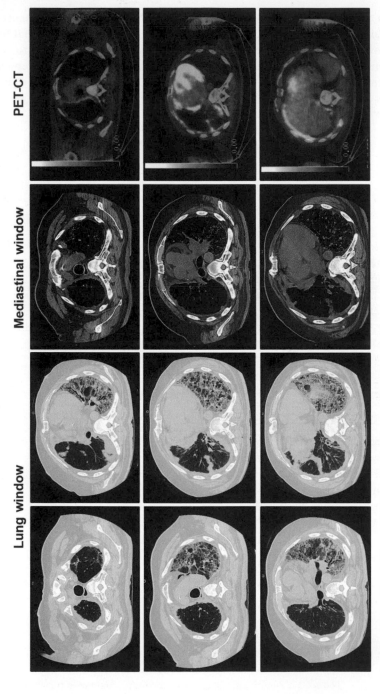

Image 47-6 • Chest CT and PET-CT for the patient in **Question 47-9**.

ANSWERS

Q47-1: B
Blunting of the left costophrenic angle

Rationale: One can see blunting of the left costophrenic angle, with a typical fluid meniscus sign. This is also apparent on the lateral film, consistent with the likely presence of a pleural effusion. There is also a linear opacity on the left; however, there are lung markings lateral to this change in density, and thus there is no pneumothorax. There are no bilateral masses or nodules.

Q47-2: B; C
Left-sided pleural effusion; Left-sided atelectasis

Rationale: Here, one can see the presence of a homogenous pleural effusion on the left (more clearly seen on the mediastinal windows), which is associated with left lower lobe atelectasis. The lack of significant air bronchograms and the loss of volume help to differentiate atelectasis from the consolidation seen in pneumonia. Also, note that the atelectatic portion of the lung is not linear but rather rounded in shape. There are no pleural plaques on the mediastinal windows. There is no free air in the pleural space, so there is no hydropneumothorax. There is a hiatal or diaphragmatic hernia. The right lung and pleural space are within normal limits.

Q47-3: D
Asbestos

Rationale: The patient has a benign pleural effusion, which is exudative with some blood present. All culture data are negative. The patient is asymptomatic. He reported no actual chest trauma during the accident and no recent falls. He has no medical condition for which he would take anticoagulant medications. The shape of the atelectatic lung (round) is adjacent to the pleural surface and is also associated with some mild pleural thickening. The most inferior image of the lung CT window also shows the "crow feet" sign. This is consistent with rounded atelectasis and associated benign asbestos-related pleural effusion (BAPE). The posterior lower lobes are most frequently involved. Up to 25% of patients with rounded atelectasis and BAPE have associated pleural plaques. These are common findings in patients with prior asbestos exposure, and this patient's long-term employment in a textile mill places him at high risk for prior asbestos exposure. Beryllium is associated with both an acute (inhalation fever) and a chronic (interstitial lung disease) process. Bird dander and mold are most commonly associated with hypersensitivity pneumonitis. Radon exposure is associated with an increased risk of malignancy but not with the development of lung or pleural disease. Radiation-associated lung disease is more commonly associated with prior radiation therapy, not incidental occupational exposure, which is more likely to affect the skin, thyroid gland, and reproductive organs. BAPE and rounded atelectasis are often found in combination; however, patients may develop either condition independently.

Q47-4: D
15 to 45 years

Rationale: The typical latency period between the first asbestos exposure and the development of BAPE is 15 to 45 years. Patients are usually asymptomatic, with the effusions discovered incidentally. Rarely, patients will present with pleuritic chest pain or cough. Dyspnea may also be present if the effusion is of considerable size or the patient has underlying lung disease that reduces pulmonary reserve. The risk of BAPE likely increases with the duration of exposure, though only 1 to 2 years of exposure may be sufficient (particularly if the exposure load is high). BAPE typically presents as a unilateral pleural effusion, and up to 90% of patients will have associated pleural plaques. Only about 50% of patients will have rounded atelectasis, which may demonstrate a "comet tail" or "crow's feet" pattern. Up to a quarter of patients will have evidence of pleural thickening. The pleural fluid is often serosanguinous or sanguineous, and as a result, there is typically some degree of eosinophilia. BAPE typically resolves spontaneously over the course of weeks to months, though it may persist if the patient develops rounded atelectasis or if rounded atelectasis preceded the development of BAPE. When BAPE does resolve, it typically leaves blunting of the costophrenic angles and pleural thickening.

Rounded atelectasis most commonly develops in patients with prior asbestos exposure; however, it may also develop in patients with any type of pleural inflammation.

Q47-5: E
Mesothelioma

Rationale: The differential diagnosis for BAPE includes rheumatoid pleuritis, *Mycobacterium tuberculosis* infection with effusion, and malignancy. The patient's asbestos exposure history places him at higher risk for the development of mesothelioma. Although the first thoracentesis demonstrated normal cytology, the sensitivity of cytology for a malignant pleural effusion is about 60%, and typically three independent cytology specimens are required to rule out malignancy. Additionally, due to the associated rounded atelectasis, patients may also have underlying primary lung malignancy that is not visualized on CT. It would be important to rule out sarcoidosis and histoplasmosis, both of which may cause pleural inflammation, but these are much less common causes of isolated rounded atelectasis and pleural effusions. IPF and AAT are not associated with rounded atelectasis or pleural effusions.

Q47-6: A
PET-CT

Rationale: Although the patient has many of the features of rounded atelectasis (rounded shape of the atelectatic lung, subpleural location, local pleural thickening), the patient lacks pleural plaques. The next step in the evaluation of this patient would be to rule out malignancy mesothelioma and primary lung cancer. A PET-CT scan would be particularly useful to determine if there is evidence of malignancy in the pleura or the atelectatic lung. MRI of the brain with contrast is commonly used to rule out metastatic lung cancer, but it would not help determine if malignancy was present. An echocardiogram would potentially help to rule out the presence of overt heart failure leading to a pleural effusion; however, with a normal BNP, this is unlikely. A PE-protocol CT scan would help rule out a pulmonary infarction as the cause of the rounded atelectasis and associated effusion, but again, this does not rule out malignancy. A contrasted CT scan of the sinuses and neck would not be helpful unless there is suspicion of possible thymoma or thyroid cancer. Bronchoscopy with transbronchial biopsy or CT-guided transthoracic needle aspiration may be useful to rule out malignancy in the atelectatic lung, but a bronchoalveolar lavage alone would not be particularly useful here. Ultimately, a pleural biopsy is the only way to rule out mesothelioma.

Q47-7: B
Observation only with repeat CT scan in 3 to 6 months

Rationale: This PET-CT scan demonstrates only physiologic uptake of fluorodeoxyglucose in the pleura, pleural effusion, and the atelectatic portion of the lung. Coupled with the negative cytology from the thoracentesis, this would be inconsistent with mesothelioma or an advanced stage primary lung cancer. There is no increased uptake in the hilar or mediastinal lymph nodes as well. Therefore, the most appropriate next step would be a repeat CT scan in 3 to 6 months to evaluate for a change. If the patient were adamant to obtain a definitive diagnosis, a VATS biopsy could be considered; however, this carries the inherent risk associated with major thoracic surgery. As there is no evidence of malignancy, there is no role for an indwelling pleural catheter (eg, PleurX). A course of antibiotics would be appropriate if the patient had a pulmonary abscess; however, that is not the case here. Extrapleural pneumonectomy and pleurectomy with decortication are surgical treatment options for mesothelioma.

Q47-8: A; D
Asbestosis; Focal pleural thickening

Rationale: The images in **Image 47-4** demonstrate changes consistent with pleural thickening and asbestosis. The lung windows show a lower lobe–predominant interstitial pneumonia, while the mediastinal windows demonstrate evidence of pleural thickening. Pleural thickening is another potential complication of asbestos exposure. Patients may have either focal pleural thickening or diffuse thickening, which is defined as a pleural thickness greater than 3 mm extending at least 8 cm in the craniocaudal dimension and 5 cm axially. Here, there are areas of focal pleural thickening, particularly in the right upper lobe area, but this does not meet the criteria for diffuse pleural thickening. There is no evidence of a pleural effusion or pleural plaques.

Q47-9: F
Mesothelioma

Rationale: The patient had early-stage primary lung cancer 5 years ago that was treated with definitive radiation therapy. He has extensive fibrotic changes in the left lung, possibly related to radiation fibrosis and treatment changes. However, on the right, there is evidence of diffuse pleural thickening, and the pleura has increased fluorodeoxyglucose uptake on the PET-CT scan. Malignant pleural mesothelioma is classically associated with prior asbestos exposure, with up to 80% of patients having some recorded exposure. Most patients have prior occupational exposure to asbestos; however, patients with simply environmental or second-hand exposure have also been reported. The latency periods may be between 30 and 45 years from the initial exposure, and the risk of developing mesothelioma may increase with concomitant smoking tobacco exposure. Mesothelioma is also more prevalent in patients with prior radiation exposure to the lung, including lymphoma, breast cancer, and lung cancer. A detailed discussion regarding the management of mesothelioma is outside the scope of this text. Patients are generally classified according to resectable and nonresectable disease. The overall life expectancy ranges from 6 to 24 months from the time of diagnosis.

References

Husain AN, Colby TV, Ordóñez NG, et al. Guidelines for pathologic diagnosis of malignant mesothelioma 2017 update of the consensus statement from the International Mesothelioma Interest Group. Arch Pathol Lab Med. 2018;142:89.

Kindler HL, Ismaila N, Armato SG 3rd, et al. Treatment of malignant pleural mesothelioma: American Society of Clinical Oncology Clinical Practice Guideline. J Clin Oncol. 2018;36:1343.

Marsh GM, Riordan AS, Keeton KA, Benson SM. Non-occupational exposure to asbestos and risk of pleural mesothelioma: review and meta-analysis. Occup Environ Med. 2017;74:838.

Mintzer RA, Cugell DW. The association of asbestos-induced pleural disease and rounded atelectasis. Chest. 1982;81:457.

Partap VA. The comet tail sign. Radiology. 1999;213:553.

Scherpereel A, Opitz I, Berghmans T, et al. ERS/ESTS/EACTS/ESTRO guidelines for the management of malignant pleural mesothelioma. Eur Respir J. 2020;55.

Schwartz DA, Fuortes LJ, Galvin JR, et al. Asbestos-induced pleural fibrosis and impaired lung function. Am Rev Respir Dis. 1990;141:321.

Stathopoulos GT, Karamessini MT, Sotiriadi AE, Pastromas VG. Rounded atelectasis of the lung. Respir Med. 2005;99:615.

Voisin C, Fisekci F, Voisin-Saltiel S, et al. Asbestos-related rounded atelectasis. Radiologic and mineralogic data in 23 cases. Chest. 1995;107:477.

CASE 48

You are asked to provide pulmonary consultation on a 34-year-old man who is day +18 from an allogenic, sibling-matched identical hematopoietic stem cell transplantation (HSCT) who developed scant blood-tinged sputum, tachypnea, dyspnea, cough, and hypoxia over the last 24 hours. The patient had non-Hodgkin lymphoma, which was treated with R-CHOP therapy (cyclophosphamide, doxorubicin, vincristine, and prednisone, plus the monoclonal antibody rituximab) and underwent nonmyeloablative preparation with fludarabine, cyclophosphamide, antithymocyte globulin, and total body irradiation to 2 Gy. He had no known pulmonary disease prior to transplantation, and his pulmonary function testing prior to transplantation demonstrated normal spirometry, lung volumes, and DLCO. The patient has yet to achieve engraftment with an absolute neutrophil count (ANC) of 450/µL. The patient has been maintained on acyclovir and posaconazole for prophylaxis, in addition to tacrolimus, prednisone, and mycophenolate mofetil for maintenance immunosuppression. The patient has not experienced a fever during the last 72 hours. The patient's vital signs are T 97.6°F, HR 110, BP 100/65, RR 22, O_2 saturation 94% on 4 L/min supplemental O_2. The patient was empirically started on vancomycin and piperacillin-tazobactam antibiotics the day prior.

The patient's chest radiograph is shown below in Image 48-1.

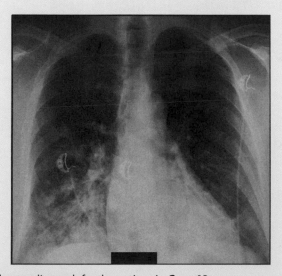

Image 48-1 • Chest radiograph for the patient in **Case 48**.

QUESTIONS

Q48-1: What is the best description of the patient's chest radiograph?

A. Normal chest radiograph
B. Diffuse, lower lobe–predominant alveolar opacities
C. Diffuse interstitial opacities, mixed linear and reticular
D. Reticulonodular opacities
E. Cavitary and cystic lung lesions

Q48-2: The patient undergoes a noncontrasted CT scan of the chest, which is shown in Image 48-2.

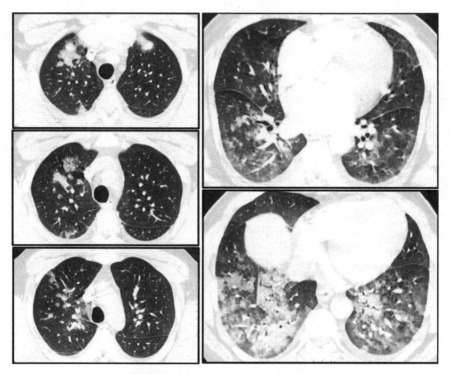

Image 48-2 • Noncontrasted CT of the chest for the patient in **Case 48**.

Which abnormalities are present on the CT scan of the chest shown in Image 48-2? Select all that apply.

A. Ground-glass opacities
B. Interlobular septal thickening
C. Large pleural effusion
D. Consolidative/nodular opacities
E. Plate-like atelectasis
F. Cavitary lung lesions
G. Reverse halo sign
H. Halo sign

Q48-3: The patient has a recent echocardiogram that demonstrates no abnormalities, and the patient's cardiovascular examination demonstrates no murmurs, rubs, or clicks. The patient's platelet count is currently 9 ×10^9/mL. What is the next step in the management of this patient?

A. Procalcitonin serum study
B. Serum beta-D-glucan study
C. Histoplasma urine antigen study
D. Cryptococcal serum antigen study
E. Bronchoscopy with bronchoalveolar lavage
F. Bronchoscopy with serial bronchoalveolar lavage
G. Bronchoscopy with bronchoalveolar lavage and transbronchial biopsy

Q48-4: The patient's serial lavage returns consistent with diffuse alveolar hemorrhage. The patient has an ANCA panel and antiglomerular basement membrane antibody, and the ANA returns negative. What are the most common causes of DAH in patients who underwent HSCT?

A. Infection, trauma, and radiation
B. Drug interaction, radiation, and infection
C. Infection, graft-versus-host disease, and idiopathic
D. Idiopathic, graft-versus-host disease, and anticoagulation adverse effect
E. Graft-versus-host disease, malignancy recurrence, and pulmonary cytolytic thrombi

Q48-5: The patient deteriorates rapidly over the next several hours and requires intubation with mechanical ventilation. The patient is loaded with voriconazole in addition to the aforementioned antibiotics, and additional infectious disease studies are pending. The patient's PCP polymerase chain reaction from bronchoscopy returns negative. What is the next step in management for the patient?

A. High-dose trimethoprim/sulfamethoxazole with systemic glucocorticoids, 0.5 mg/kg/day
B. Azithromycin
C. Plasmapheresis, intravenous immunoglobulin (IVIG), and rituximab
D. Plasmapheresis and IVIG
E. Systemic glucocorticoids, 1 mg/kg/day

ANSWERS

Q48-1: B
Diffuse, lower lobe–predominant alveolar opacities

Rationale: This is likely AP film because there is no lateral film provided. The cardiac silhouette is relatively crisp, the heart borders are within normal limits, the airway is midline with no deviation noted, and the carina is visible. The aortic knob is within normal limits. Some prominence and mild haziness of the pulmonary vasculature at the hilum is visible. There are bilateral, lower lobe–predominant, and right-greater-than-left hazy alveolar opacities, which are also present to a lesser degree in the upper lobes. There is some sparing of the periphery in the upper lobes as well. There are possibly some reticulonodular opacities underlying this, but the predominant finding is the alveolar consolidative opacities. There is no apparent cavitation or cystic lesions present.

Q48-2: A; B; D
Ground-glass opacities; Interlobular septal thickening; Consolidative/nodular opacities

Rationale: On the CT scan, the abnormalities are predominantly in the lower lobes, though the upper lobes are not spared. There are areas of interlobular septal thickening with associated ground-glass opacities as well as areas of consolidation (which may also be termed "nodular"). There may be trace left-greater-than-right pleural effusions, but it is difficult to tell without the mediastinal windows. There are some areas with air bronchograms, but these are not clearly demonstrated here. There is no plate-like atelectasis, and none of the consolidative or nodular opacities has evidence of cavitation. There is no obvious halo or reverse halo sign (area of consolidation surrounding an area of ground-glass opacities or vice-versa), with a relatively random distribution of the ground-glass opacities and consolidation.

Q48-3: F
Bronchoscopy with serial bronchoalveolar lavage

Rationale: The patient is immunocompromised and underwent a haplotype-identical allogeneic bone marrow transplant. The differential diagnosis for the patient's acute respiratory failure is quite broad and would include infection (including opportunistic infections, such as cytomegalovirus, *Pneumocystis jiroveci* pneumonia [PCP], fungal infection, and *Nocardia*), diffuse alveolar hemorrhage (more common in autologous than allogeneic transplant), idiopathic pneumonia syndrome (similar to acute interstitial pneumonia but occurs in the immediate post-transplantation period, typically within 30 days of transplantation), new connective tissue disease (rare, but more likely to occur with myeloablative preparation regimens), organizing pneumonia, drug toxicity, radiation pneumonitis, recurrent malignancy with lymphangitic dissemination, pulmonary edema (cardiogenic and noncardiogenic), and pulmonary alveolar proteinosis (PAP). Although options A, B, C, and D are all reasonable approaches, bronchoscopy with bronchoalveolar lavage will not only help evaluate for the presence of infection, it will also help diagnose diffuse alveolar hemorrhage (DAH) and PAP. A diagnosis of DAH requires serial lavage. In diffuse alveolar hemorrhage, one would expect to see progressively more bloody lavage samples with sequential injections in the same subsegment, as well as hemosiderin-laden macrophages on cytology. The samples become more sanguineous as more fluid reaches the alveolar spaces. Transbronchial biopsy could certainly help not only in identifying an infectious agent but also in ruling out organizing pneumonia and drug toxicity, but the patient's platelet count is too low (40-50 $\times 10^6$/mL minimum required). Assuming the patient's respiratory status is safe for bronchoscopy, this would be the most appropriate study. Options A, B, C, D could also be ordered to supplement this workup.

Q48-4: C
Infection, graft-versus-host disease, and idiopathic

Rationale: DAH consists of bleeding into the alveoli due to disruption of the basement membrane. A variety of diseases are associated with the development of DAH, and it is generally classified according to histopathologic findings. For this case, we will focus on HSCT-associated DAH. DAH is relatively rare following transplantation, occurring two to five times more frequently in autologous than allogeneic stem cell transplantation. The most common cause of DAH in patients who underwent HSCT is infection. Infection can be due to any type of infection (bacterial, fungal, mycobacterial, viral). Graft-versus-host disease is also a common cause of DAH. When these two etiologies are ruled out, the diagnosis is considered idiopathic. Very rarely will a patient develop a new connective disease/vasculitis following transplantation, and this has largely been ruled out by the additional serologies. Patients on anticoagulation can develop bland pulmonary hemorrhage; however, most patients are not anticoagulated after transplantation due to thrombocytopenia, such as in this case. Radiation and drug toxicity are not associated with DAH. Trauma can lead to DAH or pulmonary hemorrhage, but this is uncommon after transplantation. The pathogenesis for DAH after transplantation remains unclear. It is not thought to result solely from thrombocytopenia.

The clinical presentation of DAH in HSCT is rather acute, typically with a rapid progression. Patients rarely present with frank hemoptysis. Patients may have a cough, dyspnea, tachypnea, and hypoxia but do not usually have pleuritic pain. The chest imaging findings in this case are very common for patients with DAH with diffuse alveolar consolidations or airspace disease.

Q48-5: E
Systemic glucocorticoids, 1 mg/kg/day

Rationale: Assuming infection has been adequately evaluated and treated, current guidelines recommend treatment of DAH with systemic glucocorticoids, 0.5 to 1 mg/kg/day, for several days. This is recommended treatment for either graft-versus-host disease–associated DAH or idiopathic DAH. Although survival has been poor in patients with DAH who progress to respiratory failure (approaching 60%-90%), anecdotal evidence suggests that treatment with high-dose methylprednisolone is associated with a threefold increase in ICU survival. For patients with significant blood loss due to alveolar hemorrhage, the use of recombinant factor VII has been reported. High-dose trimethoprim/sulfamethoxazole in combination with gluco-corticoids would be appropriate for patients with PCP pneumonia. Plasmapheresis, IVIG, and rituximab—in addition to systemic glucocorticoids—may be appropriate for patients with severe DAH due to pulmonary-renal syndromes or vasculitis. As DAH following HSCT is not believed to be antibody mediated, this treatment regimen would not be appropriate.

Diffuse alveolar hemorrhage in patients who have not undergone HSCT will be covered separately.

References

Blatt J, Gold SH, Wiley JM, et al. Off-label use of recombinant factor VIIa in patients following bone marrow transplantation. Bone Marrow Transplant. 2001;28:405.

Gupta S, Jain A, Warneke CL, et al. Outcome of alveolar hemorrhage in hematopoietic stem cell transplant recipients. Bone Marrow Transplant. 2007;40:71.

Hicks K, Peng D, Gajewski JL. Treatment of diffuse alveolar hemorrhage after allogeneic bone marrow transplant with recombinant factor VIIa. Bone Marrow Transplant. 2002;30:975.

Kotloff RM, Ahya VN, Crawford SW. Pulmonary complications of solid organ and hematopoietic stem cell transplantation. Am J Respir Crit Care. Med 2004;170:22.

Leung AN, Gosselin MV, Napper CH, et al. Pulmonary infections after bone marrow transplantation: clinical and radiographic findings. Radiology. 1999;210:699.

Pastores SM, Papadopoulos E, Voigt L, Halpern NA. Diffuse alveolar hemorrhage after allogeneic hematopoietic stem-cell transplantation: treatment with recombinant factor VIIa. Chest. 2003;124:2400.

Raptis A, Mavroudis D, Suffredini A, et al. High-dose corticosteroid therapy for diffuse alveolar hemorrhage in allogeneic bone marrow stem cell transplant recipients. Bone Marrow Transplant. 1999;24:879.

Roychowdhury M, Pambuccian SE, Aslan DL, et al. Pulmonary complications after bone marrow transplantation: an autopsy study from a large transplantation center. Arch Pathol Lab Med. 2005;129:366.

Weinstock DM, Feinstein MB, Sepkowitz KA, Jakubowski A. High rates of infection and colonization by nontuberculous mycobacteria after allogeneic hematopoietic stem cell transplantation. Bone Marrow Transplant. 2003;31:1015.

Yen KT, Lee AS, Krowka MJ, Burger CD. Pulmonary complications in bone marrow transplantation: a practical approach to diagnosis and treatment. Clin Chest Med. 2004;25:189.

CASE 49

A 72-year-old woman is admitted to the hospital with several weeks of fatigue, fevers, drenching night sweats, a 20-lb weight loss (unintentional), maxillary and frontal sinus tenderness, diffuse arthralgias without effusions or redness, and a dry cough. She reports that the symptoms started gradually about 8 weeks ago and accelerated significantly over the last 4 weeks. She also has some increased dyspnea on exertion. She has never smoked tobacco or used illicit drugs. She worked as a nurse for 35 years before retiring a few years ago. She has not had any pulmonary or rheumatologic conditions. She takes escitalopram for anxiety and depression but reports no issues with anhedonia, poor appetite, sleep disturbances, or depressed mood in the last 10 years. She also takes omeprazole for gastroesophageal reflux disease (GERD) and uses acetaminophen intermittently for headaches. She reports an increase in headache frequency with these fevers recently but no other neurologic symptoms. She reports no diarrhea, abdominal pain, lightheadedness, dizziness, chest pain, or hemoptysis. She has a family history of cardiovascular disease and chronic obstructive pulmonary disease (COPD), which is smoking related in first-degree relatives. The patient's vital signs are T 102.5°F, HR 103, BP 155/79, RR 18, and O_2 saturation 96% on 2 L/min supplemental O_2. On examination, the patient has no apparent cardiopulmonary findings, with a clear lung examination bilaterally with good air movement. There are no joint deformities, effusions, or areas of redness or tenderness. There is no abdominal tenderness or distention. She is alert and oriented to person, place, time, and situation, with no deficits on examination. Her skin examination is unremarkable. There is no flank tenderness.

The patient's chest radiograph is shown in Image 49-1.

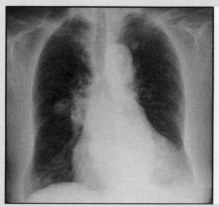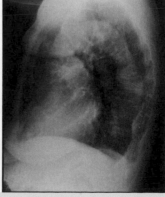

Image 49-1 • Chest radiograph for the patient in **Question 49-1**.

QUESTIONS

Q49-1: Which abnormalities are present in the chest radiograph in Image 49-1?
Select all that apply.

A. Lung nodules and masses without cavitation
B. Lung nodules and masses with cavitation
C. Cystic lung mass
D. Right hilar prominence
E. Left hilar prominence
F. Bilateral hilar prominence

Q49-2: The patient undergoes a chest CT scan, which is shown in Image 49-2.

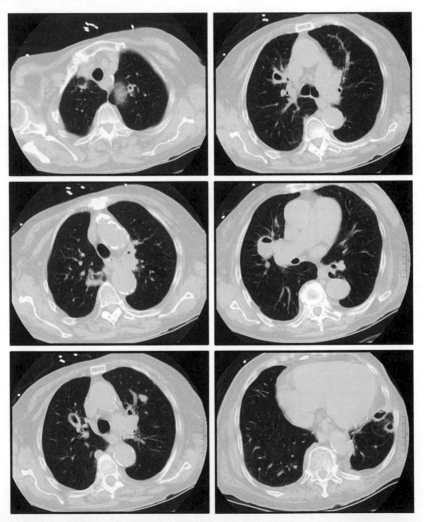

Image 49-2 • CT scan (noncontrasted) of the chest for the patient in **Question 49-2**.

Which abnormalities are present on the CT scan of the chest shown in Image 49-2? Select all that apply.

A. Cavitary lung lesions
B. Lung nodules
C. Ground-glass opacities
D. Cystic lung lesions
E. Centrilobular emphysematous changes
F. Panlobular emphysematous changes
G. Pleural effusion

Q49-3: Which additional abnormalities are demonstrated in Image 49-3?

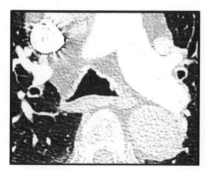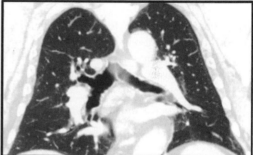

Image 49-3 • CT scan of the chest for the patient in **Question 49-3**.

A. External compression of the central airways
B. Airway nodularity and tracheal wall thickening
C. Saddle pulmonary embolism
D. Aortic dissection
E. Hilar adenopathy

Q49-4: The patient has additional laboratory work on admission that includes the following: a negative QuantiFERON Gold *Mycobacterium tuberculosis* test, a WBC count of 17.6 ×10⁹/L with a slight neutrophilic predominance and no peripheral eosinophils. The patient's rheumatoid factor (Rf) is within normal limits. An antinuclear antibody test is mildly positive with a titer of 1:40. An anti-double-stranded DNA (dsDNA) antibody test is less than 25 IU/mL. An anti-cyclic citrullinated peptide (anti-CCP) antibody test is normal. The erythrocyte sedimentation rate is greater than 140 mm/h. She has a sputum culture for bacteria, fungus, and acid-fast bacillus (AFB) pending, and the patient has three AFB smears over 24 hours reported as negative. The sputum Gram stain demonstrates only significant polymorphonuclear leukocytes with no organisms. The patient's procalcitonin level is 0.10 pg/mL. The urinalysis demonstrates 2+ protein, 2+ blood, negative leukocyte esterase, negative nitrates, and 3 WBCs per high-powered field. The patient's creatinine level is 1.8 mg/dL, with a baseline of 0.8 mg/dL 3 months ago at a primary care appointment. The patient's urinalysis performed 18 months ago demonstrated no protein or RBCs.

What is the top differential diagnosis for this patient?

A. Disseminated *M. tuberculosis* infection
B. Latent *M. tuberculosis* infection
C. Rheumatoid arthritis (RA)
D. ANCA-associated vasculitides
E. Systemic lupus erythematosus (SLE)
F. Eosinophilic pneumonia

Q49-5: **Which laboratory study would you anticipate returning positive in this patient?**

A. MPO antineutrophil cytoplasmic antibodies
B. Anti-Jo-1 antibodies
C. Anti-Scl70 antibodies
D. PR3 antineutrophil cytoplasmic antibodies
E. Antihistone antibodies
F. Elevated serum aldolase
G. Elevated serum creatinine kinase (CK)

Q49-6: **What is the most appropriate next step in the patient's management?**

A. Echocardiogram to evaluate for pericardial effusion
B. Pulmonary function testing, including a DLCO
C. MRI of the brain
D. Nerve conduction study and electromyography
E. Skin biopsy
F. Temporal artery biopsy
G. Transbronchial lung biopsy
H. Kidney biopsy

Q49-7: **The patient's kidney biopsy and ANCA testing confirmed a diagnosis of GPA with PR3 antibodies. What is the most appropriate treatment regimen for the patient at this point?**

A. Systemic glucocorticoids alone
B. Systemic glucocorticoids with methotrexate
C. Rituximab alone
D. Systemic glucocorticoids, cyclophosphamide, and rituximab
E. Mycophenolate or azathioprine
F. Plasmapheresis and intravenous immunoglobulin therapy (IVIG)

Q49-8: A 45-year-old man presents with shortness of breath, cough, and non-massive hemoptysis. He requires 50% FIO_2 via a heated, high-flow nasal cannula. His urinalysis is positive for 3+ hematuria and trace protein, no glucose, and less than 5 WBCs per high-powered field. The nephrology team centrifuged the patient's urine and identified cellular casts. The patient denies any constitutional symptoms and rather feels like he has gained 3 to 5 lb of water weight recently. The patient's creatinine level is 5.4 mg/dL, from a baseline of 1.1 mg/dL 6 months ago. He has no medical history aside from stage 1 essential hypertension. The patient's chest imaging is shown in Images 49-4 and 49-5.

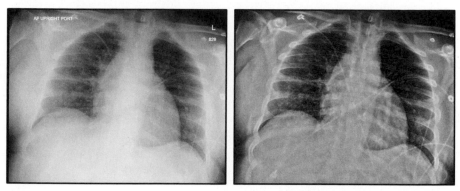

Image 49-4 • Chest radiograph (and enhanced chest radiograph, right) for the patient in **Question 49-8**.

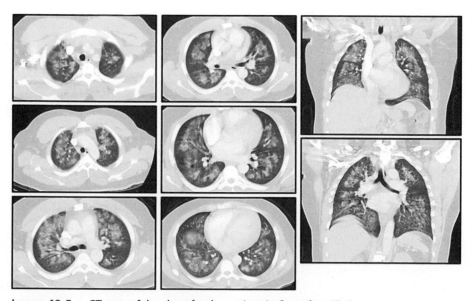

Image 49-5 • CT scan of the chest for the patient in **Question 49-8**.

The patient undergoes a kidney biopsy that returns with linear deposition of IgG antibodies along the capillaries. What is the most appropriate treatment for this patient?

A. Systemic glucocorticoids alone
B. Systemic glucocorticoids, rituximab, and plasmapheresis
C. Anti-thymocyte globulin (ATG)
D. Alemtuzumab (anti-CD52 antibody)
E. Mycophenolate alone
F. Plasmapheresis, dexamethasone, and carfilzomib (proteasome inhibitor)

ANSWERS

Q49-1: B; D
Lung nodules and masses with cavitation; Right hilar prominence

Rationale: This is a PA and lateral chest film. There is a good inspiratory effort with possibly some hyperinflation (note the slight flattening of the diaphragms). The chest radiograph shows several lung nodules and masses (recall that consolidations less than 3 cm are classified as nodules and greater than 3 cm are masses). These masses have clear cavitation present, visible on both the PA and lateral films and particularly in the upper lobes. There is also prominence of the right hilum with some increased haziness. The aortic knob and left hilum are relatively normal in appearance, with some calcification in the knob. The heart silhouette appears overall slightly enlarged, with some blunting of the left costophrenic angle on the PA film, with a possible small effusion. There are no cystic lung nodules.

Q49-2: A; B; C; G
Cavitary lung lesions; Lung nodules; Ground-glass opacities; Pleural effusion

Rationale: There are ground-glass opacities, solid nodules, and cavitary nodules present bilaterally on the CT scan of the chest, distributed throughout the upper and lower lobes. The largest such lesion abuts the right hilum. It is difficult to exclude adenopathy here. These lesions are thick walled, and therefore they are cavitary rather than cystic. Some of the nodules have not cavitated. There are no significant emphysematous changes throughout the lung. There is possible a trace pleural effusion present in the left pleural space, though this may also be pleural thickening.

Q49-3: B
Airway nodularity and tracheal wall thickening

Rationale: Here (**Image 49-6**), one can see nodularity along the central airways (trachea, bronchus intermedius, left main stem bronchi). There is also some degree of tracheal and bronchial wall thickening. There is no apparent external compression of the airway, nor is there evidence of aortic dissection. The pulmonary artery demonstrates a normal contrasted pattern with no evidence of a saddle embolus. There is also no overt hilar adenopathy, which will be discussed in more detail later in the case.

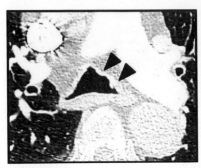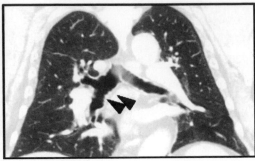

Image 49-6 • Annotated CT scan for the patient in **Question 49-3**. Note the airway nodularity demonstrated on CT images (*black arrows*).

Q49-4: D
ANCA-associated vasculitides

Rationale: The patient presents with constitutional symptoms, fatigue, arthralgias, and a dry cough, which developed over a subacute period of approximately 8 weeks. The patient has new-onset acute kidney injury with new proteinuria and hematuria. The chest imaging demonstrates lung nodules that are not only cavitary. This may raise a question for a number of possible conditions, including infection (particularly *M. tuberculosis* or fungal infections), malignancy (without prior imaging for comparison, this is difficult to exclude), RA, SLE, sarcoidosis, pulmonary amyloidosis, ANCA-associated vasculitis, and pulmonary-renal syndromes. The involvement of the lower respiratory tract/subglottic airway with nodularity and thickening potentially helps narrow the diagnosis, which would include amyloidosis, ANCA-associated vasculitides, sarcoidosis, RA, relapsing polychondritis, and inflammatory bowel disease. The patient's lack of bowel symptoms makes an inflammatory bowel disease less likely, particularly at this patient's age. The negative AFB smears and QuantiFERON Gold study suggest that the patient does not have active or latent *M. tuberculosis*. The negative Rf and anti-CCP studies suggest that RA is not likely (though seronegative RA is possible). The ANA is very low titer (typically anticipate an ANA titer of greater than 1:256 for active disease), and dsDNA is negative, suggesting no evidence of SLE. Of the available answers, the patient's presentation is most consistent with ANCA-associated vasculitis. Additional consideration could be given to anti–glomerular basement membrane (GBM) disease, which may also present with pulmonary and kidney disease.

Q49-5: D
PR3 antineutrophil cytoplasmic antibodies

Rationale: There are numerous classification systems for the ANCA-associated vasculitides, which traditionally include granulomatosis with polyangiitis (GPA; previously Wegener granulomatosis), microscopic polyangiitis (MPA; previously pauci-immune vasculitis), and eosinophilic granulomatosis with polyangiitis (EGPA; previously Churg-Strauss syndrome). The Chapel Hill Consensus Conference classified these disease processes based on histopathologic findings. GPA is defined as a necrotizing small/medium vessel vasculitis that lacks immune deposits but has granulomas present on biopsy, while MPA lacks granuloma formation. Under this classification system, the ANCA serologies are not considered. GPA is classically PR3 (cytoplasmic, cANCA) positive, while MPA is classically MPO (perinuclear, pANCA) positive, and some clinicians have called for the ANCA-associated vasculitides (AAV) to be redefined by serology and termed MPO-AAV and PR3-AAV. The ANCA serologies are generally better predictors of response to therapy and risk of relapse than the histopathologic classifications alone (PR3-AAV is more likely to experience disease recurrence or flares). Approximately 10% of patients will have a negative ANCA test.

The Jo-1 antibody test is used in the diagnosis of antisynthetase syndrome/myositis, Scl70 in scleroderma, and antihistone antibodies in drug-induced SLE. Aldolase and creatine-kinase levels are nonspecific, but elevated levels may be seen in myositis.

MPA (MPO-AAV) more commonly manifests with fibrosing interstitial lung disease, commonly in a usual interstitial pneumonia pattern. Only about 20% of patients with GPA present with ground-glass opacities, reticular interstitial abnormalities, bronchiectasis, fibrotic lung disease with honeycombing, and pleural effusions (rare). An example of a patient with MPA is shown in **Image 49-7**. GPA is most commonly associated with cavitary parenchymal lung nodules and subglottic airway involvement, such as that seen in this case. Multiple nodules may be present, but they are generally not numerous (less than 10-15). One may also see the "vasculitis" sign (large, irregular, potentially nodule-studded pulmonary arteries/arterioles) or even wedge-shaped areas of infarction. Therefore, one would expect the PR3 antineutrophil cytoplasmic antibodies to be positive here rather than the MPO antibodies. Nearly 100% of patients with GPA have involvement of upper airways as well. Here, the patient presented with maxillary and frontal sinus involvement, consistent with likely nasal/sinus tract disease. GPA may also manifest with tracheal/bronchial stenosis, airway malacia, or ulceration. Both MPO- and PR3-AAVs may present with diffuse alveolar hemorrhage as well. Kidney involvement is very common in both of the AAVs, manifesting as hematuria, proteinuria, and a reduced glomerular filtration rate. Patients may also have cutaneous manifestations, such as leukocytoclastic angiitis, urticaria, and painful nodules. Ocular, neurologic, GI, and cardiac involvement is also possible.

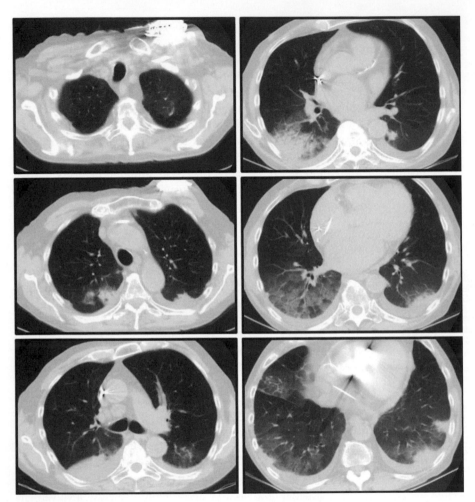

Image 49-7 • CT scan of the chest for a patient with MPO ANCA-associated vasculitis, with ground-glass opacities, consolidation, and pleural effusions.

A few things should be noted about ANCA testing: (1) this is largely not standardized and relies on subjective interpretation of antibody staining; (2) a positive test is not specific for vasculitis, so a strong pretest probability is necessary; and (3) a negative test does not rule out vasculitis because up to 10% of patients may be ANCA-negative.

EGPA is small/medium vessel vasculitis that is associated with eosinophilia, asthma, and vasculitis. Patients may also present with polyneuropathy, sinus disease, pulmonary infiltrates, GI symptoms (pancreatitis, gastrointestinal bleeding), cardiomyopathy, proteinuria, and kidney failure. Hematuria, however, is rare. EGPA typically stains positive for MPO (perinuclear) antineutrophilic cytoplasmic antibodies. The classic ANCA vasculitides are MPA and GPA. Another vasculitis, polyarteritis nodosa (PAN), typically spares the lungs.

Q49-6: H
Kidney biopsy

Rationale: Whenever possible, a diagnosis of ANCA-associated vasculitis should be confirmed with a tissue biopsy. As discussed previously, ANCA is not specific for a diagnosis of ANCA-vasculitis and can be seen in almost any other subacute or chronic inflammatory/autoimmune condition, including drug-induced vasculitis (eg, hydralazine), cocaine-induced vasculitis, RA, SLE, scleroderma, ulcerative colitis, cystic fibrosis, and even in some infectious conditions. If a patient presents with severe disease, it may not be possible to obtain a biopsy before initiation of treatment, or it may be necessary to initiate treatment before histopathologic analysis can be performed and resulted. Here, the patient is clinically stable, so obtaining a biopsy before the initiation of treatment would be appropriate. A tissue sample should be obtained from the affected tissue. There is no skin involvement, and the temporal artery is a large vessel and would not be appropriate for biopsy here. Generally, skin, kidney, or nasal biopsies are preferred because they are associated with less procedural risk. MRI of the brain would be useful if there were a concern for central nervous system involvement. Pulmonary function tests (PFTs) would not be particularly helpful here. PFT abnormalities in ANCA vasculitis will vary with the type and degree of airway and parenchymal involvement. Here, we may expect to see some evidence of obstruction due to airway involvement and possibly a reduced DLCO. In patients with more parenchymal involvement, there may be a more restrictive pattern. A nerve conduction study and electromyography may be useful if there is concern for polyneuropathy or myopathy.

If a kidney biopsy is not possible, nasal imaging and possible biopsy or a lung biopsy via bronchoscopy could be considered. Both suffer from a high rate of false-negative findings because it may be difficult to target affected tissue. However, bronchoscopy has the added benefit of allowing for direct airway examination, and endobronchial lesions are a more viable biopsy option. Occasionally, video-assisted thoracoscopic surgery (VATS) biopsy is required. Importantly, note that we have ruled out active *Mycobacterium tuberculosis* (TB) infection. As the clinical symptoms of TB infection are very difficult to distinguish from ANCA-vasculitis, this is a necessary step in the evaluation of the patient to prevent aerosolization of spores and possible transmission to staff members during either procedure.

Q49-7: D
Systemic glucocorticoids, cyclophosphamide, and rituximab

Rationale: Treatment for GPA and MPA involve both induction and maintenance phases. The first step is to identify if the patient has a severe or life-threatening disease, such as acute respiratory failure, diffuse alveolar hemorrhage, central nervous system vasculitis, glomerulonephritis, or pericarditis. As this patient has evidence of acute glomerulonephritis, she would require a more aggressive treatment course. These patients generally receive induction therapy with systemic glucocorticoids (pulse dosing, typically about 500-1000 mg a day) with cyclophosphamide or rituximab. The use of plasmapheresis remains controversial but is often employed in patients with more severe clinical presentations, and IVIG may also be used. However, these are adjuvant therapies and the use of plasmapheresis and IVIG alone are not recommended. This is continued until remission is achieved and maintenance therapy can be initiated. Maintenance therapy typically includes a taper of glucocorticoids and a steroid-sparing agent, most commonly methotrexate, azathioprine, or mycophenolate. The decision when to taper off maintenance therapy requires close monitoring for disease recurrence and should only be performed by a rheumatologist or pulmonologist with considerable experience. Patients are typically maintained on maintenance therapy for several years. Patients with non–life-threatening disease are generally treated with lower doses of glucocorticoids (0.5-1 mg/kg/day) in combination with a steroid-sparing agent, though oral cyclophosphamide or rituximab have also been used.

Q49-8: B
Systemic glucocorticoids, rituximab, and plasmapheresis

Rationale: This is a classic presentation of anti-GBM disease (formerly Goodpasture disease), another pulmonary-renal disease. The patient presented with likely diffuse alveolar hemorrhage in combination with nephritic syndrome but without the constitutional symptoms typically seen in vasculitis. The biopsy demonstrates linear deposition of IgG antibodies along the glomerular capillaries consistent with anti-GBM disease. The treatment for anti-GBM disease is systemic glucocorticoids and cyclophosphamide or rituximab, typically in combination with plasmapheresis to expedite removal of the offending antibodies. ATG is more commonly used to remove B and T cells, which would not affect the existing auto-antibody levels present. Campath is a treatment used in CLL and for chronic rejection in certain types of solid organ transplantation and would not affect B-cell function. Mycophenolate or glucocorticoid therapy alone would be insufficient. Dexamethasone and carfilzomib are used in the treatment of multiple myeloma and have not been used in the treatment of anti-GBM disease.

References

Cartin-Ceba R, Diaz-Caballero L, Al-Qadi MO, et al. Diffuse alveolar hemorrhage secondary to antineutrophil cytoplasmic antibody-associated vasculitis: predictors of respiratory failure and clinical outcomes. Arthritis Rheumatol. 2016;68:1467.

Casal Moura M, Irazabal MV, Eirin A, et al. Efficacy of rituximab and plasma exchange in antineutrophil cytoplasmic antibody-associated vasculitis with severe kidney disease. J Am Soc Nephrol. 2020;31:2688.

Charles P, Perrodeau É, Samson M, et al. Long-term rituximab use to maintain remission of antineutrophil cytoplasmic antibody-associated vasculitis: a randomized trial. Ann Intern Med. 2020;173:179.

Daum TE, Specks U, Colby TV, et al. Tracheobronchial involvement in Wegener's granulomatosis. Am J Respir Crit Care Med. 1995;151:522.

De Groot K, Rasmussen N, Bacon PA, et al. Randomized trial of cyclophosphamide versus methotrexate for induction of remission in early systemic antineutrophil cytoplasmic antibody-associated vasculitis. Arthritis Rheum. 2005;52:2461.

Falk RJ, Gross WL, Guillevin L, et al. Granulomatosis with polyangiitis (Wegener's): an alternative name for Wegener's granulomatosis. Arthritis Rheum. 2011;63:863.

Feragalli B, Mantini C, Sperandeo M, et al. The lung in systemic vasculitis: radiological patterns and differential diagnosis. Br J Radiol. 2016;89:20150992.

Geetha D, Specks U, Stone JH, et al. Rituximab versus cyclophosphamide for ANCA-associated vasculitis with renal involvement. J Am Soc Nephrol. 2015;26:976.

Guillevin L, Cordier JF, Lhote F, et al. A prospective, multicenter, randomized trial comparing steroids and pulse cyclophosphamide versus steroids and oral cyclophosphamide in the treatment of generalized Wegener's granulomatosis. Arthritis Rheum. 1997;40:2187.

Hruskova Z, Stel VS, Jayne D, et al. Characteristics and outcomes of granulomatosis with polyangiitis (Wegener) and microscopic polyangiitis requiring renal replacement therapy: results from the European Renal Association-European Dialysis and Transplant Association Registry. Am J Kidney Dis. 2015;66:613.

Iatrou C, Zerbala S, Revela I, et al. Mycophenolate mofetil as maintenance therapy in patients with vasculitis and renal involvement. Clin Nephrol. 2009;72:31.

Jayne D, Rasmussen N, Andrassy K, et al. A randomized trial of maintenance therapy for vasculitis associated with antineutrophil cytoplasmic autoantibodies. N Engl J Med. 2003;349:36.

Lally L, Spiera RF. Pulmonary vasculitis. Rheum Dis Clin North Am. 2015;41:315.

Langford CA, Talar-Williams C, Sneller MC. Mycophenolate mofetil for remission maintenance in the treatment of Wegener's granulomatosis. Arthritis Rheum. 2004;51:278.

Mukhtyar C, Guillevin L, Cid MC, et al. EULAR recommendations for the management of primary small and medium vessel vasculitis. Ann Rheum Dis. 2009;68:310.

Pendergraft WF 3rd, Cortazar FB, Wenger J, et al. Long-term maintenance therapy using rituximab-induced continuous B-cell depletion in patients with ANCA vasculitis. Clin J Am Soc Nephrol. 2014;9:736.

Polychronopoulos VS, Prakash UB, Golbin JM, et al. Airway involvement in Wegener's granulomatosis. Rheum Dis Clin North Am. 2007;33:755.

Screaton NJ, Sivasothy P, Flower CD, Lockwood CM. Tracheal involvement in Wegener's granulomatosis: evaluation using spiral CT. Clin Radiol. 1998;53:809.

Sebastiani M, Manfredi A, Vacchi C, et al. Epidemiology and management of interstitial lung disease in ANCA-associated vasculitis. Clin Exp Rheumatol. 2020;38 Suppl 124:221.

Specks U, Merkel PA, Seo P, et al. Efficacy of remission-induction regimens for ANCA-associated vasculitis. N Engl J Med. 2013;369:417.

Stassen PM, Tervaert JW, Stegeman CA. Induction of remission in active anti-neutrophil cytoplasmic antibody-associated vasculitis with mycophenolate mofetil in patients who cannot be treated with cyclophosphamide. Ann Rheum Dis. 2007;66:798.

Stone JH, Hoffman GS, Merkel PA, et al. A disease-specific activity index for Wegener's granulomatosis: modification of the Birmingham Vasculitis Activity Score. International Network for the Study of the Systemic Vasculitides (INSSYS). Arthritis Rheum. 2001;44:912.

Stone JH, Merkel PA, Spiera R, et al. Rituximab versus cyclophosphamide for ANCA-associated vasculitis. N Engl J Med. 2010;363:221.

Travis WD, Hunninghake G, King TE Jr, et al. Idiopathic nonspecific interstitial pneumonia: report of an American Thoracic Society project. Am J Respir Crit Care Med. 2008;177:1338.

Walsh M, Merkel PA, Peh CA, et al. Plasma exchange and glucocorticoids in severe ANCA-associated vasculitis. N Engl J Med. 2020;382:622.

Yamada H. ANCA: associated lung fibrosis. Semin Respir Crit Care Med. 2011;32:322.

CASE 50

A 77-year-old man presents to the pulmonology clinic for evaluation after an abnormal lung cancer screening chest CT scan. He is a long-time smoker, 50 to 75 pack-years, who currently smokes four to five cigarettes a day. He does not drink or use illicit drugs. He worked for an automotive company on the manufacturing line for 22 years and then worked as an automotive mechanic in a small local shop for another 10 years before retiring. He has no travel or exposure history otherwise. He has diabetes mellitus type 2, non–insulin dependent, for which he is on metformin and glipizide, and hypertension, for which he is on amlodipine-HCTZ. He had an appendectomy and cholecystectomy but no chest surgery. He reports no pulmonary issues aside from a cough that is productive in the early morning but clears by the time he has showered. He denies any constitutional symptoms, chest pain, dyspnea, orthopnea, paroxysmal nocturnal dyspnea, or hemoptysis. His cough in the morning is productive of clear-white sputum, which is sometimes yellow. He walks three to five miles every other day. He can walk at least three or four flights of stairs before becoming short of breath and needing to rest. His vital signs on presentation to the clinic are T 98.1°F, BP 138/91, HR 66, RR 13, and O_2 saturation 97% on room air. He was entered into a lung cancer screening program 1 month ago after a lengthy discussion with his primary care provider. After his initial CT scan, he was referred to the pulmonary clinic for further evaluation and discussion.

The patient's CT scan is shown in Image 50-1.

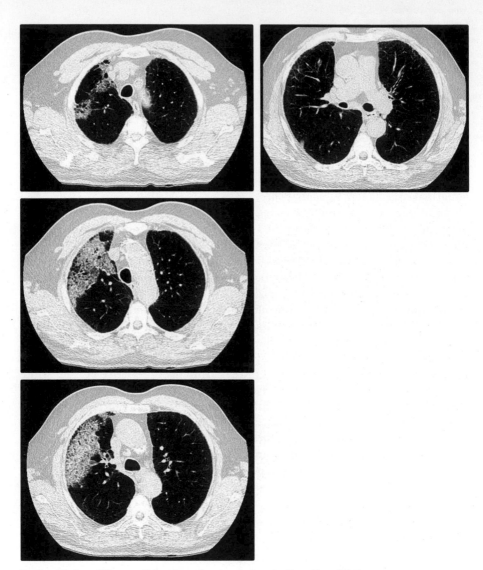

Image 50-1 • CT scan of the chest for the patient in **Question 50-1**.

QUESTIONS

Q50-1: How would you describe the abnormalities in the chest CT scan in Image 50-1?

A. Cystic and cavitary lesions in the right upper lobe
B. Subpleural reticulations in the right upper lobe
C. Centrilobular emphysematous changes with a focal bleb in the right upper lobe
D. Areas of ground glass and consolidation with interlobular septal thickening in the right upper lobe with associated cavitation
E. Right upper lobe pneumothorax
F. Diffuse crazy paving

Q50-2: What would be the next step in this patient's evaluation?

A. Referral to hospice
B. Referral to thoracic surgery for resection
C. MRI of the brain
D. PET-CT scan
E. Cardiopulmonary exercise testing (CPET)
F. Pulmonary function testing (PFT)
G. Referral to radiation oncology for palliative radiation
H. Bronchoscopy with BAL and transbronchial biopsy

Q50-3: The patient undergoes a PET-CT that demonstrates a fluorodeoxyglucose (FDG)-avid mass in the right upper lobe, but with no evidence of distant disease or uptake of FDG in the hilar or mediastinal lymph nodes. There is no uptake of FDG in the pleura or pericardium, and there is no pleural effusion. The primary lesion is 6.7 cm in the largest diameter. What is the patient's radiographic lung cancer stage?

A. T1cN0M1a, stage IVA
B. T2aN0M0, stage IB
C. T2bN0M0, stage IIB
D. T4N0M0, stage IIIA
E. T3N0M0, stage IIB

Q50-4: The patient undergoes bronchoscopy with bronchoalveolar lavage, transbronchial lung biopsy of the lesion in the right upper lobe, and endobronchial ultrasound assessment of mediastinal and hilar lymph nodes. All lymph nodes are found to be normal in size (less than 0.5 cm), and the biopsy of the lesion is shown in Image 50-2 below. What is the likely diagnosis?

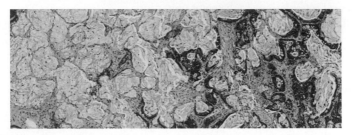

Image 50-2 • Histopathology for the patient in **Case 50**.

A. Squamous cell carcinoma
B. Small cell carcinoma
C. Adenocarcinoma
D. Clear cell carcinoma
E. Carcinoid tumor

Q50-4: The patient elects not to undergo resection of the malignancy and elects for only radiation therapy. He has a good response to radiation therapy. Approximately 12 to 18 months after treatment, the patient returns to the pulmonary clinic as a referral from the radiation oncology follow-up clinic for complaints of worsening dyspnea on exertion and a dry cough. He denies any constitutional symptoms, and he has had no hemoptysis, chest pain, pleuritic pain, or productive cough. The patient's CT scans performed before and after treatment are shown in Image 50-3 below.

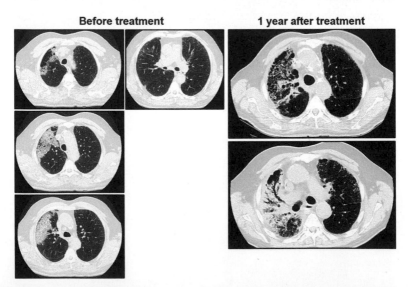

Image 50-3 • Pre- and postradiation therapy CT scan images for the patient in **Case 50**.

What is the likely cause of the patient's worsening dyspnea and cough?

A. Radiation pneumonitis
B. Lung cancer metastatic to the opposite lung
C. Radiation fibrosis and treatment effect
D. Fungal infection
E. Idiopathic pulmonary fibrosis (IPF)
F. Nonspecific interstitial pneumonitis (NSIP)

Q50-5: Another patient presents with the following chest imaging findings shown in image 50-4.

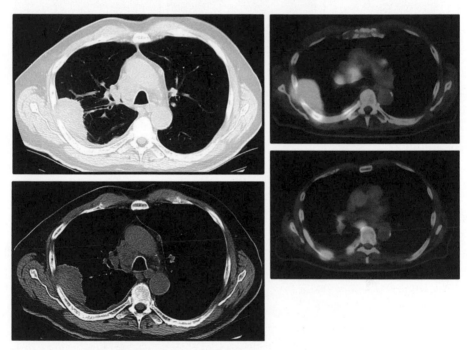

Image 50-4 • Chest imaging for the patient in Question **50-5**.

Which lymph node stations are shown to be involved in this patient? Select all that apply.

A. Station 2
B. Station 4R
C. Station 4L
D. Station 7
E. Station 10R
F. Station 5

Q50-6: Which lymph node stations are concerning in the following imaging study shown in Image 50-5? Select all that apply.

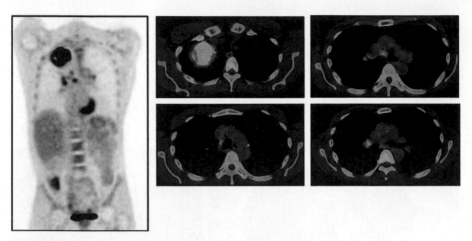

Image 50-5 • PET-CT images for the patient in **Question 50-6**.

A. Station 2R
B. Station 4R
C. Station 4L
D. Station 6
E. Station 7
F. Station 10R
G. Station 11L

Q50-7: Which lymph node is pathologically enlarged in the Image 50-6 below?

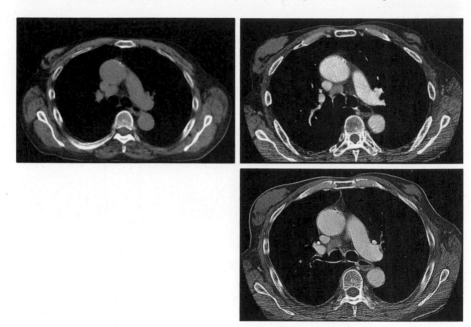

Image 50-6 • CT scan of the chest for the patient in **Question 50-7**.

A. Station 2R
B. Station 2L
C. Station 4R
D. Station 4L
E. Station 7
F. Station 10R
G. Station 11R
H. Station 13R

Q50-8: What is the minimum size of a nodule that is considered amenable to a PET-CT scan?

A. Less than 4 mm
B. 4 to 6 mm
C. 6 to 8 mm
D. Greater than 8 mm

ANSWERS

Q50-1: D
Areas of ground glass and consolidation with interlobular septal thickening in the right upper lobe with associated cavitation

Rationale: Here, one can see an irregularly shaped area consisting of ground glass, consolidation, and interlobular septal thickening in the right upper lobe. There is a possible cystic area in the more apical portion of the lung, though this may also be consistent with the presence of a bleb. There is no overt evidence of centrilobular emphysema or and pneumothorax. The changes seen could be described as crazy paving, but in a focal rather than typically diffuse or mosaic pattern. There are no isolated subpleural reticulations.

Q50-2: D
PET-CT scan

Rationale: This patient has a lesion that is highly suspicious for primary lung cancer. The primary suspicion would be for a non-small cell lung cancer given the tumor's location, though the radiographic pattern is not reliable to differentiate between adenocarcinoma and squamous cell carcinoma. The lesion is not a typical solid nodule seen in most cases but rather a likely mixed component lesion. The lesion itself is well over 3 cm in the largest diameter (30 mm). As such, the patient should undergo complete radiographic staging, including a PET-CT scan (primary) and MRI of the brain. The PET-CT is the priority because it will help identify potentially metastatic lymphadenopathy or distant sites of disease that may be more amenable to biopsy. Although MRI of the brain is required to complete staging, a lack of any hilar or mediastinal adenopathy on a PET-CT scan would suggest a low likelihood of metastatic disease to the CNS. A CPET and PFTs may be helpful to assess a patient's suitability for thoracic surgery; however, we are not yet at that stage. Complete radiographic staging followed by pathologic staging is required to develop an adequate treatment strategy. Bronchoscopy with BAL and transbronchial biopsy is likely insufficient; endobronchial ultrasound and potential transbronchial needle aspiration of pathologically enlarged lymph nodes would be needed. Additionally, if metastatic disease was identified elsewhere (eg, liver, adrenal glands), this site would be more appropriate because a biopsy should be obtained from the site that provides the most accurate disease staging. Referral to hospice without staging and pathologic results would be inappropriate unless the patient refused further evaluation. Even if the patient was deemed too high risk for biopsy or surgical intervention, palliative radiation therapy could be considered. In this case, the patient is fully functional and without apparent exercise limitation.

Although not an option, a CT-guided transthoracic needle aspiration would be plausible in this patient since there is no hilar/mediastinal adenopathy on PET-CT and no metastatic disease has been identified.

Q50-3: E
T3N0M0, stage IIB

Rationale: The patient's radiographic staging would be a primary lesion between 5 and 7 cm in largest diameter, with no active lymph node disease and no distant metastatic disease. This would be a T3 lesion on the current eighth edition of the non-small cell lung cancer TMN staging, with N0, M0 designation and would therefore be consistent with stage IIB disease and a 53% 5-year survival. Aside from prognostic information, the current TMN staging system provides guidelines as to which patients are surgical candidates, which patients require neoadjuvant chemotherapy before consideration for surgery, and which patients are only candidates for chemotherapy/immunotherapy/radiation therapy. Patients with limited-stage disease may also be candidates for definite radiation therapy. This patient would still need to undergo pathologic staging to ensure his treatment plan is clinically appropriate. Please refer to Detterbeck et al, (2017) for complete details regarding non-small cell lung cancer staging.

It should be noted that a PET-CT scan is neither 100% sensitive nor specific for lung cancer. Other inflammatory processes, such as rheumatologic disease, sarcoidosis, or infection can cause a false positive on PET-CT, while slow-growing lung cancers (adenocarcinoma in situ/lepidic growth tumors) may also cause a false negative. This will be further addressed below.

Q50-4: C
Adenocarcinoma

Rationale: Note the complete effacement of the alveolar spaces with a well-differentiated glandular structure, including areas with columnar cells and production of mucin throughout the image. This sample stained positive for TTF-1 and CK-7 but negative for CK-5/6, consistent with a diagnosis of adenocarcinoma. Examples of squamous cell and small cell carcinoma are shown in **Images 50-7** and **50-8** below. Squamous cell carcinoma of the lung stains positive for CK-5/6 and p63 but negative for TTF-1. Small cell lung cancer typically stains positive for chromogranin, CD56, TTF-1, and p16. Carcinoid tumors may present in a number of morphologies but typically stain positive for Ki-67, chromogranin, synaptophysin, and CD56. Although differentiating small and non-small cell lung cancer is relatively straightforward, differentiating the subtypes of non-small cell lung cancer becomes exceeding more difficult as the cells become more poorly differentiated. Immunohistochemistry is often required in this setting, but again, it may not be able to differentiate the underlying pathology. A complete examination of lung cancer histopathology is out of the scope of this case series, so we will focus primarily on diagnostic procedures and staging.

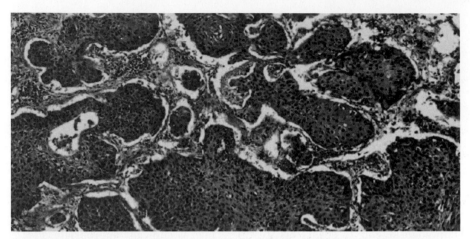

Image 50-7 • Example of squamous cell carcinoma of the lung. Note the presence of polygonal cells, intracellular bridges, and crisp cytoplasm. The nuclei are hyperchromatic and angular. Also note the lack of any columnar structures.

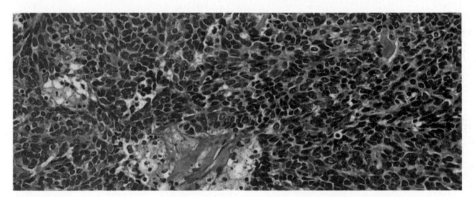

Image 50-8 • Example of small cell carcinoma of the lung, with oval cells, minimal cytoplasm, and finely dispersed chromatin. The cells are the predominant feature, with scant stroma underlying the cells. The cells appear in sheets (palisading).

Q50-4: C
Radiation fibrosis and treatment effect

Rationale: There are two forms of radiation-induced lung injury. The subacute form of injury is termed *radiation pneumonitis*, while the chronic form of injury is termed *radiation fibrosis*. This is determined primarily by the dose of radiation delivered to the lung tissue and surrounding pleura, though it may be modulated by concurrent or subsequent chemotherapy or immunotherapy. Radiation pneumonitis can be difficult to differentiate from pure drug toxicity, atypical/viral infection, and edema. Radiation fibrosis is generally more straightforward to identify if dosing mapping is available from the patient's treatment planning/report. Although this patient's lung cancer staging calls for resection of the primary tumor and adjuvant chemotherapy, the patient elected for definitive radiation therapy alone. The patient's current CT demonstrates extensive fibrosis, consolidation, and septal thickening within and extending beyond the initial tumor bed. The changes within the tumor bed itself are considered treatment effects, but the more extensive fibrosis presenting now would be consistent with radiation fibrosis. The patient is certainly at risk for opportunistic infections such as MAI with his structural lung disease; however, he lacks any productive cough or constitutional symptoms to suggest an infectious etiology at this point. The focal nature of the structural lung disease is not consistent with either NSIP or IPF.

Radiation fibrosis is more likely to present gradually, with the development of dyspnea and reduced exercise tolerance and perhaps a dry cough. The examination findings are likely to demonstrate inspiratory crackles over the affected area, and effusions are less likely. Pulmonary function testing may demonstrate restriction and a reduced DLCO. Chest radiographs in radiation fibrosis may demonstrate dense consolidations or reticular interstitial opacities in the affected areas. Prior to the introduction of CRT, the "straight-line" sign—affected tissue limited to that between the lines representing the treatment area and ignoring anatomic boundaries (fissures)—was diagnostic of radiation pneumonitis and particular fibrosis. Now that modern treatment methods feature multiple low-dose beams at multiple angles in three-dimensional space, this effect is not commonly seen. However, it may still be seen in cases where the primary lesions allow for only one or two beam paths without causing significant damage to bystander organs or tissue. This may yield any number of topographic dosimetry maps. This is why obtaining dosimetric information in the form of isodose or dose delivery maps overlayed on CT imaging before treatment is essential for diagnosis. This allows one to compare the current and pretreatment scans to determine if the pattern of lung injury observed matches the treatment or delivery-dose maps. CT imaging typically shows ground-glass opacities surrounding the lesion. As the disease shifts from inflammatory/exudative to organizing/proliferative, consolidations may then form. This may yield a patchy pattern of consolidations, an inside-out pattern in which there is a halo of consolidation surrounding central GGO (ie, halo sign), oran "outside-in" pattern in which there is a halo of ground-glass opacities surrounding a central area of consolidation (ie, reverse halo sign). Patients may also have nodules, tree-in-bud opacities, or septal thickening (the latter, in combination with ground-glass opacities, can lead to a "crazy paving" pattern). Pulmonary effusions are almost exclusively ipsilateral. As the disease progresses to a fibrotic phase, one may see septal thickening, architectural distortion, traction bronchiectasis, consolidation, and volume loss. Honeycomb changes may also be seen. Patients may have small linear opacities as well that conform to individual beam paths but ignore anatomic boundaries, depending on the radiation delivery technique.

Q50-5: B; D; E; F
Station 4R; Station 7; Station 10R; Station 5

Rationale: This patient's PET-CT scan shown in **Image 50-9** demonstrates a peripheral lung mass with likely involvement of the pleura on the right. There is increased FDG uptake in the right hilum as well as at the right 4R nodal station, in addition to the station 7 node. The station 4R and 7 nodes are N2 (mediastinal nodes), while the station 10R node is an N1 node. This is significant because N2 disease places a patient at stage IIIA or above and would necessitate neoadjuvant chemotherapy in stage IIIA disease (while anything beyond stage IIIA disease is generally nonresectable). N1 disease may be associated with stage IIB disease. All these lymph nodes could be biopsied during endobronchial ultrasound-guided transbronchial needle aspiration to provide an adequate pathologic stage before deciding on a treatment option.

There are 14 different lymph node stations for lung cancer screening. The N2 nodes include: station 1, highest mediastinal (not accessible via flexible bronchoscopy); station 2, upper paratracheal (accessible), station 3, prevascular (not accessible); station 4R/L with right/left determined by a position relative to the *left* border of the trachea, lower paratracheal (accessible); station 5 (subaortic) and station 6 (para-aortic; both generally not accessible); station 7, sub-carinal (accessible); station 8, paraesophageal (approachable via endoscopic ultrasound); station 9, pulmonary ligament (not accessible). The N1 nodes are: station 10, hilar (accessible); station 11, interlobar (accessible); station 12, lobar, (accessible); station 13, segmental (generally not accessible); and station 14, subsegmental (generally not accessible).

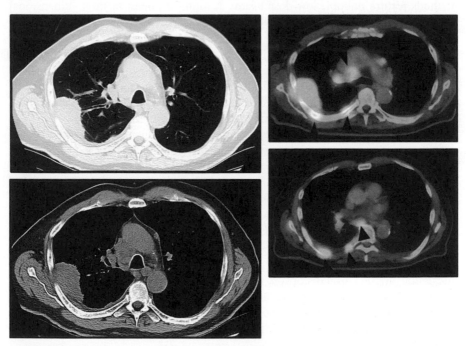

Image 50-9 • Note the increased fluorodeoxyglucose uptake in the primary lesions and along the pleura (as denoted by the black arrows) as well as in the following positions: station 10R (N1), station 4R (N2), station 5 (far right of top right image), and station 7 nodes.

Q50-6: A; B; F
Station 2R; Station 4R; and Station 10R

Rationale: See the annotated **Image 50-10** below.

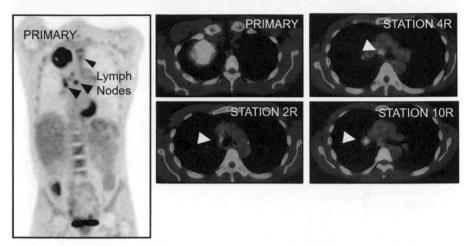

Image 50-10 • Annotated PET-CT scan for the patient in **Question 50-6**. (Left image) Note the increased fluorodeoxyglucose (FDG) uptake (shown in black) in the primary mass as well as mediastinal and hilar lymph nodes (black arrows). (Right image). Here, the increased FDG uptake is indicated by the white arrows at the specified lymph node stations.

Q50-7: C
Station 4R

Rationale: The lymph node at station 4R (lower paratracheal) is pathologically enlarged in this patient as shown in **Image 50-11**. Note the image on the left is noncontrasted, while the images on the right are contrasted. Note the radiodense lymph node located between the ascending aorta anteriorly, the pulmonary arteries on the left, and the dividing mainstem bronchi posteriorly. As the lymph node is situated to the *left* of the left border of the trachea, the lymph node is considered a 4R rather than a 4L lymph node. A station 2R or L node would be more cranial in location, while a station 7 node would be caudal to the carina. The hilar nodes (10, 11, 12, 13, and 14) would be more lateral/peripheral.

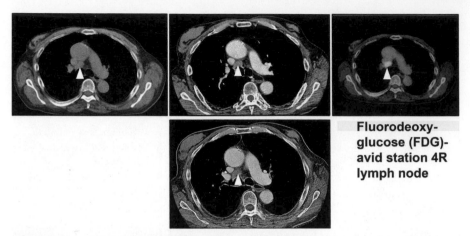

Fluorodeoxy-
glucose (FDG)-
avid station 4R
lymph node

Image 50-11 • Annotated chest CT and PET-CT scan for the patient in **Question 50-7**. The presence of this N2 node (indicated by the white arrow) altered this patient's treatment plan from resection to neoadjuvant chemotherapy with reconsideration for resection pending tumor response.

Q50-8: D
Greater than 8 mm

Rationale: PET-CT lacks appropriate sensitivity for nodules below 8 mm (and more conservatively, less than 10 mm). Additionally, slow-growing tumors (eg, lepidic adenocarcinomas, previously known as *bronchoalveolar carcinomas*, [BACs]) may also demonstrate no significant increase in FDG uptake, even at larger nodule size. Therefore, most lung cancer screening or incidental pulmonary nodule guidelines use a cutoff of 0.8 cm (8 mm) as the minimal size to consider a PET-CT. Even with a negative finding, a nodule that continues to grow should be considered suspicious for adenocarcinoma.

References

American Thoracic Society. Implementation guide for lung cancer screening. https://www.lung-cancerscreeningguide.org/ Accessed April 16, 2021.

Black WC, Gareen IF, Soneji SS, et al. Cost-effectiveness of CT screening in the National Lung Screening Trial. N Engl J Med. 2014;371:1793.

Canadian Task Force on Preventive Health Care. Recommendations on screening for lung cancer. CMAJ. 2016;188:425.

Chansky K, Detterbeck FC, Nicholson AG, et al. IASLC Staging and Prognostic Factors Committee, Advisory Boards, and Participating Institutions. The IASLC Lung Cancer Staging Project: external validation of the revision of the TNM stage groupings in the eighth edition of the TNM classification of lung cancer. J Thorac Oncol. 2017;12:1109.

Detterbeck FC, Boffa DJ, Kim AW, Tanoue LT. The eighth edition lung cancer stage classification. Chest. 2017;151:193.

Detterbeck FC, Chansky K, Groome P, et al. IASLC Staging and Prognostic Factors Committee, Advisory Boards, and Participating Institutions. The IASLC Lung Cancer Staging Project: methodology and validation used in the development of proposals for revision of the stage classification of NSCLC in the forthcoming (eighth) edition of the TNM classification of lung cancer. J Thorac Oncol. 2016;11:1433.

Etzel CJ, Bach PB. Estimating individual risk for lung cancer. Semin Respir Crit Care Med. 2011;32:3.

Flehinger BJ, Kimmel M, Polyak T, Melamed MR. Screening for lung cancer. The Mayo Lung Project revisited. Cancer. 1993;72:1573.

Goldstraw P, Chansky K, Crowley J, et al. The IASLC Lung Cancer Staging Project: proposals for revision of the TNM stage groupings in the forthcoming (eighth) edition of the TNM classification for lung cancer. J Thorac Oncol. 2016;11:39.

Gould MK, Donington J, Lynch WR, et al. Evaluation of individuals with pulmonary nodules: when is it lung cancer? Diagnosis and management of lung cancer, 3rd ed: American College of Chest Physicians evidence-based clinical practice guidelines. Chest. 2013;143:e93S.

Jaklitsch MT, Jacobson FL, Austin JH, et al. The American Association for Thoracic Surgery guidelines for lung cancer screening using low-dose computed tomography scans for lung cancer survivors and other high-risk groups. J Thorac Cardiovasc Surg. 2012;144:33.

Katki HA, Kovalchik SA, Berg CD, et al. Development and validation of risk models to select ever-smokers for CT lung cancer screening. JAMA. 2016;315:2300.

Kinsinger LS, Anderson C, Kim J, et al. Implementation of Lung cancer screening in the Veterans Health Administration. JAMA Intern Med. 2017;177:399.

Lindell RM, Hartman TE, Swensen SJ, et al. Five-year lung cancer screening experience: CT appearance, growth rate, location, and histologic features of 61 lung cancers. Radiology. 2007;242:555.

MacMahon H, Naidich DP, Goo JM, et al. Guidelines for management of incidental pulmonary nodules detected on CT images: from the Fleischner Society 2017. Radiology. 2017;284:228.

Mazzone PJ, Silvestri GA, Patel S, et al. Screening for lung cancer: CHEST guideline and expert panel report. Chest. 2018;153:954.

McKee BJ, Regis SM, McKee AB, et al. Performance of ACR Lung-RADS in a clinical CT lung screening program. J Am Coll Radiol. 2015;12:273.

McWilliams A, Tammemagi M, Mayo J, et al. Probability of cancer in pulmonary nodules detected on first screening computed tomography. N Engl J Med. 2013;369:910.

National Lung Screening Trial Research Team, Aberle DR, Adams AM, et al. Reduced lung-cancer mortality with low-dose computed tomographic screening. N Engl J Med. 2011;365:395.

Ost D, Fein AM, Feinsilver SH. Clinical practice. The solitary pulmonary nodule. N Engl J Med. 2003;348:2535.

Pasquinelli MM, Tammemägi CM, Kovitz KL, et al. Risk prediction model versus United States Preventive Services Task Force lung cancer screening eligibility criteria—reducing race disparities. J Thorac Oncol. 2020;15:1738.

Patz EF Jr, Greco E, Gatsonis C, et al. Lung cancer incidence and mortality in National Lung Screening Trial participants who underwent low-dose CT prevalence screening: a retrospective cohort analysis of a randomised, multicentre, diagnostic screening trial. Lancet Oncol. 2016;17:590.

Pinsky PF, Gierada DS, Black W, et al. Performance of Lung-RADS in the National Lung Screening Trial: a retrospective assessment. Ann Intern Med. 2015;162:485.

Roberts H, Walker-Dilks C, Sivjee K, et al. Screening high-risk populations for lung cancer: guideline recommendations. J Thorac Oncol. 2013;8:1232.

Spitz MR, Hong WK, Amos CI, et al. A risk model for prediction of lung cancer. J Natl Cancer Inst. 2007;99:715.

Swensen SJ, Silverstein MD, Ilstrup DM, Schleck CD, Edell ES. The probability of malignancy in solitary pulmonary nodules. Application to small radiologically indeterminate nodules. Arch Intern Med. 1997;157:849.

Tammemägi M, Church T, Hocking W, et al. Evaluation of the lung cancer risks at which to screen ever- and never-smokers: screening rules applied to the PLCO and NLST cohorts. PLoS Medicine. 2014;11: e1001764.

Tammemagi MC, Katki HA, Hocking WG, et al. Selection criteria for lung-cancer screening. N Engl J Med. 2013;368:728.

US Preventive Services Task Force. Lung cancer screening: recommendation statement. Ann Intern Med. 2004;140:738.

US Preventive Services Task Force. Screening for lung cancer: Recommendation statement 2013. www.uspreventiveservicestaskforce.org/Page/Document/UpdateSummaryFinal/lung-cancer-screening. Accessed April 16, 2021.

Veronesi G, Maisonneuve P, Spaggiari L, et al. Diagnostic performance of low-dose computed tomography screening for lung cancer over five years. J Thorac Oncol. 2014;9:935.

Wender R, Fontham ET, Barrera E Jr, et al. American Cancer Society lung cancer screening guidelines. CA Cancer J Clin. 2013;63:107.

Wood DE. National Comprehensive Cancer Network (NCCN) clinical practice guidelines for lung cancer screening. Thorac Surg Clin. 2015;25:185.

CASE 51

A 54-year-old woman is admitted to your inpatient service for worsening short-ness of breath. The patient has a history of hypertension, obesity (body mass index 44 kg/m^2), diabetes mellitus type 2, gout, hyperlipidemia, and stage 2 chronic kidney disease, with a baseline creatinine level of 1.6 mg/dL. She currently takes losartan, metformin, glipizide, allopurinol, and amlodipine. She does not smoke or use illicit drugs. She has no notable occupational exposures, having worked as a paralegal at a local law firm since graduating college 20 years ago. She has two children, both healthy. She has never been diagnosed with a pulmonary or rheumatologic condition. She has experienced a 20-lb weight loss over the past 6 months, though this was in the setting of starting a new diet. The patient denies any fevers, chills, or sweats. She has a dry cough intermittently. Her primary com-plaint is the insidious onset of dyspnea with exertion to dyspnea at rest over the last 3 to 4 months, now requiring 4 L/min supplemental O$_2$ at rest. She recently saw her primary care physician, who ordered a chest radiograph that was read as abnormal. The patient was admitted to this hospital this evening because of the increased O$_2$ requirement. Her vital signs are T 97.5°F, HR 101, BP 145/78, RR 20, and saturation 95% on 4 L/min supplemental O$_2$. When attempting to wean the supplemental O$_2$, you are unsuccessful.

The patient's chest radiograph is shown in Image 51-1.

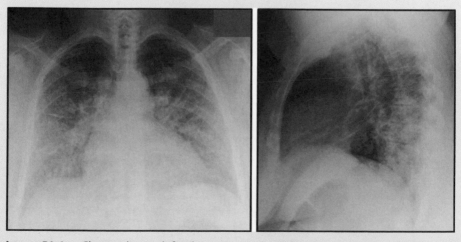

Image 51-1 • Chest radiograph for the patient in **Question 51-1**.

QUESTIONS

Q51-1: How would you describe the abnormalities in the chest radiograph in Image 51-1?

A. Miliary pattern of nodular opacities
B. Diffuse cystic lesions
C. Diffuse interstitial opacities (linear and reticular)
D. Diffuse alveolar opacities
E. Consolidation with right middle lobe atelectasis

Q51-2: The patient has a brain (B-type) natriuretic peptide that is elevated at 155 pg/mL. An echocardiogram is performed, and there is evidence of diastolic heart failure, consistent with long-standing hypertension. The patient is diuresed aggressively over the next several days, with the development of a mild contraction alkalosis. The patient's dyspnea and chest imaging findings remain largely unchanged, and her O_2 requirement is stable. A d-Dimer is performed, which is mildly elevated. The patient undergoes a CT-pulmonary embolism (PE) protocol to further evaluate for a possible source of her hypoxemia. The contrasted portion of the CT is read as negative for acute PE. The noncontrasted position of the CT is shown in Image 51-2.

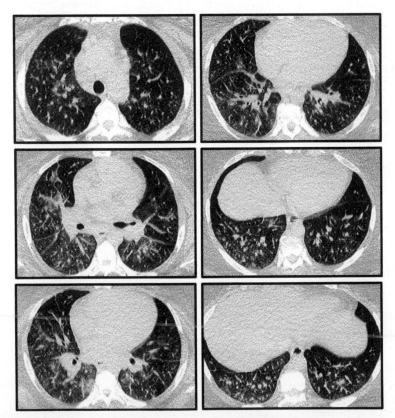

Image 51-2 • CT scan of the chest for the patient in **Question 51-2.**

How would you describe the abnormalities on the chest CT in Image 51-2?

A. Diffuse septal and interlobular interstitial thickening with ground glass
B. Diffuse cavitary lung lesions
C. Traction bronchiectasis with honeycomb changes
D. Areas of focal lung consolidation
E. Increased attenuation due to low lung volumes

Q51-3: The patient undergoes a respiratory viral panel that is negative. The patient's physical examination is difficult because of the patient's obesity, and a point-of-care ultrasound is performed, which reveals an inferior vena cava that is 1.6 cm in diameter with normal collapse. The patient also undergoes a right-heart catheterization that demonstrates a pulmonary capillary wedge pressure of 6 mm Hg, with a mean pulmonary artery pressure of 18 mm Hg and an elevated cardiac index of 3.4 L/min/m². There is no evidence of intracardiac shunt. What is the next step in the patient's evaluation?

A. Cardiac biopsy
B. Cardiac MRI
C. Abdominal fat-pad biopsy
D. Bronchoscopy with transbronchial biopsy
E. Colonoscopy, mammography, and Papanicolaou (Pap) smear

Q51-4: The patient undergoes biopsy and is found to have "abnormal-appearing cells occluding the lymphatic of the lung, with distention of the lymphatics but overall preservation of the alveolar and airway architecture." The cytology is also concerning for atypical cells. What is the next step in the patient's evaluation?

A. Colonoscopy, mammography, and Pap smear
B. PET-CT
C. Cardiac MRI
D. Abdominal fat pad biopsy
E. Diuresis
F. Lung transplantation evaluation
G. Anticoagulation

Q51-5: A 66-year-old woman is admitted to your service for intractable productive cough with copious whitish sputum. She is a former smoker, having smoked for 25 years, 1 pack per day, from the ages of 32 to 57. She denies any fevers, chills, sweats, or weight loss. She denies any chest pain or hemoptysis. She has some dyspnea on exertion. She has no family history of cardiovascular, pulmonary, or rheumatologic disease. She and her husband own a series of gas stations, but she primarily works as the business administrator and accountant while her husband handles business at the actual business locations. She recalls no obvious exposures at work or at home, and they have a cat in the house that has lived with them for 14 years. She has two children, both healthy, with only a history of uterine fibroids in her daughter and hypertension in her son. She takes no medications and only has some mild osteoarthritis in her left knee. The knee is not red, swollen, or tender, and there is good range of motion. On examination, she has a wet cough with bronchial breath sounds throughout. There is no dullness to percussion. Her vital signs are T 99.3°F. HR 88, BP 104/57, RR 17, and O₂ saturation 94% on room air.

Her radiograph and CT scan of the chest from admission are shown in Images 51-3 and 51-4, respectively.

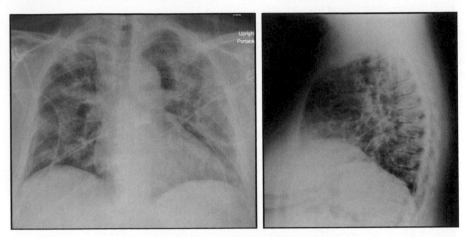

Image 51-3 • Radiograph of the chest for the patient in **Question 51-5**.

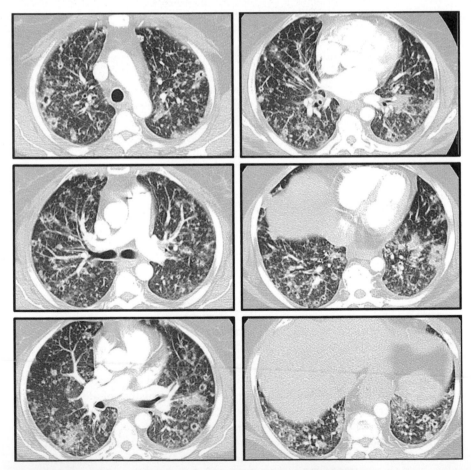

Image 51-4 • CT scan of the chest for the patient in **Question 51-5**.

Which differential diagnoses would you consider? Select all that apply.

A. Pulmonary Langerhans cell histiocytosis (PLCH)
B. Disseminated fungal infection
C. Disseminated invasive mucinous adenocarcinoma
D. Sarcoidosis
E. Pulmonary alveolar proteinosis

Q51-6: A 72-year-old man is admitted to your service with worsening hypoxemia and dyspnea. He also complains of a cough that is nonproductive. He denies any chest pain, hemoptysis, nausea, emesis, or aspiration events. He denies any fevers, chills, or sweats but endorses recent weight loss and generalized fatigue. His chest radiograph and CT images are shown in Images 51-5 and 51-6, respectively.

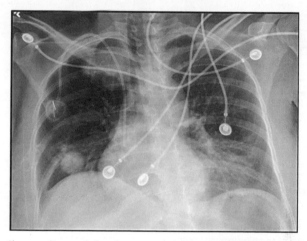

Image 51-5 • Chest radiograph for the patient in **Question 51-6**.

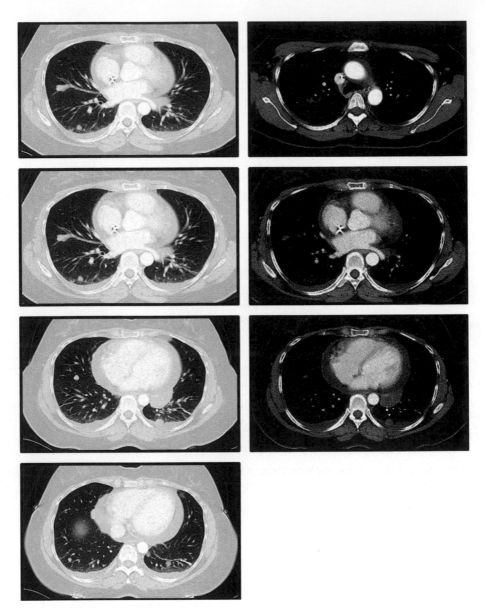

Image 51-6 • CT scan of the chest for the patient in **Question 51-6**.

Which underlying condition do you most suspect in this patient, despite the limited history provided?

A. Renal cell carcinoma
B. Sarcoidosis
C. Pulmonary hamartomas
D. Lymphangioleiomyomatosis (LAM)
E. Primary lung cancer

Q51-7: Match the following paraneoplastic syndromes to the most common primary lung malignancy.

A. Adenocarcinoma
B. Squamous cell carcinoma
C. Small cell lung cancer (SCLC)

Q51-7-1: Syndrome of inappropriate antidiuretic hormone (SIADH). _____

Q51-7-2: Hypercalcemia of malignancy. _____

Q51-7-3: Hypertrophic pulmonary osteoarthropathy. _____

Q51-7-4: Trousseau syndrome. _____

Q51-7-5: Lambert-Eaton syndrome. _____

Q51-7-6: Cushing syndrome. _____

Q51-8: Assume for the following question that a patient is referred for evaluation of a solid pulmonary nodule that is 6.5 mm in largest dimension found incidentally on CT of the chest performed for minor trauma. For which patient is the use of the Fleischner 2017 guidelines for evaluation and management of an incidental pulmonary nodule appropriate?

A. A 23-year-old man with no medical history and no smoking history
B. A 55-year-old woman with cervical cancer who underwent resection and adjuvant chemotherapy last year
C. A 65-year-old man with common variable immune deficiency
D. A 57-year-old man with a 30–pack-year smoking history, ongoing, and no family history of cancer
E. A 60-year-old man with no smoking history and a history of hypertension and hyperlipidemia
F. A 60-year-old man with no smoking history and new-onset hemoptysis

Q51-9: For the patient in Question 51-8, a 60-year-old man with hypertension, hyperlipidemia, no smoking history, and no first-degree relative with lung cancer, what is the most appropriate next step in evaluation?

A. Determine the risk of malignancy based on the characteristics of the lesion.
B. Obtain a follow-up CT scan in 6 to 12 months.
C. No further follow-up is needed.
D. Obtain prior chest imaging for comparison.
E. Obtain a follow-up CT scan in 3 to 6 months.
F. Order a PET-CT scan.

Q51-10: Assume the patient has the following lesion identified on CT (Image 51-7).

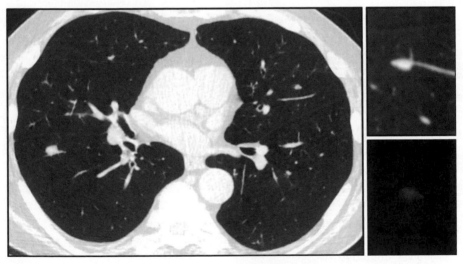

Image 51-7 • CT scan of the chest for the patient in **Question 51-10**.

Also assume the following characteristics: lower lobe, a diameter of 6.5 mm, and the characteristics seen here. Determine the patient's malignancy risk score using Dr. Stephen Swensen's Mayo Clinic Model, available at (https://www.mdcalc.com/solitary-pulmonary-nodule-spn-malignancy-risk-score-mayo-clinic-model#use-cases). Then determine the patient's appropriate next step in evaluation according to the guidelines.

Risk:

A. 1.0%
B. 2.5%
C. 5.4%
D. 11.1%
E. 26.2%

Q51-11: A 65-year-old man presents with a history of smoking, 20–pack-years in total, and he quit 25 years ago. He has no family history of malignancy. A 7-mm nodule is identified on CT with the characteristics shown in Image 51-8 below. He has no history of malignancy.

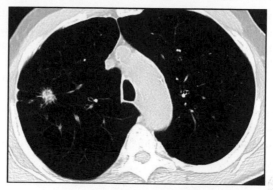

Image 51-8 • CT image of the chest for the patient in **Question 51-11**.

What is the patient's risk of malignancy, assuming the lesion is solid and using the Mayo Clinic Model?

A. 1.0%
B. 2.5%
C. 5.4%
D. 11.1%
E. 26.2%
F. 32.9%

Q51-12: A patient presents with the following CT scan (Image 51-9).

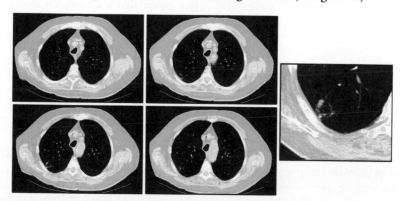

Image 51-9 • CT of the chest for the patient in **Question 51-12**.

How would you describe the lesion in this image?

A. Solid
B. Subsolid
C. Pure ground-glass opacity
D. Cystic lesion

ANSWERS

Q51-1: C
Diffuse interstitial opacities

Rationale: This is a PA and lateral chest film. There is a slight deviation of the airway toward the right, but this is likely positional. The carina is identifiable. Overall, the heart borders are distinct, as is the diaphragm. The costophrenic angles are visible, though there is some haziness. There is no apparent pneumothorax or pleural effusion. The mediastinal borders appear normal. There are diffuse linear and reticular opacities, and there is no overt or cavitary nodules. There is some perihilar fullness. The fissure on the right is quite thickened. There is a diffuse haziness, but in the pattern typically described as "alveolar." Overall, this is a nonspecific chest radiograph finding that could be consistent with infection or pulmonary edema, among other possibilities.

Q51-2: A
Diffuse septal and interlobular interstitial thickening with ground-glass opacities

Rationale: The patient's CT scan likely demonstrates a reduction in overall lung volume and mildly increased attenuation of the lung parenchyma as a result, but this is not the primary abnormality identified. The CT shows a diffuse pattern of interlobular thickening with septal thickening and scattered ground glass. The thickening of the interstitium is somewhat nodular. This thickening extends from the hilum. This is not quite a crazy paving pattern. There are overt cavitary nodules. There is no traction bronchiectasis or honeycomb changes. There are no focal areas of consolidation, though there is perhaps some hilar fullness on the right that is greater than on the left. There is no evidence of a pleural effusion. Again, this is a relatively nonspecific finding.

Q51-3: D
Bronchoscopy with transbronchial biopsy

Rationale: The patient's evaluation has effectively ruled out cardiogenic pulmonary edema, with a normal pulmonary capillary wedge pressure, a borderline normal mean pulmonary arterial pressure, and an elevated cardiac index. The elevated index may be related to obesity. The other primary consideration in the differential diagnosis would include viral pneumonia, atypical pneumonia, sarcoidosis, radiation pneumonitis, lymphocytic interstitial pneumonia (as there may be a lack of cystic changes early in the disease process), and lymphangitic carcinomatosis. The patient has no recent radiation exposure and no history of malignancy, so radiation pneumonitis is not likely. The remaining diagnoses can be differentiated with bronchoscopy with transbronchial biopsy and bronchoalveolar lavage. A cardiac biopsy, abdominal fat pad biopsy, or MRI would be helpful if the diagnosis was thought to be sarcoidosis or amyloidosis; however, there is no apparent abnormality on the echocardiogram or evidence of a primary cardiac pathology to pursue this route first. A colonoscopy, mammography, and a Pap smear represent age-appropriate cancer screenings, but these are not indicated at this point in the evaluation because a diagnosis has not been obtained.

Q51-4: B
PET-CT

Rationale: The patient's findings on histopathology suggest a diagnosis of lymphangitic carcinomatosis. This occurs when tumors spread through and occlude the lymphatic of the lung, most commonly seen in adenocarcinoma of the breast, lung, colon, and prostate/cervical origin. The tumor most likely undergoes hematogenous spread to the lung, with extension to the lymphatics. The entire lymphatics of the secondary lobule may be involved, yielding thickening not only of the bronchovascular bundles but also the interlobular septa. The tumors are seen in the lymphatics and possibly the interstitium, with preservation of the underlying lung architecture. Therefore, the next step for this patient is a PET-CT scan to identify the primary site of the malignancy. In rare cases, this may arise from the lung itself (formerly termed *bronchoalveolar carcinoma*, now termed either *adenocarcinoma in situ, minimally invasive adenocarcinoma,* or *invasive mucinous adenocarcinoma,* depending on the stage of disease). A colonoscopy, mammography, and Pap smear would not account for all possible sources of the malignancy, which can also arise from the stomach, pancreas, thyroid, and esophagus. All the remaining answers would be inappropriate. This patient's PET-CT scan returned positive for primary colon adenocarcinoma.

Lymphangitic carcinomatosis often presents with progressive dyspnea over several months if the patient does not have a previous diagnosis of cancer. On chest CT, there is interlobular and septal thickening, which is often smooth initially and progresses to a more nodular approach as the lymphatics become overwhelmed and congested. Eventually, this can lead to fluid leaking into the interstitium, yielding ground-glass opacities. This is important to differentiate from a tumor embolism, in which tumors block the pulmonary arteries. PET-CT is also very effective at helping confirm a diagnosis of lymphangitic carcinomatosis. Overall, the prognosis is very poor, as this represents metastatic disease in many cases. Attempts at chemotherapy or radiation to the primary tumor can be considered, but treatment is otherwise supportive, including O_2 therapy.

Q51-5: Answers A through D

Rationale: The patient has a diffusely distributed disease process, with diffuse pulmonary nodules, some of which have cavitary changes. There are also some surrounding ground-glass opacities. The primary differential diagnosis would include a disseminated fungal (or mycobacterial infection) or disseminated adenocarcinoma, most likely an invasive mucinous adenocarcinoma. Although the findings are somewhat atypical for PLCH in terms of the distribution of lesions and the clinical course, it could still be considered, and while the findings are atypical for sarcoidosis, this should not be ruled out either. Pulmonary vasculitis could be considered, but the number of nodules (more than 10) is quite atypical. Rheumatoid arthritis can produce nodules that cavitate as well, but the distribution and number present here would be atypical. This finding is not consistent with pulmonary alveolar proteinosis unless there was a superinfection present.

This is an example of a patient with lepidic growth adenocarcinoma, formerly termed *bronchoalveolar carcinoma*. This is a very slow-growing malignancy that may present as adenocarcinoma in situ, minimally invasive adenocarcinoma, lepidic growth adenocarcinoma, or invasive mucinous adenocarcinoma. This patient presents with bronchorrhea, a classic finding in invasive mucinous adenocarcinoma. This is a relatively rare subtype of adenocarcinoma, which arises in the periphery of the lung and grows along the alveolar walls with little destruction of the underlying parenchyma. It may present as multicentric or diffuse disease, or it may arise from an area of prior scarring. On lung screening, this is often found as a pure ground-glass or mixed component nodule in early disease stages (approximately 50% of cases). Another 30% of cases present as pneumonia mimics, with findings of poor organizing consolidative opacities. Only 15% to 20% of patients present with the multinodular form seen here. This CT scan demonstrates evidence of cavitating pulmonary metastases termed the "Cheerio" sign (**Image 51-10**). The prognosis depends on the stage at which the cancer is diagnosed.

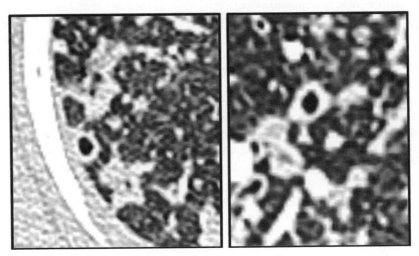

Image 51-10 • Example of the "Cheerio" sign seen in lepidic growth adenocarcinomas (formerly termed *bronchoalveolar carcinoma*). This is an example of a patient with invasive mucinous adenocarcinoma of the lung.

Q51-6: A
Renal cell carcinoma

Rationale: The images above reveal classic findings of "cannonball" metastases in the lung parenchyma. These lesions are typically large, well circumscribed, homogenous, and round, with a relatively random distribution. On the chest radiograph, there is a large nodule in the right lower lobe as well as several well-circumscribed but overlapping lesions in the right upper lobe. The CT shows numerous well-circumscribed lesions throughout the lung, in close approximation to the bronchovascular bundle in some cases. There are also bilateral pleural effusions. This is most commonly seen in renal cell carcinoma, sarcoma, and choriocarcinoma, though it can also be seen in prostate adenocarcinoma. This is unlikely to be a primary lung malignancy given the lack of a clear primary lesion. This would be an atypical presentation of sarcoidosis. Hamartomas have a heterogeneous appearance. This presentation is not consistent with LAM in multiple ways (patient sex, age, radiographic presentation).

Q51-7-1: C
Small cell lung cancer

Rationale: This occurs most commonly with SCLC but may occur with any pulmonary pathology.

Q51-7-2: B
Squamous cell carcinoma

Rationale: This is classically associated with squamous cell carcinoma, but it may also be seen in adenocarcinoma or SCLC.

Q51-7-3: A
Adenocarcinoma

Q51-7-4: A
Adenocarcinoma

Rationale: This is migratory superficial thrombophlebitis. Hypercoagulable states are most commonly seen in adenocarcinomas.

Q51-7-5: C
Small cell lung cancer

Rationale: The neurologic paraneoplastic syndromes, including Lambert-Eaton syndrome, limbic encephalopathy, cerebellar degeneration, and autonomic neuropathy, are all associated with SCLC.

Q51-7-6: C
Small cell lung cancer

Rationale: This may also be seen in either adenocarcinoma or squamous cell carcinoma.

Q51-8: E
A 60-year-old man with no smoking history and a history of hypertension and hyperlipidemia

Rationale: The Fleischner guidelines for evaluation and management of incidental pulmonary nodules should *not* be confused with lung cancer screening. The Fleischner guidelines are intended for patients 35 years of age or older with the finding of an incidental pulmonary nodule on CT of the chest and none of the following exclusion criteria: (1) immunosuppression, (2) active or prior malignancy, (3) signs or symptoms potentially attributable to the lesion in question, and (4) baseline cancer risk equivalent to that of the general population (ie, not a candidate for lung cancer screening). Although the lung cancer screening guidelines vary slightly between organizations, the general principles for inclusion are (1) age 50 to 55 through 74 to 80, (2) 20- to 30–pack-year smoking history, and (3) current use or quit use within the last 15 years. The patient in option A is younger than 35 years of age, and the risk of lung cancer is exceedingly small at this age. The patient in option B has a recent malignancy, and there would be a concern for metastatic disease that would change the evaluation and management. The patient in option C is immunocompromised, and infectious causes would be high on the differentiation and necessitate a different evaluation path. The patient in option D is appropriate for lung cancer screening because his risk factors place him at a higher risk than the general population. The patient in option F is experiencing symptoms that could be due to a pulmonary lesion and would necessitate a more urgent evaluation.

Q51-9: D
Obtain prior chest imaging for comparison

Rationale: For this patient who meets the criteria for the Fleischner guidelines, the most appropriate first step is to compare the film with any prior chest imaging. If the lesion was present on a CT scan from 3 years ago and is stable in appearance, it is likely benign and would not necessitate further evaluation. This is always the first step in evaluation. If the patient does not have prior chest imaging, this is considered the first scan moving forward. If the patient did not have prior imaging, his risk for malignancy would need to be assessed before determining the appropriate next step.

Q51-10: B
2.5%

Next Step:
A. Follow-up CT scan in 6 to 12 months
B. No further follow-up needed
C. Follow-up CT scan in 12 months
D. Follow-up CT scan in 3 to 6 months
E. PET-CT scan

Q51-10: A
Follow-up CT scan in 6 to 12 months

Rationale: This patient has a single pulmonary nodule, size 6.5 mm, with smooth margins, and there are no spiculations. The patient has no smoking history and no extrathoracic malignancy in 5 years, and the lesion is not in the upper lobe. Based on this information, the risk according to the Mayo clinic model is 2.5%. This places the patient in the low-risk category (less than 5% risk), and the recommendation would be for a follow-up CT scan in 6 to 12 months.

Incidental pulmonary nodules may represent primary lung cancer, metastatic disease from other sites, carcinoid tumors (particularly diffuse idiopathic pulmonary neuroendocrine cell hyperplasia [DIPNECH] if multiple nodules are present), infectious etiologies (histoplasmosis), benign tumors (hamartomas), pulmonary arteriovenous malformations (AVMs), vasculitis, rheumatoid arthritis–associated nodules, rounded atelectasis, bronchogenic cysts, pseudotumors (fluid loculated within an interlobar fissure), and perifissural nodules (PFNs). The evaluation and management of patients with incidental pulmonary nodules is highly individualized and requires clear communication between the patient and physician. The risk of malignancy is determined primarily by the size and characteristics of the lesions (margins, density, presence of calcifications or fat, location, enhancement on CT, fluorodeoxyglucose [FDG] uptake on PET-CT) as well as patient risk factors (smoking history, history of extrathoracic malignancy, family history of lung cancer, sex assigned at birth and, most importantly, age). There are a number of risk calculators available to estimate the risk of malignancy, including the Mayo Clinic model developed by Swensen and the Brock University calculators (https://brocku.ca/lung-cancer-screening-and-risk-prediction/risk-calculators/). As these calculators become more focused on specific populations, some may be applicable only to lung cancer screening patients and others to incidental pulmonary nodule patients, so care should be taken in selecting the appropriate screening tool. According to the Mayo Clinic model, the risk is 2.5%. According to the full model from the Brock University calculator, the risk is 1%. Also, it is important to understand what the calculator provides. It may indicate a lifetime risk or a 6- to 10-year risk of a nodule being cancer, or it may indicate the chance a patient will be diagnosed with cancer during a standard follow-up period of the nodule (2-4 years).

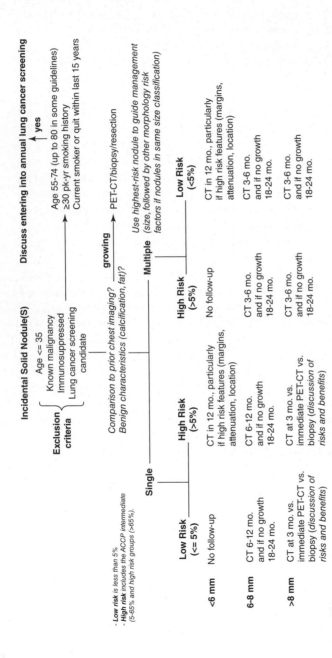

Image 51-11 • Fleischner 2017 Guidelines for evaluation and management of incidental lung nodules. *(Data from MacMahon H, Naidich DP, Goo JM, et al: Guidelines for Management of Incidental Pulmonary Nodules Detected on CT Images: From the Fleischner Society 2017, Radiology 2017 Jul;284(1):228-243. Risk assessment per the following references: Mayo clinic model, Swensen SJ, Silverstein MD, Ilstrup DM, et al: The probability of malignancy in solitary pulmonary nodules. Application to small radiologically indeterminate nodules. Arch Intern Med. 1997 Apr 28;157(8):849-55. Brock University Full Model, McWilliams A, Tammemagi M, Mayo J, et al: Probability of cancer in pulmonary nodules detected on first screening CT, N Engl J Med 2013 Sep 5;369(10):910-919.)*

After all the information has been obtained, a patient's risk of malignancy can be calculated, and a plan can be formulated that is based not only on the guideline recommendations but also on a discussion of the risks and benefits of each option, including early diagnostic procedures and surgical resection.

Q51-11: F
32.9%

Rationale: The patient has a spiculated, 7.5-mm nodule in the right upper lobe. He is a prior smoker at age 65. There was no PET-CT performed because the lesion is less than 8 mm and PET-CT loses sensitivity below 8 mm. With no history of extra-thoracic malignancy, the risk is 32.9%. The Brock calculator would assign a 6.1% risk of being diagnosable as cancer in a standard 2- to 4-year follow-up. This patient's lesion grew and was FDG-avid on follow-up (**Image 51-11** and additional examples in **Images 51-12** and **51-13**). The lesion was resected, and the patient had stage IA1 adenocarcinoma.

Several terms are used to describe pulmonary nodules, and these are detailed in **Image 51-14**. First, one must determine if the nodule is solitary or multiple. Next, if there are multiple nodules, the decision is based primarily on the nodule with the highest risk factor. For solitary nodules, the next step is to determine if the density is solid, subsolid (mixed solid and ground-glass opacities), or pure ground-glass opacities. Subsolid nodules have the highest risk, followed by solid nodules, followed by pure ground-glass opacities. Next, the size is determined, and this is the primary risk factor. Nodules less than 5 mm have a less than 1% chance of being malignant; those 5 to 9 mm have a 2% to 6% chance; those 9 to 20 mm have an 18% chance; and those greater than 20 mm (2 cm) have a 50% chance. The presence of any of the calcification patterns seen below suggests a more benign lesion, likely resulting from prior infection or granulomatous disease. Similarly, the presence of fat suggests a hamartoma. In terms of margins, smooth and round or polygonal lesions have the lowest risk, lobulated lesions have an intermediate risk, and spiculated and coarse lesions have the highest risk. Spiculations are thought to represent an extension of the tumor into the interlobular interstitium, while lobulations represent different growth rates within a nodule. In terms of location, upper-lobe lesions are higher risk than lower-lobe lesions (additional examples of spiculation are shown in **Images 51-12** and **51-13**). A lesion that does not enhance on contrasted CT is less likely to be malignant. Similarly, if a lesion is larger than 8 mm in diameter, a negative PET-CT makes it less likely that the lesion is malignant. The sensitivity and specificity of PET-CT is 91% and 76%, respectively, for lesions greater than 8 mm. False positives occur because of FDG-uptake in inflammatory lesions (sarcoid, vasculitis, infection), and false negatives may occur in slow-growing, less metabolically active lesions (adenocarcinoma in situ, minimally invasive adenocarcinoma).

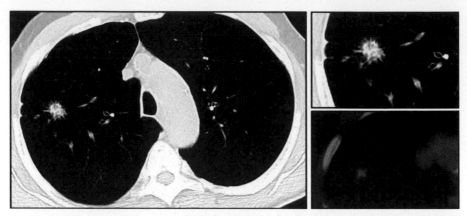

Image 51-12 • CT of the chest and PET imaging studies for the patient in **Question 51-11**.

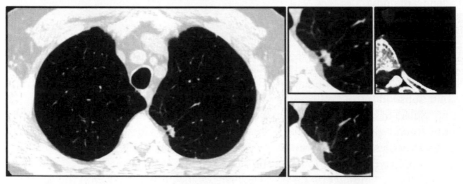

Image 51-13 • Another example of an upper-lobe pulmonary nodule.

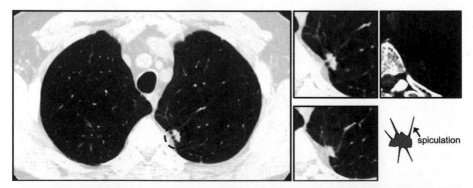

Image 51-14 • Spiculated pulmonary nodules demonstrated in **Image 51-13**. Note the spioulations (black arrows) identified in the solitary pulmonary nodule (black circle).

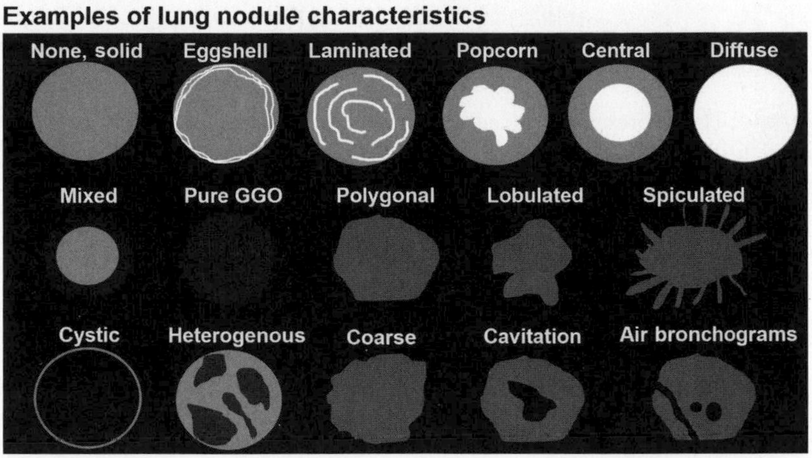

Examples of lung nodule characteristics

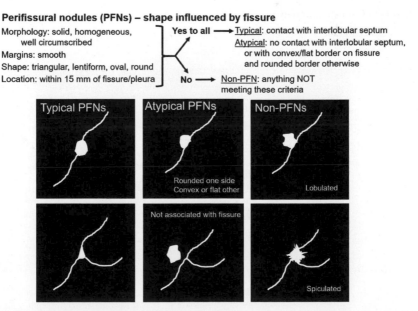

Image 51-15 · Characteristic descriptors of lung nodules. Characteristics of interest include attenuation (density; solid, mixed component, pure ground glass, or cystic), margins (well circumscribed/smooth, coarse), shape (round, polygonal, lobulated, spiculated, cavitary, with/without air bronchograms), consistency (homogeneous, heterogeneous, fat containing), calcifications (eggshell, laminated or lamellated, popcorn, central, or diffuse), size (in mm or cm in largest dimension), volume, and growth (greater than 2 mm change in size). GGO, ground-glass opacities.

Additionally, CT scanning may identify PFNs. There are nodules that occur along interlobular fissures and are benign lesions if they have the typical findings (**Image 51-16**).

Image 51-16 · Perifissural nodules (PFNs). Definitions of typical, atypical, and non-PFNs are provided. Typical PFNs require no follow-up, while atypical and non-PFN nodules should be treated as standard pulmonary nodules.

Q51-12: B
Subsolid

Rationale: This represents a mixed component or subsolid lesion. The primary risk factor is the size of the solid component. Growth is defined as a greater than 2-mm increase in the size of the lesion *or* growth of the solid component of the lesion. The flow chart for pure ground-glass lesions and subsolid or mixed lesions is shown in **Image 51-17**. An additional example of a mixed lesion is shown in **Image 51-18**.

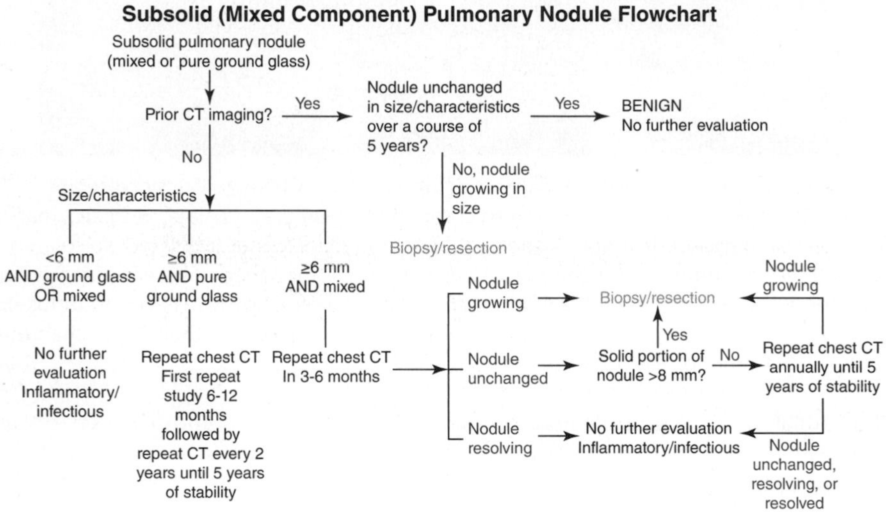

Subsolid (Mixed Component) Pulmonary Nodule Flowchart

Image 51-17 • Evaluation of pure ground-glass and subsolid pulmonary nodules.

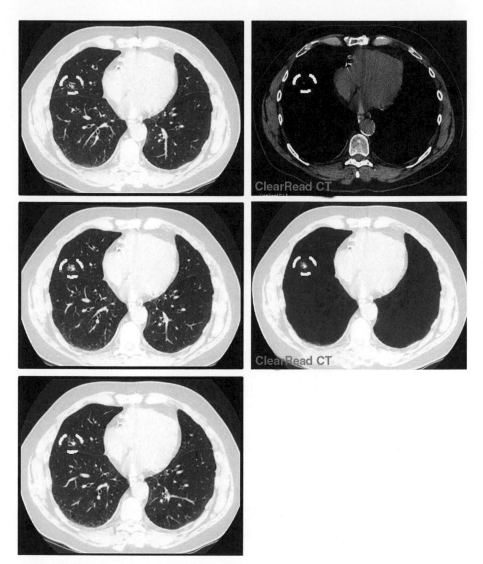

Image 51-18 • An additional example of a subsolid pulmonary nodule, with the Clear-Read CT enhancement demonstrating mixed component density.

A quick word on lung cancer screening: The overall approach to lung cancer screening is evolving and is beyond the scope of this case series; however, some discussion is appropriate. The inclusion criteria for lung cancer screening vary between organizations but are provided above. It is estimated that smoking accounts for up to 90% of lung cancer cases, and approximately 15% to 17% of the US population are active smokers. Rates are highest between the ages of 65 and 85. The prevalence is slightly higher in men than women and is equal between White and Black patients; however, the mortality rate remains highest in the Black population. The prevalence of lung cancer ranges from 0.5% to 0.8% in the US population, and lung cancer remains the leading cause of cancer deaths in men and women, with more than 150,000 deaths annually.

The clinical outcomes in lung cancer are most closely related to the patient's lung cancer stage at the time of diagnosis. The current staging guidelines (TMN 8th edition) were last updated in January 2017 to update the staging to more accurately reflect available prognostic information. Although 5-year survival rates are as high as 92% for patients with stage IA1 disease, most (approximately 75%) patients present with advanced-stage disease, and the overall 5-year survival rate remains around 20%. The TMN staging is shown in **Table 51-1**, as are the intrathoracic lymph node stations.

TABLE 51-1 • NSCLC Clinical Staging Guidelines (TMN 8th Edition) – TMN Definitions		
Tumor (T) Stage		Definition (size of the tumor refers to the tumor's greatest dimension)
Tx		Tumor in sputum or bronchoalveolar lavage/wash sample, but the tumor is not evident on imaging and not visible on a flexible bronchoscopic examination
T0		No evidence of tumor
Tis		Carcinoma in situ
T1		Tumor ≤ 3 cm, surrounded by lung parenchyma or visceral pleura only and not involving the main bronchus
	T1a(mi)	Minimally invasive carcinoma
	T1a	Tumor ≤ 1 cm
	T1b	Tumor > 1 cm but ≤ 2 cm
.	T1c	Tumor > 2 cm but ≤ 3 cm
T2		Tumor > 3 but ≤ 5 cm; *or* Tumor of any size ≤ 5 cm that meets any of the following criteria: • Tumor involves the main bronchus without involvement of the carina; *or* • Invasion of the visceral pleura; *or* • Atelectasis or postobstructive pneumonitis extending to the hilum
	T2a	Tumor > 3 but ≤ 4 cm
	T2b	Tumor > 4 but ≤ 5 cm
T3		Tumor > 5 cm but ≤ 7 cm; *or* Tumor of any size ≤ 7 cm that meets any of the following criteria: Tumor directly invades the chest wall, pericardium, or phrenic nerve; *or* Presence of satellite nodules *within the same lobe*
T4		Tumor > 7 cm; *or* Tumor meets any of the following criteria: Tumor invades the mediastinum, diaphragm, heart, great vessels, recurrent laryngeal nerve, carina, trachea, esophagus, or spine; *or* Separate smaller tumor present in a *different lobe* in *the ipsilateral lung*
Lymph Node (N)		
NX		Lymph nodes cannot be accessed
N0		No regional lymph nodes
N1		*Ipsilateral* peribronchial or ipsilateral hilar lymph nodes and intrapulmonary nodes, including by direct invasion of the primary tumor

(Continued)

TABLE 51-1 • NSCLC Clinical Staging Guidelines (TMN 8th Edition) – TMN Definitions (*Continued*)		
Tumor (T) Stage		Definition (size of the tumor refers to the tumor's greatest dimension)
N2		*Ipsilateral* mediastinal or subcarinal lymph nodes
N3		Any of the following nodes positive for disease: Contralateral mediastinal or hilar nodes Ipsilateral or contralateral scalene Ipsilateral or contralateral supraclavicular nodes
Metastatic (M)		
M0		No distant metastases
M1		Distant metastases
	M1a	Tumor in contralateral lung believed to originate from primary lesion defined in T classification; *or* Malignant pleural effusion; *or* Malignant pericardial effusion; *or* Pleural or pericardial nodules
	M1b	Single extrathoracic metastasis, including nonregional lymph nodes
	M1c	Multiple extrathoracic metastases, independent of involved regions
NSCLC, non-small cell lung cancer.		

TABLE 51-2 • NSCLC Clinical Staging (TMN 8th Edition) and Associated 5-Year Survival Rates								
T or M stage	N0		N1		N2		N3	
T1a T1b T1c	IA1 IA2 IA3	92% 83% 77%	IIB	53%	IIIA	36%	IIIB	26%
T2a	IB	68%	IIB	53%	IIIA	36%	IIIB	26%
T2b	IIA	60%	IIB	53%	IIIA	36%	IIIB	26%
T3	IIB	53%	IIIA	36%	IIIB	26%	IIIC	13%
T4	IIIA	36%	IIIA	36%	IIIB	26%	IIIC	13%
M1a	IVA	10%	IVA	10%	IVA	10%	IVA	10%
M1b	IVA	10%	IVA	10%	IVA	10%	IVA	10%
M1c	IVB	0%	IVB	0%	IVB	0%	IVB	0%
NSCLC, non-small cell lung cancer.								

TABLE 51-3 • Intrathoracic Lymph Node Stations
Thoracic lymph node stations:
• **N3 nodes (independent of laterality):**
• Scalene
• Supraclavicular
• **MEDIASTINAL, N2 Is ipsilateral, N3 if contralateral:**
• (Station 1) highest mediastinal
• (2) upper paratracheal
• (3) prevascular and retrotracheal
• (4) lower paratracheal
• (5) subaortic
• (6) para-aortic
• (7) subcarinal
• (8) paraesophageal
• (9) pulmonary ligament
• **HILAR or INTRAPULMONARY NODES, N1 if ipsilateral, N3 is contralateral:**
• (10) hilar
• (11) interlobar
• (12) lobar
• (13) segmental
• (14) subsegmental
• **METASTATIC (M1b is single; M1c is multiple):**
• any other extrathoracic node

Lung cancer screening offers plenty of potential benefits, and because low-dose CT (LDCT) scans are performed annually in a selected high-risk population, a 20% to 25% lung cancer mortality benefit and an up to 7% all-cause mortality benefit has been realized. Additionally, annual LDCT screening may positively impact smoking cessation. Currently, the incidence rate is about 0.5% to 1% overall. Studies to date suggest that for every 250 people screened for a duration of 3 years, one death will be prevented over the course of 6 years. Roughly, given the prevalence of smoking in the United States, it is predicted that up to 12,000 lives could be saved every year by LDCT screening. However, there are potential complications, including false positives, radiation exposure, patient distress, and overdiagnosis. False positives occur in 25% to 50% of patients, most of whom require some additional diagnostic procedure. About 5% of patients overall undergo invasive procedures, with about 1.5% experiencing complications, so this is something to be considered. The radiation exposure of LDCT is about one-fifth that of a standard CT scan and about one-tenth of a PET-CT scan. It is estimated that for every 100 cancers detected, one cancer will be caused by the added radiation exposure. Patient distress is considerable, particularly in light of a 96% false-positive rate. Overdiagnosis, meaning that the early diagnosis of lung cancer not impacting a patient's life expectancy due to age or comorbid medical conditions that either will cause death or prevent the patient from receiving treatment, is estimated to account for 15% to 25% of diagnoses. These are important factors to consider when discussing lung cancer screening with patients. Currently, screening is only recommended by annual LDCT scanning and not by chest radiograph or sputum cytology. The LUNG-RADS criteria are the most commonly used screening criteria for LDCT and are provided in **Image 51-19**. The most important aspect of a successful lung cancer screening program is the establishment of a multidisciplinary team consisting of thoracic surgeons, medical and radiation oncologists, pulmonologists, pathologists, and radiologists (including intervention or procedural radiologists).

Category	Risk	Definitions (LUNG-RADS for LDCT Screening)				Follow-up
0	NA	NA—incompletely imaged (sections too thick or incomplete chest imaging) or known prior chest imaging (CT) which has not yet been obtained for comparison				• If incomplete current imaging, obtain current low-dose screening CT • If prior imaging available, obtain and compare to current
1	<1%	No nodules or nodules with findings that highly favor a benign condition (fat-containing nodule–hamartomas; popcorn calcifications, complete calcification, etc)				• Continue annual screening as long as patient meets inclusion criteria
		Solid	**Mixed Attenuation**	**GGO**	**Prior Nodules**	
2	<1%	Baseline: <6mm New: <4mm	Baseline: <6mm	Baseline: <30mm or >30mm and unchanged new <30 mm	Cat. 3 or 4 with no growth over at least 3 mo. period	• Continue annual screening as long as patient meets inclusion criteria
3	1-2%	Baseline: 6-8 mm New: 4-6 mm	Baseline: >6 mm w/solid component <6 mm New: <6 mm total diameter	Baseline: >30 mm or new >30 mm		• 6-month follow-up CT
4A	5-15%	Baseline: 8-15 mm Nodule: <8 and growth New: 6-8 mm Endobronchial nodule	Baseline: >6 mm w/solid component 6-8 mm New: 6-8 mm total diameter			• 3-month follow-up CT or PET-CT if solid component >8 mm
4B	5-15%	Baseline: >15 mm Prior Nodule: >8 and growth New: >8 mm	Baseline: >8 mm Prior with solid component >4 mm and growing New with solid component >4 mm			• PET-CT if solid component >8 mm • Tissue sampling, • Counseling, MDC
4X		Cat. 3 or 4 nodules with high-risk features (spiculations, enlarged regional lymph nodes, etc). If new large nodules and concern for either inflammatory (eg, vasculitis) or infectious etiology, a 1-2 month follow-up CT may be appropriate				• PET-CT if solid component >8 mm • Tissue sampling • Counseling, MDC

MDC—multidisciplinary conference

Image 51-19 • Lung-RADS definitions and risk stratification for patients in lung cancer screening. (*Data from Pinsky PF, Gierada DS, Black W, et al: Performance of Lung-RADS in the National Lung Screening Trial: a retrospective assessment, Ann Intern Med 2015 Apr 7;162(7):485-491.*)

References

American Thoracic Society. Implementation guide for lung cancer screening. https://www.lungcancerscreeningguide.org/ Accessed April 16, 2021.

Black WC, Gareen IF, Soneji SS, et al. Cost-effectiveness of CT screening in the National Lung Screening Trial. N Engl J Med. 2014;371:1793.

Canadian Task Force on Preventive Health Care. Recommendations on screening for lung cancer. CMAJ. 2016;188:425.

Chansky K, Detterbeck FC, Nicholson AG, et al. IASLC Staging and Prognostic Factors Committee, Advisory Boards, and Participating Institutions. The IASLC Lung Cancer Staging Project: external validation of the revision of the TNM stage groupings in the eighth edition of the TNM classification of lung cancer. J Thorac Oncol. 2017;12:1109.

Detterbeck FC, Boffa DJ, Kim AW, Tanoue LT. The eighth edition lung cancer stage classification. Chest. 2017;151:193.

Detterbeck FC, Chansky K, Groome P, et al. IASLC Staging and Prognostic Factors Committee, Advisory Boards, and Participating Institutions. The IASLC Lung Cancer Staging Project: methodology and validation used in the development of proposals for revision of the stage classification of NSCLC in the forthcoming (eighth) edition of the TNM classification of lung cancer. J Thorac Oncol. 2016;11:1433.

Etzel CJ, Bach PB. Estimating individual risk for lung cancer. Semin Respir Crit Care Med. 2011;32:3.

Flehinger BJ, Kimmel M, Polyak T, Melamed MR. Screening for lung cancer. The Mayo Lung Project revisited. Cancer. 1993;72:1573.

Goldstraw P, Chansky K, Crowley J, et al. The IASLC Lung Cancer Staging Project: proposals for revision of the TNM stage groupings in the forthcoming (eighth) edition of the TNM classification for lung cancer. J Thorac Oncol. 2016;11:39.

Gould MK, Donington J, Lynch WR, et al. Evaluation of individuals with pulmonary nodules: when is it lung cancer? Diagnosis and management of lung cancer, 3rd ed: American College of Chest Physicians evidence-based clinical practice guidelines. Chest. 2013;143:e93S.

Jaklitsch MT, Jacobson FL, Austin JH, et al. The American Association for Thoracic Surgery guidelines for lung cancer screening using low-dose computed tomography scans for lung cancer survivors and other high-risk groups. J Thorac Cardiovasc Surg. 2012;144:33.

Katki HA, Kovalchik SA, Berg CD, et al. Development and validation of risk models to select ever-smokers for CT lung cancer screening. JAMA. 2016;315:2300.

Kinsinger LS, Anderson C, Kim J, et al. Implementation of lung cancer screening in the Veterans Health Administration. JAMA Intern Med. 2017;177:399.

Lindell RM, Hartman TE, Swensen SJ, et al. Five-year lung cancer screening experience: CT appearance, growth rate, location, and histologic features of 61 lung cancers. Radiology. 2007;242:555.

MacMahon H, Naidich DP, Goo JM, et al. Guidelines for management of incidental pulmonary nodules detected on CT images: from the Fleischner Society 2017. Radiology. 2017;284:228.

Mazzone PJ, Silvestri GA, Patel S, et al. Screening for lung cancer: CHEST guideline and expert panel report. Chest. 2018;153:954.

McKee BJ, Regis SM, McKee AB, et al. Performance of ACR Lung-RADS in a clinical CT lung screening program. J Am Coll Radiol. 2015;12:273.

McWilliams A, Tammemagi M, Mayo J, et al. Probability of cancer in pulmonary nodules detected on first screening computed tomography. N Engl J Med. 2013;369:910.

National Lung Screening Trial Research Team, Aberle DR, Adams AM, et al. Reduced lung-cancer mortality with low-dose computed tomographic screening. N Engl J Med. 2011;365:395.

Ost D, Fein AM, Feinsilver SH. Clinical practice. The solitary pulmonary nodule. N Engl J Med. 2003;348:2535.

Pasquinelli MM, Tammemägi CM, Kovitz KL, et al. Risk prediction model versus United States Preventive Services Task Force lung cancer screening eligibility criteria—reducing race disparities. J Thorac Oncol. 2020;15:1738.

Patz EF Jr, Greco E, Gatsonis C, et al. Lung cancer incidence and mortality in National Lung Screening Trial participants who underwent low-dose CT prevalence screening: a retrospective cohort analysis of a randomised, multicentre, diagnostic screening trial. Lancet Oncol. 2016;17:590.

Pinsky PF, Gierada DS, Black W, et al. Performance of Lung-RADS in the National Lung Screening Trial: a retrospective assessment. Ann Intern Med. 2015;162:485.

Roberts H, Walker-Dilks C, Sivjee K, et al. Screening high-risk populations for lung cancer: guideline recommendations. J Thorac Oncol. 2013;8:1232.

Spitz MR, Hong WK, Amos CI, et al. A risk model for prediction of lung cancer. J Natl Cancer Inst. 2007;99:715.

Swensen SJ, Silverstein MD, Ilstrup DM, Schleck CD, Edell ES. The probability of malignancy in solitary pulmonary nodules. Application to small radiologically indeterminate nodules. Arch Intern Med. 1997;157:849.

Tammemägi M, Church T, Hocking W, et al. Evaluation of the lung cancer risks at which to screen ever- and never-smokers: screening rules applied to the PLCO and NLST cohorts. PLoS Medicine. 2014;11:e1001764.

Tammemagi MC, Katki HA, Hocking WG, et al. Selection criteria for lung-cancer screening. N Engl J Med. 2013;368:728.

US Preventive Services Task Force. Lung cancer screening: recommendation statement. Ann Intern Med. 2004;140:738.

US Preventive Services Task Force. Screening for lung cancer: recommendation statement 2013. www.uspreventiveservicestaskforce.org/Page/Document/UpdateSummaryFinal/lung-cancer-screening. Accessed April 16, 2021.

Veronesi G, Maisonneuve P, Spaggiari L, et al. Diagnostic performance of low-dose computed tomography screening for lung cancer over five years. J Thorac Oncol. 2014;9:935.

Wender R, Fontham ET, Barrera E Jr, et al. American Cancer Society lung cancer screening guidelines. CA Cancer J Clin. 2013;63:107.

Wood DE. National Comprehensive Cancer Network (NCCN) clinical practice guidelines for lung cancer screening. Thorac Surg Clin. 2015;25:185.

INDEX

Page numbers followed by "f" denote figures; those followed by "t" denote tables.

A

A-a gradient, 292
ABPA. *See* Allergic bronchopulmonary
    aspergillosis
Acid-base disorders, 213–214
Acid-fast bacillus, 336, 343, 568
Acneiform papules/pustules, 308f, 312
Acro-osteolysis, 407
Acute berylliosis, 108
Acute chemical pneumonitis, 497
Acute eosinophilic pneumonia
    clinical presentation of, 379
    corticosteroids for, 379–380
    description of, 130
    pathology of, 374f, 379
    treatment of, 374
Acute hypersensitivity pneumonitis
    antigen avoidance for, 131, 132t, 561t–562t
    characteristics of, 132t, 561t
    description of, 126–127
    diagnosis of, 130
    laboratory studies for, 557–558
    occupational exposure as cause of,
        129–130, 607
    symptoms of, 128, 132t
    transbronchial biopsy for, 558
    treatment of, 131, 132t
Acute interstitial pneumonia
    age of onset, 216
    corticosteroids for, 216
    definition of, 215
    ground-glass opacities in, 216
    imaging of, 207f–208f, 216
    mortality rates for, 212, 218
    stages of, 215
    survival rates for, 212, 218
    treatment of, 211, 217–218
Acute lupus pneumonitis
    corticosteroids for, 330
    rash associated with, 322f
    in systemic lupus erythematosus, 327
    treatment of, 323
Acute pancreatitis, 520
Acute pulmonary blastomycosis, 354

Acute pulmonary histoplasmosis,
    347–348
Acute respiratory distress syndrome
    acid-base disorder in, 213–214
    Berlin criteria for, 213
    in blastomycosis, 356
    description of, 74
    diagnosis of, 213
    Pneumocystis jiroveci pneumonia as cause
        of, 289
    treatment of, 348
Acute respiratory failure, 323, 327
Acute reversible hypoxia syndrome, 331
Acute silicosis, 118–119
Adenocarcinoma, 639, 640f
    invasive mucinous, 657
    lepidic growth, 650f, 658
    minimally invasive, 657
Adenocarcinoma in situ, 657
Adhesive atelectasis, 74
AEP. *See* Acute eosinophilic pneumonia
AIP. *See* Acute interstitial pneumonia
Air bronchograms, 614
    with consolidation, 4f, 465
    definition of, 465
Air-crescent sign, 302–303
Air trapping, 10, 186, 453f, 553
Airspace opacities, 6
Airway
    abnormalities of, 13
    central, 2
    diameter of, at tracheal level, 576, 581
    distal, 2–4
    nodularity of, 13, 623
Airway clearance, 73
Airway collaterals, 66, 73
Airway malacia, 579, 580f, 595
Airway obstruction
    central. *See* Central airway obstruction
    expiratory, 588f, 593
    extrathoracic, 579, 594
    intrathoracic, 595
    lower, 578
    upper. *See* Upper airway obstruction

Alemtuzumab, 344
Allergic bronchopulmonary aspergillosis
  aspergilloma versus, 300
  Aspergillus fumigatus associated with,
    257–258
  central bronchiectasis, 254
  chest radiographic findings in, 258
  computed tomography findings in,
    258
  corticosteroids for, 255, 259–260
  definition of, 235
  diagnostic criteria for, 254, 257
  glucocorticoids for, 259
  immunoglobulin E levels, 257, 260
  itraconazole for, 259–260
  laboratory studies for, 257
  staging of, 255, 258
  treatment of, 255
ALP. *See* Acute lupus pneumonitis
Alpha-1-antitrypsin
  deficiency of, 456
  definition of, 456
  description of, 166, 427
  enzyme level, 455–456, 456f
Alveolar opacities, 6, 286f, 290, 553f, 614
American Thoracic Society/Infectious
    Disease Society of America, 469
Amiodarone toxicity
  corticosteroids for, 97
  onset of, 96
  pulmonary function testing for, 92
  risk factors for, 92
  signs and symptoms of, 96
Amphotericin B, 315, 347
  blastomycosis treated with, 357
  liposomal, 357
Ampicillin-sulbactam, 495–497
ANA test. *See* Antinuclear antibody test
ANCA. *See* Antineutrophilic cytoplasmic
    antibody
ANCA-associated vasculitides
  computed tomography of, 626f
  description of, 624–626
  glucocorticoids for, 627–628
  kidney biopsy for, 627
  treatment of, 627–628
  types of, 626
Angioinvasive disease, 303
Angiolipomas, renal, 167
Anterior mediastinum
  illustration of, 39f
  masses of, 47, 48f, 62
  structures of, 45, 50, 61, 581
Anthracosis, 118
Anti-acetylcholinesterase receptor
    antibodies, 50

Anti-glomerular basement membrane
    disease, 624, 628
Anti-Jo1 antibody, 388
Anti-ribonucleoprotein antibodies, 405
Anti-Ro/anti-La antibodies, 178
Anti-Scl70 antibody, 405
Anti-thymocyte globulin, 628
Antifungal therapy, 310
Antigen avoidance, for hypersensitivity
    pneumonitis, 131, 132t, 561t–562t
Antineutrophilic cytoplasmic antibody, 117
Antinuclear antibody test, 117, 327, 624
Aortic arch, 28
Aortic calcifications, 85
Aortic knob, 26
ARDS. *See* Acute respiratory distress
    syndrome
Asbestos bodies, 86
Asbestos exposure
  benign asbestos-related pleural effusions
    and, 602, 608
  description of, 86
  mesothelioma secondary to, 609–610
  pleural thickening secondary to, 609
Asbestosis
  characteristics of, 83f, 86
  computed tomography of, 604f
  end-stage lung disease as cause of, 88
  glucocorticoids for, 84, 87–88
  latency period for development of, 83, 87
  pulmonary function testing for, 84
  risk factors for, 84, 87
  rounded atelectasis and, 607–608
  smoking and, 87
  treatment of, 84, 87–88
Ascending aorta, 28
Ascites, 519
Aspergilloma
  allergic bronchopulmonary aspergillosis
    versus, 300
  definition of, 300
  laboratory studies for, 296
  surgical resection of, 301
  treatment of, 296
Aspergillosis
  chronic necrotizing pulmonary, 303
  chronic pulmonary, 303–304
  disseminated central nervous system, 301
  invasive bronchial, 302
  invasive pulmonary, 298, 301–303
Aspergillus fumigatus, 257–258, 297, 299–300
Aspergillus-related lung disease, 300–301,
    304f
Aspiration pneumonia
  bacteria that cause, 496
  chest radiographs of, 495f

description of, 72, 406
risk factors for, 488, 497
treatment of, 495–497
Atelectasis
adhesive, 74
causes of, 66
chest computed tomography of,
69f–71f
chest radiograph of, 67f–68f, 71f
compressive, 73–74, 493f
computed tomography of, 4f
definition of, 72, 243
left-sided, 607
left upper lobe, 76
middle mediastinal mass associated with,
37–38
obstructive, 72, 76, 76f
passive, 73–74, 74f
persistent, 15
plate-like, 74, 346f
pneumonia consolidation versus, 607
replacement, 74
right middle lobe, 429
right-sided relaxation, 73–74
right upper lobe, 76
rounded, 78, 243, 607–609
subtypes of, 66
treatment of, 66, 73
ATG. *See* Anti-thymocyte globulin
Atovaquone, 292
Atrium
left, 28
right, 26, 28
ATS/IDSA. *See* American Thoracic Society/
Infectious Disease Society of America
Attenuation
decreased, 6, 11f, 11–12
increased, 10f, 10–11
mosaic pattern of, 416, 451, 453f, 554
perfusion pattern of, 417
Azathioprine, 147
Azithromycin, 281, 291, 455, 466–467
Azygous vein, 61

B
B-type natriuretic peptide, 440
BAC. *See* Bronchoalveolar carcinomas
Bactrim, 249
BAL. *See* Bronchoalveolar lavage
BAPE. *See* Benign asbestos-related pleural
effusions
Bcl-2 staining, 156
Belimumab, 330
Benign asbestos-related pleural effusions
asbestos exposure and, latency period
between, 602, 608

description of, 78
diagnosis of, 607
differential diagnosis of, 608
Berylliosis, 105, 107–108, 118, 559
Beryllium
exposure to, 607
hypersensitivity evaluations, 107
Beryllium dermatitis, 108
1,3-beta-D-glucan, 178
Beta-galactomannan, 178
Bibasilar crackles, 385, 397
Biopsy. *See specific biopsy*
Birbeck granules, 156
Bird fancier's disease, 557
Blastomyces, 355
Blastomycosis, 355–356, 365
Blebs, 6
Bleomycin-induced lung injury/toxicity, 90,
95f, 95–96
BNP. *See* B-type natriuretic peptide; Brain
natriuretic peptide
Bony structures, 4
Boutonniere deformity, 389
BRAF V600E, 158
Brain natriuretic peptide, 519
Bronchial artery
emboli of, 500
embolization of, 279
Bronchial stenosis, radiation-induced,
244
Bronchial stent placement, 73
Bronchial stump, 302
Bronchial wall thickening, 233, 256, 426,
431f, 623
Bronchiectasis
bacterial colonization associated with,
232, 235
corticosteroids for, 236
cylindrical, 233, 233f–234f, 256
cystic, 233f
cystic fibrosis as cause of, 235
description of, 13
flow-volume loop for, 231, 235
focal, 281
imaging of, 4f, 278f
inhaled rhDNase for, 236
laboratory studies for, 235
morphologies of, 233, 233f–234f
non-cystic fibrosis, 232, 235
Pseudomonas aeruginosa associated with,
235–236
pulmonary rehabilitation for, 236
saccular, 233f
"signet ring" finding associated with, 233,
234f, 426f, 431f
traction, 10f, 12, 176, 331, 388, 483

Bronchiectasis (*Cont.*):
　tram-track appearance, 431f
　treatment of, 232, 236, 281
　varicose, 233, 233f
Bronchiolar wall thickening, 278
Bronchiolitis obliterans, 417
Bronchoalveolar carcinomas, 644,
　　657–658
Bronchoalveolar lavage, 14, 83, 107
　for acute respiratory distress syndrome,
　　214
　bronchoscopy with, 570, 614–615
　for coccidioidomycosis, 363f
　for pulmonary alveolar proteinosis, 225
　for radiation pneumonitis, 246
　for sarcoidosis, 147
Bronchodilators, 96
Bronchogenic cysts, 41–42
Bronchomalacia, 451, 452f
Bronchoscopy
　of acute respiratory distress syndrome,
　　214
　with bronchoalveolar lavage, 570,
　　614–615
　of bronchomalacia, 452f
　complications of, 16
　description of, 13–16
　diagnostic procedures using, 13–14
　indications for, 15–16, 73
　of pulmonary alveolar proteinosis, 225
　of sarcoidosis, 142
　transbronchial biopsy with, 570, 656–657
　virtual, 14
Brugia malayi, 375, 380
Bullae, 6, 450
Byssinosis, 107, 118

C
Calcified mediastinal adenopathy, 213
Calcinosis cutis, 406
Calcium carbonate, 249
"Camel-hump" appearance, 579, 595
Campath, 628
Canals of Lambert, 73
CAO. *See* Central airway obstruction
CAP. *See* Community-acquired pneumonia
Caplan syndrome, 119
Carcinoid tumors, 50, 639
Cardiac silhouette, 438
Cardiogenic pulmonary edema
　clinical findings of, 481
　definition of, 442
　diagnosis of, 436f
　etiology of, 435, 441
　point-of-care ultrasound for, 435
　progression of, 442f

Carfilzomib, 628
Carina, 26
Cavitary abnormalities, 3f
Cavitary lesions
　computed tomography of, 165, 166f, 364,
　　487f, 492, 493f, 618f, 623
　definition of, 364
　description of, 12
　in left upper lobe, 295f, 300
Cavitary nodules, 12f, 497
Cavitary pneumonia, 492
Cavitation, nontuberculous mycobacterial
　　infections with, 280
CCPA. *See* Chronic cavitary pulmonary
　　aspergillosis
CD4 count, 315, 344
CD4+ lymphocytes, 107
CD1a, 156, 157f
Ceftriaxone, 496
　plus azithromycin, 466–467
CellCept, 560
Cellular nonspecific interstitial pneumonia,
　　200f
Central airway obstruction
　computed tomography of, 592f
　definition of, 578, 593
　diagnosis of, 582, 591–595, 592f
　flow-volume loops for, 578, 580f, 588f,
　　593
Central sparing, 85
Centrilobular cystic lung lesions, 165, 165f
Centrilobular emphysema, 388, 450f–452f,
　　450–451, 554, 570
Centrilobular structure, 9
Cephalization, 2–3, 441
Cerebrospinal fluid
　cryptococcal antigen titer, 315
　leakage of, 522
Cerebrovascular accident, 311
CFPA. *See* Chronic fibrosing pulmonary
　　aspergillosis
CFTR gene, 235
CFTR mutation. *See* Cystic fibrosis
　　transmembrane receptor mutation
CGD. *See* Chronic granulomatous disease
"Cheerio" sign, 658, 658f
Chemical pneumonitis, acute, 497
Chemotherapy
　cytotoxic, for pulmonary Langerhans cell
　　histiocytosis, 158
　for diffuse large B-cell lymphoma, 596
　radiation pneumonitis caused by, 247
Chest physiotherapy, 73
Chest radiography, 1. *See also specific
　　disorder*
Chest tube placement, 523, 525

Cholesterol effusion, 522
Chronic berylliosis, 108
Chronic cavitary pulmonary aspergillosis, 303
Chronic cavitary pulmonary histoplasmosis, 348
Chronic eosinophilic pneumonia, 380–381
Chronic fibrosing pulmonary aspergillosis, 303
Chronic granulomatous disease, 256
Chronic hypersensitivity pneumonitis
    chest imaging of, 555, 556f–557f
    definition of, 557
    description of, 199
    FEV1/FVC ratio in, 558
    ground-glass opacities with, 556f–557f
    histopathologic pattern of, 551
    laboratory studies for, 557–558
    risk reductions, 551
    transbronchial biopsy for, 558
Chronic necrotizing pulmonary aspergillosis, 303
Chronic obstructive pulmonary disease
    bronchodilators for, 455
    centrilobular, 481
    clinical findings of, 454
    description of, 73
    GOLD classification system for, 453, 454f
    risk factors for, 454
    smoking-related, 450, 456
    symptoms of, 454
    treatment of, 448, 455
Chronic pulmonary aspergillosis, 303–304
Chronic thromboembolic pulmonary hypertension, 541–542, 542f–544f
Churg-Strauss syndrome. See Eosinophilic granulomatosis with polyangiitis
Chylothorax, 166, 518, 518f, 522–523
Chylous ascites, 166
Chylous effusion, 166
Cicatrization, 74
CK7 staining, 156
Clarithromycin, 281
Clavicles, 26
"Claw sign," 492, 493f
Clindamycin, 292, 496
Coal workers' pneumoconiosis, 86, 114, 117–119
Coccidioides immitis, 365
Coccidioides posadasii, 365
Coccidioidomycosis
    bronchoalveolar lavage for, 363f
    description of, 357
    diagnosis of, 362, 364–365
    primary pulmonary, 365
    treatment of, 362
"Comet tail," 78, 608
Common variable immune deficiency, 214
Community-acquired pneumonia
    CURB-65 criteria for, 461, 466
    description of, 262
    diagnosis of, 469
    mortality risk for, 461, 466
Compressive atelectasis, 73–74, 493f
Computed tomography
    of chest, 6–7
    cine, 8
    contrasted, 8, 590
    high-resolution. See High-resolution computed tomography
    low-dose, 8
    of mediastinal masses, 51
    noncontrasted, 7–8, 590
    positron-emission tomography-computed tomography. See Positron-emission tomography-computed tomography
    protocols of, 7–8
    of pulmonary artery, 8
    pulmonary nodules on, 664f
    ultra-low-dose, 8
Computed tomography-guided transthoracic needle aspiration, 638
Conformal radiation therapy, 248
Congestive heart failure
    decompensated, 519
    pleural effusions caused by, 507
Consolidation
    air bronchograms with, 4f, 465
    ground-glass opacities and, 243, 641
    imaging of, 6, 11, 116, 203, 238f, 243
    left lower lobe, 465
    left upper lobe, 352f, 355
COP. See Cryptogenic organizing pneumonia
COPD. See Chronic obstructive pulmonary disease
Cor pulmonale, 441
Corticosteroids. See also Glucocorticoids; Prednisone
    for acute eosinophilic pneumonia, 379–380
    for acute interstitial pneumonia, 216
    for acute lupus pneumonitis, 330
    for allergic bronchopulmonary aspergillosis, 255, 259–260
    for amiodarone toxicity, 97
    for beryllium-related diseases, 108
    for bronchiectasis, 236
    for Pneumocystis jiroveci pneumonia, 292

Costophrenic angle
  blunting of, 511, 512f, 607
  description of, 4, 27, 176
Cough, 635
CPA. *See* Chronic pulmonary aspergillosis
Crazy paving, 10f, 11, 85, 224, 290, 641
CREST syndrome, 407
"Crow's feet," 78, 607
Cryobiopsy
  description of, 15
  transbronchial lung, 147
Cryptococcal infections, 312, 313f–314f
Cryptococcal meningitis, 316
Cryptococcal pneumonia, 314f
Cryptococcus gattii, 312
Cryptococcus neoformans, 312
Cryptogenic organizing pneumonia
  clinical presentation of, 243
  definition of, 204
  description of, 126, 128, 203
  differential diagnosis of, 205, 243
  treatment of, 197, 205
CTEPH. *See* Chronic thromboembolic
        pulmonary hypertension
CURB-65, 461, 466
CVA. *See* Cerebrovascular accident
CVID. *See* Common variable immune
        deficiency
CWP. *See* Coal workers' pneumoconiosis
Cyclophosphamide, 407, 627–628
Cylindrical bronchiectasis, 233, 233f–234f,
        256
Cyst
  bronchogenic, 41–42
  definition of, 6
Cystic abnormalities, 3f
Cystic bronchiectasis, 233f
Cystic fibrosis, 235, 279, 430, 432f
Cystic fibrosis transmembrane receptor
        mutation, 423, 425, 427
Cystic lung lesions
  centrilobular, 165, 165f
  computed tomography of, 12f, 165f
  lymphangioleiomyomatosis versus,
        164
Cytomegalovirus, 315
Cytotoxic chemotherapeutics, 158

D
D-dimer, 440, 537
DAD. *See* Diffuse alveolar damage
DAH. *See* Diffuse alveolar hemorrhage
Dapsone, 289, 292
Decompensated congestive heart failure,
        519
Deep sulcus sign, 32f, 176f

Delta F508, 427
Dermatitis, beryllium, 108
Dermatomyositis, 387f, 389f, 390
Descending aorta, 28
Desquamative interstitial pneumonia
  clinical presentation of, 571
  description of, 177–178
  pathology of, 570
  pulmonary function testing for, 569
  rheumatologic conditions associated with,
        571
  smoking cessation for, 571
  treatment of, 569, 571
Dexamethasone, 628
Diaphragmatic abnormalities, 6
Diethylcarbamazine, 380
Diff-Quick stains, 290
Diffuse airspace disease, 311
Diffuse alveolar abnormalities, 3f
Diffuse alveolar damage, 215
Diffuse alveolar hemorrhage
  description of, 214, 327–328, 328f–330f,
        554f
  after hematopoietic stem cell
        transplantation, 613, 615–616
Diffuse alveolar infiltrates, 327, 378, 497
Diffuse cavitary and cystic lung lesions,
        12f
Diffuse consolidation, 12f
Diffuse interstitial opacities, 647f, 656
Diffuse large B-cell lymphoma, 596
Diffuse nodular opacities, 343
Diffuse nodules, 12f
Diffuse pulmonary nodules, 657
Diffuse reticular opacities, 388
Diffusing capacity of carbon monoxide, 87,
        97, 106, 131, 156, 225, 404, 482, 571
Digital enhancement, 2
Digital gangrene/necrosis, 406
DIP. *See* Desquamative interstitial
        pneumonia
Disseminated central nervous system
        aspergillosis, 301
Disseminated cryptococcal infection, 310,
        312, 313f–314f
Disseminated histoplasmosis, 345, 346f
Disseminated *Mycobacterium avium*
        complex infection, 277, 280
DLBCL. *See* Diffuse large B-cell lymphoma
DLCO. *See* Diffusing capacity of carbon
        monoxide
DNase, 523–524
Dornase alfa, 236
"Double-hump," 593
DRESS. *See* Drug eruption with eosinophilia
        and systemic symptoms

Drug eruption with eosinophilia and systemic symptoms, 378
Drug-induced lung injury/toxicity, 94, 97–98, 243
Drug-induced pneumonitis, 248
dsDNA antibody, 388
Duplication cyst, enteric, 583
Dyspigmentation, 407
Dyspnea
    on exertion, 474
    laboratory studies for, 506
    in lung cancer patient, 635
    in lymphangitic carcinomatosis, 657
    persistent, 535
    tracheal lumen diameter and, 577, 582

E
EBUS. See Endobronchial ultrasound
EBV. See Epstein-Barr virus
Echocardiogram, 531f
ECMO. See Extracorporeal membrane oxygenation
"Eggshell" calcifications, 119
EGPA. See Eosinophilic granulomatosis with polyangiitis
Electrical alternans, 327
Electrocardiogram, 320f, 327
Electrothermal atomic absorption spectroscopy, 107
Elexacaftor/tezacaftor/ivacaftor, 430
Embolectomy, 539
Emphysema
    centrilobular, 388, 450f–452f, 450–451, 554, 570
    illustration of, 4f
    panlobular, 450, 455, 456f
    paraseptal, 450
Empyema, 74f, 492, 493f, 514f, 518, 520, 523
EN. See Erythema nodosum
End-stage lung disease, 88
Endobronchial biopsy, 14
Endobronchial mass, 77f
Endobronchial ultrasound
    description of, 14–15
    middle mediastinal masses on, 52
    transbronchial needle aspiration guided with, 147
Endocarditis, 498
Endotracheal tube, 582
Enteric duplication cyst, 583
Environmental exposures, hypersensitivity pneumonitis and, 551, 559–560
Enzyme immunoassay, 366
Eosinophilic granulomatosis with polyangiitis, 380, 625–626

Eosinophilic pneumonia
    acute. See Acute eosinophilic pneumonia
    chronic, 380–381
Epidural abscess, 40
Epstein-Barr virus, 178
Erasmus syndrome, 119
Erdheim-Chester disease, 158
Erythema nodosum, 133f, 143
Esophageal dilatation, 406
Esophagus, 28
    cystic mass of, 576f, 581
    rupture of, 520
ETASS. See Electrothermal atomic absorption spectroscopy
Ethambutol, 281
Everolimus, 168
Expiratory air flow obstruction, 106
Extracorporeal membrane oxygenation, 214, 226
Extrapulmonary sarcoidosis, 143, 147
Extrinsic allergic alveolitis, 301. See also Hypersensitivity pneumonitis
Exudative effusions, 516–518

F
Farmer's lung disease, 557, 559
[18]FDG. See Fluorodeoxyglucose
"Feeding vessel sign", 498
Fenestrae of Boren, 73
FEV1/FVC, 106, 131, 203, 404, 416, 454, 555, 558
Fibrocavitary disease, 280, 280f
Fibrosing mediastinitis, 349
Fibrotic nonspecific interstitial pneumonia, 200f–201f
Finger-in-glove sign, 259, 259f
5-HIAA, 62–63
Flash pulmonary edema, 443
Fleischner guidelines, 622f, 660
Flow-volume loops
    for bronchiectasis, 231, 235
    for central airway obstruction, 578, 580f, 588f, 593
    for obstructive lung disease, 411, 416, 445f, 449
    for restrictive lung disease, 588f, 593
    for tracheobronchomalacia, 588f, 593
    for upper airway obstruction, 573f, 574, 578–579, 580f
Fluconazole, 315, 366–367
Flucytosine, 315
Fluorodeoxyglucose, 8, 587f, 595, 604, 642f–643f
Focal consolidation, 12f
Focal opacity, 256, 378
Follicular bronchiolitis, 417, 417f

Follicular lymphoma, 596
Foreign objects, 5–6
Free-flowing pleural effusions, 511, 512f,
    515, 516f

G
G-LIP. *See* Granulomatous and lymphocytic
    interstitial pneumonia
Galactomannan, serum, 214, 293
"Galaxy" sign, 145
Ganglioneuromas, 62
Gastroesophageal reflux disease, 249
Geneva score, 536
GERD. *See* Gastroesophageal reflux disease
Germ cell tumors, 40, 50
GGOs. *See* Ground-glass opacities
Ghon complex, 269, 271, 343
Giemsa stain, 309, 312
GLILD. *See* Granulomatous and lymphocytic
    interstitial pneumonia
Glucocorticoids. *See also* Corticosteroids
    for allergic bronchopulmonary
        aspergillosis, 259
    for ANCA-associated vasculitides,
        627–628
    for asbestosis, 84, 87–88
    for diffuse alveolar hemorrhage, 615–616
    for interstitial lung diseases, 178–179
    for lymphocytic interstitial pneumonia,
        179
    for nonspecific interstitial pneumonia,
        203
    for pulmonary Langerhans cell
        histiocytosis, 158, 168
    for radiation pneumonitis, 247, 249
    for sarcoidosis, 146–147
Glucose-6-phosphate dehydrogenase
    deficiency, 289
Glycinothorax, 519
GM-CSF. *See* Granulocyte-monocyte colony
    stimulating factor
Goiter, 50, 590
GOLD COPD classification system, 453,
    454f
Gomori methenamine silver stain, 290
Goodpasture disease. *See* Anti-glomerular
    basement membrane disease
Gottron papules, 389
GPA. *See* Granulomatosis with polyangiitis
Graft-versus-host disease, 615
Granulocyte-monocyte colony stimulating
    factor, 226
Granulomatosis with polyangiitis, 620, 625,
    627
Granulomatous and lymphocytic interstitial
    pneumonia, 178

Granulomatous lung disease, 107
Ground-glass opacities
    in acute interstitial pneumonia, 216
    in amiodarone toxicity, 96
    in centrilobular emphysema, 570
    in chronic hypersensitivity pneumonitis,
        556f–557f
    computed tomography of, 176–177, 183f,
        187, 198, 278f, 431f, 554f, 618f, 623
    consolidation surrounded by, 243, 641
    diffuse consolidation with, 12f
    in disseminated histoplasmosis, 346f
    in hypersensitivity pneumonitis, 128,
        556f–557f
    imaging of, 10
    interlobular septal thickening with, 439f,
        614, 638, 648f, 656
    in lymphocytic interstitial pneumonia,
        177
    scattered areas of, 203, 379, 418

H
H bands, 348
H2-blocker, 249
HAART. *See* Highly active antiretroviral
    therapy
Haemophilus influenzae, 235, 468
Hairy cell lymphoma, 596
Halo sign, 243, 246, 302, 614, 641
Hamman-Rich syndrome, 215
Hampton hump, 538
HAP. *See* Hospital-associated pneumonia
HAPE. *See* High-altitude pulmonary edema
Hard metal pneumoconiosis, 118
HCAP. *See* Health care-associated
    pneumonia
"Head-cheese," 553
Health care-associated pneumonia, 469
Heart
    Langerhans cell histiocytosis involvement
        of, 157
    positioning of, 5
Heart border
    description of, 5
    left, 26
    right, 26, 59, 331
Heart failure with pulmonary edema, 128
Heberden nodes, 389
Hematopoietic stem cell transplantation
    acute respiratory failure after, 614
    diffuse alveolar hemorrhage after,
        613, 615
Hemidiaphragm, 26–27, 511
Hemolytic anemia, 292
Hemothorax, 522
Heparin, 537

High-altitude pulmonary edema, 443
High-resolution computed tomography
   lymphangioleiomyomatosis findings,
    167–168
   pulmonary fibrosis evaluations, 483
Highly active antiretroviral therapy, 291,
   316, 366
Hilar adenopathy
   bilateral, in sarcoidosis, 144
   illustration of, 4f
   mild, 338
   nodular interstitial opacities with,
    106
Hilum, right, 27
Histoplasma capsulatum, 337, 344,
   344f, 349
Honeycombing, 12, 85–86, 176, 224,
   331, 482
Hospital-associated pneumonia, 470–471
"Hot tub lung," 129, 281
HP. *See* Hypersensitivity pneumonitis
HRCT. *See* High-resolution computed
   tomography
HSCT. *See* Hematopoietic stem cell
   transplantation
HTLV-1. *See* Human T cell lymphotropic
   virus type 1
Human immunodeficiency virus
   description of, 178
   opportunistic infection risks, 281, 315
   Pneumocystis jiroveci pneumonia
    secondary to, 291
Human T cell lymphotropic virus type 1,
   174, 178
Hydropneumothorax, 492, 511, 515
Hypercalcemia, 50
Hyperinflation, 165, 416, 438, 449
Hypersensitivity pneumonitis
   acute/subacute
    antigen avoidance for, 131, 132t,
     561t–562t
    characteristics of, 132t, 561t
    description of, 126–127
    diagnosis of, 130
    laboratory studies for, 557–558
    occupational exposure as cause of,
     129–130, 607
    symptoms of, 128, 132t
    transbronchial biopsy for, 558
    treatment of, 131, 132t
   CellCept for, 560, 562t
   chronic
    chest imaging of, 555, 556f–557f
    definition of, 557
    description of, 199
    FEV1/FVC ratio in, 558

    ground-glass opacities with,
     556f–557f
    histopathologic pattern of, 551
    laboratory studies for, 557–558
    risk reductions, 551
    transbronchial biopsy for, 558
   environmental exposures and, 551,
    559–560
   IgG antigen-antibody complements in,
    558
   mosaic attenuation associated with,
    416
   in *Mycobacterium avium* complex, 277,
    557
   occupational exposures, 129–130, 607
   prednisone for, 560, 561t–562t
   smoking and, 559
Hypertensive emergency/urgency, 443
Hypoglycemia, 50
Hypoxemia, 92, 535

I

Idiopathic interstitial pneumonia, 108, 379
Idiopathic pulmonary fibrosis, 87, 106, 224,
   243, 408, 475f, 478, 481–484
IDSA. *See* Infectious Disease Society of
   America
IDSA/ATS. *See* Infectious Disease Society of
   America/American Thoracic Society
IgG antibodies, 622
IgG antigen-antibody complement, 558
IGRA. *See* Interferon gamma release assay
Immune reconstitution inflammatory
   syndrome, 366
Immunoglobulin E, 257, 260
Immunotherapy, 247
Incidental pulmonary nodules, 653,
   660–661, 662f
Infectious cavitary lesion, 12f
Infectious Disease Society of America,
   255
Infectious Disease Society of America/
   American Thoracic Society, 466, 469
Inferior vena cava, 440–441
Inferior vena cava filter, 539
Inflammatory pleural effusions, 245
Inhaled rhDNase, 236
Inspiratory effort, 2
Interferon gamma release assay, 266, 269,
   272, 343
Interlobular septal thickening, 12, 343, 388,
   439f, 614, 638
Interlobular septum, 9
Internal Labor Organization, 118
International Thymic Malignancy Interest
   Group, 38, 48, 59, 580

Interstitial abnormalities, 12
Interstitial lung disease(s)
    bronchoscopy of, 16
    comorbid disease processes with, 174
    computed tomography of, 198, 331, 549f, 553
    dermatomyositis and, 390
    flares of, 398
    glucocorticoids for, 178–179
    noncontrasted computed tomography of, 8
    polymyositis and, 390
    pulmonary function testing for, 182, 186
    radiographic findings for, 388
    in rheumatoid arthritis, 418
    scleroderma-associated, 403
    treatment of, 178
Interstitial lung disease-protocol CT scan, 85
Interstitial opacities, 6, 378
Intracranial pressure, elevated, 311
Intralobular septal thickening, 85–86, 388
Intrathoracic lymph node stations, 670t
Invasive bronchial aspergillosis, 302
Invasive mucinous adenocarcinoma, 657
Invasive pulmonary aspergillosis, 298, 301–303
IRIS. *See* Immune reconstitution inflammatory syndrome
Isocyanates, 557
Isoniazid, 270
ITMWG. *See* International Thymic Malignancy Interest Group
Itraconazole, 259–260, 347, 366
Ivacaftor, 429–430
IVC. *See* Inferior vena cava

J
Janeway lesions, 498
Jo-1 antibody test, 625

K
Kerley A lines, 438–441
Kerley B lines, 404, 438–441
Kerley C lines, 438–441
Klebsiella pneumoniae, 495–496

L
Lactate dehydrogenase, 50
"Lady Windermere" syndrome, 279
LAM. *See* Lymphangioleiomyomatosis
Langerhans cell histiocytosis
    heart involvement by, 157
    pulmonary. *See* Pulmonary Langerhans cell histiocytosis
Langerhans cells, 153, 156
LCH. *See* Langerhans cell histiocytosis

Left lower lobe
    anatomy of, 30, 31f
    collapse of, 75, 75f, 476f, 482
    consolidation of, 465
Left lung, 30, 30f
Left main pulmonary artery, 28
Left mainstem bronchi, 27
Left-sided atelectasis, 607
Left-sided pleural effusion, 438, 438f, 511, 607
Left upper lobe
    anatomy of, 30, 31f
    atelectasis of, 76, 77f
    consolidation of, 352f, 355
Left ventricle, 26
Left-ventricular end-diastolic pressure, 441
Legionella pneumophila, 467–469, 468f–469f
Legionnaire disease, 467
Lepidic growth adenocarcinoma, 650f, 658
Lichenification, 355
Light criteria, 516–517
Limited cutaneous scleroderma, 407
Linear interstitial abnormalities, 3f, 311
Linear interstitial opacities, 95, 95f, 286f, 290, 438–439
Lingua, 30
Lingular collapse, 75, 75f
LIP. *See* Lymphocytic interstitial pneumonia
Liposomal amphotericin B, 357
Liver, 29
Lobar pneumonia, 481
Lobe cephalization, 2–3
Lobular parenchyma, 9
Loculated pleural effusions, 512f–514f
Loeffler syndrome, 143, 378, 380. *See also* Acute eosinophilic pneumonia
Lofgren syndrome, 143
Low-dose computed tomography, 670
Lower airway obstruction
    definition of, 578, 593
    flow-volume loops for, 580f
Lower-lobe interlobular and intralobular septal thickening, 85–86
Lower pulmonary vascular bundle, 27
Lumacaftor/ivacaftor, 430
Lumbar puncture, 311–312, 337, 354
Lung biopsy
    indications for, 387
    surgical, 214–215
    video-assisted thoracoscopic surgery, 211, 558, 609
Lung cancer
    computed tomography-guided transthoracic needle aspiration in, 638
    lymph node stations, 635–637, 641–643
    pathology of, 634f

positron-emission tomography-computed tomography of, 638, 644f
prevalence of, 667
race and, 667
radiation fibrosis associated with, 245f
radiation therapy for, 240f
radiographic staging of, 633, 639
screening for, 571, 642, 644, 660, 667–668, 668t–669t, 670
small cell, 639, 659
smoking and, 667
staging of, 668, 668t–669t
TMN staging of, 668, 668t–669t
Lung malignancies, 115
Lung nodules, 623–624, 644
LUNG-RADS criteria, 670, 671f
Lung resection, 281–282
Lung transplantation
end-stage lung disease treated with, 88
invasive bronchial aspergillosis after, 302
for pulmonary alveolar proteinosis, 227
pulmonary Langerhans cell histiocytosis treated with, 158, 168
Lung-volume reduction surgery, 448, 457
Lupus pernio, 145
Lupus pleuritis, 327–328
LVEDP. *See* Left-ventricular end-diastolic pressure
LVRS. *See* Lung-volume reduction surgery
Lymph node stations, 635–637, 641–643
Lymphadenopathy, 6, 13, 41
Lymphangioleiomyomatosis, 155
cystic lung lesions versus, 164
etiology of, 167
high-resolution computed tomography findings, 167–168
pulmonary. *See* Pulmonary lymphangioleiomyomatosis
serum vascular endothelial growth factor-D levels in, 164, 168
sporadic, 168
treatment of, 168
tuberous sclerosis complex-, 163, 167–168
Lymphangitic carcinomatosis, 657
Lymphocytic interstitial pneumonia
comorbid diseases associated with, 174, 178
definition of, 166, 177
description of, 155
glucocorticoids for, 179
ground-glass opacities in, 177
polyclonal infiltrate associated with, 177
Sjogren syndrome associated with, 178
treatment of, 175
Lymphoma
description of, 50
diffuse large B-cell, 596
follicular, 596
hairy cell, 596
marginal cell, 596
non-Hodgkin, 589, 595
percutaneous core needle biopsy of, 52

M
M bands, 348
Magnetic resonance imaging
indications for, 590
of mediastinal masses, 42, 51
of posterior mediastinal masses, 60, 61f
of progressive massive fibrosis, 120
Main pulmonary artery, 28
Malignant pleural effusions, 521–522
Malignant pleural mesothelioma, 610
MALT lymphomas. *See* Mucosa-associated lymphoid tissue lymphomas
Marginal cell lymphoma, 596
Masses, 6
Mayo Clinic Model, 654–655, 661
McConnell sign, 538
Mechanic's hand, 389
Mediastinal abnormalities, 6
Mediastinal fibrosis, 267, 347
Mediastinal granulomas, 346f, 349
Mediastinal masses
anterior, 47, 48f, 583, 595
classification of, 48, 59, 580–581
clinical presentation of, 41
computed tomography of, 51, 592f
contrasted computed tomography of, 41
description of, 35, 37–38
differential diagnosis of, 40, 41t, 583, 595
imaging of, 41–42, 51
laboratory studies for, 50
magnetic resonance imaging of, 42, 51
middle. *See* Middle mediastinal masses
posterior. *See* Posterior mediastinal masses
Mediastinal shift, 4f
Mediastinal widening, 4f
Mediastinum
anatomy of, 580
anterior. *See* Anterior mediastinum
borders of, 4
compartments of, 31, 32f, 38, 39f, 40t, 48, 48f, 49t, 59f, 60, 574f, 580, 581
definition of, 38, 59
middle. *See* Middle mediastinum
posterior. *See* Posterior mediastinum
superior, 40, 49
widened, 590
Mendelson syndrome, 497
Meningocele, 40, 62

Meningoencephalitis, 315
Meniscus sign, 267, 515f
Mepolizumab, 381
Mesothelioma, 608–610
Metanephrines, serum, 62–63
Methemoglobinemia, 292
Methicillin-resistant *Staphylococcus aureus,*
    467–468, 471
Methotrexate
  pneumonitis caused by, 418
  sarcoidosis treated with, 147
Metronidazole, 496
Micronodular opacities, 183f, 187, 570
Micronodules, 108, 302
Microscopic polyangiitis, 625, 626f, 627
Middle mediastinal masses
  chest radiograph of, 574f
  computed tomography of, 576f
  description of, 35
  differential diagnosis of, 62, 583, 595
  endobronchial ultrasound of, 52
  lymphadenopathy as cause of, 41
  positron-emission tomography-computed
    tomography of, 591, 591f
Middle mediastinum
  imaging of, 39f, 48f
  posterior mediastinum and, border
    between, 59
  structures of, 40, 50, 61
Migratory superficial thrombophlebitis,
  659
Miliary pattern with reticulonodular
  opacities, 343
Miliary tuberculosis, 271, 365
Minimally invasive adenocarcinoma, 657
mMRC dyspnea scale. *See* Modified Medical
  Research Council dyspnea scale
Modified Medical Research Council dyspnea
  scale, 453
Monoclonal antibody therapy, 380
Monod sign, 302–303
Mosaic attenuation, 10, 10f, 416, 451, 453f,
  554
MPA. *See* Microscopic polyangiitis
MRSA. *See* Methicillin-resistant *Staphylococcus
  aureus*
mTOR complex, 167
Mucosa-associated lymphoid tissue
  lymphomas, 179
Mucous plug, in right mainstem bronchus,
  72
Multidetector computed tomography, 7
Multidrug-resistant organisms, 471
Multiple myeloma, 628
Myasthenia gravis, 45
Mycobacterium abscessus, 279

Mycobacterium avium complex
  description of, 129
  disseminated infection, 277, 280
  hypersensitivity pneumonitis associated
    with, 277, 557
  laboratory studies for, 277, 279
  sputum cultures for, 277, 279
Mycobacterium fortuitum, 279
Mycobacterium kansasii, 279
Mycobacterium tuberculosis
  ANCA-associated vasculitis versus, 627
  description of, 117
  interferon gamma release assay, 266, 272
  prophylactic treatment for, 263
  tuberculous pleurisy caused by, 268
  vertebral involvement of, 271
Mycophenolate mofetil, 147, 407, 560
Mycoplasma pneumonia, 468

N
N-terminal proBNP, 440, 519–520
NAA. *See* Neutron activation analysis
Nephrotic syndrome, 518–519
Neuroblastoma, 62
Neurofibroma, 62
Neurofibromatosis 1, 58, 62
Neurogenic tumors, 62
Neutron activation analysis, 107
Nintedanib, 408, 484
Nodular interstitial opacities with hilar
  adenopathy, 106
Nodular opacities, 116
Nodules
  description of, 6
  lung, 623–624, 644
  lymphatics, 12
Non-cystic fibrosis bronchiectasis, 232, 236
Non-Hodgkin lymphoma, 589, 595
Noncardiogenic pulmonary edema,
  128, 442
Noncaseating granulomas, 144, 177, 338
Noncaseating granulomatous inflammation,
  131
Nonspecific interstitial pneumonia
  cellular, 200f
  clinical presentation of, 199, 279
  definition of, 199
  description of, 129, 390
  diagnosis of, 198–199
  differential diagnosis of, 243
  fibrotic, 200f–201f
  glucocorticoids for, 203
  pathology of, 391f
  pulmonary function testing for, 195
  subtype of, 194
  treatment of, 203

Nontuberculous mycobacterial infections, 117–118, 279–280
NSIP. *See* Nonspecific interstitial pneumonia
NTM infections. *See* Nontuberculous mycobacterial infections

O

Obliterative bronchiolitis, 417
Obstructive atelectasis, 72, 76, 76f
Obstructive lung disease, flow-volume loop for, 411, 416, 445f, 449
Obstructive sleep apnea, 588f, 593, 595
Omalizumab, 381
Opacification, 238f, 243, 429
Opacities, 6, 378
  airspace, 6
  alveolar, 6, 286f, 290, 553f, 614
  diffuse interstitial, 647f, 656
  diffuse nodular, 343
  diffuse reticular, 388
  ground-glass. *See* Ground-glass opacities
  linear interstitial, 95, 95f, 286f, 290, 438–439
  micronodular, 183f, 187, 570
  nodular opacities, 116
  reticular interstitial, 3f, 198, 224, 311, 404, 481
  reticulonodular. *See* Reticulonodular opacities
  "tree-in-bud," 12, 243, 278f, 426, 431f
Ophthalmology referral, 281
Opportunistic infections, 281, 315
Organic dust toxic syndrome, 129, 559
Organizing pneumonia, 390
  conditions associated with, 204
  cryptogenic. *See* Cryptogenic organizing pneumonia
  description of, 197
Orkambi. *See* Lumacaftor/ivacaftor
"Outside-in" pattern, 641
Oxygen supplementation, 87, 457

P

Pacemaker leads, infected, 500
Palla sign, 537
Pancreaticopleural fistula, 520
Pancreatitis, acute, 520
Panlobular emphysema, 166, 450, 455, 456f
Panniculitis, 143
PaO_2/FIO_2 ratio, 213
PAP. *See* Pulmonary alveolar proteinosis
Papular sarcoidosis, 138f, 145
Papules, 145
Paracoccidioidomycosis, 367

"Paramalignant" effusion, 522
Paraneoplastic syndromes
  primary lung malignancies and, 653
  with thymomas, 45
Parapneumonic effusion, 518, 524f
Paraseptal emphysema, 450
Paraspinal mass, 61f
Parathyroid adenoma, 52
Parenchymal bands, 85–86
Parietal pleura, 494
Passive atelectasis, 73–74, 74f
Patulous esophagus, 406
Pauci-immune vasculitis. *See* Microscopic polyangiitis
PCP. *See Pneumocystis jiroveci* pneumonia
PDH. *See* Progressive disseminated histoplasmosis
PE. *See* Pulmonary embolism
Pentamidine, 292
Percutaneous core needle biopsy, 46, 51–52
Perfusion attenuation, 417
Perfusion scan, 532f
Peribronchial cuffing, 438
Peribronchial "cuffing," 2
Peribronchovascular thickening, 12
Pericardial abnormalities, 13
Pericardial effusions, 4f, 321f, 327–328
Pericarditis, 327
Pericardium
  anterior surface of, 38
  imaging of, 28
Perifissural nodules, 661, 665f
Perihilar mass, 76f
Peripheral blood smear, 256
Peripherally inserted central catheter, 26
Periungual telangiectasias, 389
Personal protective equipment, 129
PESI. *See* Pulmonary embolism severity index
PET-CT. *See* Positron-emission tomography-computed tomography
PFNs. *See* Perifissural nodules
PFT. *See* Pulmonary function testing
Pharyngeal pouch, 51
PICC. *See* Peripherally inserted central catheter
Pirfenidone, 482, 484
Plaque sarcoidosis, 145
Plasmapheresis, 330
Plate-like atelectasis, 74, 346f
PLCH. *See* Pulmonary Langerhans cell histiocytosis
Pleural abnormalities, 6, 13
Pleural biopsy, 269

Pleural effusions
anteroposterior imaging of, 32
benign asbestos-related
asbestos exposure and, latency period between, 602, 608
description of, 78
diagnosis of, 607
differential diagnosis of, 608
bilateral, 378–379
cavitation and, 314f
chest radiographs of, 267f
complex, 523
computed tomography of, 364f, 512f–513f, 515
congestive heart failure as cause of, 507
description of, 13, 72
diagnosis of, 505, 515
etiology of, 505
exudative, 516–518
free-flowing, 511, 512f, 515, 516f
imaging of, 4f, 504
inflammatory, 245
laboratory studies for, 323, 505
lateral decubitus films of, 515
left-sided, 438, 438f, 511, 607
loculated, 512f–514f
malignant, 521–522
massive, 525
meniscus sign, 267
parapneumonic, 518, 524f
passive atelectasis caused by, 74
right-sided, 513f
serosanguinous, 518f
thoracentesis for, 516
transudative, 516–518
ultrasound of, 322f, 515
Pleural fluid
albumin to serum albumin gradient, 519
tests of, 323, 507–508
Pleural meniscus sign, 511
Pleural plaques, 85, 85f
Pleural pressure, 593
Pleural thickening, 604f, 609
PMF. *See* Progressive massive fibrosis
Pneumoconiosis
coal workers', 86, 114, 117–119
definition of, 116–117
hard metal, 118
Pneumocystis jiroveci pneumonia
acute respiratory distress syndrome caused by, 289
azithromycin for, 291
corticosteroids for, 292
dapsone for, 289
description of, 225, 249
diagnosis of, 289

human immunodeficiency virus as risk factor for, 291
pathology of, 288f
polymerase chain reaction testing in, 293
prophylactic medications for, 288, 291
risk factors for, 288
treatment of, 289, 292
trimethoprim/sulfamethoxazole for, 292
Pneumomediastinum, 37
Pneumonia
acute eosinophilic. *See* Acute eosinophilic pneumonia
acute interstitial. *See* Acute interstitial pneumonia
aspiration. *See* Aspiration pneumonia
cavitary, 492
community-acquired. *See* Community-acquired pneumonia
cryptogenic organizing. *See* Cryptogenic organizing pneumonia
desquamative interstitial. *See* Desquamative interstitial pneumonia
health care-associated, 469
hospital-associated, 470–471
isolated cryptococcal, 314f
Legionella, 467–469, 468f–469f
lobar, 481
lymphocytic interstitial. *See* Lymphocytic interstitial pneumonia
Mycoplasma, 468
nonspecific interstitial. *See* Nonspecific interstitial pneumonia
Pneumocystis jiroveci. See Pneumocystis jiroveci pneumonia
Streptococcus, 467
usual interstitial. *See* Usual interstitial pneumonia
ventilator-associated, 470–471
Pneumonia severity index, 466
Pneumonitis
methotrexate, 418
risk factors for, 96
Pneumothorax, 72
anteroposterior imaging of, 32
complications of, 429
deep sulcus sign, 32f
Pneumotox.com, 98
Poikiloderma, 388
Polymerase chain reaction testing, in *Pneumocystis jiroveci* pneumonia, 293
Polymyositis, 390, 391f
Pores of Kohn, 73
Positron-emission tomography
description of, 8
pulmonary nodules on, 664f

Positron-emission tomography-computed tomography
  benign asbestos-related pleural effusion evaluations, 608–609
  description of, 8
  lung cancer evaluations, 638, 644f
  mediastinal masses on, 37–38, 42, 51, 591, 591f
  in mediastinum, 590
  middle mediastinal masses on, 591, 591f
Posterior mediastinal masses
  differential diagnoses for, 56, 62, 583, 595
  imaging of, 59f, 59–60
  magnetic resonance imaging of, 60, 61f
  neurogenic tumors as cause of, 62
Posterior mediastinum
  imaging of, 39f, 48f
  middle mediastinum and, border between, 59
  structures of, 40, 50, 56, 61
Pott disease, 271
Pouch defect, 541
PPD. *See* Purified protein derivative
PPE. *See* Personal protective equipment
Precipitins, serum, 107, 130, 214, 558
Prednisone. *See also* Corticosteroids
  for cryptogenic organizing pneumonia, 205
  for hypersensitivity pneumonitis, 560, 561t–562t
  for lymphocytic interstitial pneumonia, 179
  for radiation pneumonitis, 242, 247, 249
  for sarcoidosis, 147
Primaquine, 292
Primary pulmonary coccidioidomycosis, 365
Primary tuberculosis, 279–280
Procalcitonin, 366
Progressive disseminated histoplasmosis, 345
Progressive massive fibrosis, 114–115, 117, 120
Proton pump inhibitors, 249, 497
"Pruning," 540–542, 544f
Pseudomembranous tracheobronchitis, 302
Pseudomonas aeruginosa, 235–236, 466–467, 469–470
Pseudonormalization, 106
PSI. *See* Pneumonia severity index
Pulmonary abscess
  chest radiographs of, 495f
  definition of, 494
  description of, 492

Pulmonary alveolar proteinosis
  antibodies associated with, 223
  bronchoscopy of, 225
  causes of, 225
  clinical findings of, 225
  clinical presentation of, 279
  differential diagnosis of, 279
  pulmonary function testing for, 225
  treatment of, 223
  whole lung lavage for, 226–227
Pulmonary arterial hypertension, 531f–532f, 540. *See also* Pulmonary hypertension
Pulmonary artery, 8
Pulmonary aspergillosis, invasive, 298, 301–303
Pulmonary capillaritis, 327, 329f, 390
Pulmonary cryptococcal infection, 312, 313f–314f
Pulmonary edema, 27
  cardiogenic. *See* Cardiogenic pulmonary edema
  flash, 443
  heart failure with, 128
  high-altitude, 443
  noncardiogenic, 128, 442
Pulmonary embolism
  acute, 543f–544f
  chest radiographs of, 543f
  computed tomographic angiography for, 537, 544f
  D-dimer study for, 537
  description of, 72
  electrocardiographic findings, 536, 536f
  Hampton hump, 538
  hemodynamic stability evaluations, 536–537
  heparin for, 537
  massive, 539
  pulmonary angiography for, 544f
  pulmonary infarction caused by, 538
  saddle embolus, 538
  septic, 491, 498–500
  submassive, 540
  systemic thrombolysis for, 538–540
  ventilation-perfusion scan of, 544
  Wells criteria for, 536–538
  Westermark sign, 537
Pulmonary embolism severity index, 538
Pulmonary fibrosis
  chest radiographs of, 474f, 481
  idiopathic, 87, 106, 224, 243, 408, 475f, 478, 481–484
  lung examination findings, 474, 481

Pulmonary function testing
  for amiodarone toxicity, 92
  for asbestosis, 84
  for chronic eosinophilic pneumonia,
    381
  for desquamative interstitial pneumonia,
    569
  for hypersensitivity pneumonitis, 127
  interpretation of, 182, 186
  for interstitial lung diseases, 182, 186
  for nonspecific interstitial pneumonia,
    195
  for pulmonary alveolar proteinosis, 225
  for pulmonary Langerhans cell histiocytosis,
    156, 167
  for pulmonary lymphangioleiomyomatosis,
    163
  for radiation pneumonitis, 246
  for respiratory bronchiolitis–associated
    interstitial lung disease, 569
  for sarcoidosis, 141
Pulmonary histoplasmosis, 347–348
Pulmonary hypertension, 27, 331, 405. *See
    also* Pulmonary arterial hypertension
  chronic thromboembolic, 541–542,
    542f–544f
  diagnosis of, 531f–532f, 540
Pulmonary infarction, 538
Pulmonary Langerhans cell histiocytosis
  CD1a staining in, 156, 157f
  characteristics of, 155–156, 166
  description of, 131
  diagnosis of, 153
  genetic mutation associated with, 153
  glucocorticoids for, 158
  pneumothoraces associated with, 177
  pulmonary function testing for, 156,
    167
  pulmonary manifestation of, 166
  reticulonodular opacities in, 166
  S100 staining in, 156, 157f
  smoking cessation for, 158
  treatment of, 153, 158
Pulmonary lobule, secondary, 8–9, 9f, 29, 450f
Pulmonary lymphangioleiomyomatosis
  definition of, 166
  extrapulmonary manifestations of, 163
  genetic disorder associated with, 163
  pulmonary function testing for, 163
  signs and symptoms of, 166
  spontaneous pneumothorax associated
    with, 166
  treatment of, 164
Pulmonary nodules
  characteristics of, 665f
  incidental, 653, 660–661, 662f

perifissural, 661, 665f
  solitary, 663, 664f
  spiculated, 663, 664f
  subsolid, 663, 666f–667f
  terminology for, 663
Pulmonary rehabilitation, 236
"Pulmonary toilet," 73
Pulmonary vascular bundle, 27
Pulmonary vascular diseases, 186
Pulmozyme, 236
Purified protein derivative, 272, 276
Pyrazinamide, 270

Q
QuantiFERON Gold study/test, 276, 373, 520

R
Radial endobronchial ultrasound, 15
Radiation and drug-induced pneumonitis,
    248
Radiation-associated lung disease, 607
Radiation fibrosis, 243–244, 245f, 246,
    640–641
Radiation hypersensitivity pneumonitis, 248
Radiation-induced lung injury, 244, 247,
    640–641
Radiation pleuritis, 244
Radiation pneumonitis
  bronchoalveolar lavage for, 246
  chemotherapy as cause of, 247
  chest imaging of, 246
  definition of, 243, 245
  diagnosis of, 244–246
  differential diagnosis of, 246, 640
  glucocorticoids for, 247, 249
  grading of, 247
  immunotherapy as cause of, 247
  mean lung radiation dose and, 241,
    247–248
  prednisone for, 242, 247, 249
  pulmonary function testing for, 246
  risk factors for, 241
  severity of, 241, 247
  symptoms of, 245
  treatment of, 242
Radiation therapy
  bronchial stenosis caused by, 244
  conformal, 248
  for lung cancer, 240f
  mean lung dose from, 241, 247–248
Radon exposure, 607
Ranke complex, 269, 271
Ras oncogene, 63
Rash
  dermatologic, 322f
  in dermatomyositis, 389–390

Raynaud's phenomenon, 406–407
RB-ILD. *See* Respiratory bronchiolitis–associated interstitial lung disease
Reactivation pulmonary tuberculosis, 270–271
Reactivation tuberculosis, 269
Reactive arthritis, 143
Recall pneumonitis, 247
Recombinant factor VII, 616
Recombinant granulocyte-monocyte colony stimulating factor, 227
Red cell aplasia, 51
Renal angiolipomas, 167
Renal cell carcinoma, 652f, 658–659
Replacement atelectasis, 74
RES. *See* Reticuloendothelial system
Respiratory alkalosis, 213
Respiratory bronchiolitis
    diagnosis of, 184f, 187
    smokers' macrophages associated with, 187–188
    smoking and, 187–189
Respiratory bronchiolitis–associated interstitial lung disease
    age of onset, 188
    diagnosis of, 184, 184f, 187
    pulmonary function testing for, 569
    risk factor for, 184
    signs and symptoms of, 188
    smokers' macrophages associated with, 570
    smoking and, 187–189, 571
    treatment of, 185, 569, 571
Resting hypoxemia, 457
Restrictive lung disease, 588f, 593
Restrictive lung physiology, 106
Reticular abnormalities, 12
Reticular interstitial abnormalities, 3f
Reticular interstitial opacities, 3f, 198, 224, 311, 404, 481
Reticuloendothelial system, 108
Reticulonodular abnormalities, 3f
Reticulonodular opacities
    bilateral, in Langerhans cell histiocytosis, 155
    description of, 116, 144
    interstitial, 388
    lower-lobe predominant pattern, 176
    miliary pattern with, 343
    in pulmonary Langerhans cell histiocytosis, 166
Reverse-halo sign, 243, 246, 614, 641
Rf. *See* Rheumatoid factor
Rheumatoid arthritis-interstitial lung disease, 418
Rheumatoid effusions, 521
Rheumatoid factor, 178, 417

Rheumatoid nodules, 418–419
Rheumatoid pleurisy, 521
Rib, 28
Rifampin, 270
Right lower lobe
    anatomy of, 29
    consolidation of, 37
    mass of, 37
Right lung, 29
Right main pulmonary artery, 28
Right mainstem bronchi
    description of, 26
    mucous plug in, 72
Right middle lobe
    anatomy of, 29, 31f
    chest computed tomography of, 75f
Right-sided relaxation atelectasis, 73–74
Right upper lobe
    anatomy of, 29, 31f
    atelectasis of, 76
Right ventricular strain, 540
RILI. *See* Radiation-induced lung injury
Rituximab, 226, 330, 408, 560, 627–628
RLL. *See* Right lower lobe
RML. *See* Right middle lobe
Roflumilast, 455
Rounded atelectasis, 78, 243, 607–609
RUL. *See* Right upper lobe
RV/TLC, 167

S
S100, 156, 157f
Saber-sheath trachea, 451, 452f
Saccular bronchiectasis, 233f
Saddle embolus, 538
SAFS. *See* Severe asthma with fungal sensitivity
Sarcoidosis
    age of onset, 143
    biomarkers of, 146
    bronchoscopy of, 142
    in coal workers, 117
    cutaneous manifestations of, 136–139
    definition of, 143
    differential diagnosis of, 128, 279
    extrapulmonary, 143, 147
    noncaseating granulomas associated with, 177
    occupations at high risk for, 107
    papular, 138f, 145
    plaque, 145
    pulmonary, 147
    pulmonary function testing for, 141
    screening for, 141, 146
    staging of, 135, 144–145
    treatment of, 142, 146–147
    ulcerative, 145

Sarcoma, 50
Satellite nodules, 302
Schwannoma, 62
Sclerodactyly, 406
Scleroderma
   interstitial lung diseases associated with,
      403, 408
   silica-induced, 119, 398, 399f
Secondary pulmonary lobule, 8–9, 9f, 29f,
      450f
Septal flattening, 538
Septal thickening, 213, 343, 439f, 648f,
      656
   lower-lobe interlobular and intralobular,
      85–86
   subpleural interlobular and intralobular,
      85
Septic pulmonary emboli, 491, 498,
      498f–499f, 500
Serial lavage, 327–328
Serosanguinous effusions, 518f
Serotonin syndrome, 108
Serum precipitins, 107, 130, 214, 558
Serum soluble IL-2 receptor alpha, 146
Serum vascular endothelial growth factor-D,
      164, 168
Severe asthma with fungal sensitivity, 2457
Shawl sign, 390
Short tau inversion recovery, 389
"Shred sign", 465
Shrinking lung syndrome, 331
"Signet-ring" finding/sign, 233, 234f, 426,
      431f
Silica exposure, 114, 118
Silica-induced scleroderma, 119
Silicosis, 118–119
Simple pulmonary eosinophilia, 378
Sinus tachycardia, 327
Sirolimus, 158, 168
Sjogren syndrome
   laboratory tests for, 175
   lymphocytic interstitial pneumonia and,
      178
Skin
   blastomycosis manifestations, 356–357
   dyspigmentation of, 407
   sarcoidosis manifestations, 139
SLE. *See* Systemic lupus erythematosus
Slice increment, 7
Small airways disease, 426–427
Small cell carcinoma, 639, 640f
Small cell lung cancer, 639, 659
Smokers' macrophages, 178, 187–188, 570
Smoking
   asbestosis and, 87
   cessation of, 188–189, 448, 571

chronic obstructive pulmonary disease
      caused by, 450, 456
   desquamative interstitial pneumonia and,
      571
   hypersensitivity pneumonitis and, 559
   lung cancer and, 667
   pulmonary Langerhans cell histiocytosis
      and, 155, 158
   respiratory bronchiolitis and, 187
   respiratory bronchiolitis–associated
      interstitial lung disease and, 187–189,
      571
Solid pulmonary nodules, 653
Solitary pulmonary nodules, 12f, 663, 664f
Spiculated pulmonary nodules, 663, 664f
Spine, 26
"Spine sign", 27
"Split pleura" sign, 492, 494f, 514f
Spontaneous pneumothorax, 166
Sputum cultures, for *Mycobacterium avium*
      complex, 277, 279
Squamous cell carcinoma, 639, 640f, 659
SS. *See* Sjogren syndrome
Staphylococcus epidermidis, 235
Stellate nodules, 155
Sternal angle, 40
Sternal osteomyelitis, 47
Sternal wires, 267, 267f
Sternum, 27
STIR. *See* Short tau inversion recovery
"Straight-line sign", 246, 641
Streptococcus pneumoniae, 235, 311, 467
Streptomycin, 270
Stridor, 302
Subacute hypersensitivity pneumonitis
   antigen avoidance for, 131, 132t,
      561t–562t
   characteristics of, 132t, 561t
   description of, 126–127
   diagnosis of, 130
   laboratory studies for, 557–558
   occupational exposure as cause of,
      129–130, 607
   symptoms of, 128, 132t
   transbronchial biopsy for, 558
   treatment of, 131, 132t
Subacute pulmonary histoplasmosis, 348
Submassive pulmonary embolism, 540
Subpleural interlobular and intralobular
      septal thickening, 85
Subpleural reticulations, 86
Subsolid pulmonary nodules, 663,
      666f–667f
Substernal goiter, 590
Superior mediastinum, 40, 49
Sweat chloride test, 235, 427

Symdeko. *See* Tezacaftor/ivacaftor
Systemic lupus erythematosus, 325–327, 330f
Systemic sclerosis, 398
Systemic thrombolysis, for pulmonary embolism, 538–540

T
Talcosis, 118
TBLC. *See* Transbronchial lung cryobiopsy
Telangiectasia, 355, 407
Teratoma, 40, 50
Tezacaftor/ivacaftor, 430
Thoracentesis, 267–268, 509, 516
Thoracic inlet, 44, 49–50
Thorax, 26
Three-tcst rule, 517
Thrombolysis, systemic, 538–540
Thymic cyst, 50
Thymomas
    complications of, 45, 51
    computed tomography of, 47f, 50
    diagnosis of, 45
    imaging of, 40, 45, 50
    paraneoplastic syndromes associated with, 45
    percutaneous core needle biopsy of, 46, 51–52
    signs and symptoms of, 50
Thymus, 45, 51
Thyroid cancer, 590
Thyroid carcinoma, 50
Thyroid disease, 97
Thyroid goiter, 50
Tissue plasminogen activator, 523–524, 539
tPA. *See* Tissue plasminogen activator
TPE. *See* Tropical pulmonary eosinophilia
Trachea
    airway diameter in, 576, 581
    anatomy of, 26–27
    deviation of, 26, 47, 47f–48f
    extrathoracic, 593
    narrowing of, 26
    obstruction of, 579, 594
    saber-sheath, 451, 452f
Tracheal lumen diameter, 577, 582
Tracheal wall thickening, 623
Tracheobronchitis, 302
Tracheobronchomalacia, 588f, 593
Tracheostomy, 582
Traction bronchiectasis, 10f, 12, 176, 331, 388, 483
TRALI. *See* Transfusion-related acute lung injury
"Tram-tracks," 233, 431f
Transbronchial biopsy

bronchoscopy with, 570, 656–657
    description of, 14–15
    endobronchial ultrasound-guided, 147
    for subacute and chronic hypersensitivity pneumonitis, 558
Transbronchial lung cryobiopsy, 147
Transfusion-related acute lung injury, 442–443
Transudative effusions, 516–518
"Tree-in-bud" opacities/nodules, 12, 243, 278f, 426, 431f
Trikafta. *See* Elexacaftor/tezacaftor/ivacaftor
Trimethoprim/sulfamethoxazole, for *Pneumocystis jiroveci* pneumonia, 292
Tropical pulmonary eosinophilia, 380
TSC2 gene, 167
TSC-LAM. *See* Tuberous sclerosis complex-lymphangioleiomyomatosis
TST. *See* Tuberculin skin test
Tuberculin skin test, 272
Tuberculosis
    miliary, 271, 521f
    primary, 279–280
    reactivation, 269–271
    risk factors for, 343
Tuberculous effusions, 269, 520
Tuberculous pleurisy
    causes of, 268
    diagnosis of, 263, 269
    pleural biopsy for, 269
    treatment of, 263, 270
    tuberculosis development after, 263, 270
Tuberous sclerosis complex-lymphangioleiomyomatosis, 163, 167–168
Two-test rule, 517

U
UIP. *See* Usual interstitial pneumonia
Ulcerative sarcoidosis, 145
Ulcerative tracheobronchitis, 302
Upper airway obstruction
    definition of, 578, 593
    flow-volume loops for, 573f, 574, 578–579, 580f
    tracheostomy for, 582
Upper pulmonary vascular bundle, 27
Urinary tract infections, 97–98
Urine antigen testing, for *Histoplasma capsulatum*, 345
Urinothorax, 518
Usual interstitial pneumonia
    acute exacerbation of, 215
    definition of, 178
    diagnosis of, 224, 483–484
    pathology of, 202f
    prevalence of, 418

V

"Valley fever," 365

Valve replacement rings, 267, 267f

VAP. *See* Ventilator-associated pneumonia

Varicose bronchiectasis, 233, 233f

Vascular abnormalities, 13

Vascular endothelial growth factor-D, serum, 164, 168

Vasculitis cavitary nodule, 12f

"Vasculitis" sign, 625

Ventilation-perfusion scan, 532f, 533, 534f, 541

Ventilator-associated pneumonia, 470–471

Ventricle, 28

Verrucous lesions, 355

Video-assisted thoracoscopic surgery lung biopsy, 211, 558, 609

Viral pleurisy, 516

Virtual bronchoscopy, 14

Visceral pleura, 494

Vitamin C, 87

Voriconazole, 304

W

"Water bottle" sign, 4f, 5

"Waterbag" sign, 5

Wegener granulomatosis. *See* Granulomatosis with polyangiitis

Wells criteria, 536–538

Westermark sign, 537

Whole lung lavage, for pulmonary alveolar proteinosis, 226–227

Wolff-Parkinson-White syndrome, 327

World Health Organization pulmonary hypertension classifications, 540

WPW syndrome. *See* Wolff-Parkinson-White syndrome

Wuchereria bancrofti, 375–376, 380

X

Xpert MTB/RIF test, 269